Peter Lanzer · Martin Lipton (Eds.)
Diagnostics of Vascular Diseases: Principles and Technology

Springer
Berlin
Heidelberg
New York
Barcelona
Budapest
Hong Kong
London
Milan
Paris
Santa Clara
Singapore
Tokyo

Peter Lanzer · Martin Lipton (Eds.)

Diagnostics of Vascular Diseases

Principles and Technology

With Contributions by
A. Bauer, E. Blessing, H.J. Blom, E.G. Cape, T. Diebold, W.-R. Dix, P.J. Fitzgerald, A. Fronek, W. L. Gross, S. Grosskopf, C.W. Hamm, D. Hausmann, A. Hildebrand, V.W.M. van Hinsbergh, P.R. Hoskins, K.-F. Kamm, G. Karczmar, J.F. Keany, J. Kekow, H. Kleinholz, C. Korninger, W. Krause, W. Kupper, P. Lanzer, K. Lindström, M. Lipton, M.P.M. de Maat, M.R. Malinow, W.N. McDicken, A. Mügge, P.A. Olofsson, D.G.W. Onnasch, P.H.A. Quax, H. Refsum, J. Ricke, R.E. Roller, J.A. Rumberger, R. Schlief, M. Sturm, P.M. Ueland, J.A. Vita, T.J. Vogl, H. Wieland, J.E. Wilting, F.W. Zonneveld

With 160 Figures in 208 Parts and 47 Tables

Springer

Editors:

Dr. Peter Lanzer
Kardiologische Gemeinschaftspraxis
Saalbaustraße 27, 64283 Darmstadt, Germany

Prof. Dr. Martin Lipton
The University of Chicago Hospitals, Department of Radiology
5841 South Maryland Avenue
Chicago, IL 60637, USA

ISBN-13:978-3-642-64437-5 e-ISBN-13:978-3-642-60512-3
DOI: 10.1007/978-3-642-60512-3

Die Deutsche Bibliothek – CIP-Einheitsaufnahme

Diagnostics of Vascular Diseases. – Berlin ; Heidelberg ; New York ; Barcelona ; Budapest ; Hong Kong ; London ; Milan ; Paris ; Santa Clara ; Singapore ; Tokyo : Springer.
Literaturangaben
Principles and technology / P. Lanzer ; M. Lipton. – 1997
ISBN-13:978-3-642-64437-5
NE: Lanzer, Peter

Softcover reprint of the hardcover 1st edition 1997

Cover Design: E. Kirchner, Heidelberg
Typesetting: FotoSatz Pfeifer GmbH, Gräfelfing
SPIN: 10499730 21/3135 – 5 4 3 2 1 0 – Printed on acid-free paper

Preface

Over the past decade vascular diagnostic techniques have evolved from a collection of "low-tech" modalities (e.g. oscillometry, plethysmography, continuous wave dopper) into a complex "high-tech" enterprise (e.g. color doppler, nuclear magnetic resonance imaging, spiral computed tomography, molecular techniques). There also have been remarkable advances in radiology- and surgery-oriented vascular diagnostics, which has become a multidisciplinary endeavour involving radiologists, cardiovascular physicians (i.e. cardiac and vascular surgeons, cardiologists, and angiologists), end-organ specialists (i.e. neurologists, pulmologists, nephrologists, gastroenterologists, and dermatologists), and, more recently, lipidologists, hematologists, immunologists, laboratory and basic scientists.

Due to the rapid evolution of diagnostic technology and its multidisciplinary proliferation, an understanding of its working principles and modes of application has become mandatory for those physicians involved in caring for patients with vascular disease. The need for an optimum choice of diagnostic procedures performed by highly trained physicians has been greatly reinforced by the increasingly competitive economical environment. Resource management and cost efficiency are now important nonmedical criteria in the strategic selection of technology for individual patient treatment. Unquestionably the quality, results and costs of the vascular diagnostic evaluations directly depend upon the expertise, skills, and experience that the investigators bring to bear in utilizing the diagnostic tools of their choice.

This book has been designed to provide vasculals physicians with a comprehensive yet succint review of the scientific background and applied principles of the vascular diagnostic technology and instrumentation. Based on the knowledge used by the experts in the field and presented in this book the readers will be assisted in selecting, evaluating and applying vascular diagnostic methods to their fulliest advantage in their own clinical settings.

The text has been divided into two parts and six sections. In the first part state-of-the-art vascular diagnostic methodology is presented. The text first discusses techniques, which do not involve imaging and proceeds to noninvasive and invasive diagnostic imaging strategies. All techniques are presented in a procedure oriented manner. Individual methods are discussed under separate headings allowing both a systematic and random review of each topic. Doppler sonography and x-ray radiography have been highlighted because of their paramount clinical importance in vascular diagnosis. Due to the increasing impact of chemical analytical and laboratory methods in the evaluation and management of vascular disease, a separate section has been devoted to the assessment of hemostasis, lipoproteins, homocysteine and immune factors in patients with vascular disease. The second part of the book describes work-in-progress in imaging and reviews imaging as well as laboratory vascular diagnostic techniques Here the role of high resolution ultrasound is emphasized for early recognition of disease by detecting abnormalities of function as well as morphology. This is valuable in the context of preventive medicine for the early detection and management of cardiovascular disease. The increasingly evident need for an integrated, interdisciplinary approach to vascular diagnostics has been reflected upon in the closing chapter.

Our hope is that this textbook will serve the needs of the growing multidisciplinary community of physicians and scientists who are striving to improve the quality of modern cardiovascular diagnosis and care. We wish to thank our co-authors as well as Dr. Heilmann, Ms. Duhm, Ms. Sundell and the staff of Springer Verlag in Heidelberg, for all their hard work and outstanding talents in making this project possible.

Peter Lanzer
Martin Lipton

Contents

Part II: Diagnostics of Vascular Diseases: Work-in-Progress

Section I: Imaging Methods

Section II: Laboratory Methods

Section III: Future Perspectives

Contributors

A. Bauer, Clinical Development Diagnostics, Ultrasound Contrast Media, Schering AG, Müllerstraße 178, 13342 Berlin, Germany

B.R. Binder, Department for Vascular Biology and Thrombosis Research, University of Vienne, Schwarzspanierstraße 17, 1090 Vienna, Austria

E. Blessing, Department of Cardiology, Division of Internal Medicine, Hannover Medical School, Konstanty-Gutschow-Straße 8, 30625 Hannover, Germany

H.J. Blom, University of Bergen, Clinical Pharmacology Unit, Central Laboratory, Haukeland Hospital, 5021 Bergen, Norway

E.G. Cape, Division of Pediatric Cardiology, Children's Hospital of Pittsburgh, University of Pittsburgh, 3705 Fifth Avenue, Pittsburgh, PA 15213, USA

T. Diebold, Department of Radiology, Virchow Hospital, Humboldt University of Berlin, Augustenburger Platz 1, 13353 Berlin, Germany

W.-R. Dix, Hamburger Synchrotronstrahlungslabor HASYLAB at DESY, Noltkestraße 85, 22603 Hamburg, Germany

P.J. Fitzgerald, Stanford University Medical Center, Center for Research in Cardiovascular Interventions, 300 Pasteur Drive, Stanford, CA 94305, USA

A. Fronek, Department of Surgery and Bioengineering, University of California, San Diego, and Veteran's Medical Center, Basic Science Building, RM 5028, La Jolla, CA 92093-0643, USA

W.L. Gross, Department of Rheumatology, Medical University of Lübeck, Ratzeburger Allee 160, 23538 Lübeck, and Rheumaklinik Bad Bramstedt GmbH, Oskar-Alexander-Straße 26, 24572 Bad Bramstedt, Germany

S. Grosskopf, Fraunhofer Institute for Computer Graphics, Wilhelminenstraße 7, 64283 Darmstadt, Germany

C.W. Hamm, Division of Cardiology, University Hamburg, University Hospitals Eppendorf, Martinistraße 52, 20246 Hamburg, Germany

D. Hausmann, Department of Cardiology, Division of Internal Medicine, Hannover Medical School, Konstanty-Gutschow-Straße 8, 30625 Hannover, Germany

A. Hildebrand, Fraunhofer Institute for Computer Graphics,
Wilhelminenstraße 7, 64283 Darmstadt, Germany

V.W.M. van Hinsbergh, TNO Health Research, Vascular Research,
Gaubius Laboratory, Zernikedreef 9, 2300 AK Leiden, The Netherlands

P.R. Hoskins, Department of Medical Physics and Medical Engineering,
Royal Infirmary, The University of Edinburgh, 1 Lauriston Place,
Edinburgh EH3 9YW, UK

K.-F. Kamm, Philips GmbH, Philips Medical Systems, Röntgenstraße 24,
22335 Hamburg, Germany

G. Karczmar, The University of Chicago, Department of Radiology,
MC-2026, 5841 South Maryland Avenue, Chicago, IL 60637, USA

J.F. Keany, Evans Memorial Department of Medicine, and Whitaker
Cardiovascular Institute, Boston University Medical Center, 88 East Newton
Street, Boston, MA 02118, USA

J. Kekow, Städtisches Klinikum Magdeburg, Clinic of Rheumatology
Vogelsang, 39245 Vogelsang/Gommern, Germany

H. Kleinholz, Department of Radiology, Virchow Hospital, Humboldt
University of Berlin, Augustenburger Platz 1, 13353 Berlin, Germany

C. Korninger, Department of Vascular Biology and Thrombosis Research,
University of Vienne, Schwarzspanierstraße 17, 1090 Vienna, Austria

W. Krause, Clinical Development Diagnostics, Ultrasound Contrast Media,
Schering AG, Müllerstraße 170–178, 13342 Berlin, Germany

W. Kupper, Herz-Kreislauf-Klinik, Röhmerstätterstraße 25,
29549 Bad Bevensen, Germany

P. Lanzer, Kardiologische Gemeinschaftspraxis, Saalbaustraße 27,
64238 Darmstadt, Germany

K. Lindström, Department of Electrical Measurements, Lund Institute of
Technology, P.O. Box 118, 22100 Lund, Sweden

M. Lipton, The University of Chicago, Department of Radiology, MC-2026,
5841 South Maryland Avenue, Chicago, Illinois 60637, USA

M.P.M. de Maat, TNO Health Research, Vascular Research, Gaubius
Laboratory, Zernikedreef 9, 2300 AK Leiden, The Netherlands

M.R. Malinow, Oregon Regional Primate Research Center, 505 NW 185th
Avenue, Beaverton, Oregon 97006, USA

W.N. McDicken, Department of Medical Physics and Medical Engineering,
Royal Infirmary, The University of Edinburgh, 2 Lauriston Place, Edinburgh
EH3 9YW, UK

A. Mügge, Department of Cardiology, Division of Internal Medicine, Hannover Medical School, Konstanty-Gutschow-Straße 8, 30625 Hannover, Germany

P.A. Olofsson, Department of Biomedical Engineering, Malmö University Hospital MAS, 20502 Malmö, Sweden

D.G.W. Onnasch, Clinic for Pediatric Cardiology, Pediatric Hospital, Christian-Albrechts-University Hospitals, Schwanenweg 20, 24105 Kiel, Germany

P.H.A. Quax, TNO Health Research, Vascular Research, Gaubius Laboratory, Zernikedreef 9, 2300 AK Leiden, The Netherlands

H. Refsum, University of Bergen. Clinical Pharmacology Unit, Central Laboratory, Haukeland Hospital, 5021 Bergen, Norway

J. Ricke, Department of Radiology, Virchow Hospital, Humboldt University of Berlin, Augustenburger Platz 1, 13353 Berlin, Germany

R.E. Roller, Department for Vascular Biology and Thrombosis Research, University of Vienne, Schwarzspanierstraße 17, 1090 Vienna, Austria

J.A. Rumberger, Department of Cardiovascular Diseases and Internal Medicine, Mayo Clinic and Foundation, 200 First St. S.W., Rochester, MN 55905, USA

R. Schlief, Clinical Development Diagnostics, Ultrasound Contrast Media, Schering AG, Müllerstraße 178, 13342 Berlin, Germany

M. Sturm, Department of Cardiology, Division of Internal Medicine, Hannover Medical School, Konstanty-Gutschow-Straße 8, 30625 Hannover, Germany

P.M. Ueland, University of Bergen. Clinical Pharmacology Unit, Central Laboratory, Haukeland Hospital, 5021 Bergen, Norway

J.A. Vita, Evans Memorial Department of Medicine, and Whitaker Cardiovascular Institute, Boston University Medical Center, 88 East Newton Street, Boston, MA 02118, USA

T.J. Vogl, Department of Radiology, Virchow Hospital, Humboldt University of Berlin, Augustenburger Platz 1, 13353 Berlin, Germany

H. Wieland, Division of Clinical Chemistry, University Hospital Freiburg, Hugstetter Straße 55, 79106 Freiburg, Germany

J.E. Wilting, Philips Medical Systems Nederland b.v., Veenpluis 4–6, Building QG-119, 5680 DA Best, The Netherlands

F.W. Zonneveld, Department of Radiology, E01-132, Utrecht University Hospital, P.O. Box 85500, 3508 GA Utrecht, The Netherlands

Part I: Diagnostics of Vascular Diseases: State-of-the-Art

Section I: Nonimaging Vascular Diagnostic Methods

Principles and Clinical Applications

A. Fronek

The introduction of duplex scanning has significantly affected our use of various noninvasive methods to diagnose arterial and venous disease. Some methods have become outdated, some have more limited application, and some still maintain their importance, escpecially when cost-effectiveness is considered.

The types of methods described below have been selected with these considerations in mind.

Diagnosis of Arterial Disease

Pressure Measurement

Introduction

Pressure measurements of different segments of the extremity (upper or lower) have become the most widely used and also the most useful method in the diagnosis of peripheral arterial occlusive disease (PAOD). In contrast to the routine arm pressure measurement that is based on the Korotkoff phenomenon, pressure measurement of the lower extremity has to utilize the sphygmomanometric principle.

Basic Principle

The Basic principle of the sphygmomanometric method ist that a pneumatic cuff encircling the limb is connected to a source of variable pressure. The peripheral pulse or Doppler velocity signal is monitored while the cuff pressure is increased to a slightly suprasytolic value. The cuff pressure is slowly released and the pressure at which the first pulse is recorded is equated to the systolic pressure.

Description of the method

Cuff size
It is well known that an undersized cuff leads to erroneously high blood pressure values. The original American Heart Association Committee recommendation can be applied to the lower extremities as well, namely cuff width = 1.2 x diameter [28]. Considering the above-described relationship, the following cuff blader width dimensions are recommended: arm: 13.0 cm; thigh: 18 cm; above knee: 16.0 cm; below knee: 15.0 cm; above ankle: 13.0 cm; toe: 2 cm. In many laboratories, however, for the sake of simplicity, a uniform cuff width of 13 cm is used except for the toe, where a 2-cm cuff width is recommended.

Sensing devices
Monitoring the Doppler velocity signal ist the most widely used method to sense the presence, absence, and reappearance of the peripheral pulse after gradually reducing cuff pressure. Usually the posterior tibial or dorsalis pedis artery is selected for pulse monitoring. The advantage is the simplicity and portability of the hand-held Doppler device. The disadvantage is the unreliability of toe pulse velocity monitoring, which precludes toe pressure measurement.

Possible Sources of Error

Rate of Cuff Pressure Reduction
Too rapid a reduction in cuff pressure may lead to erroneously low pressure values. Generally 2 mmHG per heart beat is recommended [2].

Increased Arterial Wall Stiffness
The reappearance of the arterial pulse depends not only on the intra-arterial pressure but also on the elasticity of the arterial wall. An increase of the modulus of elasticity (increased stiffness) leads to erroneously high blood pressure values (ankle/bra-

chial pressure index >1.2), and is found most often in patients with diabetes mellitus, but may also be seen in patients who have undergone repeated renal dialysis.

Inadequate Accuracy of the Manometer
Although the conventional aneroid manometer is more convenient in daily practice, its accuracy is inferior to that of the mercury manometer, which must still be considered the "gold standard." It is, therefore, advisable to check the aneroid against a mercury manometer regularly (at least once a year).

Improper Cuff Placement
Loose application of the cuff may lead to erroneously high pressure readings. A snug application at 0 mmHG without compromising the circulation is recommended.

Type and Site of Sensing
The most frequently used site of sensing is the posterior tibial or the dorsalis pedis artery when Doppler velocity monitoring is used or the toe pulse when photoplethysmography is deployed. The advantage of Doppler velocity signal monitoring is its simplicity and mobility, especially when using the handheld device. However, as mentioned above, it precludes the measurement of toe pressure because of the usually weak Doppler signal at the toe.

Photoplethysmographic sensing permits toe pressure recording as well as simultaneous recording from both legs. A wider acceptance of this type of sensing was impeded until recently because a recorder was needed. This relative disadvantage can be remedied by using a photoplethomographic instrument with an audio output [17], the photoelectric signal being transformed into an acoustic one.

Clinical Applications

Lower-extremity blood pressure measurement is the most informative method in the diagnosis of peripheral arterial occlusive disease. The full value of this simple method is utilized when pressure is determined at different levels (segmental pressure measurement). This approach increases the accuracy and helps to localize the site of the obstruction (Fig. 1). It is useful to relate the segmental pressures to the brachial pressure (A/B index); this ist most helpful in patients with hypertensive disease.

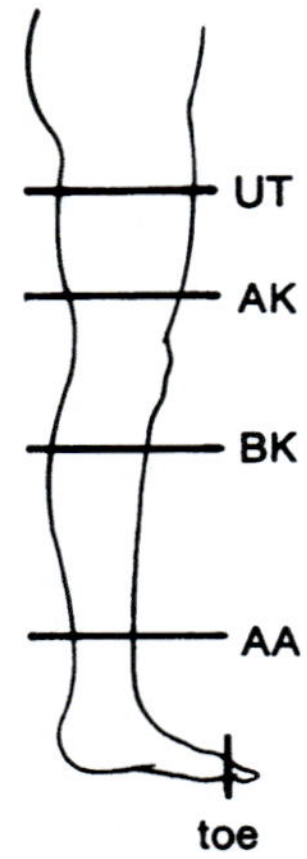

Fig. 1. Segmental arterial pressure measurement. Cuff positions: *UT*, upper thigh; *AK*, above knee; *BK*, below knee; *AA*, above ankle. (From [13], p. 89)

Examination at the following levels is recommended: upper thigh (UT), above knee (AK), below knee (BK), above ankle (AA), and toe. The segment/brachial artery index depends on the size of the cuffs. Under normal conditions, the larger cuffs (15 cm width) at the UT, AK, and BK levels and a 13-cm cuff at the AA level yield a ratio of 1.0 ± 0.15. Many laboratories use uniform cuffs of 13 cm width which yield a ratio of 1.1 ± 0.15. The smaller width of 13 cm permits a slightly more accurate topographic diagnosis on the thigh since the large "thigh" cuffs may overlap.

UT/Arm Pressure Index
A reduced index (usually less than 0.85) points to an aortoiliac obstruction. This diagnosis has to be confirmed by the finding of a significantly reduced common femoral velocity (Doppler) signal (see below). A reduced UT/arm pressure ratio with a normal Doppler velocity signal reflects a proximal superficial femoral artery stenosis. This set of data virtually rules out a hemodynamically significant aortoiliac artery disease.

AK/Arm Pressure Index
A reduced AK/arm index (≤0.8) in the presence of a normal UT/arm pressure index or a normal common femoral artery Doppler signal strongly suggests the presence of superficial femoral artery stenosis. A ratio of ≤0.55 is indicative of a complete occlusion of the superficial femoral arery (usually confirmed by an extremely low popliteal artery Doppler signal).

BK/Arm Pressure Index

A reduced BK/arm index ($\leq$0.80) usually reflects the presence of a distal obstruction of the superficial femoral artery (especially if the AK/arm ratio is not conclusive).

AA/Arm Pressure Index

This is the most widely used pressure parameter. A reduced ratio ($\leq$0.80) suggests that there is a hemodynamically significant obstruction in the calf or thigh, but this measurement alone does not permit a more detailed identification of the site of the obstruction. A normal AA/arm index, however, strongly suggests the absence of a significant arterial lesion, although there are at least two sources of error in this regard: (1) increased rigidity of the arterial wall may obscure the correct pressure reading (see above); and (2) it is possible that under resting conditions the pressure drop may be minimal, but it may become significant under increased metabolic requirements (e.g., exercise). It is, therefore, advisable to add some type of stress test in patients with claudication but with a normal resting AA/arm pressure ratio (exercise or postocclusive reactive hyperemia test – see below).

Toe/Arm Pressure Index

A toe/arm pressure ratio of 0.65 or lower in the presence of a normal AA/arm index suggests an arterial obstructive disease either in the foot or in the toes. Usually, if a significantly reduced toe pressure ratio is found in the great toe, similar reductions are observed in the remaining toes. However, it is not unusual to find significant differences between individual toes, implying the presence of selective small artery disease.

Penile/Arm Pressure Index

Penile pressure can be determined by using a 2.5-cm cuff placed at the base of the penis and the same criteria are used as for the leg segmental oscillographic presure measurement. Doppler velocity signal or PPG signals can be used as monitoring modes. A reduced penile/arm pressure ratio (usually $\leq$ 0.6) is considered pathologic and may explain sexual impotence due to a significant stenosis of the internal or common iliac artery. The effect of age, however, has to be considered. On the basis of Kempzinski's [26] findings, in patients less than 40 years old an index of 0.80 or above is considered normal, while above 40 years old a penile/arm index of 0.75 is considered normal. Naturally, if the UT/arm pressure index is reduced and the common femoral artery velocity signal is reduced, a common iliac artery obstruction has to be considered. This may explain the patient's symptoms (if the take-off of the internal iliac artery is distal to the site of obstruction).

Stress Test

A mild degree of arterial stenosis need not, under resting conditions, cause a measurable drop in AA/arm pressure index. A significant pressure drop may, however, develop if arterial flow through the stenotic portion is increased. This may be induced either by exercise or by postocclusive reactive hyperemia.

Exercise Test. The most reliable exercise test utilizes a treadmill forcing the patient to walk at 3 km/h at a 12% incline for 5 min [47]. Although this method can be considered to be the standard stress test, it has limitations, mainly in the examination of patients with various neuromuscular impairments. Furthermore, an electrically driven treadmill test has to be closely monitored, especially during examination of patients with coronary heart disease. Patient-driven treadmills have the advantage of stopping immediately when the patient feels any type of discomfort. Various alternatives for exercise testing have been devised: ankle flexion, tiptoeing, standardized knee bending, or simply walking. The tests are usually performed for 5 min, after which the patient resumes the supine position and ankle and arm pressures are measured at 1-min intervals. A significant AA/arm pressure index drop (compared to the resting value) persisting for 2 min or more is consistent with a hemodynamically significant arterial occlusive disease. The extent of pressure drop and its duration are related to the severity of the disease [13].

Postocclusive Reactive Hyperemia. This test requires the measurement of ankle pressure after a 4-min suprasystolic occlusion, usually performed at the BK level (AK cuff placement seems to be slightly more effective but may be poorly tolerated). The evaluation criteria are similar to those described above (exercise/pressure test), but the pressure drop is usually smaller and the duration shorter [58]. This disadvantage is to some extend outweighed by excellent patient compliance, even in those who suffer from some type of neuromuscular impairment or coronary heart disease. The ability to measure the pressure immediately after cuff pressure release and to measure both legs simultaneously represents an additional advantage in this select group of patients.

Pulse Reappearance Time. This test is based on the well-known clinical phenomenon that in patients with severe peripheral arterial occlusive disease, pedal pulses disappear after exercise. To obtain objective and permanent results, the toe pulse volume is recorded (PPG strain gauge or air plethysmography). Similarly, as in the above-described postocclusive reactive hyperemia test, a suprasystolic pressure cuff is applied at the BK level for 4 min. The time is marked at which the postocclusive pulse amplitudes reach 50% of the preocclusion value (pulse reappearance half-time (PRT2) [16]. Under normal conditions, the PRT/2 value is close to zero, i.e., it reaches the 50% level immediately after cuff pressure release. PRT/2 values up to 10 s are still within the normal range; values between 10–20 s represent a gray zone. PRT/2 values above 20 s document a significant arterial obstruction, while values above 40 s usually reflect multilevel disease. A normal PRT/2 in the presence of a reduced segment/arm pressure ratio suggests good collateralization. If a BK suprasystolic occlusion induces a significantly delayed PRT/2, it is helpful to repeat the test with an AA-induced PRT/2. If the second test is also highly positive, there is significant occlusive disease in the foot. This was recently corroborated by Willeke et al. [59], who found a good correlation between the number of occluded foot arteries and PRT/2.

Doppler Velocity Determination

Basic Principle

As discussed in more detail in Section II under "Vascular Ultrasonography", Doppler velocity determination uses the Doppler shift effect in which ultrasonic energy is reflected from moving particles. The well-known formula

$$\Delta f = \frac{2fv\cos\vartheta}{c}$$

(Δf = Doppler-shifted frequency; f = transmitted frequency; v = blood flow velocity; ϑ = angle of incidence of the ultrasonic beam; c = propagagation speed of ultrasound) has significant practical implications. Δf: The frequency shift is within the ear's sensitivity range and is therefore audible. f: The lower the transmitter frequency, the deeper the penetration of the ultrasonic beam. The inverse is true when resolution is considered. cos ϑ: Usually the best results are obtained if the probe is held at an angle of about 60°. c: In order to optimize the transmission conditions, an aqueous gel is used to exclude air between the probe and skin (air presents a very high resistance to the transmission of ultrasonic energy).

Basically, two types of ultrasonic energy delivery are used: continuous-wave (CW) and pulsed-gated wave. The latter is used mainly in imaging-associated systems (see Section II under "Vascular Ultrasonography"), while most Doppler velocity systems used in nonimaging methods use the CW system. Although the latter does not permit the precise separation and identification of the insonated sites which is the hallmark of the pulsed-gated system, the CW system permits easier and faster identification of the selected site by cross-insonating the vessel.

Description of the Method

There are three methods utilizing the Doppler shift phenomenon: acoustic, semiquantitative, and quantitative evaluation. The acoustic mode has the advantage of high mobility (no recorder is needed), but the evaluation is subjective. The latter two modes offer a more objective examination, as well as a permanent copy which is useful especially for future comparison.

The most useful frequencies are 5–9 MHz, 9 MHz being reserved for more superficial vessels.

Clinical Application

Acoustic Analysis
An Absence of a Doppler velocity signal confirms the occlusion of the examined artery, except in the dorsalis pedis artery, which may be missing in 5%–10% of young normal subjects. A strong triphasic signal from the femoral and popliteal artery usually rules out a hemodynamically significant obstruction, while the negative component may be missing in the normal posterior tibial artery.

The proper frequency (pitch), intensity, and presence or absence of the negative component can be judged with some training and is very helpful for quick evaluation, especially under outpatient clinic conditions.

Semiquantitative Evaluation

This is the most widely used mode of application since it offers a permanent record. It is essentially a "pattern recognition" method. A triphasic common femoral and popliteal artery tracing (with a well-developed negative component) usually rules out a significant obstruction. On the other hand, a biphasic tracing of reduced amplitude suggests a significant obstruction.

Gosling's pulsatility index (peak/mean velocity ratio; Fig. 2) [21] is a very useful semiquantitative index because it offers objective evaluation without requiring calibration of the Doppler velocity system. The peak and mean values are the same units and the result is, therefore, a dimensionless number which expresses fairly well the state of circulation in the examined artery. The normal range of pulsatility index values for the common femoral artery are 5–10, and for the posterior tibial artery, 7–15. This index is most reliable in advanced degrees of obstruction.

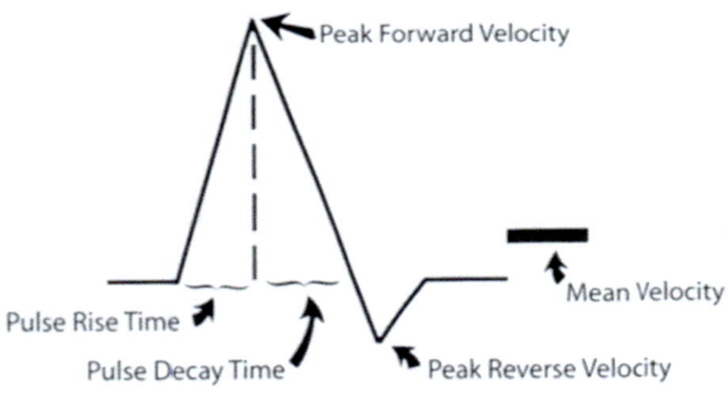

$$\text{Acceleration} = \frac{\text{Peak Velocity}}{\text{Pulse Rise Time}}$$

$$\text{Deceleration} = \frac{\text{Peak Velocity}}{\text{Pulse Decay Time}}$$

Fig. 2. Presentation of femoral artery velocity signal with various indices. (From [13], p. 107)

Quantitative Evaluation

The most reliable and accurate flow velocity determination can be obtained with the Doppler circuitry representing part of the duplex system (see Section II under "Vascular Ultrasonography"). It takes into account the actual angle of insonation and uses the fast Fourier transform system for processing. The most widely used Doppler velocity meters employ the simpler and less expensive "zero-crossing" system to process the Doppler frequency shift. It is impossible to calibrate these systems either using a 0.5% Sephadex suspension or comparing the results with those obtained with a duplex system. Since the insonation angle is not known, the principle of "maximum amplitude search" is recommended [15]. For this, the artery is first scanned horizontally until the maximum aplituted is reached. At this point the angle of the Doppler probe is changed until a maximum amplitude is reached again. The same procedure is used during calibration [49].

The most informative parameters are the peak velocity, decay time, and deceleration, which is a calculated value: peak velocity/decay time. Peak velocities for the femoral, popliteal, and posterior tibial arteries are 40.7 ± 10.9, 29.3 ± 5.9, 16 ± 10.0 cm/s respectively. Decay times are 163 ± 40, 157 ± 48, and 124 ± 52 ms respectively. The calculated values for deceleratin are 250.0 ± 60.0, 186.3 ± 47.0, and 129.8 ± 75.7 cm/s^2 respectively.

Decay time has the advantage of being independent of calibration and can be read off directly from the tracing. A common femoral artery decay time longer than 230 ms is strongly suggestive of a significant obstruction.

It has to be pointed out that the peak values are lower than those obtained with the duplex system. There may be several reasons for this discrepancy. First, duplex peak velocities are usually expressed in "peak" values at the time of peak systole, in addition to the so-called "average" duplex value which is closer to the "zero-crossing" values obtained with the standard Doppler velocity meters. Secondly, duplex systems use the pulsed system, in contrast to the CW system used in the commercially available Doppler intruments.

The quantitative Doppler evaluation is especially helpful in the diagnosis of borderline stenoses, in conjunction with segmental pressure measurements. Specifically, it helps in the diagnosis of iliac artery, superficial femora., and posterior tibial artery stenoses if pressure measurements offer borderline results.

Plethysmography

Introduction

Plethysmographic methods measure changes in the volume of organs. In the present context this means volume changes of the lower and upper extremities. Plethysmographic systems consist of (1) a sensing unit which translates volume changes into another form of energy; (2) a modifying unit that processes the received signal to a reliably recordable level, and (3) a recorder. Differences between plethysmographic methods are related to the type of sensor.

Basic Principles

Currently, the most widely used plethysmographic systems are based on the following sensing units:

1. Air plethysmography. This is one of the oldest methods used in the early stages of vascular physiology and has been revived by Winsor [60] and later modified by Raines [43].
2. Strain gauge plethysmography. Originally described by Whitney [57], the fine silicone tubing filled with mercury has been replaced by gallium and indium for improved sturdiness and reliability. This system detects even minute oscillatory volume changes (e.g., from the toe) which change the electrical resistance of the gauge.
3. Impedance plethysmography. Changes in local blood volume induce changes in electrical impedance of the examined section of the extremity. Currently, this method is used infreqeuently in the diagnosis of arterial disease, but it is still used in the diagnosis of venous disease (see below).
4. Photoplethysmography. A ligth illuminates a circumscribed part of the tissue and the reflected light is picked up by a photoelectric sensor. Since part of the absorption is related to the local blood volume, pulsatile changes (arterial pulse) or positional changes, as utilized in venous diagnostics (see below), induce changes in sensor output.

Description of the Method

Plethysmography is used in the examination of the arterial system in two different ways: to record the oscillatory part of the arterial pulse (AC component), and to record slow volume changes induced by transient outflow obstruction (DC component) – in venous occlusion plethysmography – recording arterial inflow rate).

Clinical Application

Arterial Pulse Plethysmography
Arterial pulse recording is used mainly as a sensing method in conjunction with segmental arterial pressure measurements (as an alternative to Doppler velocity monitoring – see above). Photoplethysmography (AC component) is used more often than strain gauge plethysmography, mainly because of the durability of the former. Raines [43], using air plethysmography, developed criteria to quantify the pulse volume, permitting a more quantitative evaluation of the lower extremity arterial circulation. Photoplethysmography or strain gauge plethysmography can also be utilized in the pulse reappearance time test (see above).

Venous Occlusion Plethysmography
Outflow from the examined vascular region is blocked suddenly by inflating a cuff to about 40 mmHg so as not to interfere with the inflow. The rate of volume increase is equal to blood flow. It is important to emphasize that volume changes recorded from the calf (using strain gauge or air plethysmography) essentially reflect muscle blood flow, because skin circulation represents only about 1/10 of the recorded inflow. On the other hand, venous occlusion volume changes recorded from the toes or digits do represent skin blood flow, because at the site of sensing there are only tendons and bony tissue in addition to the skin.

Diagnosis of Venous Disease

Introduction

While pathologies of the arterial system result mainly from obstruction to flow, in the venous system there are additional complexities related to changes in compliance and competency of the valvular system (reflux) in addition to outflow obstruction. The noninvasive diagnosis of venous disease has in recent years experienced a substantial improvement as a result of the introduction of the duplex system which combines the analysis of Doppler velocity signals with imaging of the examined vessels (see Section II under "Vascular Ultrasonography").

In view of this advance, some of the nonimaging diagnostic methods described below have lost some of their usefulness. There are, however, certain conditions in which their application is still fully justified and not replaceable.

Basic Principles

In contrast to the analysis of the arterial system, where the oscillating component (AC) is utilized, methods analyzing the hemodynamics of the venous system use the slow (or DC) component, usually induced by some standardized maneuvers. Standardized changes are also used in conjunction with the Doppler velocity examination of the venous system.

Description of the Methods

Doppler Velocity Examination

Complete absence of the venous Doppler signal at a well-defined examination site (e.g., common femoral, popliteal, or posterior tibial vein) confirms the obliteration of the respective vessel. In addition, several maneuvers are used to evaluate especially the state of the venous valvular system.

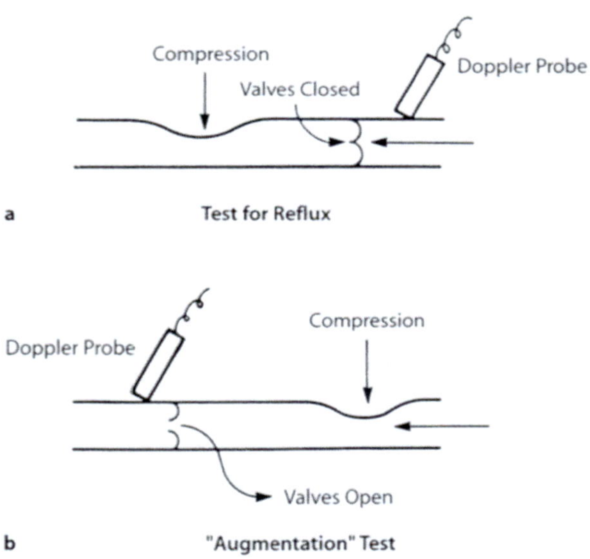

Fig. 3 a, b. Venous velocity signals and external compression. **a** Compression above the probe (valves closed: no reflux, normal); **b** Compression below the probe (augmentation: fast velocity, no obstruction). (From [13], p. 134)

Compression Maneuvers
The most widely used test, employing either a hand-held Doppler system or bidirectional system connected to a recorder, consists of selectively compressing the calf or the foot while the ultrasonic probe is positioned at a proximal site (augmentation test; (Fig 3). A clear and brisk Doppler velocity signal induced by hand compression rules out a significant outflow obstruction, at least in the close proximity of the test area. A reversed velocity signal, after release of compression, is usually due to an incompetent valvular system. If the Doppler probe is placed distal to the site of compression, absence of immediate response followed by Doppler response after release of the compression confirms the integrity of the valvular system (reflux test) (Fig. 3b).

Respiratory Changes
An additional mode of examination using the venous Doppler velocity signals is the respiratory response (Fig. 4). Increased intraabdominal pressure during inspiration reduces and sometimes even stops common femoral vein flow, while the opposite is observed (or recorded) during expiration.

Valsalva Maneuver
The exxaggerated increase in intra-abdominal pressure caused by the Valsalva maneuver leads to an immediate cessation of flow, followed by a compensatory increase in flow velocity at the termination of the maneuver (Fig. 5). This is one of the most sensitive tests for the detection of possible venous valvular insufficiency. To some degree it also helps to rule out a significant obstruction in the pelvic venous circulation (absence or presence of compensatory increase of flow velocity at the termination of the Valsalva maneuver).

Fig. 4 a–c. Effect of respiration on femoral vein flow velocity. **a** Velocity changes are synchronous with respiration. **b** Continuous velocity pattern (proximal obstruction). **c** Absent or extremely low velocity (occlusion). (From [13], p. 131)

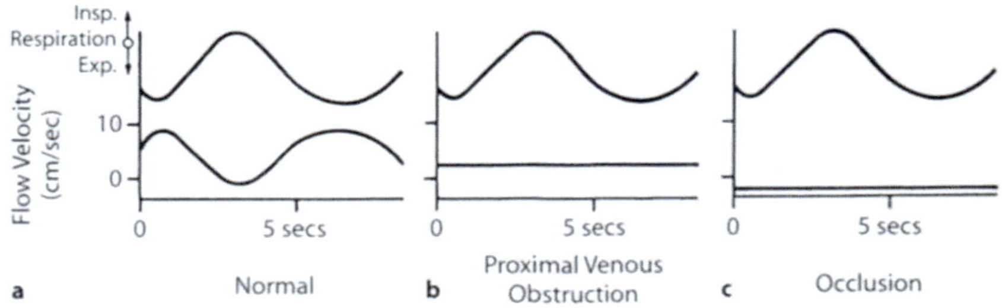

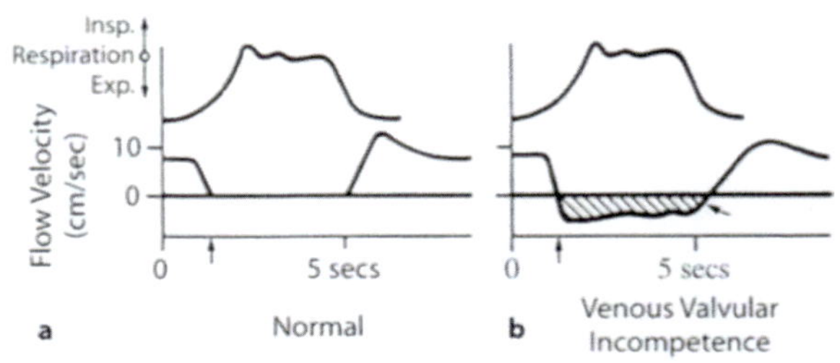

Fig. 5 a, b. Valsalva test and femoral vein velocity. **a** Complete stop (normal); **b** Reversal of velocity: reflux (venous valvular insufficiency). (From [13], p. 131)

Plethysmography

Plethysmography is more widely used in the diagnosis of venous than of arterial disease. As discussed above, several different sensing systems are used, each with some specific advantages and disadvantages.

Air Plethysmography

One of the oldest types of plethysmography, this has been revived in recent years by Nicolaides et al. [36] by combining the exercise test with volume changes induced by changes in limb position. The described method evaluates calf volume changes induced by hydrostatics (venous volume, VV) from the supine to the erect position, and the amount of blood volume displaced by exercise. In addition, calf filling time is recorded. The displacement after ten tiptoe movements yields the residual volume (RV) and a residual volume fraction (RVF) can be calculated: (RV/VV) x 100.

The advantage of this method is the quantification of displaced volume in milliliters per leg volume. Findings by this method have been well correlated with obstructive venous disease of the thigh; however, more data are still needed to determine the accuracy of the method in calf obstructive disease.

Strain Gauge Plethysmography

This type of plethysmography has been used mainly to measure the decrease in calf volume during exercise (usually tip toeing) and the outflow rate after release of thigh compression [29].

Impedance Plethysmography

As described above under "Basic Principles of the Different Sensors," a standardized outflow compression (usually 60 mmHg) causes a decrease in electrical impedance, which returns rapidly to the precompression value after the obstructing cuff pressure is released. This method has been thoroughly developed and correlated with phlebography by a number of investigators [55], although false negative and false positive findings are not unusual. The method is simple to use and is suitable as a quick prescreening test to rule out deep venous thrombosis. It does not, however, offer any information about valve competency.

Photoplethysmography

In the diagnosis of venous disease, photoplethysmographic systems use the DC mode (in contrast to the AC mode used in arterial disease studies), since changes in local blood volume induced by orthostasis or exercise are relatively slow. The method was revived by the introduction of "light reflection rheography" (LRR) [5]. Quantitative photoplethysmography was achieved by using computer-controlled light intensity [5a] or by manually calibrating the light intensity [14]. In both cases displacement of blood volume can be expressed as a percentage of optical density, which is linearly related to local blood volume changes [23]. Both systems permit quantitative recording of blood volume changes in addition to the very useful postexercise "recovery time" (see below).

Foot Volumetry

Foot volume changes, induced by knee bending, are recorded by monitoring the water level in an open container in which the feet are immersed up to the ankle [50]. The system can be easily calibrated and is quite rugged. The only limitation to a wider use of this method is the hygienic compromise one has to accept when immersing the unprotected feet in the bath.

Clinical Application

As mentioned previously, the advantage of the combined imaging and Doppler velocity analysis offered by the duplex system has displaced some of the nonimaging diagnostic methods from their dominant position. These methods will now be discussed from the viewpoint of their applicability and cost-effectiveness.

Doppler Velocity Examination

As has been mentioned before, the advantage of this method is its mobility and cost-effectiveness. It is an ideal examination tool at the bedside or under outpatient clinical conditions, especially if a handheld, portable systeme is used.

The described augmentation and reflux compression tests are especially useful in the diagnosis of venous valvular insufficiency of the common femoral, popliteal, and posterior tibial vein, as well as the long and short saphenous veins. In addition, the search for insufficient perforator (communicating) veins should not be neglected, especially in patients with poorly healing venous ulcers. Reflux documented during the Valsalva maneuver or after the release of distal compression (monitored from the common femoral vein with and without the additional application of a tourniquet) can be considered a highly specific and sensitive test to confirm or to rule out venous valvular insufficiency in the deep or superficial venous system. This strong endorsement applies a little less to the diagnosis of obstructive venous disease (deep venous thrombosis), where the changes may be more subtle unless the Doppler signal is completely absent at a well-described vein location (e.g., common femoral, popliteal, or posterior tibial vein).

From a practical point of view, the chart shown in Fig. 6 is quite helpful when performing the Doppler study.

Plethysmography

Plethysmographic methods utilize three maneuvers to study venous hemodynamics: orthostatic changes, exercise-induced volume displacement and transient venous outflow compression causing venous congestion, with monitoring of the rate of change during decongestion.

Air Plethysmography

As mentioned above, the test is performed in the supine position. After a stable baseline is reached, the patient is asked to stand up with the weight placed on the contralateral leg. The following are determined [35]:

Venous filling index (*VFI*) =

$$\frac{90\,\%\ \mathrm{VV}}{\text{time to reach } 90\,\% \text{ of filling } (\mathrm{VFT}^{90})}$$

A VFI below 2 ml/s confirms the absence of significant venous reflux. The application of a tourniquet helps to distinguish deep from superficial valvular insufficiency.

The volume decrease after one tiptoe movement (ejected volume, EV) can be normalized by VV and is expressed as ejection fraction (EF) = (EV/VV) x 100. The normal range is 60 % – 90 %. EF is significantly reduced with deep venous obstruction, in which case the highest value is about 40 %.

After ten tiptoes, the RV can be determined and again normalized by VV. Therefore, RVF = (RV/

	RIGHT					LEFT				
Signal	Common femoral	Popliteal	Post. tibial	Long saphenous	Short saphenous	Common femoral	Popliteal	Post. tibial	Long saphenous	Short saphenous
Present										
Spontaneous										
Pitch										
Response fluctuation										
Augmentation compression										
Reflux compression										
Valsalva without tourniquet										
Valsalva with tourniquet										
Post-Valsalva response										
Pulsatile										

Notes: Response amplitude: 0 = absent, 1 = weak, 2 = normal.
Pulsati e venous signal: if a stray arterial signal can be ruled out (change the angle of the probe), right heart failure should be considered.

Fig. 6. Record chart for results of venous Doppler velocity examination

VV) x 100. Under normal conditions RVF is not higher than 40%. Although there is a wide variation, especially in patients with varicose veins, the mean value is around 45% and increases with decreasing efficiency of the musculovenous pump. There is also a good correlation between RVF and the incidence of venous ulceration.

Strain Gauge Plethysmography

This method is used infrequently, although in the past it served as a basis for quantitative evaluation of other plethysmographic methods. The original apporach was to monitor the calf volume increase induced by a 60-mmHg cuff pressure applied to the thigh. Normal values (after reaching a steady state, usually 2–3 min) range between 2 to 3 ml/100 ml calf volume. Postphlebotic limbs yield a low value, as low as 1 ml/100 ml. Maximum venous outflow (MVF; ml/100 ml min), obtained from the outflow tangent after sudden cuff pressure release, seems to have a higher sensitivity and specificity. In normal subjects MVF may vary from 80 to 40 ml/100 ml min, but a value below 35 ml/100 ml min is usually found in limbs with acute venous obstruction [51].

Impedance Plethysmography

Like strain gauge plethysmography, impedance plethysmography provides an evaluation of the rate of volume change after cuff pressure release. Several investigators, primarily Wheeler et al. [56] and Hull et al. [25], identified a dependable discriminant line separating normal subjects from patients when the final steady-state volume is plotted against the volume drop 3 s after cuff pressure release. To increase "user friendliness," a fully automated impedance plethysmographic system is now available which prints out the results with a separating demarcation line.

Although the method is quite sensitive in detecting deep venous obstruction above the knee, the results are rather unreliable below the knee. That venous valvular insufficiency cannot be diagnosed with this method is an additional disadvantage.

Photoplethysmography

The usual application of the photoplethysmographic probe to the medical aspect of the ankle makes it possible to evaluate local blood volume changes in the distal portion of the calf, the usual site of trophic changes of the skin induced by increased venous pressure.

Quantitative photoplethysmography can be applied in two forms: manual calibrated photoplethysmography (C-PPG) and computer-assisted digital photoplethysmography (D-PPG), as mentioned above. Figure 7 describes the changes in optical

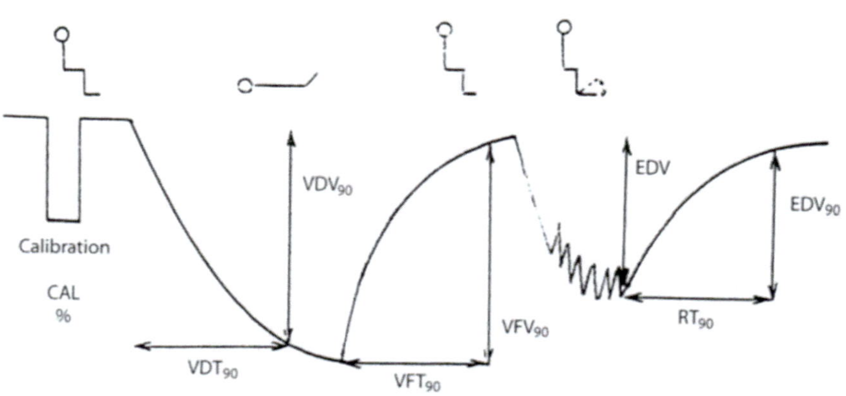

VDV = Venous Drainage Volume
VDT = Venous Drainage Time
VFV = Venous Filling Volume
VFT = Venous Filling Time
RV = Residual Volume
EDV = Exercise Drainage Volume
RT = Recovery Time

VDI = Venous Drainage Index = $\frac{\text{VDV 90 \%}}{\text{VDT 90 \%}}$

VFI = Venous Filling Index = $\frac{\text{VFV 90\%}}{\text{VFT 90\%}}$

PE = Pump Effiency = $\frac{\text{EDV}}{\text{VFV}}$

Fig. 7. Calibrated photoplethysmography (C-PPG). The effect of limb position and exercise on leg blood volume. (From [14], p. 931)

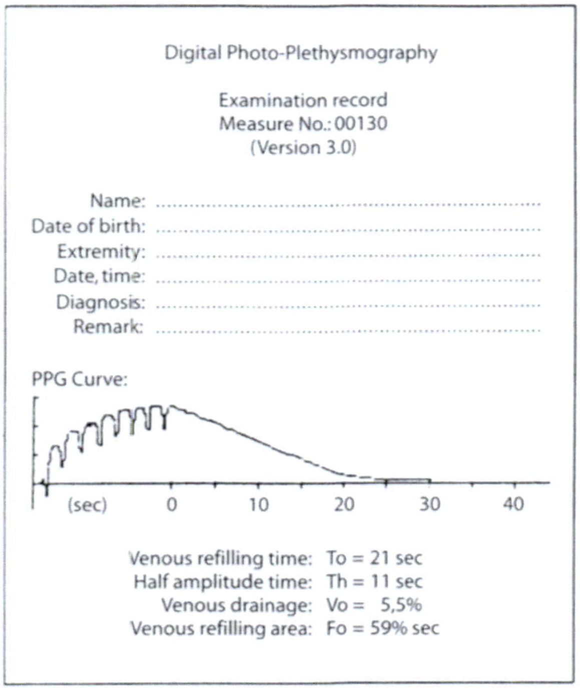

Fig. 8. Digital photoplethysmography (D-PPG). Actual tracing and recorded values. (From [14], p. 932)

density (OD) induced by orthostasis and exercise, including the parameters whch are directly obtained and those that are derived. The percentage of optical density change observed in normal subjects after changing from sitting to supine position is about 9 OD% and that after exercise about 3 OD%. The exercise-induced optical density percentage change recorded with the D-PPG system is about 6 OD% [27] (Fig. 8).

Recovery time (RT) is considered pathologic if it is less than 20 s, which was already established by Abramowitz et al. [1] as a reliable index of venous valvular insufficiency. Further correlation studies will have to confirm the reliability of both methods in the diagnosis of proximal venous obstruction.

Foot Volumetry

The advantage of this method is that foot blood volume displacement induced by exercise is recorded directly (see above). A number of parameters can be directly measured and some important hemodynamic information can be derived. The most important variables are the expelled volume (EV) and refilling flow (F). Normal mean EV values are about 17 ml and normal F = 2.3 ml/100 ml min. A good correlation was also found with direct venous pressure measurement [40]. More detailed studies evaluating the accuracy of this method in patients with different types of venous disease are still needed.

Analysis of the Cutaneous Circulation

Introduction

Although the skin is an ideal organ for noninvasive examination of blood flow, this fact is still not fully exploited in routine laboratory studies. There are several reasons for this. One is the high vasomotor activity of the cutaneous circulation – increasing the range of normal values regardless of the method used. In addition, some older methods in clinical microvascular studies used mainly subjective or semisubjective evaluation criteria (e.g., capillaroscopy). Finally, the stimulus to investigate the cutaneous circulation from the viewpoint of arterial occlusive disease has been dampened to some extent by the realization that impaired blood supply to the extremities often does not significantly affect the cutaneous circulation at a time when other methods already document a significant change (e.g., segmental pressure, Doppler velocity).

Here, we shall only discuss methods with proven clinical application.

Skin Temperature Measurement

Basic Principles

Skin temperature is the final result of a number of different factors: skin blood flow, the state of nervous and metabolic activity, ambient temperature and humidity, exposure to nicotine, type of food ingested, etc. This array of factors shows why it is necessary to maintain standardized examination conditions.

Direct Contact Thermometry

Two types of sensors are used: thermocouples and thermistors. *Thermocouples* (two different metals joined together) develop a voltage dependent on the applied temperature [19]. They are experiencing a comeback because of significant improvement and miniaturizing of DC amplifiers which are needed because of the relatively low voltage output. *Thermistors* utilize the temperature dependence of some alloys, their specific resistance decreasing with increasing temperature.

Infrared Thermometry
The skin continuously emits a certain amount of infrared (invisible) energy which is related to the temperature of the skin and of the underlying tissues.

Thermography
This method combines temperature measurement based on the emission of infrared energy, similarly to the simple version described above, with a scanning system which produces a display of the "visualized" temperatures [53]. This is displayed either in black and white with different shades of gray or in color, coded against different temperatures.

Liquid Crystals
Special cholesteric substances change color depending on temperature. Plastic films impregnated with these crystals are placed in close contact with the examined area and after a steady state is reached, color pictures are taken [18].

Description of the Methods

Depending on the method used, the sensing probe is either in close contact with the examined portion of the skin (thermocouples, thermistors, liquid crystals) or at some distance from the site of examination (infrared thermometry, thermography). In the latter case the distance is not critical; however, the closer the sensor and the smaller the radius of the examined area, the more reliably will the measured temperature represent the center of the examined area.

The advantage of the thermocouple and thermistor systems is their simplicity. However, it takes some time to reach a steady state and this may slow down the procedure, especially if several sites are measured (e.g., fingers and toes). Devices based on the principle of infrared energy sensing are more complex but offer a virtually immediate readout.

In view of the fact that skin temperature is readily influenced by a number of factors in addition to skin perfusion, as discussed above, steps have to be taken to minimize this influence. The examination room has to be a quiet place, with a controlled temperature (~25°C). The patient should be advised to refrain from smoking or drinking alcohol for at least 2 h before the examination.

Clinical Application

Reductions in skin temperature by more than 1°C (compared to a similar or contralateral measurement site, e.g., adjacent finger or toe) are indicative of a significantly reduced blood flow. On the other hand, increased temperature is suggestive of an inflammatory process (e.g., phlebitis).

The efficacy of vasodilatory drugs can be tested by comparing skin temperature before and after administration of these drugs.

Temperature stress (increasing or decreasing ambient temperature) can be used to examine the vasomotor response of the cutaneous circulation. Increased temperature can be achieved either by immersing the examined extremity in warm water (44°C). Decreased temperature (cooling) can be achieved by immersing the extremity (usually the hand) into ice-cold water. An immersion for 15 s is usually sufficient to induce a significant vasoconstriction even in normal subjects. Patients with extreme cold sensitivity (e.g., Raynaud's phenomenon, combined nerve and artery injuries) will respond not only with a painful reaction but also with significantly delayed normalization of skin temperature (>4 min) [20].

Capillaroscopy

Introduction

The morphology of capillary loops, best observed on the nailfold of fingers or toes, offers direct information on some underlying diseases, e.g., scleroderma [33]. A different type of image is obtained from the dorsum of the foot, which can be prognostic of trophic changes of the skin [7, 8].

Basic Principles and Description of the Methods

Static Capillaroscopy
Static capillaroscopy is best conducted on the nailfold of the finger or toe using a microscope, first at low magnification (x~12) followed by a wide-angle lens to permit a rapid overview. This is followed by a more detailed evaluation using a higher magnification (x25–50). A very useful simplification was described by Mahler [31] using a conventional ophthalmoscope (with a 50-diopter built-in lens, a magnification x10 can be achieved).

Dynamic Capillaroscopy

This approach represents a combination of microscopy with video monitoring in conjunction with electronic evaluation of recorded red blood cell movement [9]. The previously tedious evaluation has been simplified by the introduction of computer analysis [10], which brings this method closer to clinical application.

Clinical Application

Static Capillaroscopy

Normal nail-fold capillary pattern is characterized by parallel capillary loops. In contrast, patients with scleroderma exhibit either significant patches of hypo- or avascular areas or "giant" capillaries [33]. Mahler's method using a standard ophthalmoscope (with a green filter) offers a similar picture for a quick office evaluation, although with less detail [31]. Fagrell [7] extended the application of static capillaroscopy to the skin of the foot and ankle by introducing a classificatin of capillary morphology. Three stages are described: (a) with normal or very few "micropools" through (b) with capillary hemorrhages and (c) only few visible capillaries or complete absence of capillaries. The last stage is found in patients who develop skin ulceration within 3 months [7].

Dynamic Capillaroscopy

Direct observation of a complete cessation of red blood cell movement, especially in response to local cooling, can be considered as reliable confirmation of increased cold sensitivity of the microvasculature. This can be observed, for instance, in patients with Raynaud's phnenomenon.

Transcutaneous PO_2 Measurement

Basic Principle

Transcutaneous PO_2 (TcPO_2) is the partial oxygen tension which can be measured on the surface of the skin using a modified Clark-type platinum electrode. Under normal conditions, tcPO_2 on the surface of the skin is close to zero. Usable results can be obtained after vasodilation has been induced, usually by activating a built-in heater.

Method

It is important to remove the most superficial cell layers of the skin by repeatedly placing and removing a piece of heavy duty adhesive tape. The optimal probe temperature is 43°C; a higher temperature may lead to unnecessary irritation of the skin, especially in patients with severely compromised skin blood flow.

Clinical Application

TcPO_2 monitoring is widely used in neonatology, the area in which it was first applied after being developed by Huch and Huch [24]. Although there is a relationship between tcPO_2 and skin blood flow, it is not linear. In effect, a moderate degree of peripheral arterial occlusive disease has very little effect on the resulting tcPO_2, but a severe degree leads to a significant decrease from about 40 mmHg to 20 mmHg or less. One of the most useful application areas is in determination of optimal level for an amputation. It could be shown that a tcPO_2 level $\leq$10 mmHg is incompatible with per primam amputation stump healing. The reliability of this test can be increased by a combination with oxygen inhalation: if the 20 mmHg tcPO_2 value is not increased after 5 min of oxygen inhalation, there is a very low probability that the amputation stump will heal [22, 41].

A variety of different tcPO_2 values has been observed in patients with venous disease. tcPO_2 was reduced in patients who developed trophic changes of the skin including ulcer [32, 42]. On the other hand, values close to zero have been found in atrophie blanche [12], not necessarily leading to the development of an ulcer. The findings of Nemeth et al. [34], that tcPO_2 values are markedly reduced in ulcerated and edematous skin are also of interest, as ist the fact that reduction of edema had no effect on the tcPO_2 values.

Laser Doppler Flux Metering

Basic Principle

The detection of the Doppler shift signal from the cutaneous microcirculation utilizes a very narrow monochromatic light source (laser) to monitor the red blood cell movement in the microvasculature. The incident light source reaches the capillaries and red blood cells at a variety of angles. The recorded Doppler-shifted signal corresponds therefore to the average velocity obtained under an average angle. All these conditions are in contrast to the far more simple conditions when flow velocity is measured in an exactly defined vessel by ultrasound. To complicate the situation, the resulting signal depends not only upon the velocity, but also on the number of red blood cells (again, in contrast to Doppler ultrasound velocity determination in a simple vessel utilizing ultrasound). The resulting signal is, therefore, the product of red blood cell volume fraction (RBC) and the mean velocity (V) of the moving red blood cells. Since it is neither velocity nor flow, the term flux is used: flux = RBC x V [37].

Description of the Method

Although the electronic system is rather complex, the mode of application of Laser Doppler flux (LDF) metering is simple. Depending upon the site of examination, the probe holder is attached to the skin with double-faced tape and the probe is placed in the holder. It is also possible to simultaneously monitor red blood cell movement in the capillaries using a combined probe for laser Doppler fluxmetry and video microscopy [11].

Clinical Application

The most useful mode of application is the relative perfusion estimate – i.e., determination of the effect of a stimulus before, during, and after its application – in combination with standardized tests, e.g., inspiratory gasp, Valsalva maneuver [30], the effect of cold and heat [38], and the effect of post-occlusive reactive hyperemia [39]. Belcaro and co-workers [3, 4] documented reduction and even disappearance of the venoarteriolar response to orthostasis in patients with venous insufficiency. Currently, evaluation of relative changes, as described above, seems to be the most reliable application of LDF metering, because of difficulties with absolute calibration. This circumstance also explains the usefulness of monitoring the short-term effect of pharmacologic agents [6], the monitoring of vasomotor responses in patients with Raynaud's phenomenon [61], and the effect of orthostasis on skin perfusion in diabetics [52]. The discriminative value of LDF values in patients with peripheral arterial occlusive disease is lower for several reasons: (1) overlapping with normal values, (2) the presence of significantly reduced values mainly in advanced stages of diseases, and (3) last, but not least, the availability of only "relative units," which makes it difficult to compare different subjects, or even the same subject on different days, due to significant temporal and spatial fluctuations [48].

Flux motion (periodic changes of LDF signal) is an interesting flow-related phenomenon and at the same time an ideal object of observation for the LDF method, because absolute calibration is not of primary importance. Three different types of flux motion can be identified: low-frequency (2–10 cycles/min), high-frequency (15–25 c/min), and heart-rate-corresponding frequency [46]. In patients with peripheral arterial occlusive disease, the prevalence of high-frequency waves increased with the severity of ischemia. In contrast, recently Schmidt et al. [45] reported an increased incidence of slow wave flow motion with increased severity of peripheral arterial occlusive disease.

Laser Doppler Perfusion Imaging

A significantly new level of application possibilities is opened by the combination of LDF metering with perfusion color coding and surface scanning, which results in a very useful display of perfusion over an approximate area of 144 cm^2 [54]. Although systematic clinical evaluation is not yet available, the technical specifications and performance promise a significant enrichment of the research and diagnostic armamentarium.

References

1. Abramowitz HB, Queral LA, Finn WR, Nora PF, Peterson LK, Bergan JJ, Yao JST (1979) The use of photoplethysmography in the assessment of venous insufficiency. Surgery 86: 434
2. American Heart Association (1939) Standardization of blood pressure readings. Am Heart J 18: 95
3. Belcaro G, Nicolaides AN (1993) Laser doppler, oxygen and CO_2 tension in venous hypertension. In: Bernstein EF (ed) Vascular diagnosis. Mosby, St Louis, p 934
4. Belcaro G, Christopoulos D, Nicolaides AN (1989) Skin flow and swelling in postphlebitic limbs. Vasa 18: 136
5. Blazek V (1984) Medizinisch-technische Grundlagen der „Licht-Reflexions-Rheographie". In: May R, Stemmer R (eds) Die Licht-Reflexions-Rheographie. Perimed, Erlangen, p 15

5a. Blazek V, Schmitt HJ, Schultz-Ehrenburg O, Kerner J (1989) Digitale Photoplethysmographie D-PPG für die Beinvenendiagnostik. Phlebol Proktol 18:91

6. Creutzig A (1994) Evaluation of pharmacologic effects. In: Belcaro GV, Hoffmann U, Bollinger A, Nicolaides AN (eds) Laser doppler. Med-Orion, London, p 149
7. Fagrell B (1973) Vital capillary microscopy - a clinical method for studying changes of the nutritional skin capillaries in legs with arteriosclerosis obliterans. Scand J Clin Lab Invest Suppl: 133
8. Fagrell B (1979) Local microcirculation in chronic venous incompetence and leg ulcers. Vasc Surg 13: 217
9. Fagrell B, Fronek A, Intaglietta M (1977) A microscope television system for studying flow velocity in human skin capillaries. Am J Physiol 233: H318
10. Fagrell B, Eriksson SE, Malmström S, Sjölund A (1988) Computerized data analysis of capillary blood cell velocity. Int J Microcirc Clin Exp 7: 276
11. Franzeck UK (1994) Combined probes for laser doppler fluxmetry, transcutaneous oxygen tension measurements and video microscopy. In: Belcaro GV, Hoffmann U, Bollinger A, Nicolaides AN (eds) Laser doppler. Med-Orion, London, p 73
12. Franzek UK, Bollinger A, Huch R, Huch A (1984) Transcutaneous oxygen tension and capillary morphologic characteristics and density in patients with chronic venous incompetence. Circulation 70: 806
13. Fronek A (1989) Noninvasive diagnostics in vascular disease. McGraw-Hill, New York, 293
14. Fronek A (1993) Recent developments in venous photoplethysmography. In: Bernstein EF (ed) Noninvasive diagnostic techniques in vascular disease, 4th edn. Mosby, St Louis, p 930
15. Fronek A, Coel M, Bernstein EF (1976) Quantitative ultrasonographic studies of lower extremity flow velocities in health and disease. Circulation 53: 953
16. Fronek A, Coel M, Bernstein EF (1977) The pulse reappearance time, an index of the overall blood impairment in the ischemic extremity. Surgery 81: 37
17. Fronek A, Blazek V, Curran B (1994) Toe pressure determined by audio-photoplethysmography. J Vasc Surg 30: 267-270
18. Gautherie M, Quenenneville Y, Gross C (1974) Thermographic cholesterique. Pathol Biol (Paris) 22: 553
19. Geddes LA, Baker LE (1975) Principles of applied biomedical instrumentation, 2nd edn. Wiley, New York, p 156
20. Gelberman RH, Blasingame JP, Fronek A, Dimick MP (1979) Forearm arterial injuries. J Hand Surg 4: 401
21. Gosling RG, King DH (1974) Arterial assessment by doppler-shift ultrasound. Proc Soc Med 67: 447
22. Harward T, Volny J. Golbranson F, Bernstein EF, Fronek A (1985) Oxygen inhalation-induced transcutaneous PO_2 changes as a predictor of amputation level. J Vasc Surg 2: 220
23. Higgins JL (1988) Photoplethysmography: theoretical and experimental considerations in the diagnosis of venous disease. Thesis, University of California, San Diego
24. Huch A, Huch R (1977) Technical, physiological and clinical aspects of transcutaneous PO_2 measurements. In: Taylor DEM, Whamond J (eds) Noninvasive clinical measurement. University Park Press, Baltimore, p 171
25. Hull R, Hirsch J, Sackett DL, Powers P, Turpie AGG, Walker I (1977) Combined use of leg scanning and impedance plethysmography in suspected venous thrombosis - an alternate to venography. N Engl J Med 298: 1497
26. Kempcznski RF (1979) Role of the vascular diagnostic laboratory in the evaluation of male impotence. Am J Surg 138: 278
27. Kerner J, Schultz-Ehrenburg U, Blazek V (1989) Digitale Photoplethysmographie (D-PPG) - klinische Eignung der neuen Messmethode zur venösen Funktionsdiagnostik. Phlebol Proktol 18: 98
28. Kirkendall WM, Burton AC, Epstein FH et al (1967) Recommendations for human blood pressure determinations by sphygmomanometers. Circulation 36: 980
29. Kuiper JP, Brakkee RJM (1971) Unblutige Venendruckmessung. Hautarzt 22: 153
30. Low PA et al (1983) Evaluation of skin vasomotor reflexes by using laser doppler velocimetry. Mayo Clin Proc 58: 592
31. Mahler F (1981) Kapillarmikroskopie mit dem Augenspiegel. Vasa 10: 18
32. Mani R, White JE, Barrett DF, Weaver PF (1989) Tissue oxygenation, venous ulcers and fibrin cuffs. J. R Soc Med 82: 345
33. Maricq HR, Le Roy EC, D'Angelo WA, Medzger TA et al (1980) Diagnostic potential of in vivo capillary microscopy in scleroderma and related disorders. Arthritis Rheum 23: 183
34. Nemeth A, Falanga V, Altstadt SP, Eaglstein WH (1989) Ulcerated edematous limbs: effect of edema removal on transcutaneous oxygen measurements. J Am Acad Dermatol 20: 191
35. Nicolaides AN, Christopoulos D (1993) Quantitation of venous reflux and outflow obstruction with air-plethysmography. In: Bernstein EF (ed) Noninvasive diagnostic techniques in vascular disease, 4th edn. Mosby, St Louis, p 915
36. Nicolaides AN, Christopoulos D, Vadekis S (1989) Progress in the investigations of chronic venous insufficiency. Ann Vasc Surg 3: 278
37. Nilsson GE, Tenland T, Oberg PA (1980) A new instrument for continuous measurement of tissue blood flow by light heating spectroscopy. IEEE Trans Biomed Eng 27: 12
38. Ninet J, Fronek A (1985a) Cutaneous postocclusive reactive hyperema monitored by laser doppler flux metering and skin temperature. Microcirc Res 30: 125
39. Ninet J, Fronek A (1985b) Laser doppler flux monitored cutaneous response to local cooling and heating. Vasa 14: 38
40. Norgren L, Thulesius O, Gjores JE, Soderlund S (1974) Foot-volumetry and simultaneous pressure measurements for evaluation of venous insufficiency. Vasa 3: 140
41. Oishi C, Fronek A, Golbranson F (1988) The role of noninvasive vascular studies in determining levels of amputation. J Bone Joint Surg [Am] 70: 1520
42. Partsch H (1984) Hyperaemic hypoxia in venous ulceration. Br Med J 110: 249
43. Raines JK (1985) The pulse volume recorder in peripheral arterial disease. In: Bernstein EF (ed) Noninvasive diagnostic techniques in vascular disease, 3rd ed. Mosby, St Louis, p 563
44. Sandeman DD, Pym CA, Green EM, Seamark C, Shore AC, Tooke JE (1991) Microvascular vasodilation in feet of newly diagnosed non-insulin dependent diabetic patients. Br Med J 302: 1122
45. Schmidt JA, Borgström P, Firestone GP et al (1993) Peri-

odic hemodynamics (flow motion) in peripheral arterial occlusive disease. J Vasc Surg 18: 207
46. Seifert H, Jäger K, Bollinger A (1988) Analysis of the flow motion by the laser doppler technique in patients with peripheral arterial occlusive disease. Int J Microcirc Clin Exp 7: 223
47. Strandness DE Jr, Sumner DS (1972) Non-invasive methods of studying peripheral arterial function. J Surg Res 12: 419
48. Tenland T, Salerud GG, Nilsson GE, Oberg PA (1983) Spatial and temporal variations in human skin blood flow. Int J Microcirc Clin Exp 2: 81
49. Thangavelu M, Fronek A, Morgan R (1977) Simple calibration of doppler velocity metering. Proc San Diego Biomed Symp 16: 1
50. Thulesius O (1985) Foot volumetry. In: Bernstein EF (ed) Noninvasive diagnostic techniques in vascular disease, 3rd ed. Mosby, St Louis, p 828
51. Thulesius O et al (1978) Diagnostik bei akuter Venenthrombose der unteren Extremitäten. In: Kriessmann A, Bollinger A (eds) Ultraschall-Doppler-Diagnostik in der Angiologie. Thieme, Stuttgart
52. Tooke JE, Lins P-E, Ostergren J, Fagrell B (1985) Skin microvascular autoregulatory response in type I diabetes: the influence of duration and control. Int J Microcirc Clin Exp 4: 249
53. Wallace JD, Cade CM (1975) Clinical thermography. CRC Press, Clevelan
54. Wardell K, Jakobsson A, Nilsson GE (1993) Laser doppler perfusion imaging by dynamic light scattering. IEEE Trans Biomed Eng 40: 316
55. Wheeler HB, Anderson FA Jr (1985) The diagnosis of venous thrombosis by impedance plethysmography. In: Bernstein EF (ed) Noninvasive diagnostic techniques in vascular disease, 3rd edn. Mosby, St Louis, p 775
56. Wheeler HB, Pearson D, O'Connell D, Mullick S (1972) Impedance phlebography: technique, interpretation and results. Arch Surg 104: 164
57. Whitney RJ (1949) The measurement of changes in human limb volume by means of a mercury-in-rubber strain gauge. J Physiol (Lond) 109: 5
58. Wilbur BG, Olcott C (1977) A comparison of three modes of stress on doppler ankle pressures. In: Dietrich EB (ed) Noninvasive cardiovascular diagnosis. University Park Press, Baltimore, p 137
59. Willeke A, Wuppermann T, Fronek A (1995) Pulse reappearance time and foot vascularization in patients with peripheral arterial occlusive disease. J VAsc Invest 1: 75
60. Winsor T (1953) Clinical plethysmography. I. An improved direct writing plethysmograph. Angiology 4: 134
61. Wollersheim H, Thien T (1994) The evaluation of Raynaud's phenomenon. In: Belcaro GV, Hoffmann U, Bollinger A, Nicolaides AN (eds) Laser doppler. Med-Orion, London, p 103

Part I: Diagnostics of Vascular Diseases: State-of-the-Art

Section II: Imaging Vascular Methods

Vascular Ultrasonography

Physics and Instrumentation of Doppler Ultrasound

P.R. Hoskins and W.N. McDicken

Doppler Effect

Imaging of soft tissue is performed using B-scan ultrasound in which the ultrasound echo amplitude is measured and displayed. Information about blood flow is acquired by measurement of the Doppler shift of the transmitted ultrasound after it is scattered by moving blood. The essential quantities of interest in Doppler ultrasound are shown in Fig. 1. Blood of velocity v flows in a vessel. Ultrasound is transmitted with frequency F, and the angle between the ultrasound beam and the direction of motion of the blood flow is θ. Ultrasound is scattered in all directions from the moving blood. The ultrasound backscattered towards the transducer is received. This now has a frequency of $F+\delta F$. The frequency shift is the Doppler shift. The Doppler effect is a general effect which occurs when there is relative motion between a source of waves and an observer. The most common situation in which the

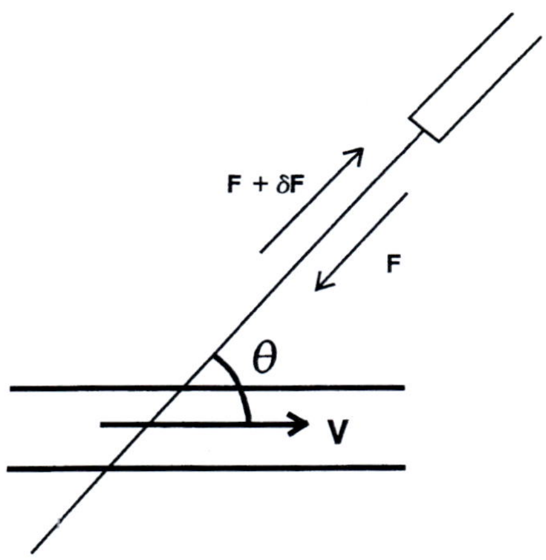

Fig. 1. Essential quantities relevant to the Doppler equation. Blood of velocity v flow in a vessel. Ultrasound of centre frequency F is incident on the vessel, and the angle between the ultrasound beam and the direction of blood flow is θ. The frequency of the ultrasound wave received by the transducer has been shifted by an amount δF

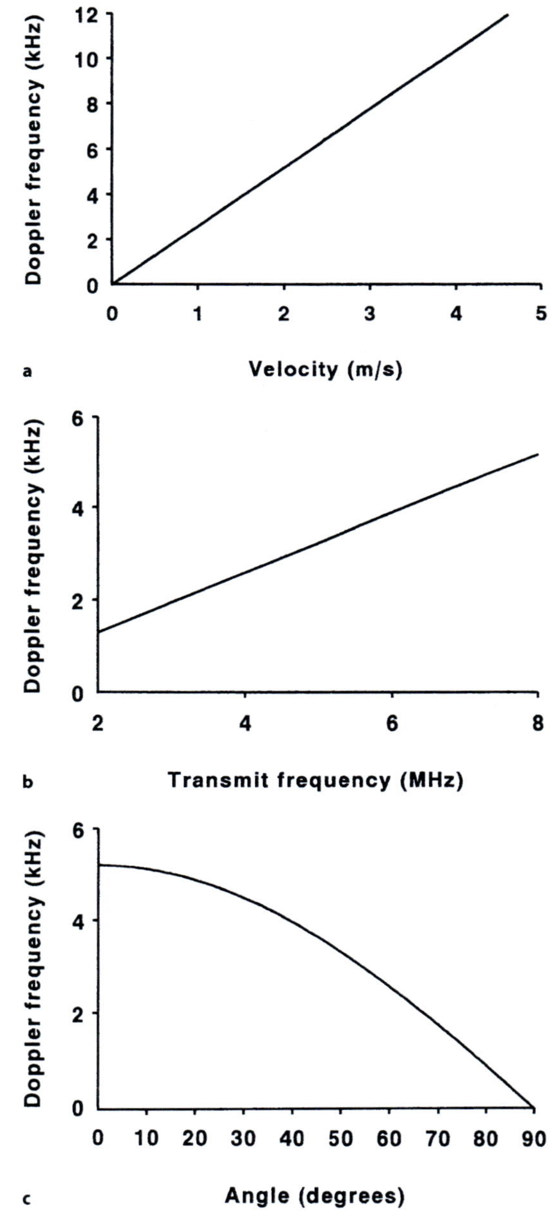

Fig. 2. Doppler shift as calculated from Eq. 1 (see text). The assumed acoustic velocity is 1540 m/s.
a Effect of variation of velocity; F=4 MHz, θ=60°. **b** Effect of variation of transmit frequency; θ=60°, v=1 m/s. **c** Effect of variation of angle; F=4 MHz, v=1 m/s

Doppler effect is present is in the change in tone which is heard as an ambulance or police car passes by. The pitch of the siren is higher as the ambulance moves towards the observer compared with the pitch heard as it moves away from the observer. In medical ultrasound, the Doppler shift equation is:

$$\delta F = 2F(v/c)\cos\theta$$

where c is the velocity of ultrasound in tissue.

The Doppler equation is probably the most important equation in Doppler ultrasound. There are two features of this equation which are worth noting. Firstly, δF is proportional to the velocity, and secondly, δF is proportional to the cosine of θ (cosine is written as cos for short). The Doppler shift is maximum when θ is zero, i.e. when the beam and the direction of the velocity vector are aligned. The Doppler shift, according to the equation, falls to zero as the angle approaches 90°. In fact, the Doppler shift is not exactly zero at 90°, but has a small finite value. This will be discusscd later in this chapter in relationship to geometric spectral broadening. It is therefore necessary for the vessel to be angled with respect to the Doppler beam.

The value of the Doppler shifts arising from specific situations may be estimated by inserting appropriate values into Eq. 1, as shown in Fig. 2. The Doppler shift typically varies between 0 and 20 kHz. Most of the time, except for very high velocities, the Doppler shift is within the audio range. The Doppler shift signal can therefore be heard simply by playing it through loudspeakers.

Sonogram-Based Doppler Systems

The Sonogram

The Doppler ultrasound signal is usually displayed in the form of a real-time sonogram (Fig. 3). This is a Doppler frequency shift versus time display in which the average brightness level at a particular Doppler shift frequency is related approximately to the corresponding number of red cells travelling with the corresponding blood velocity. The sonogram consists of consecutive lines in which the spectral content of the Doppler signal has been analysed. This is illustrated in Fig. 4. The Doppler signal is split into equal time intervals of approximately 10 ms. The frequency content of each one of these is analysed in turn and displayed as a single line on the sonogram. The difference between the spectrum

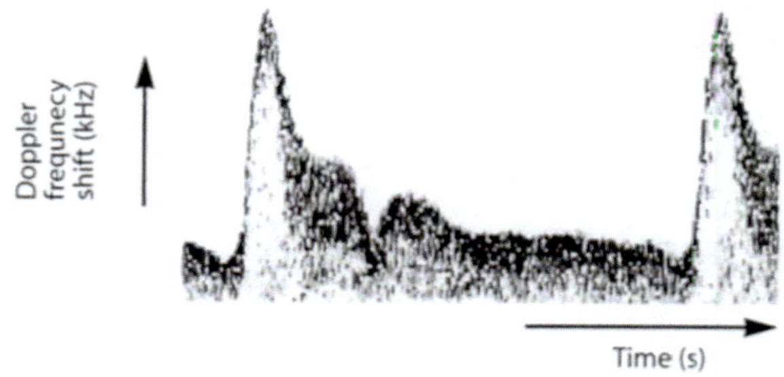

Fig. 3. Sonogram from the internal carotid artery obtained using a continuous wave probe

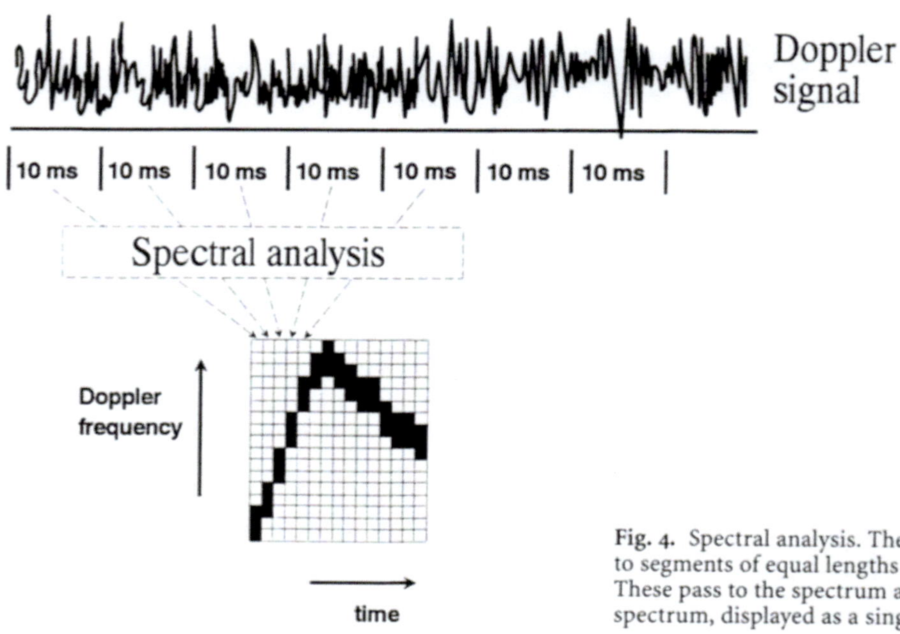

Fig. 4. Spectral analysis. The Doppler signal is broken into segments of equal lengths of approximately 10 ms. These pass to the spectrum analyser, which calculates the spectrum, displayed as a single line on the sonogram

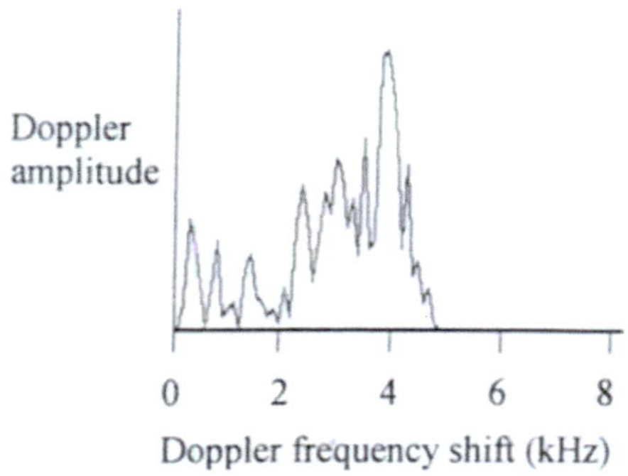

Fig. 5. Single spectral line showing high variations in amplitude

and the sonogram should be appreciated. The spectrum is estimated approximately every 10 ms. The sonogram consists of consecutive spectra. Virtually all modern Doppler systems perform spectral analysis by use of the Fourier transform. A computationally efficient version of this transform is used in practice called the fast Fourier transform (FFT). Detailed examination of the sonogram reveals that it is very noisy; the extent of this noise may be appreciated by examination of one spectral line (Fig. 5). This has similar origins to the speckle seen on B-scan images, i.e. fluctuations in the amplitude of the received ultrasound arising as a result of changes in the number and location of red cells in the ultrasound beam. The observer must therefore "edit" the noise to reveal the underlying brightness level. Other methods of speckle reduction are available as research tools, including image processing [14] and other methods of spectral estimation [6, 11, 24]. In practice, the limitations of FFT-based spectral analysis do not appear to be great. FFT estimation of the Doppler spectrum has been widely accepted, and there is no move on the part of manufacturers to use other spectral estimation methods.

Continuous-Wave

The earliest and most simple Doppler ultrasound device is the continuous-wave (CW) system. The probe consists of two adjacent piezoelectric crystals mounted in the end of a pencil probe. One crystal continuously transmits ultrasound, and the other continuously receives ultrasound. The sensitive region in space is the region in which the transmission and reception beams overlap. Focusing may be applied by shaping the end of the probe to form an acoustic lens. The width of the ultrasound beam is dependent on the ratio of the crystal diameter to the wavelength of the transmitted ultrasound. This explains why 8-MHz probes have a diameter in the range of 6–8 mm, while the diameter of 2-MHz probes is typically 15–20 mm.

The detection of the Doppler signal may be most easily understood by considering the CW Doppler system (Fig. 6). The received ultrasound signal consists of three components (Fig. 7): (1) high-intensity ultrasound signals from stationary tissue, (2) high-intensity signals from slowly moving tissue and (3) low-intensity signals from blood. The high-intensity signals from tissue, useful for formation of the B-scan image, are of no use in the estimation of the sonogram and must be removed. This is usually performed by application of the "phase-quadrature" technique. The details of this are unimportant for this book, but are described in other sources (e.g. [8]).

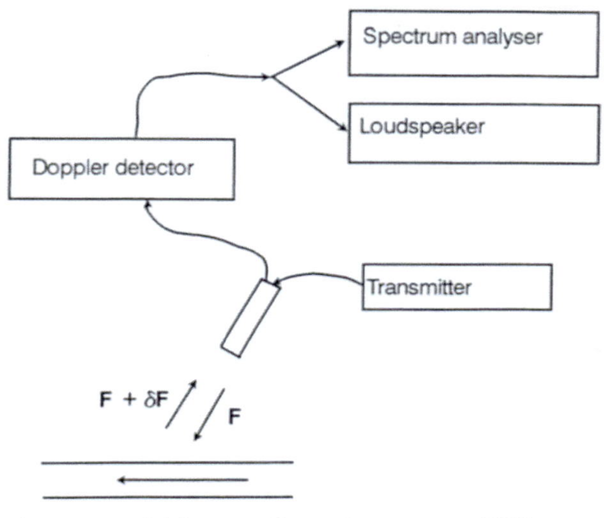

Fig. 6. Essential features of a continuous-wave (CW) Doppler system

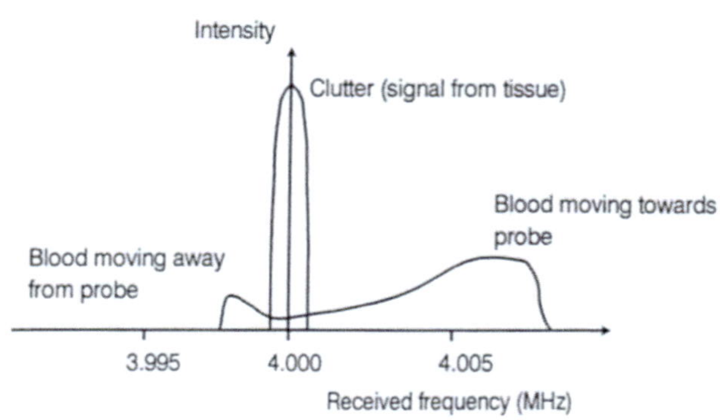

Fig. 7. The three components of the received ultrasound signal

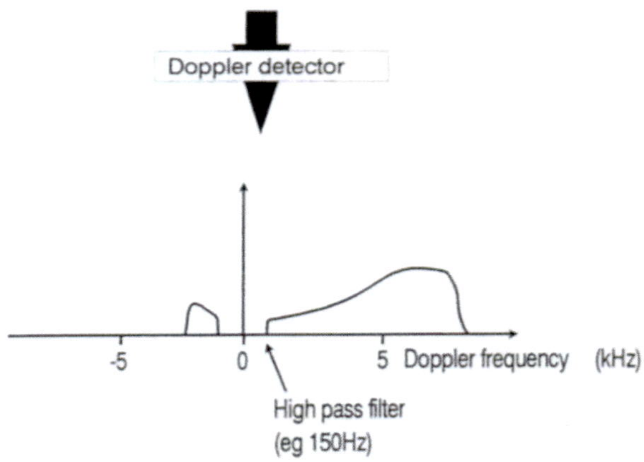

Fig. 8. Doppler detection and filtering by the wall thump filter remove the high-intensity component, revealing the Doppler signal

The high-intensity signals from slowly moving tissue are suppressed by the use of a filter, commonly referred to as the "wall thump filter", "cut-off filter", or simply "filter". The final detected Doppler signal, which is now suitable for spectral analysis, is shown in Fig. 8. It should be noted that application of the wall thump filter has removed the low-frequency components of the Doppler signal. In practice, the lowest possible value of the wall thump filter is used in order to visualise as much of the Doppler signal as possible. This is particularly relevant in obstetrics, where the degree of diastolic flow of the umbilical artery is used as an indicator of fetal well-being. In this case, typical filter levels are 50–100 Hz. In peripheral vascular applications, higher filter levels of 100–200 Hz may be necessary, and in cardiology levels of 300 Hz are not uncommon.

The features of the CW Doppler system which influence practice are the following:

- Doppler shift cos θ dependence
- Ultrasound transmitted and received continuously
- No depth discrimination
- No aliasing (no upper limit to detected velocity)
- No B-scan image
- Use for vessels with well-defined locations
- Use for vessels with well-defined waveform shape

CW Doppler systems are available as stand-alone systems without B-scan imaging. As such, they are inexpensive, but they do have limitations. They can only be used for vessels which have well-defined locations and/or well-defined waveform shapes. They are particularly suited to the application of umbilical artery Doppler waveforms and are also used in the lower limb and carotid artery. They are unsuitable for those areas in which there are a number of vessels which have similar waveform shapes, such as the abdomen, the fetus or the placenta.

Pulsed-Wave Doppler Devices

Pulsed-wave (PW) Doppler systems are very similar to CW Doppler systems apart from one main feature, namely the ultrasound is transmitted as a series of regularly spaced pulses. This enables depth discrimination in the same way as is performed for B-scan imaging, i.e. measurement of the time between transmission of the pulse and reception of echoes. The Doppler signal arises from a small region called the sample volume. The operator selects the depth of interes and also the range of depths for which ultrasound signals are reccived (Fig. 9). This latter aspect is generally referred to as the 'gate'. This refers to the electronic implementation whereby, from the point of transmission, the received ultrasound signal is blocked, i.e. the gate is closed, until the appropriate depth has been reached, when the gate is opened. The length of time the gate is open is the main factor which dictates the range of depths from which Doppler signals are received. Typical gate lengths vary from 1 to 10 mm. The other factor is the pulse length, so that the sample volume length is slightly larger than the gate length.

The main advantage of PW Doppler systems is their ability to sample Doppler signals from a known depth. The main disadvantage is that the use of PW (rather than CW) places an upper limit on the

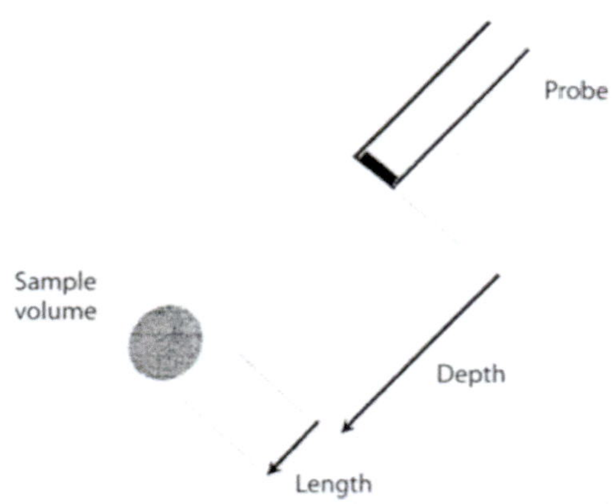

Fig. 9. The Doppler signal from a pulsed-wave (PW) Doppler system originates from a sample volume. The depth and length of this are under the control of the operator

maximum detectable Doppler shift δF_{max}. The number of pulses that are transmitted per second is known as the puls repetition frequency (prf). The maximum detectable Doppler frequency shift is:

$$\delta F_{max} = prf/2$$

This is a general restriction placed on sampled signals. Frequencies above half of the prf are not estimated correctly, and the sonogram demonstrates 'aliasing'. Figure 10 shows a sonogram from a PW system. Aliasing is demonstrated, whereby Doppler shift frequencies greater than prf/2 are displayed in the incorrect channel.

For a PW system, the aliasing frequency will decrease for greater depths. This follows from the fact that a greater time must elapse for the capture of ultrasound signals from greater depths, and hence the prf must fall. PW Doppler systems transmit in one of two ways. The first is that the prf is fixed and is determined by the greatest depth which may be of interest. In these systems, the maximum detectable Doppler frequency is very limited. Many PW systems now operate in "high-prf" mode, i. e. as soon as the echo information from the depth of interest is received, the next pulse is transmitted. Attempts to overcome the aliasing limit by signal processing are in an early stage of development and are not yet commercially available.

The features of PW Doppler which influence practice are the following:

- Ultrasound transmitted as pulses (prf = 1–10 kHz)
- Depth discrimination
- Sample volume depth and gate length set by user
- Aliasing
- Doppler shift cos θ dependence
- Use for vessels with well-defined locations
- Use for vessels with well-defined waveform shape

In modern usage, stand-alone PW Doppler systems are largely restricted to transcranial applications.

Duplex Devices

A duplex system usually refers to a combination of a real-time B-scanner with a PW Doppler system. The basic features of PW Doppler as described above apply to the duplex system. The great advantage of these systems over the stand-alone PW system is that there is knowledge, from the B-scan image, of the vessel and the location within the vessel, from which Doppler signals are acquired. This means that there is more confidence in the acquisition of data from the peripheral arteries, and Doppler signals may now be acquired from the abdomen and the fetus. The other great advantage of duplex stems is that an attempt may be made to measure the angle θ between the beam and the velocity vector (Fig. 11). This is done by manual alignment of a cursor with the vessel wall. The duplex system then

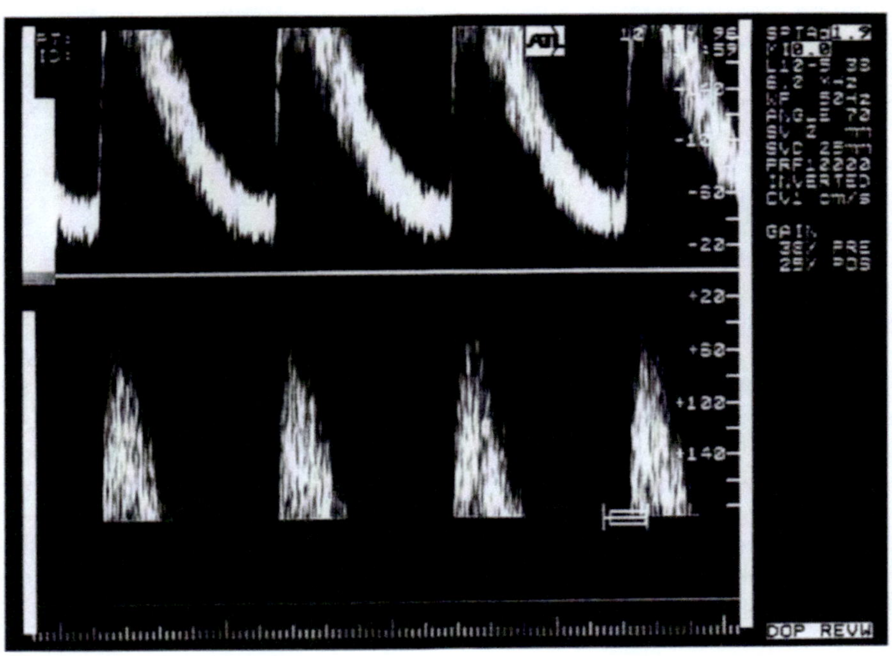

Fig. 10. Effect of aliasing. Use of a pulsed-wave (PW) system gives rise to an upper limit on the detectable frequency shift. Frequencies above this are displayed in the opposite channel

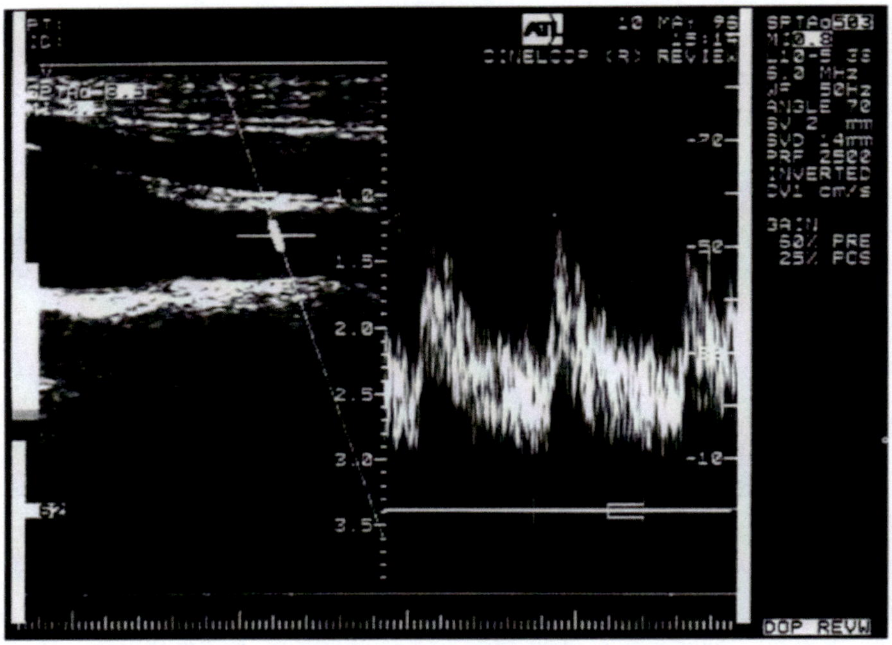

Fig. 11. Using a duplex system it is possible to obtain an estimate of the angle θ by alignment of the cursor with the vessel wall

automatically displays the sonogram in units of velocity. This method of angle measurement has lead to the use of the phrase "beam-vessel angle". This is misleading, since it is the angle with respect to the velocity vector that is of interest. This is considered in more detail later in this chapter in relation to the accuracy of measurement of velocity.

All the available types of transducers used for B-scanning may be used for duplex scanning. For transducers which produce sector images (phased array, mechanical sector and annular array), the Doppler beam is angled in the same direction as the B-scan beam. For the linear array, the Doppler beam is formed by use of elements from part of the array. Steering of the Doppler beam is performed by delayed excitation of the array elements, in the same way that beam steering is performed for phased arrays. The direction of the B-scan beam and of the Doppler beam are then different. Early linear-array duplex systems did not steer the Doppler beam. There are problems with the use of such an array, as the optimum angle for display of the arterial wall,i.e. 90°, is the angle which is the worst for acquisition of Doppler signals. Most modern linear-array systems use steering of the Doppler beam, which enables good visualisation of the vessel wall on the B-scan image, along with a sufficiently small angle for acquisition of good Doppler signals.

It is most desirable that there is simultaneous real-time B-scan imaging and real-time sonogram display. The other commonly used option is real-time display of the sonogram with update of the B-scan image at regular intervals. For this latter case, there are gaps in the sonogram display while the B-scan image is updated. Updating is mostly used for mechanical sector devices where the mechanical vibrations produced by the transducer would be picked up and displayed as Doppler signals. Some mechanical sector devices are sufficiently low noise to enable simultaneous display of the B-scan image and the sonogram.

The transmission of ultrasound pulses is time shared between the B-scan image and the Doppler sonogram. Only one ultrasound pulse is used to generate each B-scan line, whereas 80–100 pulses are typically used to produce each spectral line of the sonogram. In duplex mode, the majority of pulses are used for production of the Doppler sonogram. In practice, the frame rate and line density of the B-scan image may be reduced in order to obtain the maximum prf for production of the Doppler sonogram. Further increase in the prf may be obtained by switching off the B-scan image so that all pulses are allocated to the Doppler system. In this case, the maximum detectable Doppler frequency (the aliasing frequency) is also increased, so that switching off the B-scan image may sometimes be useful.

The features of a duplex system may be summarised as follows:
- Real-time B-scan and PW Doppler
- Sonogram from known vessel and location within vessel
- Use angle correction to convert to velocity

Physical Factors Affecting the Sonogram

The impact of various physical factors may be explored using a simple idealised model, i.e. insonation of steady flow in a long, straight tube far from the entrance to the tube. The velocity profile in this situation is parabolic. The distribution of red cells in the tube is shown in Fig. 12; it can be seen that the distribution is flat and there are equal numbers of red cells flowing in each velocity increment. The spectrum from the vessel is shown in Fig. 13. The presence of speckle would obscure any trend, so that speckle has been removed by averaging over 1000 consecutive spectra from the sonogram. The effect of the cut off high-pass filter on the smoothed spectrum is shown, along with two other features. Firstly, the spectrum is not flat, and secondly, it does not have a sharp cut-off at the maximum frequency. These are related to two physical effects: (1) the interaction between the ultrasound beam and the velocity profile and (2) geometric spectral broadening.

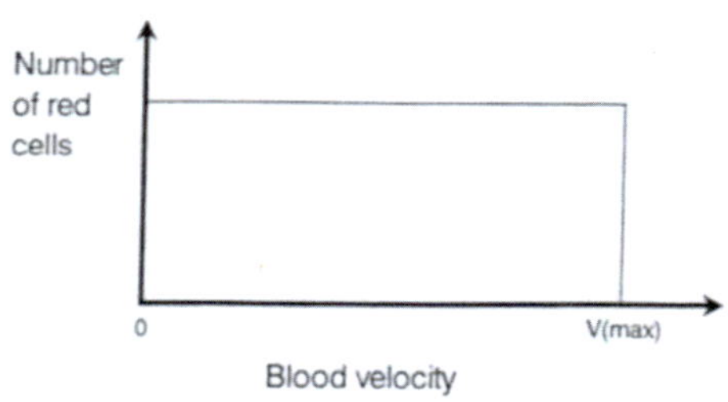

Fig. 12. Distribution of velocities during steady flow in a long, straight vessel

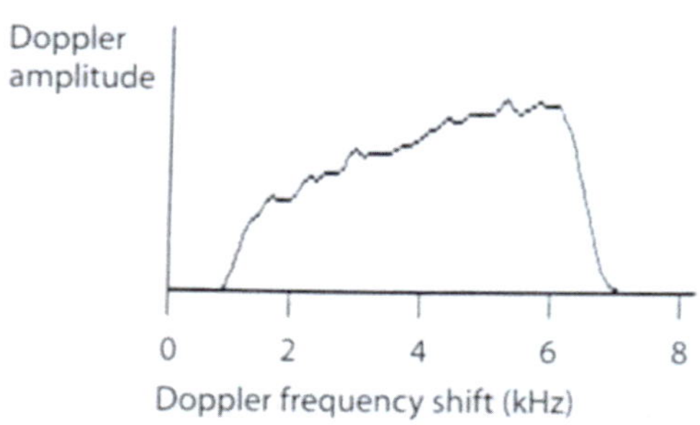

Fig. 13. Spectral line from steady flow; the average of 1000 spectra has been taken to reduce variations arising from Doppler speckle

If the ultrasound beam is broad and uniformly insonates the vessel, then all the velocity components in the vessel will be equally represented in the Doppler signal. In this case, the spectrum is largely flat. Non-uniform insonation has been studied for the case of alignment of beam and vessel using computer simulation by Evans [7] and for the case

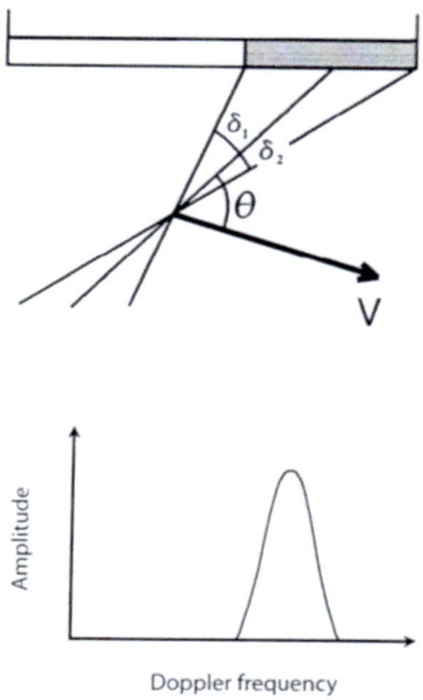

Fig. 14. Origin of geometrical spectral broadening. The velocity vector subtends a range of angles, from $\theta - \delta_2$ to $\theta + \delta_1$ at the transducer, which in turn leads to a range of Doppler shift frequencies

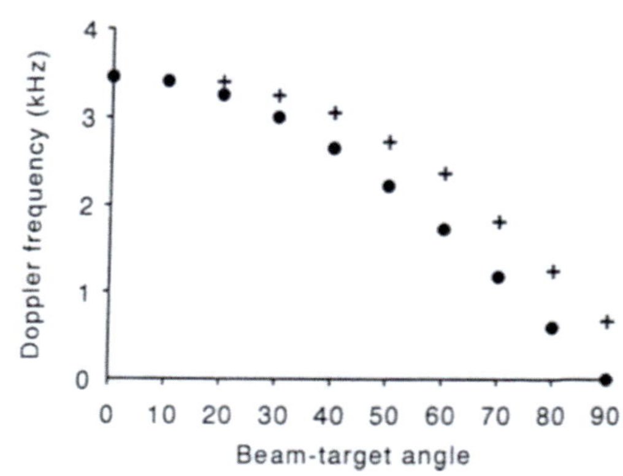

Fig. 15. Variation of detected Doppler frequency with the angle between the beam and the velocity vector. The data indicated by *crosses* were obtained from a string phantom with a constant speed of 50 cm/s and demonstrate a finite Doppler shift at 90°. The data indicated by *circles* were calculated from the Doppler equation, which assumes a cos θ dependence

of misalignment by Cobbold et al. [5]. If the beam and vessel are aligned, but the beam width is less than the vessel diameter, then the sides of the vessel do not contribute to the Doppler signal, and there is loss of low frequencies from the spectrum; this is the case in Fig. 13. Misalignment of the beam and vessel results in some reduction in height of the maximum frequency, but not complete loss unless the misalignment is severe. It can be seen that the mean frequency will be very strongly affected by the ratio of beam width to vessel diameter and by the degree of beam-vessel alignment. Though the intensity of the maximum frequency is affected to some extent, the maximum frequency itself is not so affected. In practice, the maximum frequency is used rather than the mean frequency for analysis of Doppler waveforms because of its relative resistance to the beam width and alignment effects.

The rounded nature of the spectrum near to the maximum frequency is due to geometrical spectral broadening. This can be understood with reference to Fig. 14. The Doppler frequency is dependent on the cosine of the angle between the beam and the blood flow direction. In practice, a range of angles is subtended rather than a single angle. This will give rise to a range of Doppler frequency shifts. Figure 14 shows that, for a single velocity, the resulting spectrum has the same rounded appearance as the spectrum from the vessel with steady flow in Fig. 13. Geometrical spectral broadening has been explored in several studies [4, 19]. The variation of Doppler frequency shift with angle for one linear array is shown in Fig. 15. In this figure, a string phantom has been used as the target. This has a single velocity. This is of interest in the measurement of velocity from the sonogram (see below), where it is noted that geometrical spectral broadening gives rise to errors in maximum velocity estimation, which increase as the beam-blood vector angle approaches 90°.

Maximum Frequency Envelope

It is often the maximum frequency envelope that is of interest. Velocities may be derived from the envelope at particular points, such as the peak systolic velocity and the end diastolic velocity. Alternatively, the shape of the waveform may be quantitated by the use of various indices calculated from the maximum frequency envelope (see below). The maximum frequency envelope tends to be relatively resistant to alignment of the beam and the vessel and is thus used in preference to the mean frequency. A common task performed in Doppler ultrasound studies is identification of the maximum frequency envelope. Manual methods usually involve tracing using a trackerball. This is time consuming, and in practice the operator obtains waveform index values from only two or three waveforms. Methods may be used in which the maximum frequency envelope is traced automatically. With these methods, the operator can obtain in real time the average waveform index values for several waveforms, typically five to 15. Such systems are most used in obstetrics and in transcranial Doppler. Two of the techniques used for detection of the maximum frequency envelope are the percentile method and the threshold method. In the percentile method, the total value T of pixels of a single spectral line is calculated. The maximum frequency is that point at which the sum of pixel values below that frequency just exceeds a specified percentage of T, say 7/8 or 15/16 expressed in percentage terms. In the threshold method, the maximum frequency follower algorithm starts from the high-frequency end of a spectral line and works to the lower frequencies, comparing each pixel value with the threshold value. The highest frequency at which the pixel value exceeds the threshold is called the maximum frequency. The detection algorithms must perform several tasks: (a) identify the start (and end) of each waveform, (b) identify the maximum frequency envelope and (c) calculate the waveform index. Maximum frequency followers tend to work reasonably well provided that there is no noise of any kind above the maximum frequency. Electronic noise, either random background noise or spurious electronic signals of various kinds, and signals from overlying vessels tend to upset the algorithm, and in general the maximum frequency is inaccurate (Fig. 16). In practice, good results may be obtained using automated estimation of waveform indices; however, care is needed. The best use of such devices is to display simultaneously the sonogram and the estimated maximum frequency. The operator adjusts the probe position and Doppler gain to obtain good waveforms as judged from the sonogram, and a representative maximum frequency trace. Some commercial machines display the sonogram and the real-time waveform index values, but omit to display the estimated maximum frequency envelope. It may be very difficult to know with this type of system whether the detected maximum frequency is accurate, and hence the index reliable.

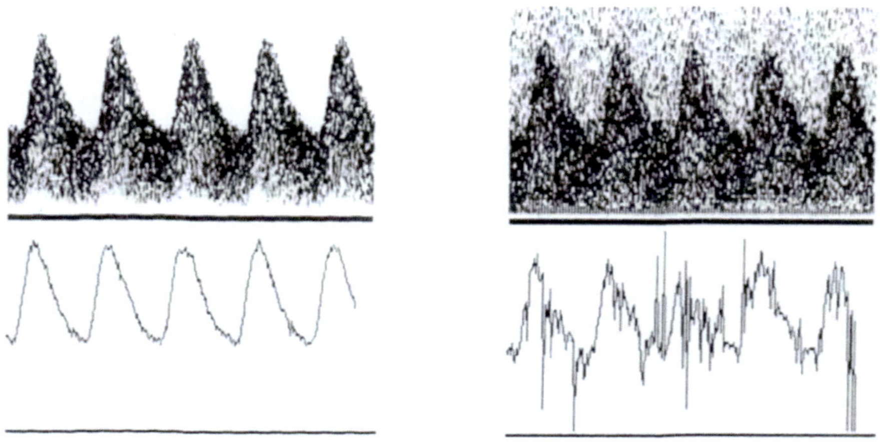

Fig. 16. Maximum frequency detected automatically from sonograms with no noise (*left*) and with noise (*right*)

Effect of Different Flow States

Laminar flow involves ordered motion, whereby blood flows along well-defined stream lines. Laminar flow occurs at low velocities. Turbulence occurs at higher velocities and is associated with random changes of blood speed and direction, superimposed on the average speed and direction. Disturbed flow is concerned with the generation and motion of vortices or eddies. These may be generated when there is a change in the geometrical shape of the containing vessel and may occur in the region distal to a stenosis. Disturbed and turbulent flow produce a broadening of the spectrum. The vortices generated in disturbed flow will exhibit a wide range of angles as the vortex passes through the sample volume. Similarly, randomly moving blood elements during turbulent flow will exhibit a wide range of angles. Spectral broadening of the sonogram arising from disturbed flow and turbulence therefore has two causes: one is the increased range of speeds within the sample volume, and the second is the increased range of angles between the beam and the direction of motion of the blood.

Measurement of Velocity from the Sonogram

One of the most common measurements made using Doppler ultrasound systems is that of maximum velocity. In order to convert the Doppler frequency shift to velocity using Eq. 1, knowledge is required of the angle between the beam and the direction of motion of the blood. With a duplex system, the angle is manually measured using the angle cursor, by alignment of the cursor with the vessel, and as noted above it is common to refer to this angle as the beam-vessel angle. Narrowing of the vessel lumen by atherosclerosis results in increase in blood velocity. Tables are used to convert the maximum velocity reading to a percentage stenosis [2, 22]. There are two potential sources of error, both related to knowledge of the angle between the beam and blood direction.

First let us return to geometric spectral broadening. It was noted that geometric spectral broadening is related to the spread of angles which the blood will subtend at the transducer. The accuracy of the maximum velocity estimation may be checked using a string phantom. Figure 17 shows typical results for a linear array. The maximum velocity is overestimated at all angles by the duplex device. It is noted that there is no critical angle such as 60° below which the error is acceptably small. Overestimation of velocities typically varies between 10% and 60% [13, 27]; however, if angles near to 90° are used, errors of over 100% may be produced. The optimum method of reduction of this source of error is correction of Doppler frequency shifts by the use of the angle at the edge of the Doppler aperture. At the time of writing, there is to our knowledge only one manufacturer (Diasonics, California, USA) which adopts this practice. These errors would seem to be large. The impact on the assessment of the degree of stenosis and on consequent patient management may be of clinical relevance. An error of ± 20% in estimated maximum velocity may mean the categorisation of a normal artery as abnormal. An individual hospital may adjust the values in the tables to suit their own practice. The problem seems to arise when a machine is replaced, or a second machine is bought. It may then be no-

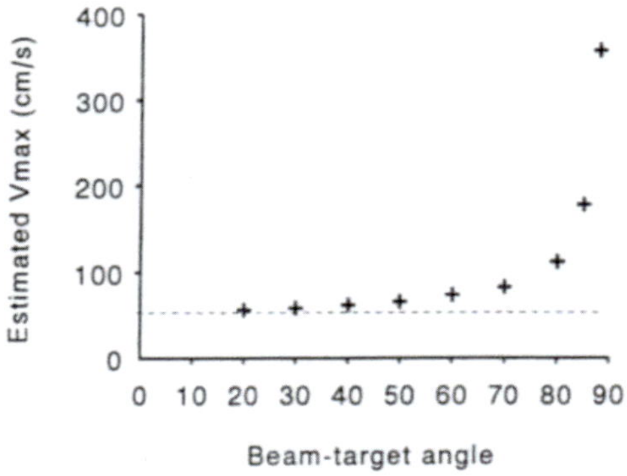

Fig. 17. Estimated maximum velocity as a function of beam-target angle. The data were acquired from a string phantom using an Acuson L7384 linear-array probe at a depth of 5 cm. The maximum velocity increases as the angle approaches 90°

ticed that the maximum velocity values are not the same between the machines. Though there is no direct evidence, it seems to be the case that use of one machine produces little error in practice, provided that the values in published tables can be adjusted. The problems arise mainly on introduction of a second machine when tables are used from the literature without adjustment.

The second source or error in maximum velocity estimation is associated with knowledge of the angle between the beam and the blood velocity vector. The blood velocity will change direction as it passes through the stenosis, and the blood velocity vector will not be aligned with the vessel wall. Correct measurement of the magnitude and direction of blood flow cannot be performed with Doppler systems used in the standard way in this situation. All Doppler systems derive Doppler frequency shift information only from the component of velocity in the direction of the beam, i.e. they are one-dimensional systems. Correct estimation of the magnitude and direction of blood velocities would require a system capable of measuring all three components of blood velocity (along the x, y and z axes). Two- and three-dimensional Doppler systems have been described in the literature [9, 20], but are not available commercially. Three-dimensional systems involve the use of specialist transducers, whereas current linear arrays could be adapted for two-dimensional vector Doppler.

Measurement of Indices of Waveform Shape from the Sonogram

It would be desirable to relate the location and extent of disease to the shape of the Doppler waveform. Various factors will influence the Doppler waveform. These factors can be explored in relation to their effect on the Doppler waveform from an artery supplying musculature:

- *Normal artery:* waveform is pulsatile with a period of reverse flow.
- *Proximal disease:* the degree of pulsatility is reduced, and the loss of pulsatility will depend on the severity of disease and the degree of collateral supply.
- *Compliance:* the time to peak is reduced if vessel stiffness increases (e.g. in diabetes).
- *Distal disease:* severe disease downstream may cause a shoulder to be seen on the downslope of the waveform.

This is a complex state of affairs, and in general the relation between a particular waveform feature and disease must be investigated separately for each artery [12]. The most commonly used approach has been characterisation of the degree of pulsatility by the use of simple indices of the maximum frequency envelope (Fig. 18), such as resistance index (RI) [21] and pulsatility index (PI) [10]. In some circumstances these indices are related to the degree of distal resistance to flow. This is true for arteries supplying normal musculature, in which a marked decrease in pulsatility occurs as a result of vasodilatation occurring during exercise or during reactive hyperaemia. There is good evidence to suggest that the increase in the RI and PI of umbilical artery waveforms is related to increased placental resistance [1, 26]. The use of advanced methods of waveform analysis has been attempted based on feature extraction (principal component analysis) [18] or mathematical modelling (Laplace transform analysis)

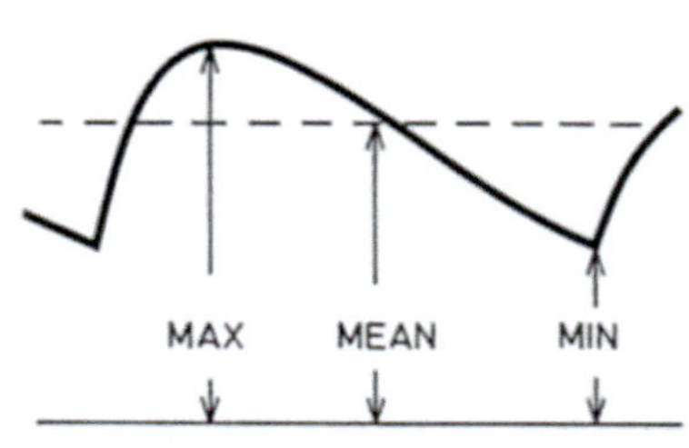

Fig. 18. Commonly used waveform indices derived from the Doppler waveform. A/B = max/min; resistance index (RI) = (max – min)/max; pulsability index (PI) = (max – min)/mean

[25]. These methods have never entered routine use, possibly because they do not add any more useful information than very simple indices.

Color Flow Devices

Color Velocity Imaging

A color velocity image is a real-time B-scan image upon which is superimposed a real-time two-dimensional display of the mean Doppler frequency coded at each point with an appropriate color (Fig. 19). The elements of a color flow scanner are shown in Fig. 20. The function of these elements will be briefly considered below.

Clutter Filter

Clutter is a term originating from radar and refers to signals from stationary targets. In medical ultrasound, clutter refers to the high-amplitude signals from tissue. The echo pattern from such targets does not change with time, so that subtraction of the echoes received from successive pulses will to a large extent remove these signals. In practice, the design of the clutter filter is central to the performance of color velocity imaging devices. The ability of modern systems to image low velocities, compared with the first systems that were introduced, which could only detect the high velocities found in cardiology, is linked to the use of sophisticated clutter filters.

Autocorrelator

The mean Doppler frequency is not obtained by performing spectral analysis at each point followed by calculation of the mean frequency. If this was performed, then the color flow frame rate would be 1 or 2 s^{-1}. Instead, the mean frequency is estimated directly using a device called an autocorrelator [15]. It was noted above that generation of a sonogram requires 80–100 pulses. The autocorrelator typically uses three to 20 pulses, enabling the production of real-time color velocity images. The autocorrelation technique was the first to be introduced, and is still the method adopted by virtually all manufacturers. Other methods of production of the color flow image have been tested in the laboratory, but have not been commercially adopted by manufacturers (the one exception is the 'time domain' method described in 1986 by Bonnefous and Pesque [3] and used by the Dutch company Philips). The autocorrelator produces two other quantities, variance and power. The variance is related to the variability of the Doppler signal. During laminar flow, variance is small; however, it increases in regions of turbulence. The power of the Doppler signal is discussed in the next section. Variance may occasionally be displayed mixed in with the mean frequency image; however, in general the simple mean frequency image is adequate.

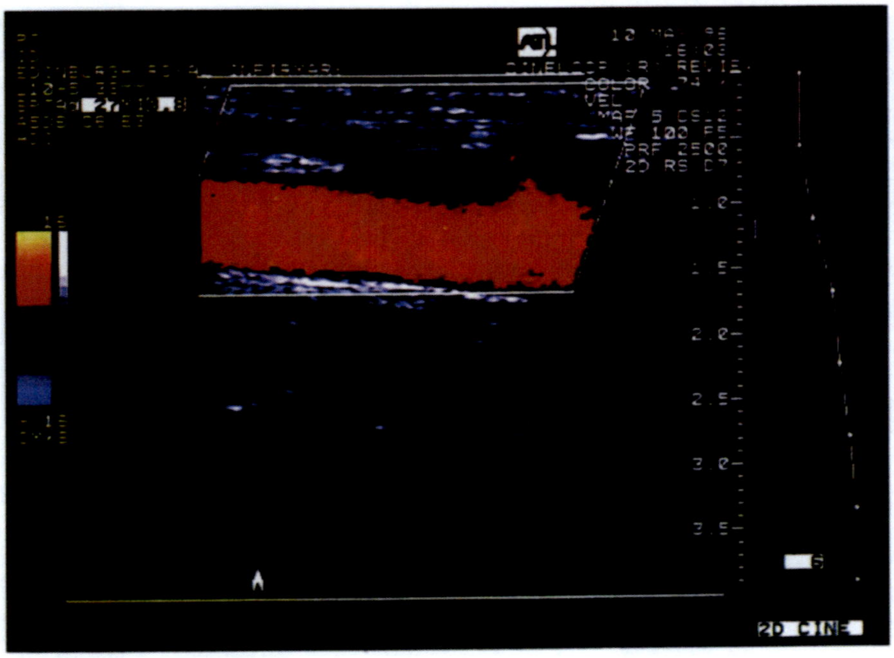

Fig. 19. Color velocity image from the carotid arteries

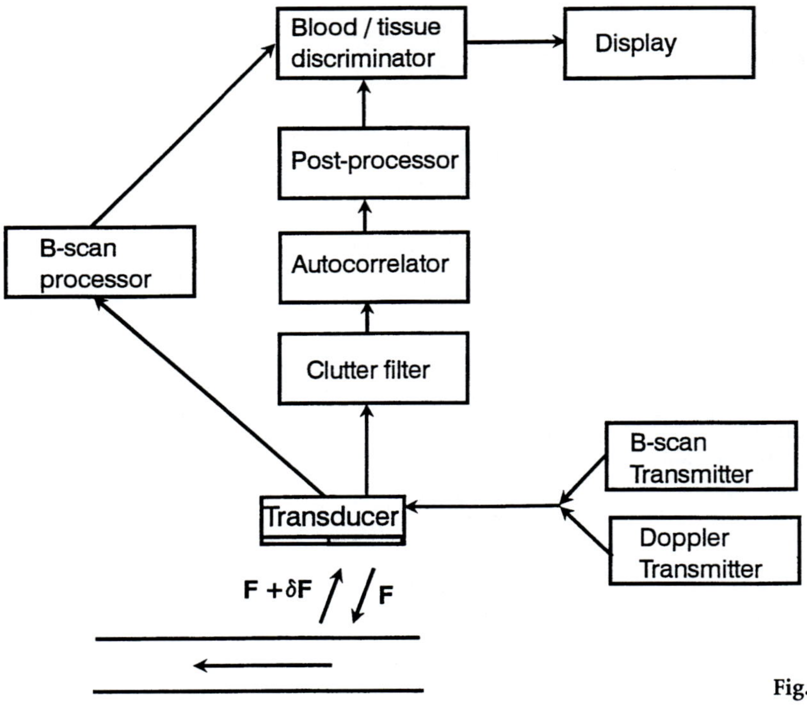

Fig. 20. Elements of a color flow scanner

Blood Tissue Discriminator

It is necessary for the color velocity system to display for each pixel of the image either the B-scan value coded with an appropriate grey level or the mean frequency coded with an appropriate color. A feature of early color systems was the appearance of color in regions of tissue. The design of the blood tissue discriminator is very important; however, there is very little information available from manufacturers. One method of performing this task is to write color on the final display dependent on the power of the detected ultrasound signal using a two-stage process based on the B-scan echo amplitude and the Doppler echo amplitude, as illustrated in Table 1. On most systems, the operator can alter the degree of coloration with respect to the B-scan image by use of the "color write priority" control.

Table 1. The blood tissue discriminator may operate by use of a combination of the B-scan echo amplitude and the Doppler amplitude.

	B-scan amplitude less than threshold	B-scan amplitude greater than threshold
Doppler amplitude less than threshold	Write color (blood)	Write B-scan (stationary tissue)
Doppler amplitude greater than threshold	Write B-scan (moving tissue)	Write B-scan (moving tissue)

Post-processor

Most color velocity systems provide a persistence facility whereby the color image is averaged over several frames to reduce color noise. If consecutive frames are averaged and the flow is stable over the averaging period, then the color noise will be reduced, enabling better visualisation of the true flow pattern. Rapidly changing flow patterns will, however, not be properly visualised if the persistence is too high.

The color velocity image, though strictly speaking of mean Doppler frequency, is commonly displayed in units of velocity. The mean frequency has been converted to velocity under the assumption that the angle θ is zero. Velocity may be coded in a variety of color scales. A red-based color scale is commonly used to display flow in one direction, while a blue based scale is used for the opposite direction. If shades of red and blue are used, then the very dark shades may be difficult to distinguish from black at low velocities. This problem is overcome by the use of a color scale based on bright shades of red and blue, with admixture of a second color or of white at higher values of mean frequency.

We will now examine in more detail the constraints on color velocity spatial resolution and frame rate. For a B-scan image, only one ultrasound pulse is needed for production of one scan line, enabling high frame rates of 25–50 s^{-1} to be produced. Three to 20 pulses are typically used per line for color flow. If the same image area were used as for the B-scan image, then the frame rate would be only 2 or 3 s^{-1}. Restriction of the field of view of the color velocity image is performed in order to increase the frame rate. Color is displayed within a color box for which the operator is able to control the shape and position. The frame rate may be increased by narrowing the color box and also by decreasing its depth. In order to further increase the frame rate, the line density may be reduced. In color velocity imaging of tissue [17], the large Doppler signal size enables the use of multiple simultaneous beams and fewer pulses (three or four), so that a higher frame rate and a larger box size may be used.

The lateral resolution is determined by beam shape and by line density. The axial resolution is determined by pulse length and by the gate length over which the mean frequency estimation is performed. In practice, the user has very little direct control over these quantities. In general, spatial resolution is optimised by restriction of the size of the color box.

The color velocity image is obtained using a pulsed Doppler technique and hence suffers from aliasing. Adjustment of the color scale is performed in order to display unaliased signals in the same way that the frequency range scale is adjusted for display of the sonogram.

The features of color velocity imaging may be summarized as follows:

- Real-time B-scan image and image of blood fow.
- Mean Doppler frequency is color coded.
- Mean frequency calculated using an autocorrelator, not by FFT.
- Color image displayed in units of velocity (this assumes that $\theta=0°$).
- The displayed color velocity has a cos θ dependence.
- This is a PW technique, and there is therefore aliasing.

Power Doppler Imaging

In power Doppler images, the power of the Doppler signal is color coded (Fig. 21) [23]. The power Doppler image may be considered to be an image of the blood pool.

The power of the Doppler signals from small vessels may only be marginally above the noise level. In a color velocity image, adjustment of the color gain in order to visualise a small vessel leads to production of color noise in the surrounding region. The mean frequency of the noise may assume a value over the entire range of possible displayed values. The estimated mean frequency values change randomly and are comparable with the displayed mean frequencies from the small vessel. Noise on a

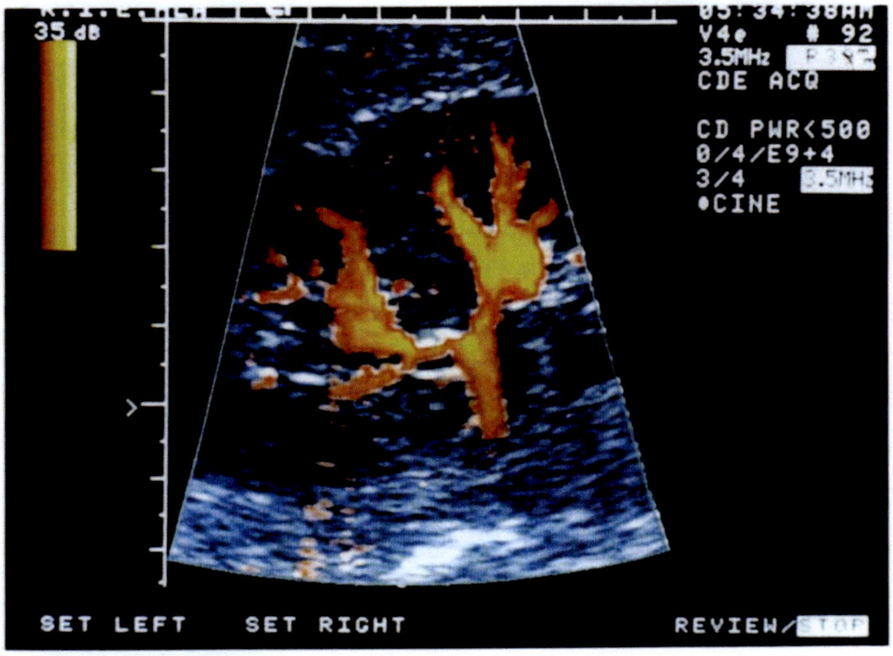

Fig. 21. Color power from the kidney

color velocity image therefore consists of randomly changing colors, and in this situation it is very difficult to distinguish a small vessel from the surrounding noise. The noise in a power Doppler image is less variable than the estimated mean frequency; this and the higher power levels from vessels means that small vessels are more easily distinguishable from the noise. The power Doppler image demonstrates strong persistence. This is sensible, as a high frame rate, required for the display of rapidly changing flow fields, is not necessary. This enables further reduction in noise and enhanced visualisation of small vessels.

Color power images are relatively insensitive to the angle θ and are not sensitive to the direction of flow. This may be understood with reference to Fig. 22, in which the Doppler power from blood moving with a single velocity is shown as a function of Doppler frequency for θ=60° and θ=90°. The spread of frequency shift values is due to geometric spectral broadening, as noted above. For θ=90°, the mean frequency is zero; however, the power, which is given by the area under the curve, is very similar to that for θ=60°.

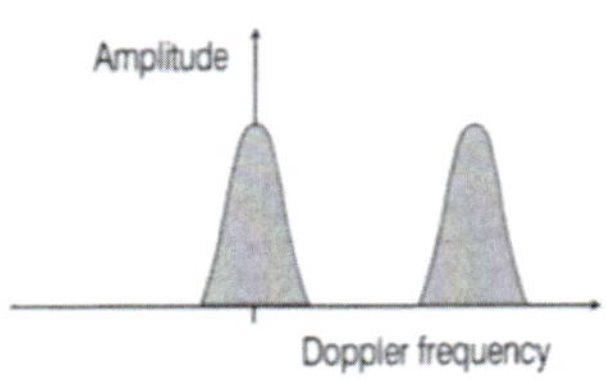

Fig. 22. Doppler spectrum from blood with a single velocity acquired at 60° and at 90°. The power is the area under the curve, which is similar for each angle

Aliasing is a phenomenon which occurs when frequency is estimated; consequently, this does not occur in power Doppler images. This can be understood with reference to Fig. 23, in which again the Doppler spectrum from a single velocity is shown. In this case, the spectrum demonstrates aliasing. The power of the signal, given by the area under the curve, remains similar to that from the previous example shown in Fig. 22.

The backscattered power from blood does not depend on blood velocity during laminar flow. This explains why power Doppler images tend to be of a single uniform color. The change in color seen at the edge of vessels is due to part of the beam being outside the vessel.

In many ways, the color power image mode is easier to use than the color velocity mode. There is

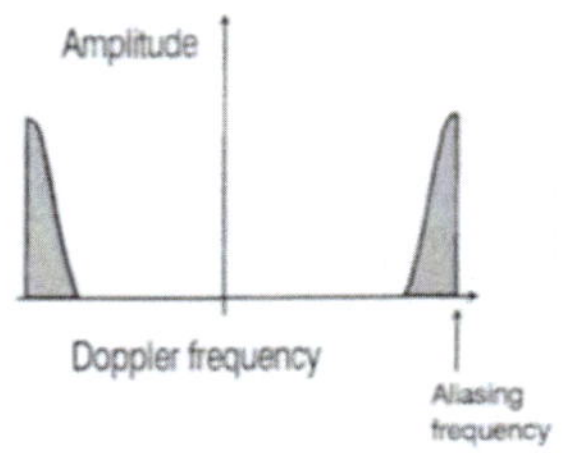

Fig. 23. Doppler spectrum from blood with a single velocity demonstrating aliasing. The total power consists of the area under the two separate curves

no color gain, no aliasing, no cos θ dependence and improved sensitivity. There is also no information on blood velocity, so that color power imaging cannot replace color velocity imaging in all circumstances. The recent flood of interest in power Doppler arises from the supposed superior visualisation of small vessels. The technique is very sensitive to movement, so that in superficial arteries where there is substantial wall thump it is difficult to use. In transcranial applications, the superior visualisation of small vessels makes this technique preferable to color velocity imaging [16].

The features of color power imaging can be summarised as follows:
- Real-time B-scan and image of blood pool.
- The power of the Doppler signal is color coded.
- No directional discrimination.
- No aliasing.
- Little dependence on cos θ.

References

1. Adamson SL, Morrow RJ, Langille BL et al (1989) Site dependent effect of increases in placental vascular resistance on the umbilical arterial velocity waveform in fetal sheep. Ultrasound Med Biol 16: 19–27
2. Bluth EI, Stavros AT, Marich KW et al (1988) Carotid duplex sonography: a multicenter recommendation for standardised imaging and Doppler criteria. Radiographics 8: 487–506
3. Bonnefous O, Pesque P (1986) Time domain formulation of pulse-Doppler ultrasound and blood velocity estimation by cross correlation. Ultrasonic Imaging 8: 73–85
4. Censor D, Newhouse VL, Vantz T, Ortega HV (1988) Theory of ultrasound Doppler-spectra velocimetry for arbitrary beam and flow configuration. IEEE Trans Biomed Eng 35: 740–751
5. Cobbold RSC, Veltink PH, Johnston KW (1983) Influence of beam profile and degree of insonation on the CW Doppler ultrasound spectrum and mean velocity. IEEE Trans Son Ultrason 30: 364–370
6. David JY, Jones S, Giddens D (1991) Modern spectral analysis techniques for blood velocity and spectral meas-

urements with pulsed Doppler ultrasound. IEEE Trans Biomed Eng 38: 589–596
7. Evans DH (1982) Some aspects of the relationship between instantaneous volumetric blood flow and continuous wave Doppler ultrasound recordings. I. The effect of ultrasonic beam width on the output of maximum frequency, mean frequency and RMS processors. Ultrasound Med Biol 8: 605–609
8. Evans DH, McDicken WN, Skidmore R, Woodcock JP (1989) Doppler ultrasound: physics, instrumentation and clinical applications. Wiley, Chichester
9. Fox MD, Gardiner WM (1988) Three-dimensional Doppler velocimetry of flow jets. IEEE Trans Biomed Eng 35: 834–841
10. Gosling RC, King DH (1974) Continuos wave ultrasound as an alternative and complement to X-rays. In: Reneman RS (ed) Cardiovascular applications of ultrasound. North Holland, Amsterdam, pp 266–282
11. Guo Z, Durand LG, Lee HC (1994) Comparison of time-frequency distribution techniques for analysis of simulated Doppler ultrasound signals of the femoral artery. IEEE Trans Biomed Eng 41: 332–342
12. Hoskins PR (1990) Measurement of arterial blood flow by Doppler ultrasound. Clin Phys Physiol Meas 11: 1–26
13. Hoskins PR (1996) Measurement of maximum velocity using duplex ultrasound systems. Br J Radiol 69: 172–177
14. Hoskins PR, Loupas T, McDicken WN (1991) A comparison of three difficult filters for speckle reduction of Doppler spectra. Ultrasound Med Biol 16: 375–389
15. Kasai C, Namekawa K, Koyano A, Omoto R (1985) Real-time two-dimensional blood flow imaging using an autocorrelation technique. IEEE Trans Son Ultrason 32: 458–464
16. Kenton AR, Martin PJ, Evans DH (1996) Power Doppler: an advance over colour Doppler for transcranial imaging. Ultrasound Med Biol 22: 313–317
17. McDicken WN, Sutherland GR, Moran CM, Gordon LN (1992) Colour Doppler imaging of the myocardium. Ultrasound Med Biol 18: 651–654
18. McPherson DS, Evans DH, Bell PRF (1984) Common femoral artery Doppler waveforms: a comparison of three methods of objective analysis with direct pressure measurements. Br J Surg 71: 46–49
19. Newhouse VL, Furgason ES, Johnson GF, Wolf DA (1980) The dependence of ultrasound Doppler bandwidth on beam geometry. IEEE Trans Son Ultrason 27: 50–59
20. Overbeck JR, Beach KW, Strandness DE (1992) Vector Doppler: accurate measurements of blood velocity in two dimensions. Ultrasound Med Biol 18: 19–31
21. Pourcelot L (1974) Applications cliniques de l'examen Doppler transcutane. In: Peronneau (ed) Velocimetrie ultrasonore Doppler. Seminaire INSERM, Paris, pp 213–240
22. Robinson ML, Sacks D, Perlmutter GS, Marinelli DL (1988) Diagnostic criteria for carotid duplex sonography. Am J Roentgenol 151: 1045–1049
23. Rubin JM, Bude RO, Carson PL et al (1994) Power Doppler US: a potentially useful alternative to mean-frequency based color Doppler US. Radiology 190: 853–856
24. Schlindwein FS, Evans DH (1989) A real time autoregressive spectrum analyser for Doppler signals. Ultrasound Med Biol 15: 263–272
25. Skidmore R, Woodcock JP (1980) Physiological interpretation of Doppler shift waveforms. I. Theoretical considerations. Ultrasound Med Biol 6: 7–10
26. Thomson RS, Stevens RJ (1989) Mathematical model for interpretation of Doppler velocity waveform indices. Med Biol Eng Comput 27: 269–276
27. Thrush AJ, Evans DH (1995) Intrinsic spectral broadening: a potential cause of misdiagnosis of carotid artery disease. J. Vasc Invest 1: 187–192

Applications of Doppler Ultrasound

E.G. Cape

The Link Between Principles and Technology

Traveling sound waves are characterized by minute fluctuations in pressure within the conducting medium. Waves with frequencies above 20 000 Hz are above the audible range of sound for the human ear and are classified as *ultrasound*. Advances in technology have allowed construction of transducers which can generate sound at frequencies well into the ultrasonic range and with enough power to penetrate tissue, experience reflection and scattering, and return with enough energy to be processed by the receiving apparatus of a transducer. Well understood properties of the ultrasound waves facilitate construction of images and calculation of blood cell velocities. It is the purpose of this chapter to describe the basic *principles* of physics which govern the manipulation of ultrasound to produce vascular images and measurements of blood flow, and the *basic technology* which remains relatively constant in the face of rapid updates in modalities and options. It will conclude with a discussion of three relatively new ultrasound approaches: color Doppler energy, three-dimensional imaging, and contrast sonography.

Basic Ultrasound Principles

Sound waves are characterized by local fluctuations of pressure in the medium through which they pass. The local pressure fluctuations are facilitated by particle motion parallel to the direction of wave propagation. Since the moving particles "carry" the sound, the nature of the medium can affect the speed of sound dramatically. For example, in blood the speed of sound is approximately 1560 m/s. In a medium such as air, which has a much greater distance between molecules, the speed of sound falls dramatically to 331 m/s [1]. In contrast, sound travels through the lattice structure of bone at drastically greater speeds (3360 m/s) than in blood. In vascular medical ultrasound applications, it is usually the goal to direct ultrasound into a region of interest through a path composed largely of tissue and blood. Since tissue is primarily water (which has a speed of sound similar to that of blood), it is reasonable to assume a constant speed of sound for these applications.

The following definitions, which are developed in detail by Kremkau [1]), will be useful in the remainder of this chapter. The *wavelength* of traveling sound can be calculated by dividing the speed by the frequency of sound (number of oscillations in pressure per second). The *amplitude* is the magnitude of pressure variation from its undisturbed value. The *intensity* is the power of sound divided by the area (cross-sectional) through which it passes. The *impedance* of tissue is the product of density and sound propagation speed. Sound is said to be *refracted* if it changes direction at a boundary. This phenomenon occurs when sound encounters a boundary at a non-perpendicular angle of incidence and when the speeds of sound in the two media are different. The angle of incidence will be increased if the speed of sound in the distal medium is greater than that in the proximal medium.

As traveling sound crosses a boundary between two tissues (or tissue and fluid) of different acoustic impedance, it will be absorbed, reflected, or scattered. *Absorption* is a fundamental process in which some sound is dissipated as heat in the tissue. This process is governed by conservation of energy, but for most practical purposes it is viewed as a loss of sound intensity or amplitude. That is, transducers are designed such that significant heating of the tissue does not occur, but the lost amplitude or intensity due to absorption can still be quite noticeable.

Sound which has not been absorbed will continue to pass through tissue, and as it encounters an interface between two media of different acoustic impedance, part of it will be *reflected*. No reflection will occur if a boundary is encountered between two media with equal acoustic impedance. Knowledge of the speed of sound allows proper location of tissue structures in B-mode imaging, by use of reflected waves, and this modality will be discussed in a subsequent section.

Sound which has not been absorbed or reflected may encounter structures which are similar in size to or smaller than the wavelength of the sound. Sound will be *scattered* from these structures. In contrast to reflection, scattering is characterized by multidirectional reversal of sound propagation from its original path. Knowledge of the speed of sound and the frequency shift which occurs when comparing scattered to incident sound, allows calculation of blood cell velocities using the Doppler principle, to be discussed in a subsequent section.

The process of absorption combines with reflection and scattering to produce a net loss of sound which is called *attenuation*. Attenuation effects are increased as the frequency of sound increases. Therefore, when considering transducers of different carrier frequencies, it is important to remember that high-frequency transducers will be limited in their available depths of penetration.

In summary, sound traveling through tissue may be absorbed, reflected, or scattered. All combine to produce a net attenuation of sound. Absorption is a conversion of sound into heat. Reflection of sound occurs at boundaries of structures which are large compared to the wavelength and is a uniform return of sound toward its source. It can be used to locate tissue structures in B-mode imaging. Scattering occurs at boundaries of structures which are of similar size to or smaller than the wavelength and is characterized by a multidirectional shift in direction. Scattered sound can be used to calculate blood cell velocities in Doppler ultrasound applications.

Instrumentation and Technology

Transducers

Transducers serve as the primary interface between the ultrasound instrument and the tissue being imaged. Electrical voltages are converted into ultrasound using piezoelectric principles [2]. Piezoelectric materials deform when subjected to an applied voltage and, conversely, produce a voltage when deformed. Transducers are therefore constructed of piezoelectric crystals which produce ultrasound waves at a prescribed frequency and receive scattered or reflected sound, which is converted back into voltage for further processing. After a brief discussion of image shape (which is controlled by the type of transducer), data processing and image display will be described.

In order to construct an array of scan lines for two-dimensional imaging, transducers consist of a phased array of piezoelectric crystals capable of focusing the sound beam along alternate paths, or a mechanically oscillating transducer head which moves at a frequency equal to the frame rate. Specific image shapes are determined by the transducer configuration. Most common in vascular applications are linear, vector, and sector arrays. Figure 1 displays these image shapes. Linear arrays are constructed by focusing the scan line along adjacent parallel paths to produce a rectangular-shaped image. Vector arrays are produced by scan lines emerging in a radial fashion from a semicircular locus as shown. Sector arrays are similar to vector arrays but are pie-shaped, with scan lines extending radially from a single point as shown in Fig. 1. Linear arrays are most easily analyzed, especially when Doppler applications are activated, since the beam paths all pass in a single direction and it is relatively simple to account for angle of incidence effects. Sector and vector arrays amplify angle of incidence difficulties but are useful since they require a small "footprint" (point of contact between transducer and patient) to produce a large area of interrogation.

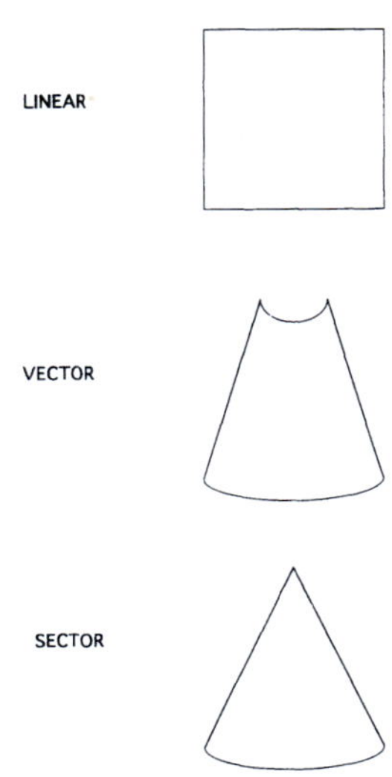

Fig. 1. Common geometries of tomographic image sectors in vascular ultrasound

Data Processing

After piezoelectric conversion of ultrasound into voltage, the electrical signals are processed to construct the desired image or velocity information. Gain is a controllable feature on the instrument which results in amplification of the basic voltages. In addition to providing an overall amplification of the signal, it is common to compensate for variations in amplitude resulting from attenuation effects in the far field. This is done by a graded increase in amplification of late-arriving signals. Data are stored in what is called a digital scan converter, which is a matrix of numbers to be converted into display. Depending on the modality, data may be tissue structure and acoustic density (for B-mode) or velocities (frequency shifts in Doppler mode). Display may be in the form of gray-scale brightness (B-mode or spectral Doppler) or shade of color (color Doppler). In B-Mode ultrasound, structure brightness is arranged on an image representing two dimensional space. Spectral Doppler intensities are placed on a velocity scale (y-axis) which scrolls across the screen with an x-axis representing time. In color Doppler, shades of color are superimposed on the B-mode image.

Image Display (Postprocessing)

Display of Doppler information is intimately connected to the modality of choice. Modern instruments exclusively use a television-type monitor for display. B-mode displays gray-scale images of solid structures. Continuous or pulsed wave spectral Doppler displays velocity distributions versus time. Color Doppler is characterized by color-encoded velocity patterns superimposed on the B-mode images. More details on each of these displays are included in the sections describing each modality.

B-Mode Sonography

Imaging of anatomic structures is possible by use of B-mode sonography. When ultrasound passes through an interface of two media with different acoustic impedance, part of the sound will be reflected back to the transducer. Transducers constructed of a phased array of piezoelectric crystals or a mechanically oscillating transducer head can acquire and allow analysis of the positions of structures within a tomographic plane and display these structures in a B-mode image. Increasing transducer carrier frequency improves image quality but limits penetration depth.

Despite widespread use for three decades, B-mode sonography retains several limitations. Structure geometries and dimensions must be carefully interpreted with attention to the tomographic nature of the image in the context of complex three-dimensional physiology. Reverberations, produced by sound traveling through two media of significant density difference, are often produced by prosthetic devices and preclude quality B-mode images from standard windows.

High-Resolution B-Mode Imaging

In applications with rapid motion of structures, conventional frame rates (determined by the speed of sound and area covered by the image) are not sufficient since critical time points can be missed. The development of parallel processing transducers has allowed significantly elevated frame rates to be achieved (two to four times higher than those obtained with conventional instruments). Images obtained using these instruments provide significant improvement in image quality but can introduce additional expense in storage of data. Conventional frame rates are approximately 30/s., which coincide with the frame rates of video tapes on which sonographic data is typically stored. Increasing the B-mode frame rate to 120/s, for example, is of little use unless the frames can be digitally stored or unless the exam is interpreted on-line. The former is not financially feasible in many centers and the latter is difficult, since sonographic exams are usually read off-line by the physician. Over the next decade, therefore, the value of high-resolution B-mode sonography will be indirectly proportional to the cost of digital storage algorithms and hardware, and directly proportional to the rate of new and more efficient systems.

Doppler Ultrasound

The Doppler principle written in the context of ultrasound is:

$$v = (cf_d)/2f_o\cos\theta$$

where c = the speed of sound in the medium (approximately 1560 m/s for tissue/blood), f_d = the Doppler shift, f_o = the frequency emitted from the

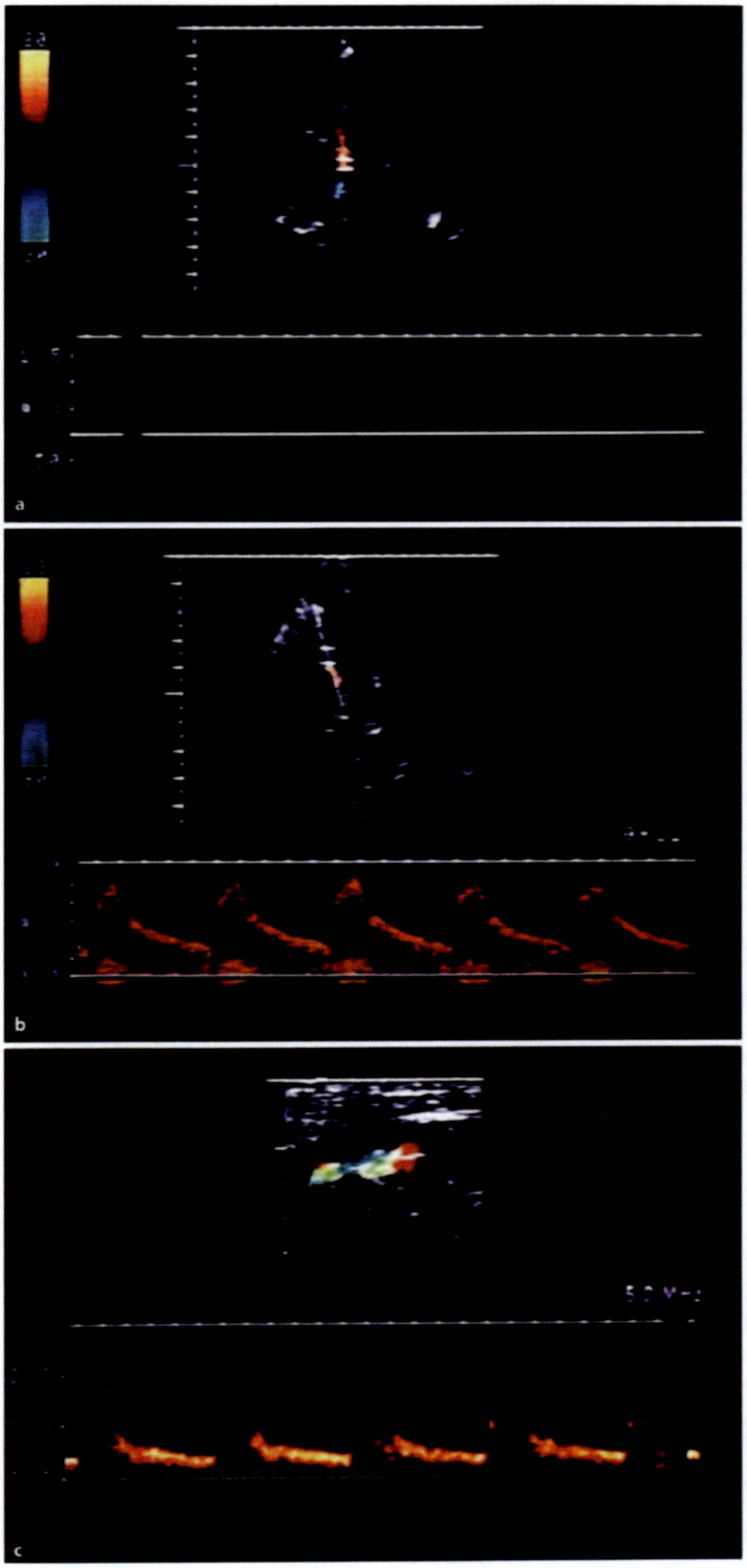

Fig. 2 a–c. Clinical example of simultaneous use of color and spectral Doppler: **a** middle cerebral artery, **b** stenosis of middle cerebral artery, **c** stenosis of internal carotid artery

ultrasound transducer, and θ = the angle between the ultrasound beam path and the velocity vector of the target. The Doppler shift, f_d is the difference in frequency between the emitted sound waves and those returning to the transducer after collision with a target. Since the emitted frequency is set for a given instrument configuration and the speed of sound is well known, target velocities can be directly calculated using this equation. Transducers are equipped to determine the returning frequency. Signal processing circuitry within the instrument converts the Doppler shifts into velocity.

Spectral Doppler vs Color Doppler

Depending upon the desired information, the Doppler equation can be implemented in several ways. These "modalities" can be divided into spectral modes and color imaging modes. Spectral Doppler is characterized by a vertically oriented spectrum of velocities as shown in Fig. 2. The vertical strip may be thought of as a histogram with increased shading within a velocity interval representing more scattering particles traveling at that velocity. The term "Color Doppler" refers to color-encoded Doppler information distributed within a tomographic slice and superimposed on the B-mode image.

Spectral Doppler

Spectral Doppler is available in two modalities: continuous wave and pulsed wave. Continuous wave is chosen to quickly obtain a maximum velocity along a line of interest and pulsed wave is chosen to obtain velocity at a specific location or depth from the transducer.

Continuous Wave Doppler

Continuous wave Doppler transducers typically consist of a transducer with two crystals. One crystal continuously emits sound while the other continuously receives returning sound. The frequency of returning sound is assessed and compared to the known emitted frequency to produce f_d in the Doppler equation, which is then used to obtain velocity. At any single point in time, numerous signals are returning to the transducer, since numerous scattering particles exist within the beam path. The velocities of all of the targets within the beam path are placed on the spectral trace. Since the transducer is continuously emitting and receiving sound, returning signals may represent velocities from any location along the beam path. The advantage of this approach is that measurement of the peak velocity of the spectral envelope automatically corresponds to the maximum velocity along the beam path. The disadvantage is that all other signals are buried beneath the envelope and are unavailable for analysis. This modality allows for quick and convenient determination of velocity along a line of interest.

Pulsed Wave Doppler

Pulsed wave Doppler transducers usually consist of a single crystal emitting and receiving sound. Sound is emitted, the transducer waits a time t, then opens a "window" to catch the returning signal. Knowing the time between emission of the sound and reception gives knowledge of the depth from which the signals must have returned. That is,

$$\text{depth} = ct/2$$

where c = speed of sound in the medium and t is time between emission and reception of the burst. The factor of 2 accounts for the round trip of the sound from the transducer, to the target, and back to the transducer, since the total distance travelled is ct. By pulsing the ultrasound in this manner, one overcomes the range ambiguity in continuous wave Doppler and is able to select the distance from the transducer at which velocities are to be measured. Signals returning from scatterers closer than the distance d from the transducer will arrive at the transducer before the window opens, while those returning from particles beyond the distance d will arrive at the transducer after the window closes.

Although pulsed wave Doppler allows one to overcome the range ambiguity problem in continuous wave Doppler, a different disadvantage is introduced. Aliasing occurs in pulsed wave Doppler if the target velocity produces a frequency shift which is more than half of the sampling frequency. For example, if the pulse repetition frequency is 4 kHz, then pulsed wave Doppler can be used to correctly calculate velocities producing frequency shifts up to 2 kHz. Those producing frequency shifts greater than 2 kHz will begin to wrap to the opposite sign of the scale. The basic law governing this limitation is the Nyquist criterion, which states that in any frequency-dependent sampling process, the sampling frequency must be at least twice the characteristic frequency of the phenomenon being sampled.

For high velocity flows, therefore, one can increase the pulse repetition frequency of the instrument and increase the Nyquist limit. However, such an action unfortunately introduces another limitation of pulsed Doppler. Taking the limit as pulse repetition frequency goes to infinity, we reapproach continuous wave Doppler. Thus, increasing pulse repetition frequency in order to increase the Nyquist limit reintroduces range ambiguity incrementally. If the time between pulses is *t*, we will have a sample depth of *ct*/2. In principle, the spectral output will display signals returning from all integer multiples of this distance.

Color Doppler Flow Mapping

Two modalities of color Doppler are available for vascular imaging. *Color Doppler velocity mode* provides a tomographic map of color-encoded velocities superimposed upon the B-mode image. *Color Doppler energy mode* provides a color map of integrated velocity signal intensity which sacrifices velocity magnitude information but is useful for assessment of perfusion.

Color Doppler Velocity Mode

The color Doppler velocity mode is an extension of the pulsed wave Doppler concept. Figure 3 depicts a string of sample volumes which can be placed along a line of interest by combining the pulsed wave Doppler concept with the process of multigating. Ultrasound is emitted, then the window which catches returning signals is opened numerous times. At each opening, a packet of ultrasound is acquired which represents velocities at a specific distance away from the transducer. This distance can again be calculated using *ct*/2. The line of sample volumes constructed in this manner is called a scan line. In conventional transducers, the scan line can be focused along adjacent parallel paths or along wedge- or pie-shaped paths (see above, p. 37). The result is a two-dimensional matrix of velocity measurements. For typical transducer configurations the number of sample sites within a sector for a single frame numbers more than a thousand. Frame rates for color Doppler velocity will typically be less than those for B-mode owing to the much larger data processing load.

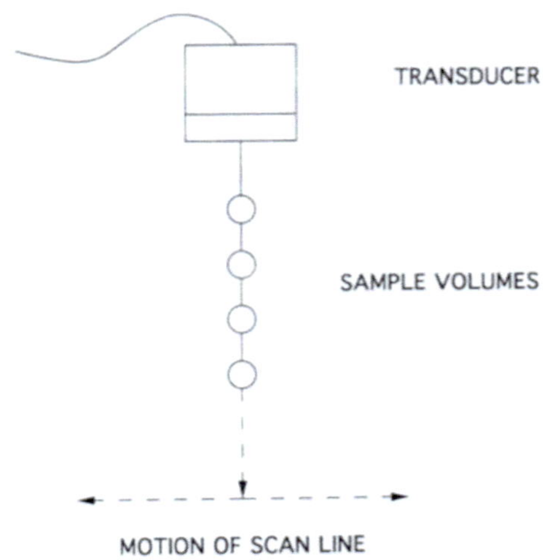

Fig. 3. Use of multigating to obtain multiple sample volumes for color Doppler imaging

Color Encoding
It is not feasible to view spectra similar to those in the lower panel of Fig. 2, for each sample volume. Instead, average velocity values for each sample volume are color-encoded. Typically, varying hues of red are used to represent velocities directed toward the transducer and varying hues of blue are used to represent velocities directed away from the transducer. A color bar representing the color encoding pattern is usually displayed alongside the image. Figure 2 shows examples of such images. The scale of the color bar will extend from positive Nyquist limit to negative Nyquist limit. A small band of no color around zero represents the wall filter. The wall filter is a high pass threshold which is incorporated into the instrument to eliminate high-amplitude signals resulting from structure or transducer motion. Blood cells producing frequency shifts which correspond to velocities below the wall filter will not receive color encoding since they will be rejected on the basis of frequency criteria.

Autocorrelation
The method used to obtain Doppler velocities in the color Doppler velocity mode actually differs profoundly from that performed to construct Doppler spectra. Owing to the large data processing load, it is difficult to directly calculate velocities by the Doppler equation for the numerous sample volumes within a sector and maintain a reasonable frame rate. In practice, the phase difference between adjacent returning waves is compared to produce an estimate of velocity. A number of these

values are obtained per sample volume per beat and these are averaged to produce the single value which is color-encoded.

Variance

Flow fields are often disturbed, especially in the vicinity of obstructions. In a jet-type flow distal to a stenosis, it is often useful to have information in addition to the elevated velocities. The variance mode is available on most conventional color Doppler instruments and can be used to indicate the possible presence of disturbed flow. In each sample volume, multiple samples are averaged to produce a single mean velocity as described above. It is then simple for the instrument to calculate a variance, by statistical definition, operating on the same data. The magnitude of variance receives a shade of green in the color encoding process and is mixed into the red and/or blue representing velocity magnitude in that region. It is important to note that variance represents a significant spatial or temporal variation in velocity within the time of frame acquisition. It does not necessarily indicate turbulent flow as defined in fluid dynamics. Significant spatial variations in velocity due to a steep velocity profile, or significant temporal variations in velocity due to elevated heart rates, can both trigger the variance algorithm and the addition of green to the color map in the absence of turbulence in the fluid mechanical sense.

Limitations

Color Doppler velocity mapping is accompanied by several critical limitations. Velocity magnitudes will almost always be underestimated in some portion of the image due to the angle dependence of the Doppler equation. In practice, one attempts to orient the transducer as parallel to the flow of interest as possible. Even in the best possible orientation, however, it is unlikely that the all of the velocity vectors will be oriented in a single direction. While it is possible to manually correct for angle of incidence, this is not always useful in two-dimensional velocity imaging. Since flow fields are often characterized by swirling and by separation zones, it is impossible to know what the required angle correction factor is by context. Furthermore, since color Doppler velocity modalities are in principle an extension of pulsed wave Doppler, all of the limitations of pulsed wave Doppler accompany color Doppler velocity mapping. The most important of course is the Nyquist limit. Velocities which can be measured using color Doppler velocity mode are limited by the pulsing frequency of the transducer. If blood cells with velocities exceeding the Nyquist limit are insonated, the signal will alias and wrap to the opposite sign of the scale. In color Doppler velocity mode this is reflected by a change in color from red to blue or vice versa. Since color Doppler is often used to detect the direction of flow (red/blue), the aliasing limitation can cause considerable confusion. Finally, the potential for range ambiguity cannot be tolerated in color flow mapping since the fundamental strength of this modality is its imaging nature. In other words, color-encoded velocities must be placed in the correct location of the B-mode image, otherwise they are useless. Therefore, pulse frequencies are set at relatively low values for color Doppler (compared to spectral pulsed wave Doppler at the same depth setting) in order to ensure that color encoded velocities are placed in the correct location.

Clinical Examples

Figure 2 shows three examples demonstrating the important method of using color and spectral Doppler in combination. Figure 2a shows a B-mode with color Doppler image of the middle cerebral artery in a patient with relatively normal flow. The color Doppler image enables visualization and localization of the flow. The color bar spans a range of velocities from -80 cm/s to +80 cm/s. A pulsed wave sample volume has been steered into the location of flow, providing the more quantitative spectral velocity output shown in the lower panel of Fig. 2a. Peak velocity just exceeds 1 m/s. In contrast, Fig. 2b shows a patient with stenosis of the middle cerebral artery. The pulsed wave sample volume is steered into the region of flow and the spectral output in the lower portion of the panel shows a velocity approaching 3 m/s. Elevated velocities correspond to increased stenosis as long as it is reasonable to assume that perfusion is being maintained. Figure 2c shows another example of elevated velocity in arterial obstruction in a patient with stenosis of the internal carotid artery.

In addition to providing guidance for the placement of spectral Doppler sample volumes, color Doppler is useful alone to identify the presence and direction of flow. Figure 4a shows the multidirectional and complex flow in the carotid bifurcation, Fig. 4b the simultaneous multidirectional flow in a renal artery and vein, Fig. 4c the flow in the circle of Willis, and Fig. 4d the large bulk flow in a single direction in the inferior vena cava.

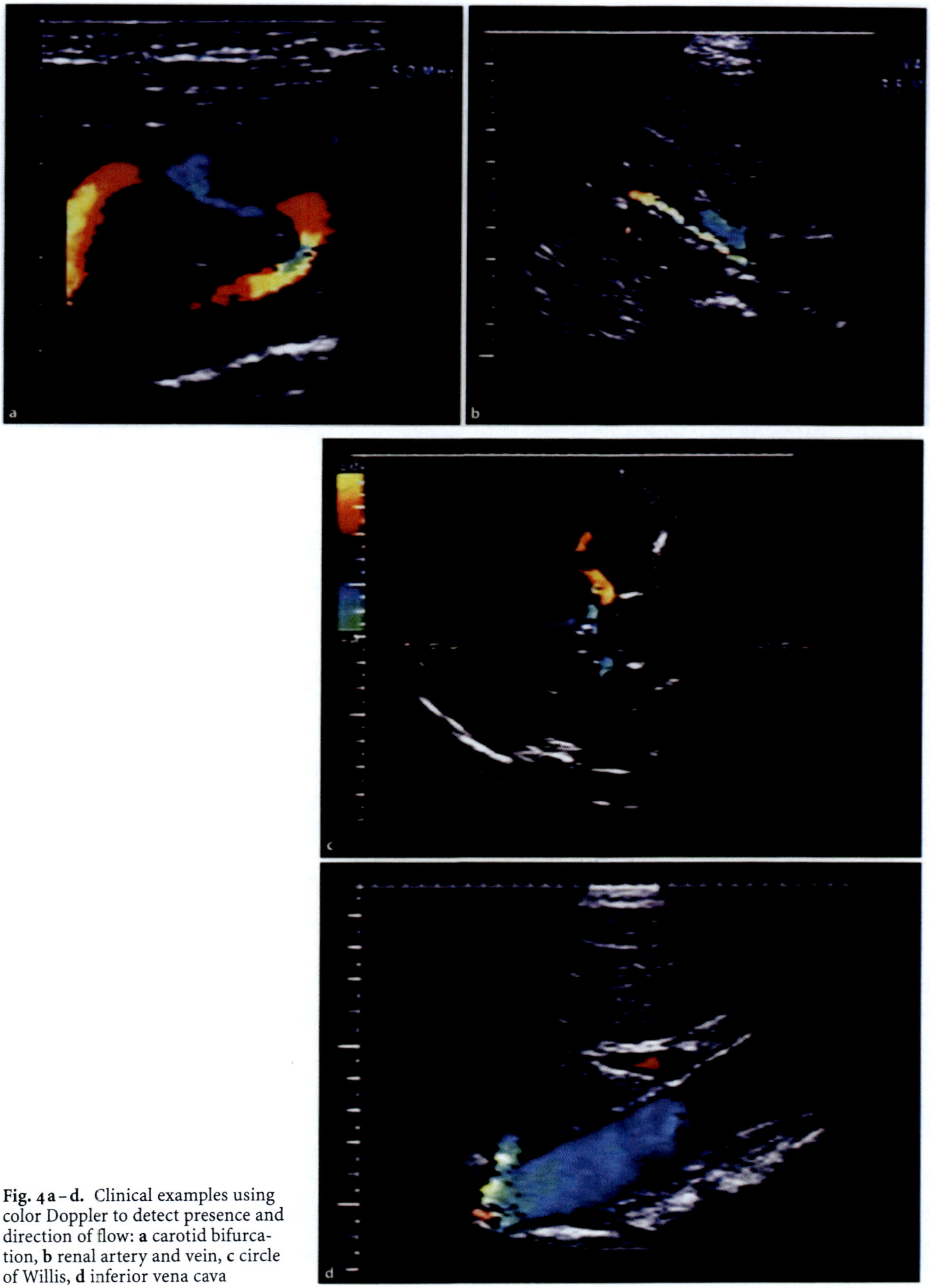

Fig. 4 a–d. Clinical examples using color Doppler to detect presence and direction of flow: **a** carotid bifurcation, **b** renal artery and vein, **c** circle of Willis, **d** inferior vena cava

Color Doppler Energy Mapping

Color Doppler energy mapping is a relatively new technology which may overcome some of the limitations of color Doppler velocity. Figure 5 demonstrates the basic theoretical principle of color Doppler energy. The curve in the upper panel represents the distribution of velocity magnitudes within a sample volume for a single frame, as obtained by a conventional color Doppler transducer. The magnitude of intensity, displayed on the y-axis, indicates the relative number of particles traveling at a specific velocity. In conventional color Doppler, these velocities are averaged to produce a single mean velocity, represented by the vertical bar, which is color encoded for display. Color Doppler energy, as shown in the lower panel, displays the integrated intensity, which is represented by the area underneath the curve.

Color Doppler energy mapping sacrifices velocity magnitude and direction to obtain "energy." Some advantages accompany this sacrifice. Color Doppler energy is in principle angle independent. Tilting of the transducer away from the axis of flow results in a shift to the left of the velocity distribution due to angle dependence of the Doppler equation, as can be seen in Fig. 6 by comparing the left and right panels. Conventional color Doppler velocities are underestimated in the righthand panel as the vertical line m_2 can shift significantly with respect to the true mean velocity m_1. The integral underneath the curve, however, should remain constant, as will the calculated color Doppler energy. The wall filter which is present as a horizontal band about zero in color Doppler velocity mapping will appear as a vertical strip of lost signal in color Doppler energy mapping. This will cause a slight decrease in the integrated value of color Doppler

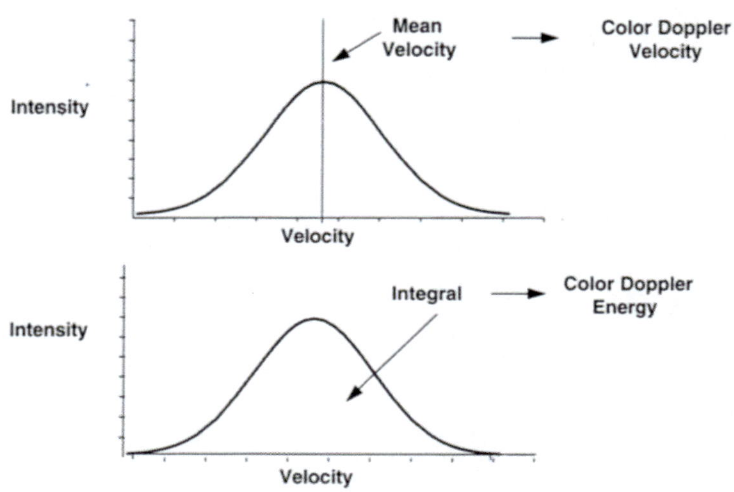

Fig. 5. Theoretical principles of color Doppler energy mapping

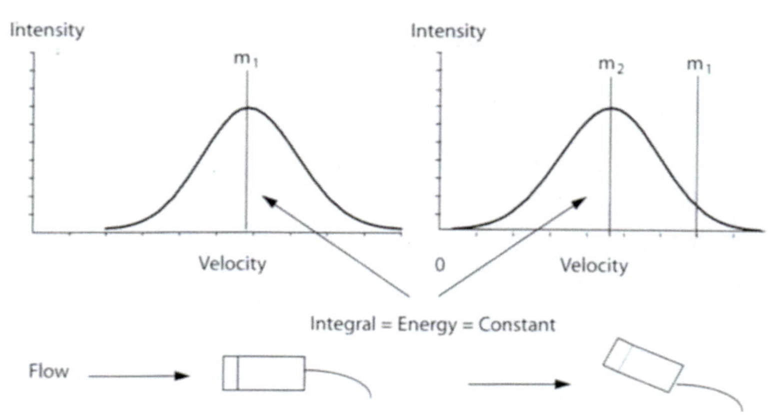

Fig. 6. Angle effects in color Doppler velocity versus color Doppler energy

energy depending on the width of the wall filter and the position of the spectrum with respect to zero.

Color Doppler energy mapping has great potential in vascular imaging as a marker of perfusion. Scatterers with very low velocity will display color on an energy map. Indeed, assuming a very low wall filter, or in cases where it can be reduced to zero, even particles with near-zero velocity will exhibit color encoding on the energy map.

Clinical Examples

Figure 7 shows some clinical examples of the application of color Doppler energy mapping. Figure 7a illustrates the ability of the color Doppler energy made to delineate flow through a tortuous internal carotid artery. Figure 7b shows the multiple vessel flow in the vicinity of the subclavian artery. Figure 7c shows flow in a carotid bifurcation. Figure 7d shows the dramatic image of renal perfusion which can be obtained using color Doppler energy mapping.

Instrument Settings

This section will describe standard instrument settings for Doppler velocimetric techniques. Since some settings such as frame rate have no meaning in spectral Doppler, the settings will be described in the context of the color Doppler velocity modality.

Gain

"Gain" is a common setting on most electrical devices and refers to an amplification of an input signal. In the context of color Doppler flow mapping, it is used to overcome attenuation of the signals caused by tissue intervening between the transducer and the region of interest. An optimum gain setting will produce a strong and clear image of colors superimposed on the B-mode image. Decreasing the gain from this point will produce gradual loss of color. If the flow field is characterized by velocities which are gradually decreasing in the vicinity of adjacent walls, a loss of signal on the edge of the flow field will usually be observed with decreases in gain. This is due to the fact that the wall filter (see below) interacts with the gain setting, such that manipulating the gain can shift the high pass filter which determines the region of no color centered about zero. Increasing gain from the optimal value will begin to amplify extraneous signals, producing an unclear signal with noise clearly apparent in the regions surrounding the flow.

Pulse Repetition Frequency

The pulse repetition frequency (PRF) determines the Nyquist limit of maximum velocity detection. The maximum detectable Doppler frequency shift is one-half of the PRF. Determination of the maximum detectable velocity can be accomplished by inserting this frequency limit into the Doppler equation. Increasing PRF allows higher velocities to be detected but introduces the possibility of range ambiguity (multiple sample volumes).

Wall Filter

The wall filter is a high pass threshold incorporated into the signal-processing algorithms of Doppler modalities. The instrumentation used to detect frequency shifts and calculate velocities by the Doppler equation is designed to provide optimal performance when the scatterers are red blood cells. Red blood cells have dimensions on the order of 3 x 8 μm. Vessel walls and other structures are also in motion and are much larger in scale than blood cells. Although these moving structures provide returning signals of relatively low frequency shift, they have very large amplitude. These high-amplitude signals can saturate the signal-processing circuitry of the instrument, resulting in a screen full of noise. Most instruments take advantage of the relatively low velocity of these structures and impose a high pass frequency filter called the wall filter; that is, returning signals with a low Doppler shift are eliminated. In practice, the wall filter is chosen to be above the typical velocities of the solid structures. This is often reflected by reduced noise as the wall filter is elevated, even if gain is held constant. Simple wall filters can be problematic in some vascular applications, since eliminating signals based on frequency alone removes not only those signals returning from solid structures such as walls, but also blood cell velocities below the wall filter threshold. More complex filtration methods which operate on frequency and amplitude are used in some conventional instruments and these are discussed in the following section.

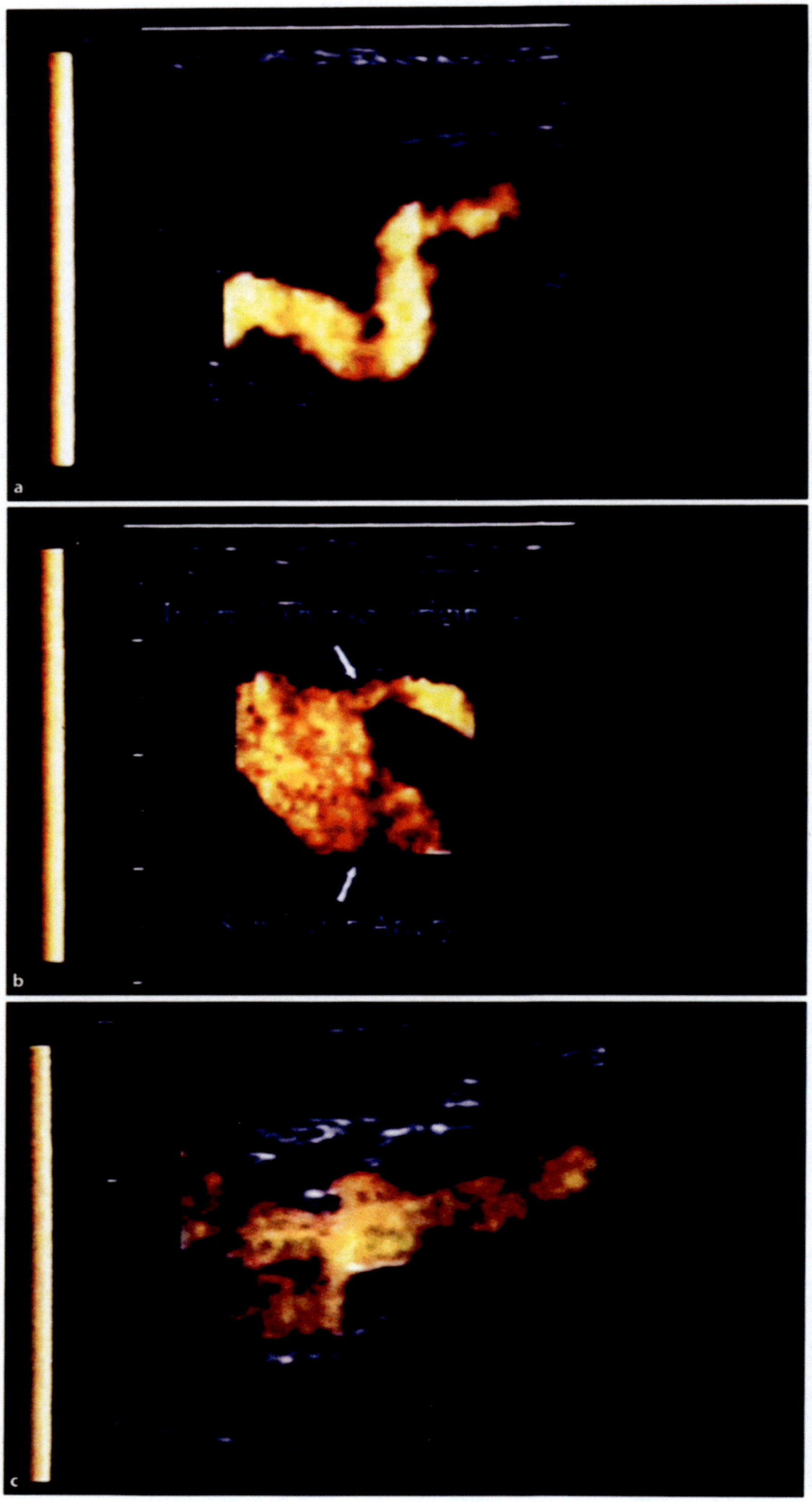

Fig. 7 a – d. Clinical images showing perfusion information obtained by color Doppler energy mapping. **a** Internal carotid artery, **b** area of subclavian artery, **c** carotid bifurcation, **d** kidney ▷

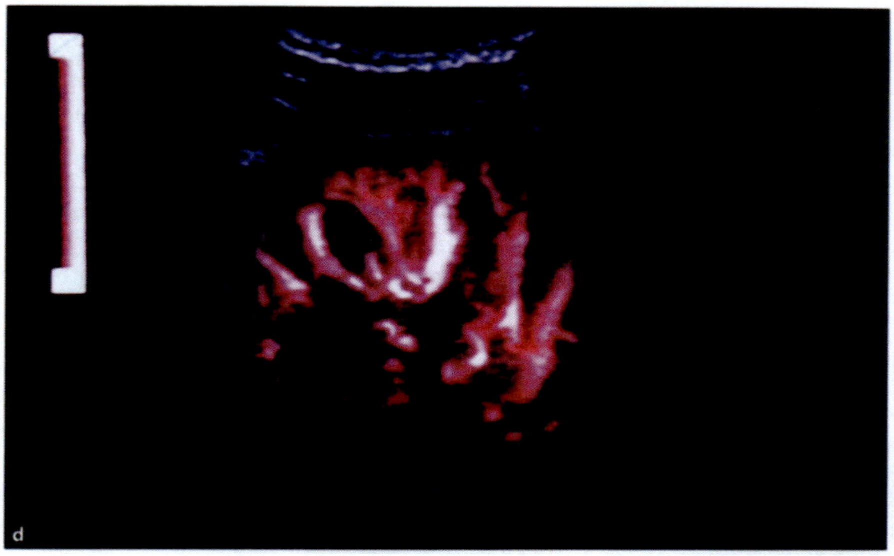

Fig. 7d

Frequency/Amplitude Filters

These filters, often called multivariate motion discriminators, allow high-amplitude signals from solid structures to be eliminated without discarding low velocity signals from blood cells. Returning signals may be classified as high-velocity/high-amplitude, high-velocity/low-amplitude, low-velocity/low-amplitude, or low-velocity/high-amplitude. High-velocity/high-amplitude signals only occur with the addition of sonographic contrast agents which move at the speed of blood cells but produce amplified signals. Blood cell velocities may be high-velocity/low-amplitude or low-velocity/low-amplitude. Structure motion is low-velocity/high-amplitude. By discriminating on the basis of amplitude rather than frequency (as in most wall filters), multivariate motion discriminators allow low-velocity/low-amplitude (blood) signals to be displayed along with high-velocity/low-amplitude signals while still eliminating low-velocity/high-amplitude signals (structures).

Carrier Frequency

The frequency of emitted ultrasound is usually referred to as the carrier frequency. This frequency is denoted f_0 in the Doppler equation given above. Lower carrier frequencies allow higher velocities to be detected for a given PRF. Higher carrier frequencies produce the opposite effect, but generally produce higher quality images. There is therefore a trade-off between image quality and velocity capabilities when choosing a carrier frequency. Higher-frequency transducers are furthermore limited to shorter depths of interrogation.

Frame Rate

The frequency with which color Doppler frames are updated is called the frame rate. These rates are necessarily equal to or less than those for B-mode images, usually considerably less. Frame rates are decreased by increasing PRF, increasing depth, increasing packet size (number of samples averaged per sarnple volume per frame), and increasing line density (density of scan lines, i.e., number of scan lines per unit width).

New Technologies

Digital Acquisition of Color Doppler Velocities

The majority of improvements in color Doppler imaging over the past decade have been in the area of image quality. The primary use of color Doppler is visualization of structure and flow. The potential of color Doppler sonography, however, promises more profound advances in the future. A method which, in principle, provides a two-dimensional matrix of velocities, is amenable to analysis by the principles of fluid dynamics and may ultimately yield a wealth of pathophysiologic information. To date this potential has been vastly underexplored.

Current Dilemma

Since color Doppler velocity modes produce a two-dimensional matrix of velocity magnitudes for superimposition on the B-mode image, it would be of great use in developing new noninvasive methods if the velocity magnitudes were available to the user. Unfortunately, such information is difficult for the average user to obtain. Economic and marketing factors have produced this situation. The ultrasound market is highly competitive and purchasing decisions are made based on familiarity with a machine and on image quality, which is certainly reasonable since the primary use of these instruments is visualization of flow presence and direction. As a result, however, color Doppler remains mostly semiquantitative due to complex postprocessing of the Doppler signals designed to produce pleasing images.

A demand for the availability of digital color Doppler data would improve this situation by allowing the user to confirm the meaning of color Doppler pixels, i.e., compare them to actual velocities. Making this information available to the user would be of long-term benefit to the manufacturers since numerous quantitation techniques which hinge upon accurate velocity maps would inevitably be produced. Some manufacturers have made such data available to the user. For example, Fig. 8 shows a color Doppler image of a low-velocity jet and the digitized matrix of velocity values. These particular data are available to the user via a commercially available software program which allows the color Doppler instrument to interface with a Macintosh computer. Other companies besides the one producing Fig. 8 have made some strides in producing digital color Doppler data, but most information is still quite proprietary.

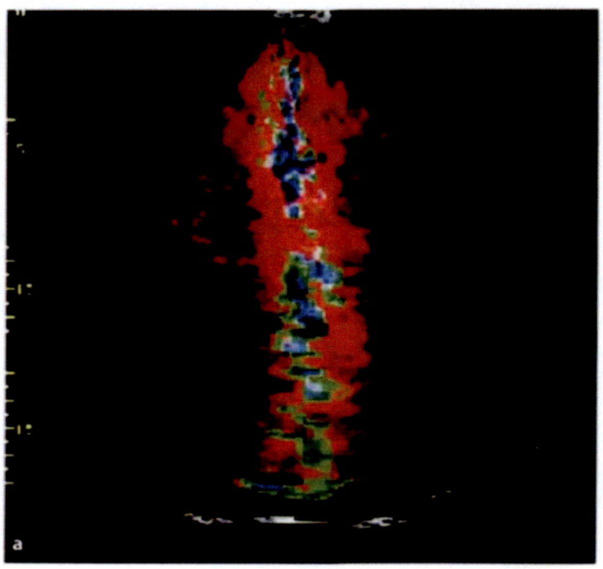

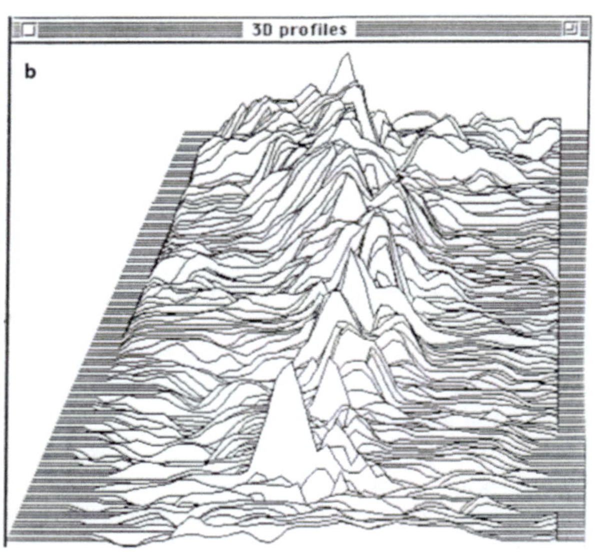

Fig. 8 a, b. Color Doppler image of jet-type flow field (**a**) and digitally acquired color Doppler velocities (**b**)

Sonographic Contrast Agents

Detection of organ perfusion has been a long-standing clinical goal. Such information is typically acquired by techniques utilizing ionizing radiation. The development of sonographic contrast agents has potentially opened the door to assessment of organ perfusion using the benign medium of ultrasound. Microbubbles injected into the blood pool will cause significant enhancement of B-mode and color Doppler images. By digitizing enhanced regions of tissue as imaged by B-mode sonography, one can potentially apply the extensive indicator dilution principles which have been developed over the years in the context of other media.

The observation that microbubbles will cause enhancement of B-mode images did not initially cause great enthusiasm. Since microbubbles have a short life span, it was difficult to have them persist in distal organs after introduction by catheter in the left heart or aorta. Contrast agents in which microbubbles were encapsulated in a carrier material required injection by catheter or intravenous injection. In the latter case, the agent would not survive pulmonary transit. Recent advances have led to the release of new contrast agents which will survive pulmonary transit and some of these agents have been approved for use in the United States and Europe. These agents have been used to enhance ultrasonic imaging of such diverse sites as coronary and carotid arteries, liver vessels and lesions, kidney vessels and renal tumors, breast masses, and ovarian tumors.

Three Dimensional Sonographic Imaging

Physiologic structures and flow are three-dimensional. Their complexity is typically increased in diseased states. Conventional methods such as B-mode and color Doppler sonography typically produce tomographic slices and are therefore fundamentally limited. Clearly, three-dimensional sonography would be an improvement. However, significant impediments currently exist which preclude true three-dimensional imaging. Transducer technology needs to be developed further before true three-dimensional reconstruction can be expected. Superimposed upon this difficulty is the basic limitation associated with the speed of sound. Actual and simultaneous interrogation of three dimensions with one transducer is most difficult to achieve while maintaining useful frame rates.

Three-dimensional imaging has been approximated, however, using new technology which combines multiple tomographic slices to show three-dimensional structures [5]. These instruments utilize existing ultrasound instruments, with the transducer positioned within a sweeping or linear translational carriage device. The translator and instrument data port are interfaced to a computer and, based on a reference point standardized to fixed points in space, multiple images are combined to produce three-dimensional images. Dynamic images can be obtained by heart beat and respiration gating. Archival of three-dimensional images is accomplished using a digital data base on a computer hard disk or laser disk.

Figure 9 shows images of a carotid arterial vessel obtained using this technology. The four panels show an axial view (Fig. 9a), views rotated 30° to either side (Fig. 9b, c), which allows viewing of the wall surface, and a face-down view of the artery (Fig. 9d). These images are quite clear and represent the cutting edge of ultrasonography. These methods have advanced significantly and rapidly over the past 5 years and further advances are expected in the near future. They are currently limited by: (1) the time required for reconstruction of images, which can obscure the basic advantage of ultrasound, which is quick acquisition of data, and

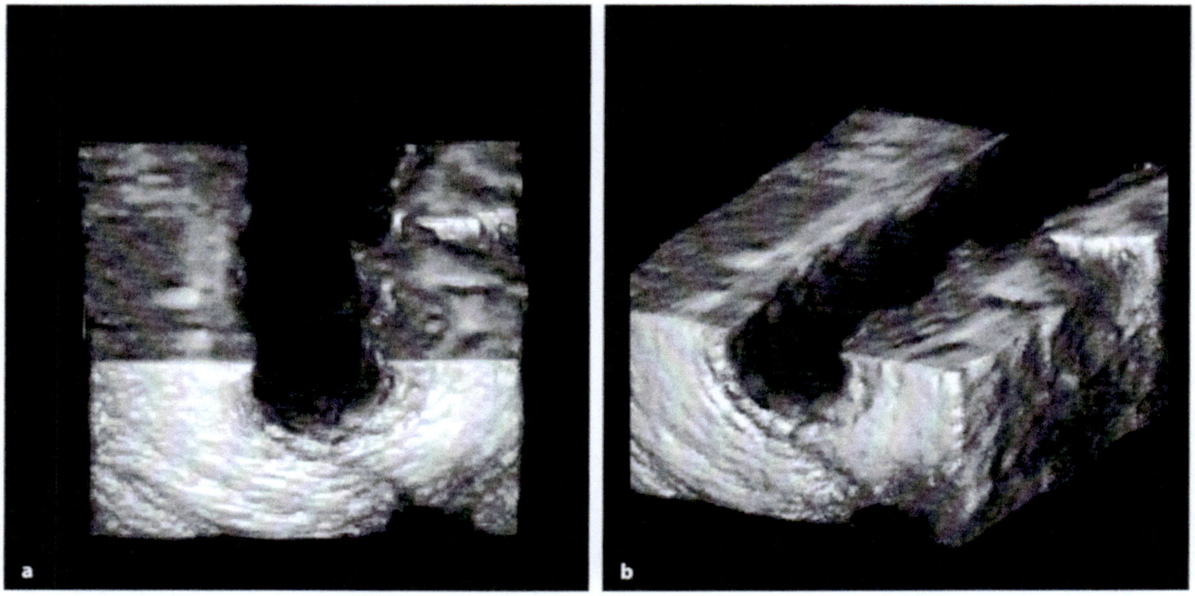

Fig. 9a, b. Three-dimensional reconstruction of carotid artery

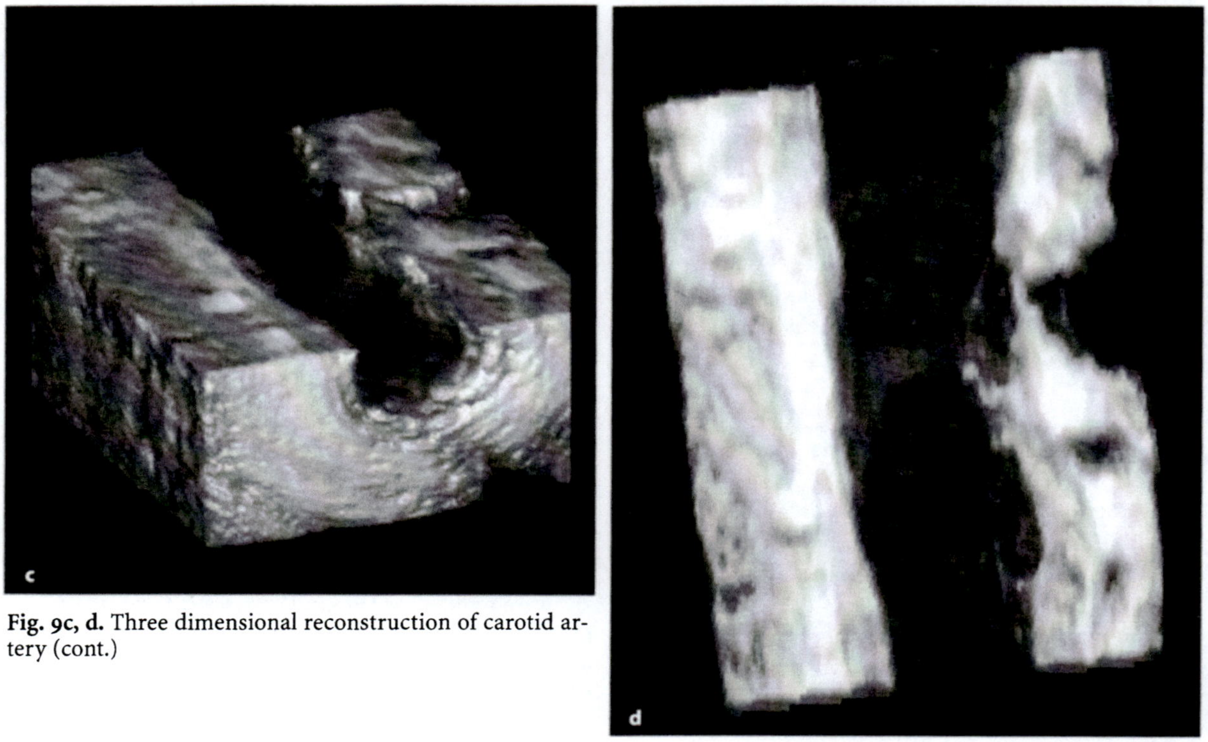

Fig. 9c, d. Three dimensional reconstruction of carotid artery (cont.)

(2) two-dimensional B-mode and color Doppler can be fraught with artifacts if care is not taken in acquisition; these artifacts can be magnified when the tomographic slices are extrapolated to produce three-dimensional images.

References

1. Kremkau FW (1990) Doppler ultrasound: principles and instruments. Saunders, Philadelphia
2. Aston R (1990) Ultrasonic equipment. In: Principles of biomedical instrumentation and measurement. Merrill Publishing Company, Columbus, pp. 489–514
3. Kremkau FW (1989) Diagnostic ultrasound: principles, instruments, exercises. Saunders, Philadelphia
4. Wells PNT (1982) Scientific basis of medical imaging. Churchill Livingstone, New York
5. Schwartz SL, Cao QL, Azevedo J, Pandian NG (1994) Simulation of intraoperative visualization of cardiac structures and study of dynamic surgical anatomy with real-time three-dimensional echocardiography. Am J Cardiol 73: 501–507

Ultrasound Contrast Agents

A. Bauer and R. Schlief

Ever since the beginnings of clinical radiology, two main factors have contributed to diagnostic progress: technological advance and the development of safe and reliable contrast agents. Often, these two factors have been inextricably linked. Many of today's accomplishments in X-ray, CT, MRI, and nuclear medicine would be unthinkable without the use of contrast agents. In medical ultrasonography, on the other hand, contrast agents are still very much an innovation. In the future, ultrasound contrast media will probably emerge as an important tool. The diagnostic advantages provided by contrast enhancement mean that clinical use of diagnostic ultrasound will dramatically expand and enhanced ultrasound may well become the imaging modality of choice in a wide range of diagnostic applications.

Enhancement of ultrasound images was pioneered in the 1960s by Gramiak and Shah [13], who credit Dr. Claude Joyner with the first observation: an increase in M-mode signals from the heart after injection of indocyanine green via a cardiac catheter. Other dyes, saline, and even X-ray contrast media, were all found to produce similar results, and it was soon recognized that the contrast effect was due to the presence of microbubbles. As the use of saline contrast became established in echocardiography, attempts were made to generate greater contrast by improving the microbubble yield. These attempts ranged from shaking the solution by hand prior to injection and varying the injection speed to the use of more elaborate devices consisting essentially of two syringes joined by a three-way stopcock, the agitated solution being obtained by repeatedly pumping the saline from one syringe to the other along with some air. In retrospect, most of these techniques can safely be described as rough and ready, however; they were only suitable for the production of very large microbubbles (>50 μm) whose size distribution was very poorly defined. It was not until 1984 that a method of producing smaller bubbles with a reasonably narrow size distribution was developed. Feinstein et al. [9] employed strong ultrasound fields to generate microbubbles. The microbubbles in these sonicated preparations were of a size suitable for contrast (e.g., 8 ± 3 μm in 70% dextrose). Their use was limited, however, as the microbubbles were unable to survive passage through the lungs after intravenous injection.

The Physics of Microbubbles

Microbubbles provide the basis for all current developments in ultrasound contrast media. The principal characteristic of microbubble-based media (and the principal mechanism of echoenhancement) is their backscatter effect. When gas-filled microbubbles are present in a region of interest, a higher proportion of the ultrasound beam is backscattered and a stronger echo is received by the transducer. The echogenicity of a medium, or the degree of backscatter, is dependent on the medium's scattering strength. This can be expressed in terms of a parameter known as its scattering cross-section: an index of the efficiency of a scattering medium defined as the power scattered from a single source (bubble) divided by the intensity of the incident ultrasound (= P/I). The scattering cross-section, σ, is given by the following equation:

$$\sigma = \left[\frac{4}{9}\,\pi r^2\left(\frac{2\pi}{\lambda}\,r\right)^4\right]\left[\left|\frac{k_s - k}{k}\right|^2 + \frac{1}{3}\left|\frac{3(\rho_s - \rho)}{2\rho_s - \rho}\right|^2\right]$$

where r = radius of scatterer, λ = ultrasound wavelength, k_S = compressibility of scatterer, k = compressibility of the embedding medium, ρ_S = density of scatterer, and ρ = density of the embedding medium.

Thus, the scattering cross-section is not only dependent on the radius of the scatterer and the wavelength of the ultrasound, but also on the difference in compressibility and density between the scatterer and its surround. Using gas-filled microbubbles, considerable differences in compressibility and density are readily obtained. Comparatively few microbubbles are required to cause a dramatic increase in backscatter. However, bubble size presents conflicting demands: larger bubbles result in increased echogenicity while the need for pulmonary transit puts a limit on their size.

Free, gas-filled microbubbles are very effective scatterers of ultrasound, but without some form of stabilization, they disintegrate rapidly and are unable to survive passage through the lungs after intravenous injection even if size requirements are met. To allow capillary passage, a thin shell sufficient to slow down diffusion of the gas – and, hence, disintegration of the bubbles – but with only a minimal effect on acoustic properties would be ideal. Attempts to produce coated microbubbles began as early as 1980 with the production of nitrogen-filled gelatin capsules [7]. The size of the bubbles (about 80 μm) made them unsuitable for practical purposes, however. It was not until some time later that the technical difficulties in manufacturing reproducibly small microbubbles were finally solved.

Pharmacokinetics

The pharmacokinetics of ultrasound contrast agents differs from that of X-ray or MRI contrast media, as they are not distributed throughout the body fluid but remain in the blood pool or in the body cavities to which they are applied. Therefore the main areas of application are echo enhancement of the blood flow in the chambers of the heart and the blood vessels (blood pool contrast agents) and imaging of body cavities.

The short life-span of microbubbles in vivo is a fundamental problem. Pulmonary transit places high demands on bubble stability, and only a very few preparations with the necessary bubble stabilization have reached the stage of clinical development. Products such as Levovist (Schering AG), a preparation based on galactose microparticles currently being launched in Europe, represent a significant breakthrough allowing echo enhancement in the left heart and the arterial system after intravenous injection. Diagnostic benefits are also shown in the venous system. Vein studies being carried out with Levovist show that enhancement is also obtained in the venous system after a secondary capillary passage.

Echo Signal Enhancement in B-Mode and Doppler Applications

Microbubbles increase the echogenicity of the blood and therefore provide a source of echogenic labeling for the blood in B-mode imaging, the brightness of the image depending on the concentration of microbubbles in the bloodstream. At high concentrations or with specific detection techniques, in the near future it should also be possible to detect signals from the blood flow in tissue, normal perfusion being characterized by homogeneous enhancement of the area in question.

Doppler applications are based on flow mapping. Depending on the velocity of the blood flow, a frequency shift is detected in the signal received by the transducer. This frequency shift, named after the physicist Christian Doppler, is the basis of all Doppler applications. In color Doppler, this frequency shift is calculated and the estimated flow velocity is visualized in color-coded form. The color-coding displays information about the direction (usually red or blue) and the apparent velocity of flow (displayed as color intensity). Recently, a new technique has been introduced: power Doppler. Rather than direction or velocity information, in power Doppler it is the amplitude of the Doppler-shifted signal that is displayed [18]. Color-coding is used to represent signal intensity as a color intensity map. Another, and perhaps the most important, Doppler application is spectral Doppler, in which the Doppler shift over time is displayed for a specific direction (CW mode) or at a specific location (PW mode). The Doppler spectrum is presented as a velocity-over-time curve with additional information on Doppler signal intensity shown in the form of grayscale brightness (Figs. 1, 2).

The significance of the use of contrast agents in clinical applications of spectral Doppler is illustrated in Fig. 1, showing the arrival of a contrast bolus in the middle cerebral artery after injection of Levovist into a peripheral vein. Clearly, no spectrum was obtained prior to arrival of the contrast agent; following its arrival, a satisfactory spectrum was obtained.

To interpret Doppler spectra, it is important to know that echo-enhancing agents such as Levovist do not alter the velocity information displayed. This has been demonstrated using a Doppler phantom [17]. A pulsatile flow model was constructed in which insufficient signal intensity can be simulated using castor oil for attenuation. The transducer is connected to a conventional ultrasound scanner,

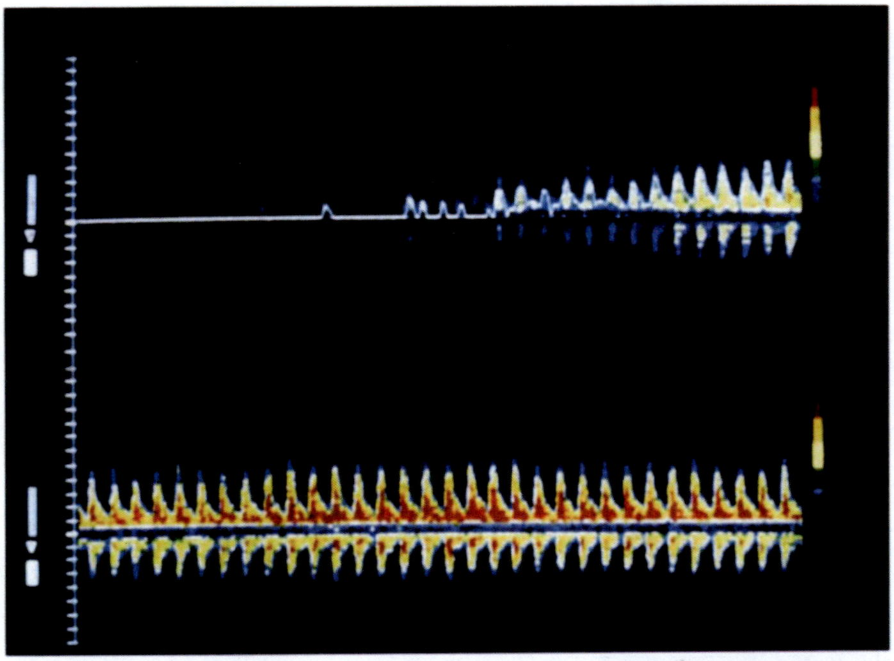

Fig. 1. Arrival of a Levovist bolus in the middle cerebral artery. Before intravenous administration of the echoenhancer no blood flow was detectable. The appearance of the contrast agent is depicted without change of transducer position, and shows optimal signal intensity for the Doppler study. (Image kindly provided by Dr. Ries)

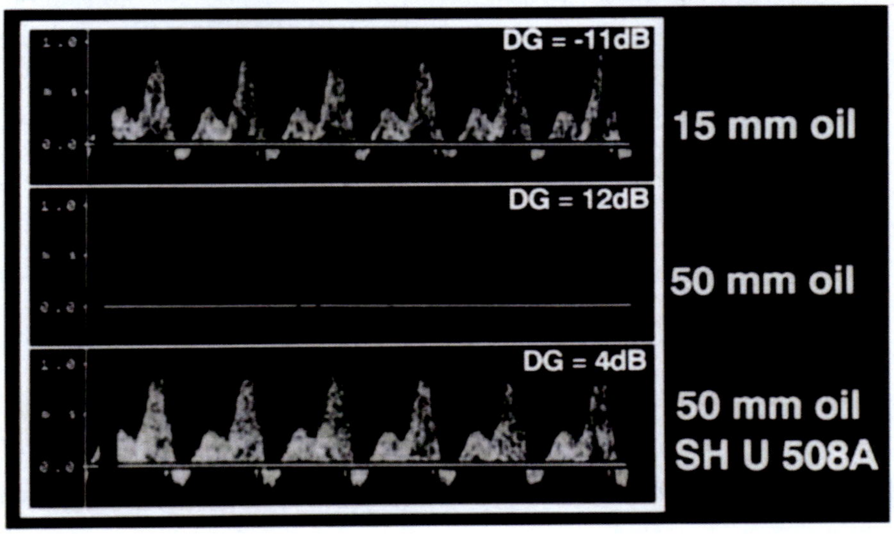

Fig. 2. Spectral Doppler recordings of identical pulsatile flow with two different attenuation layers of castor oil. The *uppermost* trace shows the correct velocity recording at low attenuation and therefore good signal intensity. After increase in attenuation (same flow conditions), the signal becomes insufficient for Doppler evaluation and is hardly visible (*middle* trace). After Levovist injection, and leaving the attenuation unchanged, the same spectrum as at the top is clearly visible and available for diagnostic evaluation (*lowermost* trace). The pulse curve is unchanged and the velocity information is not altered by the contrast agent, but the signal intensity is greatly enhanced and even the gain is reduced. Experiments were performed with a pulsatile flow model. (Image kindly provided by Dr. Petrick)

and the vessel to be scanned is represented by a tube. A computer-controlled artificial heart drives a blood-mimicking fluid through the tube. A typical experiment is illustrated in Fig. 2. The upper trace recorded with low attenuation (15 mm castor oil) shows a satisfactory Doppler spectrum: good signal intensity and a favorable signal-to-noise ratio. High attenuation (50 mm castor oil) simulates insufficient signal intensity and an inadequate Doppler signal recording is obtained (middle trace). When Levovist (SHU 508 A) is added, the increase in signal intensity enables a satisfactory spectrum to be obtained despite high attenuation (lower trace). The spectrum is qualitatively the same as that obtained without attenuation. Therefore echo contrast has no effect on velocity information or spectral content; the only parameter changed is increased signal intensity, allowing an adequate Doppler recording.

Contrast enhancement has important consequences for color Doppler applications. Detectable velocity-based color Doppler signals are unaffected by contrast agents. However, low-intensity Doppler signals are enhanced, making color Doppler visualization possible. In power Doppler, which maps the amplitude of the signals, color intensity is proportional to echo intensity. The increase in intensity by echo enhancement is proportional to the concentration of the agent. Therefore power Doppler appears well suited to asess blood flow and perfusion kinetics.

Safety

One important advantage of ultrasound is its noninvasive character that avoids exposing patients to unnecessary risk. To preserve this advantage when new equipment and techniques are introduced, various limits – particularly on power and local energy deposition – have been defined in recent years. These limits will not be affected when contrast media are employed. Ultrasound contrast agents have also been tested in cavitation studies and their safety has been confirmed for in vivo conditions [24].

Clinical trials of Levovist included 1819 patients, with up to 6 injections per patient. Approximately 10% of patients described a sensation of warmth or other transient local symptoms at the site of injection. No clinically relevant effects were observed with regard to cardiovascular function, blood or urine chemistry, or hematological or hemodynamic parameters. Consistent with the physiological nature of its constituents, Levovist is well-tolerated and safe for use in ultrasound diagnostics.

Commercial Ultrasound Contrast Media

The potential for echo-enhanced ultrasound was demonstrated experimentally at a relatively early stage, but it was several years before researchers were able to overcome all the development problems and the first ultrasound contrast medium was finally approved. Despite extensive effort and a variety of approaches being taken, many interesting ultrasound contrast media are still in the phase of comprehensive testing and development.

Echovist (SHU 454, Schering AG, Berlin)

The first commercial ultrasound contrast medium to be introduced was Echovist, a galactose based agent, which was developed as a right heart contrast medium and became clinically available in 1991. Results of the first preclinical studies with Echovist were presented as early as 1984 [22]. The effect of Echovist is based on the increased echogenicity of free gas-filled microbubbles. Essentially, Echovist acts as a vehicle to provide free bubbles of the requisite size. Echovist is supplied in the form of granules consisting of agglomerated galactose microparticles which are mixed with a specially prepared galactose solution prior to use. Granules and carrier solution are vigorously shaken, which gives rise to a homogeneous suspension with the air in the granules forming microbubbles that attach to the suspended microparticles. The size distribution of these microbubbles is wellt defined; 97% are smaller than 7 μm [11]. After intravenous administration, the galactose dissolves and the microbubbles are released into the bloodstream. The fact that the microbubbles are not stable enough to survive passage through the lungs can be exploited in one important application, the diagnosis of right-to-left shunts. With advances in scanner design and, in particular, the arrival of the transpulmonary agent Levovist, Echovist will probably play only a limited role in echocardiography. It will, however, remain an important tool in the diagnostics of body cavities, where the microbubbles do not disintegrate so rapidly and contrast effects are sufficient. Following transcervical application, Echovist has proven particularly useful in hysterosalpingo-contrast ultrasonography, where it can be used in diagnosis of patency of the fallopian tubes. It is approved for clinical use in Europe and USA.

Albunex (Molecular Biosystems, San Diego)

Albunex was the first ultrasound contrast medium with transpulmonary properties to receive approval from a regulatory authority. The microbubbles in Albunex fare enclosed in a coat of sonicated albumin. This provides the stabilization necessary for pulmonary transit. Albunex consists of three different protein fractions: a carrier fraction of 5% human serum albumin, an aqueous soluble fraction, and an aqueous insoluble fraction. It is supplied as a ready-to-use solution with a concentration of 300 to 500 x 10^6 microbubbles/ml. The mean diameter of the bubbles is about 4 μm, and 95% are smaller than 10 mm. The plasma half-life is about 1 min [3]. Albunex has been approved for use in left and right heart studies in the USA, Japan, and in some countries in Europe.

Levovist (SHU 508A, Schering AG, Berlin)

Levovist is a transpulmonary-stable, galactose-based contrast agent similar to Echovist. This new-generation ultrasound contrast medium has already been approved in a number of European countries and is commercially available. Like Echovist, Levovist is based on galactose microparticles as a vehicle for delivery of microbubbles of a defined size distribution. A microscopic view of the Levovist granules is given in Fig. 3. Two minutes prior to intravenous injection, the microbubbles are produced by mixing the galactose granules with sterile water and vigorously shaking the suspension. Levovist differs from Echovist in that it contains palmitic acid, which acts as a surfactant and forms a thin coat around the microbubbles. This fatty acid coat not only enables the bubbles to survive passage through the lungs, but also provides a high degree of stabilization in the arterial vascular bed. Depending on the concentration used (200 mg/ml, 300 mg/ml, 400 mg/ml), signal enhancement of up to 25 dB is achieved with Levovist[21]. The duration of enhancement is up to 5 min. Since Levovist is well tolerated even on multiple injection and signal enhancement is sufficient even in small peripheral arteries, Levovist is suitable and approved for use in all Doppler indications.

Future Developments in Ultrasound Contrast Media

Various avenues are being explored in the development of ultrasound contrast media, and a number of different substances with echocontrast potential have been presented in recent years. Two main possibilities emerge: fluorocarbon gas-filled microbubbles and gas-filled microbubbles with a biodegradable polymer shell.

Preparations based on perfluoro compounds offer the prospect of a marked increase in intravascular stability; perfluoro compounds are only slightly soluble in blood, such that in vivo lifespan of the contrast medium should be considerably prolonged. EchoGen (Sonus, Seattle) is a liquid perfluoro compound (dodecafluoropentane) currently undergoing clinical trials. Its boiling point is below the body temperature of 37°C. After intravenous injection the liquid starts boiling within the blood and echogenic microbubbles are formed while the liquid evaporates.

The next generation of ultrasound contrast media is likely to be based on microbubbles with biodegradable polymer shells. SHU 563 A (Schering AG, Berlin) consists of encapsulated microbubbles with a mean diameter of only 1 µm [10]. Following intravenous administration and pulmonary transit, intense, persistent vascular enhancement is achieved even at very small doses. After a blood-pool phase the particles are collected in the reticuloendothelial (RES) cells, mainly in the liver. The particles can be detected by their specific acoustic response using color Doppler. This provides a method of identifying tumors with this organ-specific compound: Since tumors do not contain any RES cells, they can easily be identified by their lack of color Doppler response.

A further polymer-based ultrasound contrast medium (NUS) has been presented by Nycomed [14], but no details of its state of development have yet been published.

The development of organ-specific and function-specific agents for ultrasound diagnostics is an exciting area. However, the full benefits, possible applications, and particular advantages of individual preparations will only become apparent in the course of clinical testing over the next few years.

Clinical Applications

Contrast Echocardiography

At present, the main diagnostic area in which ultrasound contrast media are employed is the heart. Enhanced studies can assist in all questions involving anatomical delineation of the cardiac chambers and myocardial structures as well as identification of hemodynamic phenomena. Thus, use of contrast media is indicated for clarification of pathological changes such as intracardial thrombi, septum defects, abnormal wall movement, and valvular insufficiency [16].

Hysterosalpingo-contrast Ultrasonography

Echo-enhanced ultrasound with transvaginal scanning provides an important and, above all, less invasive alternative to X-ray hysterosalpingography and laparoscopy in the diagnosis of female infertility. The method was developed with Echovist and not only permits the diagnosis of uterine anomalies but also enables tubal patency to be confirmed [19]. The advantages of the technique over conventional approaches consist in the elimination of radiation exposure, allergy-like contrast medium reactions, and/or operative risk. Hysterosealpingo-contrast ultrasonography also allows patients to observe the examination directly and to witness the results together with the physician. Clinical studies show the accuracy of diagnosis compares well with findings in X-ray hysterosalpingography or laparoscopy: B-mode scanning confirmed tubal patency with a specificity of 100% and a sensitivity of 88%. The method can thus be recommended for advance selection of patients in whom more invasive procedures may be required (Fig. 3).

Echo-Enhanced Doppler Ultrasonography

In general, the use of ultrasound contrast media indicated in Doppler ultrasonography if the precontrast signal is diagnostically insufficient (acoustic signal too "quiet" or unfavorable signal-to-noise ratio in spectral Doppler). Depending on the area being examined, insufficient signals are obtained in 5%–30% of patients. They are particularly frequent when difficult examination conditions give rise to strong attenuation, e.g., in transcranial Doppler examinations or in cases of obesity or deeply situated vessels [20].

Transpulmonary ultrasound contrast agents such as Levovist have already been investigated in relation to a number of diagnostic questions in various organ systems. Echo-enhanced Doppler applications include Doppler ultrasonography, diagnosis of the carotid arteries, cardiac applications, kidney and liver diagnostics, and peripheral studies.

Transcranial Doppler Ultrasonography

As one-dimensional (spectral) Doppler ultrasonography is still widely used, color Doppler ultrasonography is gaining increasing attention in neurology and neuroradiology. In all transcranial applications, however, the poor transmission of ultrasound through bone means that signals are often insufficient for diagnosis. Use of ultrasound contrast media can be particularly beneficial. Doppler signal enhancement is up to 25 dB [21], which offsets the loss to bone attenuation to a considerable extent. The increase in the Doppler signal following administration of Levovist is clearly illustrated in one-dimensional Doppler in Fig. 4. Transcranial duplex ultrasonography with Levovist permits complete depiction of the large intracerebral vessels; without enhancement about 15% of patients cannot be evaluated at all [6]. A particular advantage of such enhanced studies is the detection of

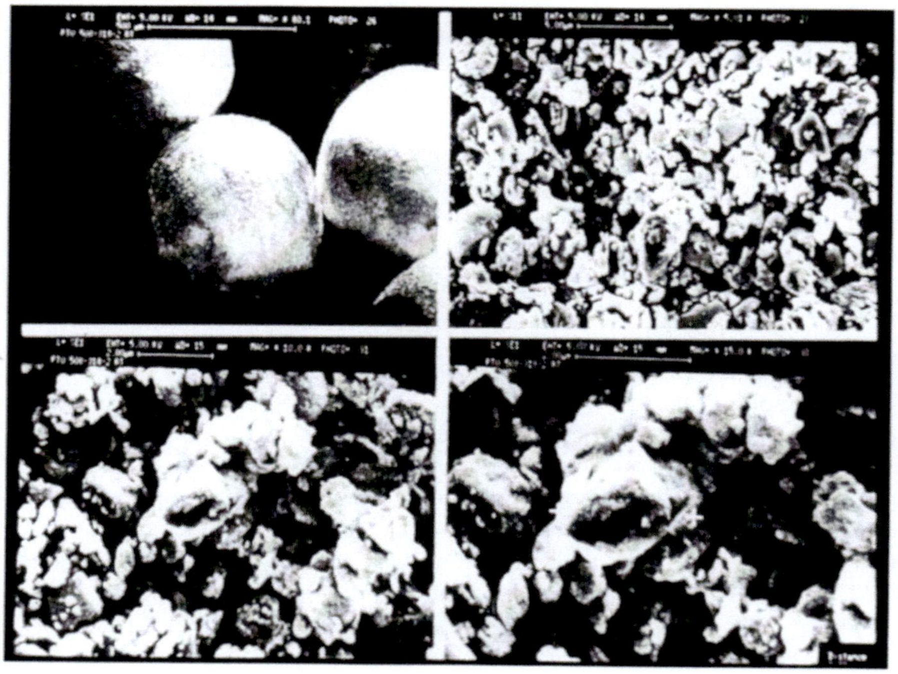

Fig. 3. Levovist granules of approx. 500 μm diameter and magnified views of the rough surface of the galactose granules (*top left*). Galactose is essential in controlling the bubble formation process and the size distribution of the microbubbles. Free bubbles covered by a thin film of palmitic acid are liberated when the galactose microparticles dissolve

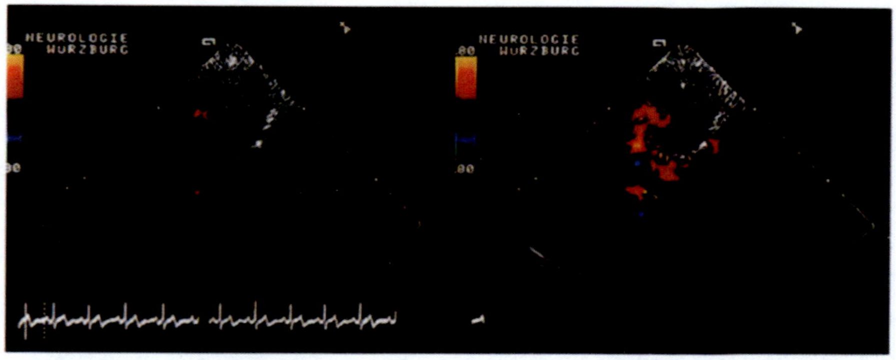

Fig. 4. Transcranial Doppler ultrasonography with Levovist, axial image plane. The precontrast scan (*left*) shows insufficient signal intensity owing to an insufficient acoustic bone window. Insufficient insonation conditions are frequently seen in transcranial Doppler recordings. Before contrast administration only the middle cerebral artery can be identified at a single point. After Levovist administration the entire circle of Willis is visualized and the segments of the anterior, middle, and posterior cerebral arteries are depicted (*right*). (Image produced by A.B. in collaboration with Prof. Bogdahn)

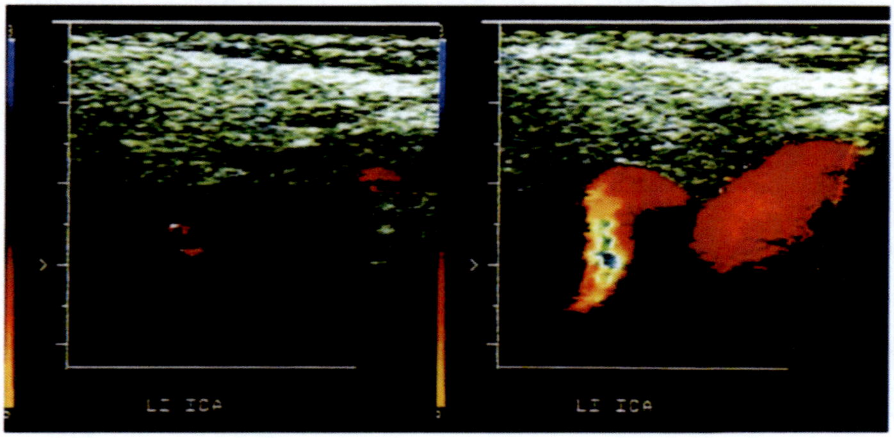

Fig. 5. Kinking of the internal carotid artery. Before contrast administration, the situation is unclear; a stenosis is suspected. After Levovist injection the bifurcation is visualized and kinking of the internal carotid with mild stenosis is seen. (Image kindly provided by Dr. Meents)

slow flow, which facilitates recognition of cavernous hemangiomas and intracerebral tumors [4] (see also Fig. 7).

Extracranial Carotid Doppler Ultrasonography

Color Doppler is widely used in the evaluation of extracranial lesions of the carotid artery, but diagnosis of high-grade stenoses (>70 %) is often difficult. Plaque calcification alters the arterial wall, and the narrowness of the residual lumen may result in very small poststenotic flow. Inadequate images are obtained in 8 % to 13 % of examinations. Levovist is expected to play an important role in such cases, particularly in grading stenoses [12]. Figure 5 shows a kinking f the left internal carotid artery, only visible after administration of Levovist.

Doppler Ultrasonography of the Renal Arteries

Insufficient signal intensity is frequent in Doppler ultrasonography of the renal arteries. The origin of the renal artery in the abdominal aorta is particularly difficult to visualize in nonenhanced studies. Use of ultrasound contrast media enables or facilitates the exclusion of renal artery stenosis in cases of hypertension and the determination of various functional indices. An important advantage of enhanced studies especially in this area is the dramatic reduction in the time taken to perform examinations compared with nonenhanced ultrasound [2]. Figure 6 shows the origin of the renal artery before and after administration of Levovist.

Doppler Ultrasonography of Peripheral Vessels

Color Doppler imaging of peripheral vessels such as leg arteries generally presents fewer problems than are encountered in other areas. Nevertheless, without the use of contrast media, signals are still

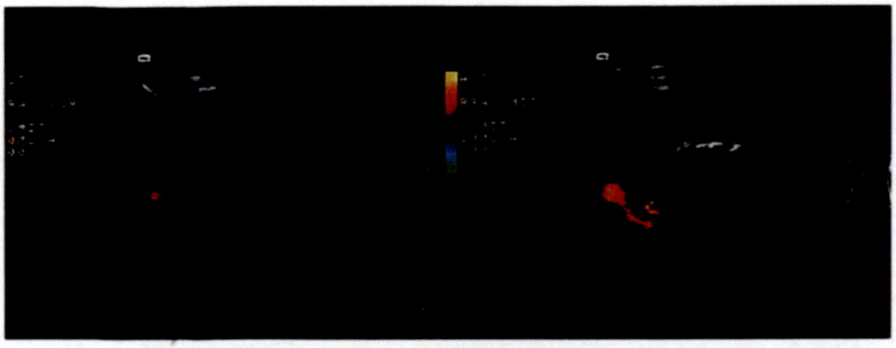

Fig. 6. Origin of the renal artery from the abdominal aorta: the renal artery could not be detected before administration of Levovist (*left*). After Levovist the origin and the continuity of the renal artery is clearly visualized (*right*). The often time-consuming process of renal studies can be shortened by the use of echoenhancers. (Image kindly provided by Dr. Bönhof)

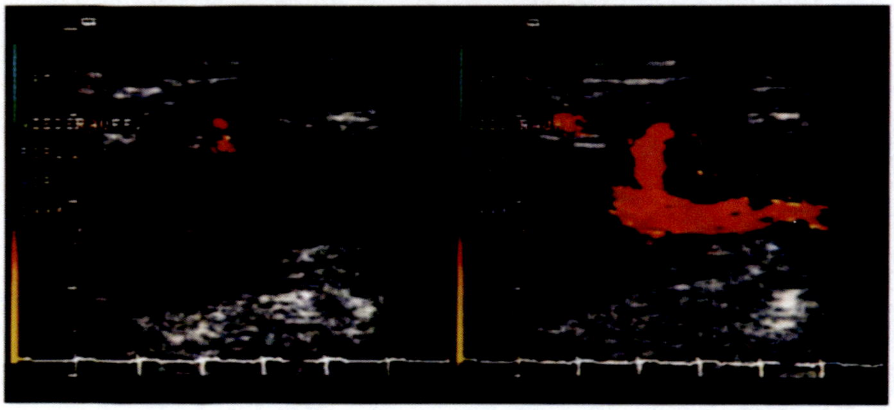

Fig. 7. Enhancement by Levovist is also important in peripheral arteries and veins; these images show a popliteal artery with insufficient signal conditions before contrast (*left*). After echo enhancement the bifurcation is clearly seen in color flow recording (*right*). (Image kindly provided by Dr. Langholz)

insufficient for diagnosis in 10%–15% of patients. In such cases, use of Levovist allows both visualization of peripheral vessels and grading of any stenosis present [15]. Echo-enhanced studies have been found to be particularly useful in iliac and lower leg vessels (Fig. 7).

Tumor Vascularization

In the absence of echo enhancement, tumor vascularization studies using spectral or color Doppler stretch ultrasound systems beyond the limits of their current capability. Sensitivity and resolution are considerably improved, however, using ultrasound contrast media such as Levovist. In particular, the increase in the intensity of the Doppler signal permits detection of slow and low-volume flow. Tumor vascularization is fundamentally different from that of normal tissue in terms of both flow characteristics and the tortuous arrangement of the neoplastic vessels [23]. Doppler enhancement allows a more complete depiction of vascular patterns and consequently an increase in diagnostic reliability. Given that all blood flows actually present in the image plane are visualized, suspect regions can be compared with normal tissue, and it also may be possible to separate benign and malignant processes in regard to specific pathologies. Tumor vascularization of a prostate is shown in Fig. 8. A number of recent studies in tumor diagnostics confirm the extent to which qualitatively new diagnostic opportunities are opened up by Levovist, e.g., in detection of gliomas [5], in breast diagnostics [8], and in various other regions [1].

Levovist does not only provide improved vascular imaging; dynamic contrast studies analogous to dynamic CT and MRI are also possible. The diagnostic potential of dynamic studies in tumor grading and in monitoring the treatment and progress of disease has yet to be demonstrated.

Outlook: Microbubble-Specific Ultrasound Scanning

Up to now, the development of contrast agents has essentially been technology-driven, with enhanced studies being employed to take full advantage of the opportunities offered by ultrasound systems and to facilitate diagnosis even when insufficient information is provided by unenhanced ultrasonography.

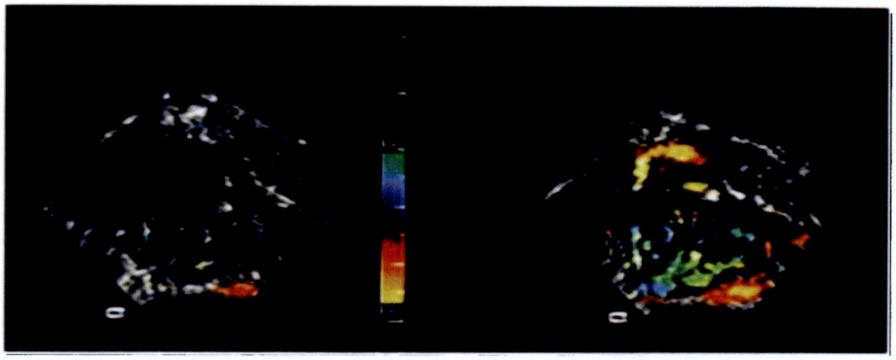

Fig. 8. Tumor vascularization of a prostatic cancer. Doppler is often limited in detection of low- and slow-flow lesions; before contrast the lesion is shown with only slight vascularization (*left*). After Levovist administration the vascularity of the tumor is clearly depicted and the tumor may be characterized as highly vascularized (*right*). (Image kindly provided by Dr. Cosgrove)

In future, however, increasing attention will be paid to the development of systems capable of fully exploiting the acoustic properties of the contrast media themselves. One important recent development, harmonic imaging, involves special scanning techniques based on the resonance behavior of the microbubbles of ultrasound contrast media. Depending on microbubble size and shell characteristics, the echo from microbubbles can contain a high proportion of harmonics (multiples of the insonating frequency) in addition to the fundamental frequency transmitted by the transducer. On insonation at a frequency of 2.5 MHz, for example, a strong echo may also be recorded at twice this frequency (5 MHz); this is termed the second harmonic. Harmonic imaging therefore exclusively shows the echo response of the contrast agent making the image information similar to that of digital subtraction angiography in the X-ray field. Further improvements in the spatial resolution of vascular Doppler imaging may be possible using this harmonic technique. Pharmaceutical developers and equipment manufacturers are collaborating closely in this field: further development of such microbubble-specific scanning techniques should lead to progress in other areas-optimized organ perfusion studies, for example.

In view of the amount of research being undertaken by all contrast medium manufacturers, a regular flow of new substances is anticipated over the next few years, offering both improved in vivo stability of the microbubbles and tissue-specific properties such as selective uptake in the RES cells of the liver. The parallel development of equipment capable of fully exploiting the acoustic properties of these microbubble media will provide a number of new opportunities for the application of ultrasound. Reductions in examination time and improvements in sensitivity and specificity are also expected, so that the efficiency and informative value of ultrasound examinations will also increase. In the near future, echo-enhanced ultrasound may well be added or preferred to other procedures in a wide range of diagnostic applications. Microbubble-based contrast media will soon be as important in ultrasound diagnostics as iodinated contrast media and gadolinium preparations are in X-radiography and MRI.

References

1. Allen CM, Lees WR (1995) Contrast enhanced ultrasound in tumour detection. BMUS Bull 3 (1): 30–32
2. Allen CM, Balen FG, Musouris C, McGregor G, Buckingham T, Lees WR (1993) Renal artery stenosis: diagnosis using contrast enhanced Doppler ultrasound. Clin Radiol 48: 5
3. Barnhart J, Levene H, Villapando E, Maniquis J, Fernandes J, Rice S, Jablonski E, Gjoen T, Tolleshaug H (1990) Characteristics of Albunex, air-filled albumin microspheres for echocardiography. Invest Radiol 25: 162–164
4. Bauer A, Becker G, Jachimczak P, Krone A, Bogdahn U (1995) Contrast enhanced transcranial duplex sonography. BMUS Bull 3 (1): 26–29
5. Bogdahn U, Becker G, Fröhlich T, Krone A, Schlief R, Schürmann J, Jachimczak P, Hofmann E, Roggendorf W, Roosen K (1994) Vascularization of primary central nervous system tumors: detection with contrast-enhanced transcranial color-coded real-time sonography. Radiology 12: 141–148
6. Bogdahn U, Becker G, Winkler J, Greiner K, Perez J, Meurers B (1990) Transcranial color-coded real-time sonography in adults. Stroke 21: 1680–168
7. Caroll BA, Turner RJ, Tickner EG, Boyle DB, Young SW (1980) Gelatine encapsuled nitrogen microbubbles as ultrasonic contrast agents. Invest Radiol 15: 260–266
8. Cosgrove DO, Kedar RP, Bamber JC (1993) Breast diseases, colour Doppler US in differential diagnosis. Radiology 189: 99–104
9. Feinstein SB, ten Cate FJ, Zwehl W, Ong K, Maurer G, Chuwa T, Shah PM, Meerbaum S, Corday E (1984) Two-

dimensional contrast echocardiography. J Am Coll Cardiol 3: 14-20
10. Fritzsch T (1995) New contrast media in ultrasound. ULTRA '95, Tampere, abstract book
11. Fritzsch T, Mützel W, Schartl M (1986) First experience with a standardized contrast medium for sonography. In: Otto RC, Higgins CB (eds). New Developments in Imaging. Thieme, Stuttgart, pp 141-149
12. Fürst G, Sitzer M, Hofer M, Steinmetz H, Hackländer T, Mödder U (1995) Kontrastmittelverstärkte farbkodierte Duplexsonographie hochgradiger Karotisstenosen. Ultraschall Med 16: 140-144
13. Gramiak R, Shah PM (1986) Echocardiography of the aortic root. Invest Radiol 3: 356-366
14. Hoff L (1995) Acoustic properties of ultrasound contrast agent particles described by viscoelastic theory. In: World Congress of Ultrasound, Berlin, 1995
15. Langholz JMW, Petry J, Schürmann R, Schlief R, Heidrich H (1993) Indikationen zur Unterschenkelarteriendarstellung mit Kontrastmittel bei der farbkodierten Duplexsonographie. Ultraschal
16. Nanda N, Schlief R (eds) (1993) Advances in echo imaging using contrast enhancement. Kluwer, Dordrecht
17. Petrick J, Schlief R, Zomack M, Langholz J, Urbank A (1992) Pulsatiles Strömungsmodell mit elastischen Gefäßen für Duplex-sonographische Untersuchungen. Ultraschall med 13: 277-282
18. Rubin JM, Bude RO, Carson PL, Bree RL, Adler RS (1994) Power Doppler US: a potentially useful alternative to mean frequency-based color Doppler US. Radiology 190: 853-856
19. Schlief R, Deichert U (1991) Hysterosalpingo-contrast sonography of the uterus and fallopian tubes: results of a clinical trial of a new contrast medium in 120 patients. Radiology 178: 213-215
20. Schlief R, Schürmann R, Balzer T, Petrick J, Urbank A, Zomack M, Niendorf HP (1993) Diagnostic value of contrast enhancement in vascular doppler ultrasound. In: Nanda N, Schlief R (eds) Advances in echo imaging using contrast enhancement. Kluwer, Dordrecht
21. Schwarz KQ, Bechar H, Schimpfky C, Vorwerk D, Bogdahn U, Schlief R (1994) A study of the magnitude of Doppler enhancement with SHU 508 A in multiple vascular regions. Radiology 193 (1): 195-201
22. Smith MD, Kwan OL, Reiser J, DeMaria AN (1984) Superior intensity and reproducibility of SHU 454, a new right heart contrast agent. J Am Coll Cardiol 3: 992-998
23. Taylor KJ, Ramos I, Carter D, Morse SS (1988) Correlation of Doppler ultrasound tumor signals with neovascular morphological features. Radiology 166: 57-62
24. Williams AR, Kubowicz G, Cramer E, Schlief R (1991) The effects of the microbubble suspension SHU 454 (Echovist) on ultrasound induced cell lysis in a rotating tube exposure system. Echocardiography 8 (4): 423-433

Part I: Diagnostics of Vascular Diseases: State-of-the-Art

Section II: Imaging Vascular Methods

Vascular Radiography

X-ray Radiography

K.-F. Kamm and D.G.W. Onnasch

Introduction

Examination of the vascular system requires sharply contrasted images taken as flash exposures in a fast sequence. Since vessels can follow any direction in space, it is of utmost importance to have a high degree of freedom in selecting the appropriate projection. The relevant section of the vessel has to be shown with minimal foreshortening.

In the early days of angiography, images were taken with standard X-ray equipment using amplifying screens, film as detector for single exposures, and film changers to record the moving heart and vessels. The large images on film showed good spatial resolution, but the main difficulties of this procedure were limited projection possibilities and limited ability to record image series. High exposures rates were impossible, since X-ray tubes with a sufficient heat storage and dissipation capacity were not available. These drawbacks were overcome by the introduction of tubes with a rotating anode in the 1920s and of X-ray image intensifiers as detectors after 1960.

Another important evolutionary process was the transition from conventional film-based systems to fully digital systems. Initially, digital image acquisition was used for real-time playback and processing. Later, it became inevitable for interventional procedures. The recent expansion of minimally invasive catheter therapies has to a large extent become possible due to the enormous progress in digital imaging. Film has also gradually been replaced as a long-term storage and exchange medium.

While current radiographic imaging systems are quite advanced, they are not yet fully automatic. Thus consistent high-quality vascular imaging requires the attention and expertise of trained staff. For optimum angiographic imaging, physicians, nurses, and technologists require at least a basic understanding of the principles of radiographic vascular imaging. In this chapter, the elementary principles of vascular X-ray radiography will be introduced and the parameters influencing image quality and radiation exposure discussed.

Physics of X-Rays

Nature of X-rays

Similar to visible and ultraviolet light or radio waves, X-rays represent a component of the continuous electromagnetic spectrum in which electric and magnetic fields vary simultaneously. The electromagnetic waves differ only in frequency. The frequency of X-rays is more than four orders of magnitude larger than that of visible light waves. Based on the dual principle of quantum physics, X-rays also behave like small energy parcels called quanta or photons (Fig. 1). The energy of the quanta increases in proportion to the frequency ν according to

$$E = h \times \nu \qquad (1)$$

with $h = 6.6256 \times 10^{-34}$ J s (Planck's constant).

There are two regions of the electromagnetic spectrum for which the human body is transparent: (1) the high-energy photon window utilized in X-ray radiography and (2) the lower-energy window utilized in magnetic resonance imaging (MRI). In the former, the X-ray beam is modulated by absorption and scattering processes, resulting in local variations in X-ray intensities by a receptor. The resulting X-ray image essentially represents a sha-

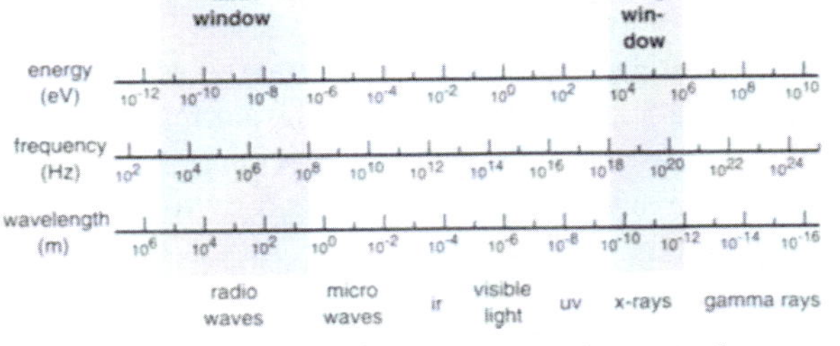

Fig. 1. The spectrum of electromagnetic waves has two windows pertinent to medical imaging, the X-ray window utilized in radiography and nuclear imaging and the low-energy window utilized in magnetic resonance imaging (*MRI*). *ir*, infrared light; *uv*, ultraviolet rays

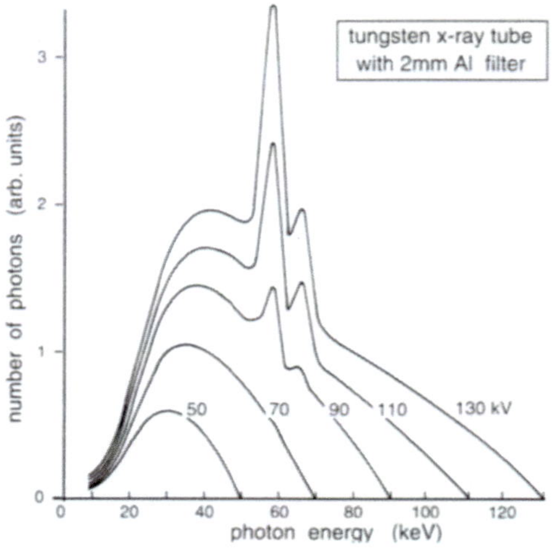

Fig. 2. The spectra of a tungsten X-ray tube with a 2-mm aluminum filter at five different tube voltages. There is rapid increase in quantum output with increasing voltage. Characteristic radiation overlaps the continuous bremsstrahlung

dowgraph reflecting the differences in X-ray absorption across the body.

To generate X-rays, electrons are thermally emitted at the cathode of the X-ray tube and accelerated by a high voltage of 60–150 kV. Loaded with high kinetic energy, they hit the anode and are decelerated in the target material. Following the collision, orbital electron transitions within the atoms of the target material are induced. This process is associated with the emission of heat (99% of the electron's energy) and two types of X-rays: (1) continuous spectrum of X-rays (bremsstrahlung) and (2) X-rays characteristic of the electron energy levels of the target atoms. For the generally used tungsten target, the characteristic radiation is emitted at four lines between 57.9 and 69 keV (Fig. 2) [1]. Its contribution can be neglected for voltages below 70 kV and increases slowly with voltage.

The number of X-ray quanta depends on the number of electrons which are released by the cathode. The resulting anode current is measured in milliampere (mA). The maximum energy $E = e \times U$ of the X-ray quantum is determined by the accelerating voltage U. The quantum energy is therefore measured in kiloelectron-volts instead of joules, where e stands for the elementary charge. Beams with higher average energy are described as being harder, and beams of lower average energy softer. The quantum output increases in proportion to the anode current and to the tube voltage by the power of two.

Interaction of X-rays with Tissue

The X-rays interacting with human tissue can be absorbed, attenuated, or scattered [2, 3]. The X-ray energy is lost as heat by photoelectric absorption and as secondary electron radiation called Compton scatter (Fig. 3).

There is an approximately exponential relationship between attenuation of the X-ray beam and the length of the pathway through the object

$$I = I_0 \times e^{-\mu\varrho x} \qquad (2)$$

where I_0 and I are the radiation doses entering and exciting the object, μ mass attenuation coefficient,

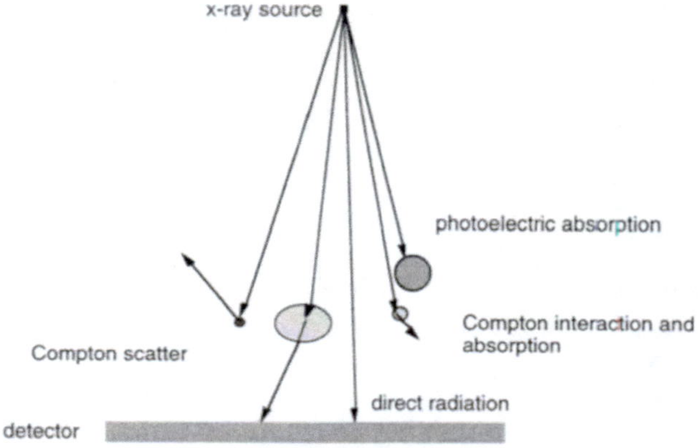

Fig. 3. Interactions of X-rays within the body

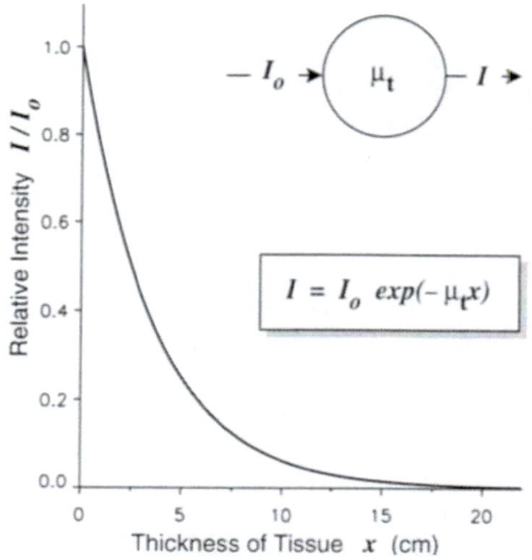

Fig. 4. Attenuation of a monoenergetic beam of X-rays along a path through homogenous tissue. In the example shown, the attenuation coefficient μ_t is set such that the X-ray intensity is decreased by half after 2.5 cm, which is typical for tissue at 77 kV

ϱ the density of the material, and x the pathway. Thus the attenuation not only increases with thickness (e.g., organ; Fig. 4), but also with density of the absorber (e.g., tissue or contrast agent). The brightness of a region containing a certain vessel reflects the amount of contrast medium deposited there.

The attenuation coefficient μ is dependent on the material and on the energy of the X-rays (Fig. 5). Thus for a broad X-ray spectrum, Eq. 2 is only an approximation. The soft part of the beam is absorbed more strongly than the hard part, which leads to the effect of beam hardening along the pathway of absorption. Low-energy photons may be absorbed totally and do not contribute anything to the information content of the image.

There is a steep decrease of μ with increasing photon energy (Fig. 5). In consequence, beam attenuation decreases with increasing voltage. The ratio of entrance to detector dose decreases approximately in proportion to the voltage to the power of -2.5. In other words, raising the voltage by 4% reduces exposure by about 10%.

Radiation that changes its direction within the patient is called scattered radiation (Fig. 3). Its amount in relation to the primary radiation depends on the kV value, the pathway in the body, and the size of the irradiated volume. In abdominal images, scattered radiation reaches 90% of the radiation arriving at the detector. In addition to the primary radiation, forward scattered radiation is used for imaging. Multidirectional or diffuse scattering is very disadvantageous. It lowers the contrast in the image considerably and is the cause of radiation exposure of the medical staff. Methods to reduce diffuse scattering in the image are described in a later section.

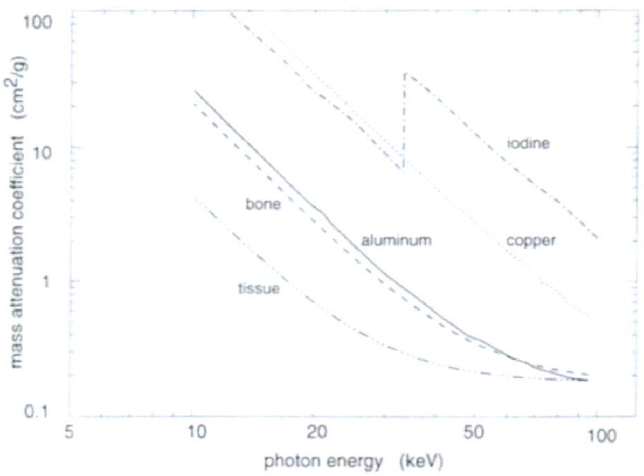

Fig. 5. The mass attenuation coefficient versus photon energy in a double-log scale for different materials. The difference between the attenuation of tissue and bone decreases as energy increases, which leads to a "soft" (low contrast) image with hard radiation. Filter materials such as aluminum and copper absorb the soft part of radiation more readily than the hard part. Contrast agents take advantage of the steep increase in the attenuation coefficient of iodine at 33 keV

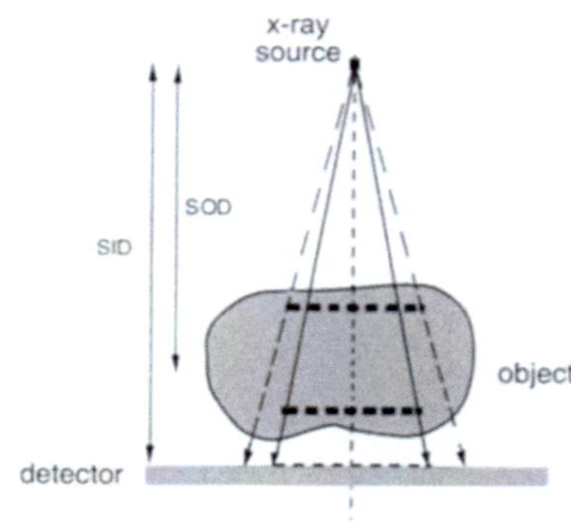

Fig. 6. Central projection and magnification. The magnification factor is obtained by dividing the source to image distance (*SID*) by the source to object distance (*SOD*)

In projection radiography, the divergent beam generates a magnified image of the object on the detector plane. Central projection means that the central X-ray beam hits the detector perpendicular to the entrance plane of the detector. In the central projection, the magnification factor m is defined by the ratio between source-to-detector and source-to-object distance (Fig. 6). Objects of the same size but with different distances to the detector are shown with different sizes in the image.

The sum of all X-ray quanta emitted from the focal spot and measured on the surface of a sphere around the spot is independent of the radius r of the sphere. The local density n of quanta is therefore inversely proportional to its surface, i.e., n is proportional to $1/r^2$ (Fig. 7). The radiation dose is inversely related to the square of the distance to the source. For a system with automatic exposure control, this means that if the magnification factor is reduced by 5%, the patient exposure is reduced by 10%.

The main source of scattered radiation is the patient, and the inverse square law also applies. Thus, at the image detector, the scattered radiation decreases as the patient-to-detector distance is enlarged while the source-to-patient distance is kept constant. Because the relative change of the source-

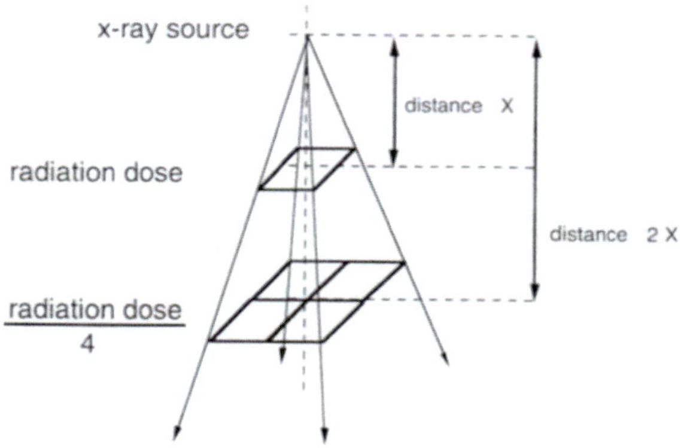

Fig. 7. Relationship between dose and distance. According to the inverse square law, radiation dose is quartered as the distance is doubled

to-detector distance is smaller than that of the object-to-detector distance in this case, the ratio between primary and detected scattered radiation improves.

Another important consequence of the inverse square law concerns the personnel working at the patient table. One or two steps back usually reduces the dose by a factor of two.

Radiographic Contrast Enhancement

Vessels containing blood and soft tissues attenuate X-rays similarly. To visualize vessels, it is therefore necessary to enhance the X-ray attenuation of vessels by injection of a contrast agent. In addition to positive contrast media, which highly attenuate the radiation, contrast media such as carbon dioxide gas, which produe negative vessel contrast are also available. The commonly employed positive contrast media use the absorption characteristic (k-edge) of iodine to create a contrast between the lumen of the contrast media-filled vessel and the surrounding tissues. The k-edge is a sudden increase in X-ray absorption at discrete energy levels. The k-edge of iodine lies at 33 keV, and the peak range of relative absorption is 33–50 keV (Fig. 5).

The contrast difference decreases with increasing tube voltage. An adequate compromise between penetration depth and iodide absorption exists between 65 and 80 kV depending on the overall thickness of the object. The concentration of the contrast agent varies between 200 mg iodine per ml blood for phlebography and 320 mg iodine per ml for arteriography. The resulting concentration in the vessel depends on injection site and hemodynamics measured as pressure, volumetric flow, and flow velocity.

If the contrast agent is highly diluted, for example in visualizing arteries by venous injection, the radiation dose has to be increased to maintain image resolution (see below). Optimum opacification of the vessel is achieved by injecting the contrast agent selectively as a short bolus.

Angiography with X-Rays

General Principles

X-ray imaging systems have the longest history of all techniques for medical imaging [4], with important technical improvements still ongoing.

As described later in detail, the complete image chain includes the high-voltage generator, the X-ray tube, filter and collimator sets, the gantry system, the antiscatter grid, the image intensifier, the automatic exposure control circuit, the television camera, a computerized acquisition system, and monitors. The central component of the angiographic equipment is the image intensifier. Here, the X-ray quanta are absorbed in the input screen and produce light by luminescence. This is converted to electrons in the photocathode, and these are accelerated and projected onto a small output phosphor screen. The electron optics of the image intensifier has two tasks, enhancement and demagnification of the input image. The light emerging from the output phosphor screen is projected by optics to recording devices such as the cine film or the video image sensor.

An ideal system can be characterized by a unextended focal spot, an adjustable monochromatic X-ray spectrum, a grid that absorbs all diffusely scattered X-rays but no primary radiation, an image intensifier with a quantum detection efficiency of 1, excellent transfer of all spatial frequencies, and no geometrical image distortion, an optical system without veiling glare, a cine film with a stable and long logarithmic characteristic curve, and a video camera with high bandwidth and no time lag. The image degradations introduced by the nonideal behavior of real components are considered in later sections. However, even in a technically ideal system, the image resolution suffers from the finite number and the stochastic nature of X-ray quanta detected at the image detector.

Quantum Noise

Independent of the equipment used, an intrinsic limitation to image quality exists because the emission, absorption, and detection processes exhibit statistical variations. The random modulation of X-ray intensity across the detector surface, present even in a homogeneous and uniformly thick absorber, is called quantum noise or quantum mottle.

The stochastic quantum fluctuations of X-ray radiation constitute a fundamental feature of the quantum mechanical emission and absorption process. If these fluctuations are too large, the image looks coarse-grained and smaller structures are not resolved.

Only approximately 1% of the electrical energy (voltage × current × exposure time) applied to the X-ray tube is used to produce X-ray photons. Let us assume that 400 000 quanta are actually emitted from the focal spot toward the central beam. The filter in the tube's housing absorbs half that quantity. Patient absorption and beam divergence according to the inverse square law further reduce the number by 97%. Finally, the antiscatter grid in front of the image intensifier reduces the beam intensity by a factor of 3. Let us further assume a detector efficiency of 60%. Then only

$$n = 400\,000 \times 0.5 \times 0.03 \times 0.3 \times 0.6 = 100 \text{ quanta}$$

are detected per picture element. All these statistical processes can be described by the Poisson distribution. Its standard deviation σ is related to the mean number of detected X-ray quanta n according to

$$\sigma = \sqrt{n} \tag{3}$$

For the given example, it is $\sqrt{100} = 10$. Therefore, there is a high probability that the number of quanta is 90 or 110 detected at adjacent picture elements, although there is no difference in absorption.

The quantum efficiency of modern image intensifiers is so high that about 200 electrons are accelerated for each absorbed quantum. By demagnification and high-voltage acceleration, the number of luminescent photons generated at the output phosphor screen are three orders of magnitude higher. Even when the detection efficiency of the camera is low, at each further stage of the image chain the number of particles carrying the image information is much higher than the number of X-ray quanta detected at the input screen.

Thus the origin of the quantum noise observed in any X-ray image is the X-ray detector. This noise is amplified and modulated by all further stages of the image chain in the same way as the signal.

Although according to Eq. 3 the absolute noise is increased, the relative noise level

$$\frac{\sigma}{n} = \frac{\sqrt{n}}{n} = \frac{1}{\sqrt{n}} \tag{4}$$

decreases as the number of detected X-rays increases. For the given example, it is 10%. Since n can be interpreted as the signal and $\sqrt{n}$ as the value of the noise, the inverse of this ratio is often called the signal-to-noise ratio (SNR).

As n is defined as X-ray intensity in terms of the number of photons per unit area, the number of detected photons associated with an object of projected square d^2 is $d^2 \times n$. Accordingly, the SNR of an object

$$\text{SNR(object)} = d\sqrt{n} \tag{5}$$

increases not only with increasing X-ray intensity, but also with its projected area. Larger arterial structures can therefore be visualized, while smaller arteries may be lost in noise.

Minimum Photon Density and Contrast Resolution

Image intensifier systems are now so sensitive that the luminous efficiency needed for exposure of the cine film or the target of the TV camera is more than sufficient. By an adjusted diaphragm in front of the camera, the light intensity is reduced to the optimum level.

The screen dose necessary for a projected image is therefore not determined by the sensitivity of the image intensifier input screen, but by the requirement of a reliable perception of small structures. The content of information given by the differential absorption of a structure is limited by the random distribution of the finite number of photons and the necessity of distinguishing between true and accidental differences in density. This limit is not only dependent on the size of the structure, but also on its contrast.

In Fig. 8, the dependence of the image spatial resolution on contrast and noise level has been visualized in nine artificial images. From top to bottom, the relative noise level is set to 5%, 10%, and 15%, respectively. From left to right, the image contrast is set to 30%, 20%, and 10%, respectively. Contrast is the change in brightness of an object relative to the background brightness. The wedge in the upper

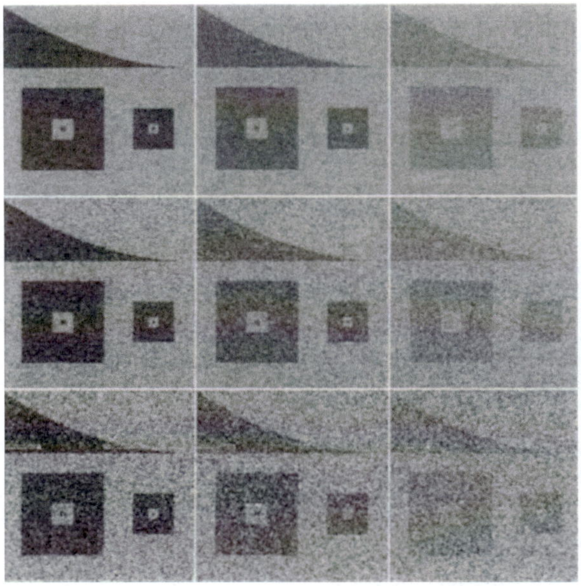

Fig. 8. Visualization of small structure dependent on image contrast and noise level. Image contrast decreases from left to right, whereas noise increases from top to bottom. The smallest object (2 × 2 pixels) can be definitely recognized only at a high contrast and low noise level

part of each subimage is shaped such that its vertical diameter decreases quadratically from left to right. Below there are two centred squares. The edge lengths of the large object are 64, 16, and 4 pixels, while the lengths of the right squares are 32, 8, and 2 pixels, respectively. (It must be borne in mind that 2 pixels correspond to 0.55 mm for a digital 512^2 image using the 14-cm field of view.)

Both a high relative noise level and a low object contrast impair visualization of small structures. For the images on the diagonal from bottom left to top right, the contrast-to-noise ratio is about 2. Below that line, only the largest objects are visible. Reliable recognition of the smallest square is only possible in the first subimage, where that ratio is larger than 5. The tail of the parabolic upper wedge is lost in noise continuously as constrast decreases and noise increases.

Albert Rose [5] estimated photon density quantitatively in its dependence on the picture content. According to his estimation, the (minimum) number n of detected quanta per mm^2 which are necessary for recognition of an object with a diameter d is

$$n = \frac{k^2}{d^2 c^2} \quad (6)$$

In this equation, the relative changes in brightness inside the picture, the *contrast*, is c, while k is the SNR which is only just enough to ensure recognizability. Generally, one has to calculate with $k = 5$ to assure that no accidental fluctuations are identified as genuine signals [5].

Example. The contrast c gives the object's brightness change in relation to the background brightness and is therefore between 0 and 1. A c value of 0.1 means 10% contrast. According to Rose's criterion, the highest dose is needed for objects with a small diameter and little contrast, for example in the presentation of the small arteries after a nonselective injection. With $d = 0.5$ mm and $c = 0.1$,

$$n = \frac{5^2}{0.5^2 \times 0.1^2}$$
$$\approx 10\ 000 \text{ photons per mm}^2$$

If we divide n by 2.8×10^4 (physical conversion factor), we get the dose in micrograys:

$$\frac{n}{2.8 \times 10^4 \,(\text{photons/mm}^2)/\mu\text{Gy}} = 0.3\ \mu\text{Gy}.$$

According to Eq. 6, in larger objects with strong contrasts such as the cardiac ventricles or the great vessels, much smaller radiation doses are sufficient. On the other hand, superposition of anatomical structures may necessitate higher vascular contrast or image dose.

Noise-Dependent Resolution. From this relationship (Eq. 6), the quantum-limited resolution R of the image can also be roughly estimated. It is defined as $1/2d$ in line pairs per millimeter (lp/mm). It increases linearly with the contrast, but only together with the root of the image dose D:

$$R \sim c \times \sqrt{D} \quad (7)$$

Doubling the contrast of the image therefore improves its resolution considerably, while improvement is slow as the dose increases.

In recognition of vascular or cardiac pathology, motion can be of critical importance. In cardiac images with diagnostic structures of low contrast, some features may not be apparent in the static views but may be readily apparent in a cine mode presentation.

Noise and Scatter. It is widely believed that scattered X-rays are the main source of noise. However, this is not true. Quantum noise is a fundamental feature of electromagnetic radiation and comes into appearance predominantly at low intensities.

Thus the primary radiation itself is noisy. Compared to primary radiation, scattered radiation can leave the patient in multiple directions (Fig. 3) and is diffuse. It degrades image quality by reducing the contrast of the image. Both the primary radiation and the scattered radiation are modulated by bones, tissue, and contrast media and are subject to statistical fluctuations. If we were to use a narrow moving slit in front of and behind the patient and exposed the image line by line, most of the scattered radiation would be removed, but nearly the same noise level would be left provided the average brightness of the image were the same. Unfortunately, moving-slit radiography cannot be used in vascular imaging because of the long total exposure time involved. Instead, the less effective antiscatter grid is used.

In addition to quantum noise, other sources of noise such as structural noise or electronic noise may degrade the image. These sources originate from technical imperfections in the components of the image chain.

Image Characteristics

The quality of medical images is intuitively described in terms of sharpness, contrast, and amount of noise in an image that is dependent on the applied X-ray dose and the biophysical properties of the examined object. From the diagnostic point of view, the structures such as small vessels, collaterals, aneurysm, guidewires, catheters, and stents should be clearly visualized during interventional procedures. Quantitative methods for specifying and evaluating the imaging capacity of angiography systems have become an important tool for users, designers, and service specialists.

Some characteristics of an X-ray image such as magnification, scattered radiation, and quantum noise have been discussed above. Image quality can be further described in terms of distortion, spatial and temporal resolution, blur, veiling glare, vignetting, dynamic range, contrast, density transfer function, modulation transfer function, and noise power spectrum. These elements are partially related to image degradations introduced by the components of the imaging chain (Fig. 9).

Geometric distortion is the relative increase in magnification at an off-axis point with respect to the magnification near the center. Resolution of an image sequence can be defined in terms of space, time, and intensity. Sources of image blur include the size of the focal spot or motion of the object during the time of exposure. Veiling glare is introduced by diffraction, scattering, and reflection of light within the optical system or of electrons within the image intensifier. It creates background luminance and reduces the large area contrast similarly to diffusely scattered radiation. Vignetting is the decrease in image luminance toward the periphery of the image.

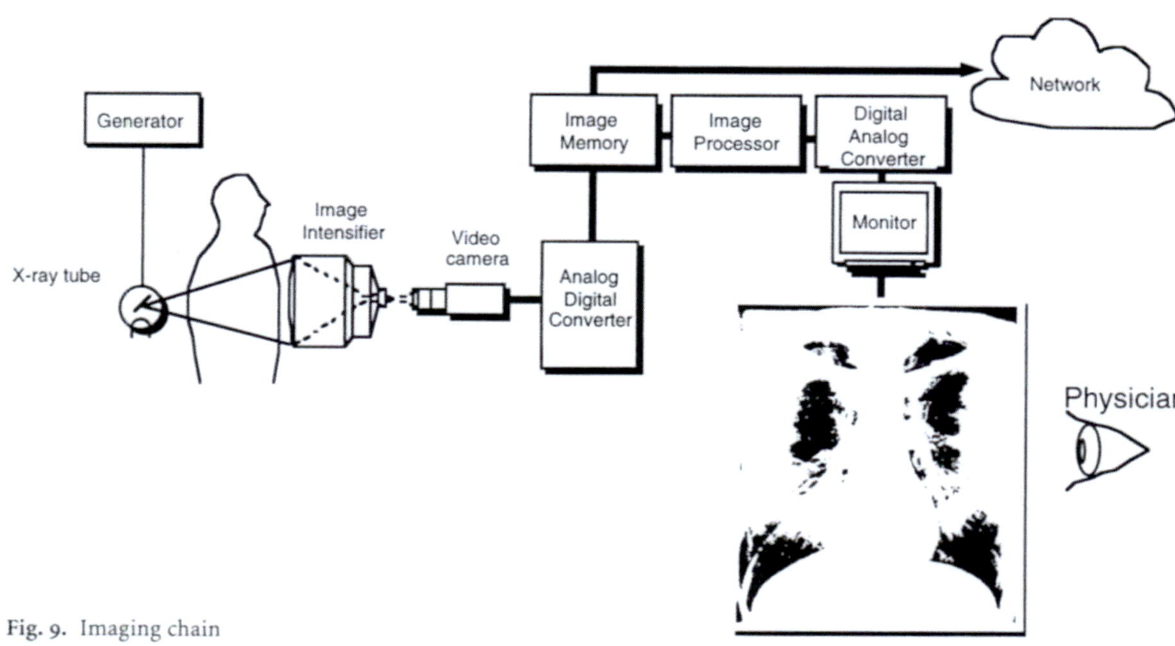

Fig. 9. Imaging chain

The characteristic curve of an angiography system describes the transformation of dose values at the detector entrance to intensity values of the resulting image on film or display. It can be easily measured as voltage, digital value, or optical density of an exposed film by using test objects with stepwise increasing attenuation. The relation between maximum and minimum dose at the detector entrance is called exposure range or dynamic range of the image chain. The first derivative of the characteristic curve is the contrast of the applied detector medium. For example, filmscreen combinations show an S-shaped characteristic and a contrast curve with a peak at specified exposure and falling contrast to higher or lower dose values. Digital systems commonly use detectors with linear characteristics to allow further contrast postprocessing. At later stages of the imaging chain, the intensity of the image is logarithmically processed or modified by white compression.

The performance of an imaging system is primarily described by sharpness and contrast rendition [6]. There are different definitions of contrast. Contrast is generally defined as the relative change in signal intensity of an object versus background. Another measure is the modulation, which is mainly used for the analysis of technical systems. Modulation is the difference between two signal values divided by the sum of the two values. In the image, the modulation of an object depends very much on the size of the object. The modulation transfer function (MTF) combines both sharpness and contrast as a model. It shows the change of contrast for details with different sizes. The MTF concept is based on the linear system analysis of electronic imaging systems and is therefore strictly only applicable to linear systems [7, 8]. For most practical systems, this requirement is fulfilled if the variations within the center of an image are kept small [9]. If the characteristic curve is nonlinear, this has to be compensated for in the MTF measurement. Using the MTF model, it is possible to characterize each component of the imaging system separately. The overall MTF results from the multiplication of each MTF of the single components. In principle, the MTF can be measured by applying sine wave intensity (luminance) patterns at the entrance of the imaging system. The intensities at the exit are measured and the contrast change is calculated. Quantifying the performance of imaging systems in terms of an MTF can prove to be a difficult task, since large amounts of data must be compared and evaluated. Therefore, simpler methods are used in practice. Lead stripes or black and white bars with varying size and distance, calibrated in line pairs per millimeter are displayed and examined with the eye. The pattern with the highest spatial frequency which is just visible is defined as the limiting spatial frequency. This corresponds to a contrast of about 4%. These test patterns allow the measurement of the maximal spatial frequency and are a good tool to adjust the sharpness of an imaging system. Practical studies show that the medically relevant frequencies range from 0 to 2 lp/mm [10]. A vessel with a diameter of 1 mm may be described by a spatial frequency of 0.5 lp/mm plus some frequencies of a higher order.

Image noise is the other main factor besides the MTF limiting the image quality in an X-ray system [11]. Noise is a technical term describing the artifacts received in the early years of electrical audio amplifiers. In modern imaging, this term is used in a figurative sense and describes all disturbances in the image which are not related to the object itself. Noise may be defined comprehensively as any perceivable signal that does not bear relevant information for the operator's task of interpreting images. Examples of noise include quantum noise of the X-ray beam, structure noise of the detector, temporal jitter and flicker of the video chain, digitization noise, spatial artifacts such as pincushion distortion, and variations in luminance of the image intensifier. In designing, selecting, and using angiography equipment, it is of paramount importance to reduce noise as much as possible.

Because the primary task of X-ray based angiography is to display objects with low contrast in such a way that they can be easily detected by the user, and because radiation exposure should be minimal, noise reduction plays a major role in the design of X-ray angiography systems. The relevant measures of noise include SNR and noise power spectrum (NPS), also called the Wiener spectrum [12, 13]. There is general agreement that the physical performance of an imaging system is best described by the intensity transfer function ($I(q)$), the MTF, and the NPS [14]. Concepts such as noise equivalent quanta (NEQ) and detective quantum efficiency (DQE) have been found useful for standardizing physical measurements on an absolute scale and for relating those measurements to the decision performance of a hypothetical "ideal observer." Thus aiming at a comprehensive measure of imaging quality, the $I(q)$, the MTF, and the NPS have to be combined. NEQ are equal to the square of the SNR at the output of the detection system. To calculate the NEQ, the $I(q)$, the MTF, and the NPS have to be measured. DQE is the relation between the SNR at the output and the SNR at the input stage of the detection system. In other words, DQE describes the percentage of the obtained SNR. An ideal detection system would have a DQE of 100%. If we assume Poisson statistics for the incoming quanta, then DQE also represents the percentage of the quanta which contribute to the SNR:

$$\mathrm{NEQ} = \frac{\mathrm{I}(q)^2\,\mathrm{MTF}(u)^2}{\mathrm{NPS}\,(q, u)}$$

q: x-ray dose
u: spatial frequency
$\mathrm{I}(q)$: Intensity Transfer Function
$\mathrm{MTF}(u)$: Modulation Transfer Function
$\mathrm{NPS}(q, u)$: Noise Power Spectrum

where q is the X-ray dose and u is the spatial frequency. DQE is a function of dose and spatial frequency. It can be defined as the NEQ in relation to the SNR of the incoming radiation [15, 16].

$$\mathrm{DQE}\,(q, u) = \frac{\mathrm{I}(q)^2\,\mathrm{MTF}(u)^2}{\Phi\,\mathrm{NPS}\,(q, u)}$$

The temporal resolution is mainly influenced by the duration of the X-ray pulses and the time lag of the image intensifier and video chain. A compromise has to be found between high temporal resolution, i.e., short exposures, and acceptable noise level in the image. Sharp images require a pulse duration of 5–8 ms to avoid blur by motion.

Angiographic Instrumentation

System Design

Competent cardiovascular diagnostics allowing both unequivocal definition of vascular pathology and safe and efficacious placement of catheters and interventional devices requires high quality equipment that has high image quality and is safe and easy to operate. The optimum system provides the highest-quality images with the least radiation exposure to patient and staff. A typical system for angiography (Fig. 10) consists of patient table, detector stand, X-ray generator and tube, image intensifier-video chain, digital image processor with large storage facilities for images, interaction devices, system controller, and several computers responsible for specific tasks (see below).

Proper tuning of each of the subsystems is coordinated by the system controller, assuring overall performance of the examination system. The first systems for angiography were a mixture of different components which were combined and adjusted for specific projects [25]. For example, image intensifiers or digital processors were add-ons to a conventional system which was not designed for this purpose. Angiographic systems are now designed as an integrated system of components which are matched to each other in their function and performance. Proper testing during production, after installation, and routinely during operation is mandatory to achieve good image quality with low radiation exposure.

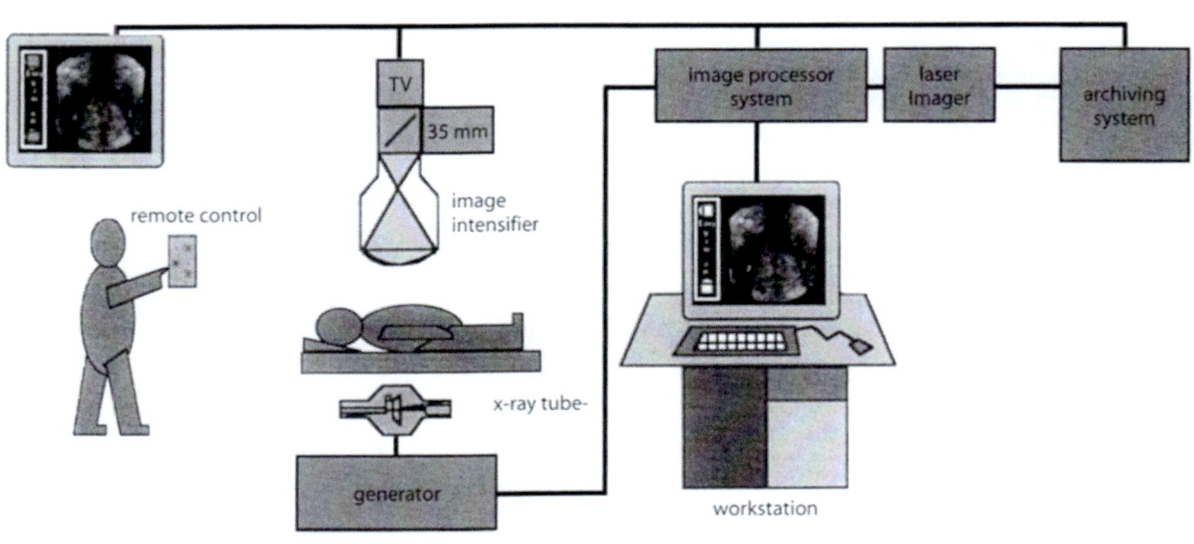

Fig. 10. Angiographic system

X-Ray Stand

X-ray stands may have a monoplane or biplane configuration. The biplane system offers the advantage of showing the passage of the contrast media in two planes, which are usually orthogonal to each other. The images in the two planes are taken independently, separated only by a short time delay. This alternating mode of acquisition is necessary to avoid interference and scattered radiation. Biplane systems are a prerequisite for three-dimensional analysis of vessels. Biplane systems have particular advantages in neurovascular and pediatric peri-interventional imaging: they shorten the procedure time, avoid motional artifacts, and reduce the risk of a second injection of contrast medium. However, radiation exposure is not reduced. The higher cost of the equipment and the restricted access to the patient are drawbacks of biplane systems. In visceral, peripheral, and coronary imaging, monoplane systems are widely used. To show the vessels without distortions and overlaying structures, a large variety of projections are needed. For example, to visualize fully the left coronary artery, extreme proximally angulated projections (craniocaudal) may be necessary in some patients. Typically, the diameter of the image intensifier (> 9 in or 23 cm) limits extreme angulations. There are several possible ways of designing the support for tube and detector. The number of pivot points defines the degree of freedom during craniocaudal angulations and rotations around the patient as utilized in ceiling- and floor-mounted U or C bows. During rotations of biplane systems, the object details should stay in the center of the image. This isocentric mode is accomplished by matching the crossing point of the central beams of each plane with the center point of the rotation. To position the equipment easily and to remove it rapidly in an emergency, the whole system is often mounted on rails at the ceiling.

Patient Table

The patient table is designed to allow easy positioning with a floating table top in the lateral and longitudinal direction. The motorized table height adjustment allows easy access for bedridden and immobile patients.

Tiltable tables are needed for special examinations such as phlebography or for use of positive contrast media such as CO_2. The table should be as homogeneous and radiolucent as possible to avoid contrast reduction in the image by X-ray scatter and structure noise. Carbon fiber table tops are recommended.

Power Injector

To obtain adequate opacification of large vessels and cardiac chambers, it is necessary to inject relatively large volumes of contrast medium through intravascular catheters. The injection of the contrast medium can be performed by hand or by a power injector. To apply a constant, well defined flow and volume of the contrast medium power injectors are used. A power injector should deliver up to 50 ml/s. In cardiology, the power injector should be an integrated part of the catheterization laboratory. Power injectors may also be used for coronary angiography, for the controlled injection of therapeutic agents with very low flow rates, and for small test injections. To guarantee a safe operation, the power injector should have a remote control to terminate the injection, an automatic detection of over-rate injection, a pressure limit control, and a mechanical stop. Electrically, the injector must provide a separate ground and an electrically isolated syringe. To optimize the timing of the injection a trigger input should allow interfacing with the film changer, cine camera, generator, and electrocardiography (ECG) equipment. Automatic injection after a predefined time interval triggered by the start of the X-ray image acquisition allows shortening of the image series. Warming the contrast medium before injection is recommended to lower its viscosity.

X-Ray Generator

To generate X-rays, the high tube voltage and the tube current are provided and controlled by the X-ray generator. The generator must stabilize the tube voltage to the programmed and automatically calculated value defined by the thickness of the object and the attenuation. High-frequency generator technology has supplanted conventional 12-pulse designs and constant potential generators. The generator should produce a power of 80–100 kW at 100 kV. A stable, high-potential wave form and constant tube current applied to the X-ray tube are of utmost importance. Fluctuations of the high tube voltage generate soft radiation, raising the radiation exposure of the patient without any contribution to the image. Cardiac angiography requires short exposure times and fast series of exposures. Exposure times of 5–8 ms for adults and 2–4 ms for children are recommended to avoid motional artifacts. In general angiography, longer exposure times are used. For intravenous digital subtraction angiography (DSA), exposure times up to 300 ms are used to achieve a high dose per image.

Several technical solutions to switch the high voltage on and off have been designed. Primary switching is achieved when the current to the tube is turned on or off by switching the primary transformer winding. Secondary switching is performed on the high voltage side of the generator. Grid-controlled switching is done by means of a grid inside the tube which controls the flow of electrons. Grid controlled switching allows very short and stable pulses with steep rise and decay. The other switching methods have disadvantages. Charge is stored in the high-voltage cables and produces additional radiation before and after the pulse. This radiation is not used for imaging and increases the patient dose. Grid-switched radiation should be used for all procedures with long duration of fluoroscopy or for exposures with a high frame rate. The generator must be prepared to perform pulsed fluoroscopy and exposures with frequencies of a few images per second to 60 images per s, depending on the application.

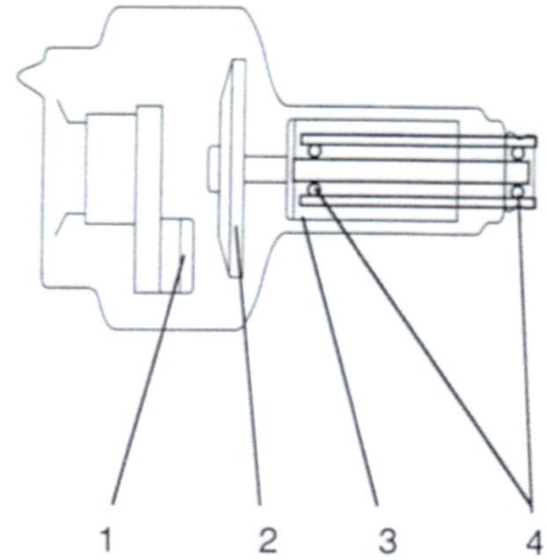

Fig. 11. Section through an X-ray tube. *1*, Cathode; *2*, rotating anode disk; *3*, rotor; *4*, bearings

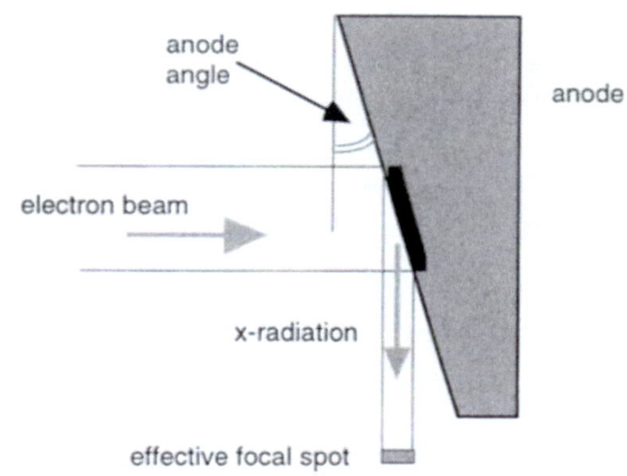

Fig. 12. Bevelled anode and line focus

X-Ray Tube and Beam Filtration

The basic function of the X-ray tube has already been described abvove. Within the vacuum of the tube, accelerated electrons hit a small area of the anode. The size of this area as seen from the perspective of the patient is called the focal spot of the X-ray tube. Because of the inefficient conversion of electrical energy into X-radiation, there is a high level of heat production within the focal spot. This heat accumulates in the anode and must be dissipated. In order to prevent melting of the anode surface, the heat is spread over the anode by enlarging and moving the focal spot. This is technically solved by a bevelled edge of anode disks, which are rotated with 1000 to over 10 000 repetitions per min during exposure.

The electrons emerge from a long, narrow-shaped cathode opposite the bevelled target area of the anode (Figs. 11, 12). X-rays are generated at this elongated focal spot, the line focus. From the perspective of the patient, the line focus appears to be nearly quadratic.

If the angle of the anode is too small, the emitted radiation will be attenuated at the edge by the surface of the anode. This is called the Heel effect and leads to a smaller irradiated field. Large fields of view with a diameter of 30 cm (12 inches) require anode angles of more than 12°, whereas for the 23-cm (9-in)) field an anode angle of 8° is large enough. The advantage of X-ray tubes with steep anode angles is their ability to produce adequate quanta during short exposures with relatively smaller focal spots.

The heat storage capacity and focal spot size are the major parameters of X-ray tube performance. To prevent damage to the X-ray tube, the examination system has to monitor the heat buildup and give a warning when the maximum permitted level is reached. The minimum recommended heat storage capacities of the anode and tube housing are 1 million HU (heat units) and 1.75 million HU, respectively. For proper working conditions, liquid cooling of the tube is necessary.

The spatial resolution of an image is largely determined by the geometrical parameters of the projection and the focal spot size. Methods of measuring the focal spot size are standardized. The blur is due to the geometrical magnification of the focal spot in projection radiography. Modern tubes offer different sizes of focal spots and two spots are selectable per tube. The smaller the effective spot size, the sharper the image. The high variability in projections of a universal angiography system requires different spot sizes. A larger size of 1–1.2 mm (50–80 kW) is optimal for high dose applications, such as steep angulations, and a small size of 0.6–0.7 mm (35–50 kW) is suitable for high spatial resolution and in particular pediatric applications. In recent years, the development of new materials and bearings has drastically changed the way X-ray tubes are constructed. To prevent melting of the focal spot due to high heat generation, the anode has to be rotated very rapidly whenever radiation is needed. The main difficulty is to bring the heat outside the tube. New bearings of the anode, such as spiral groove bearings filled with a gallium base liquid metal (Philips MRC tube), improve cooling. The liquid metal conducts heat 1000 times more efficiently than traditional ball-bearing assemblies. As a result, this tube has three times the continuous heat load of other tubes, allowing longer lengths of series and stronger filtration.

The tube is contained in a special housing designed to allow liquid cooling of the tube and shielding of the extraneous X-radiation (Fig. 13). Each tube has a typical inherent filtration expressed as a value equivalent to the filtration of aluminium. Additional filters made of aluminum or copper can be fixed to the tube housing. To adapt the lateral extension of the X-ray beam to the diagnostic field, motor-driven collimators can be moved into the beam. Straight and curved collimators are available and can be moved linearly or rotationally.

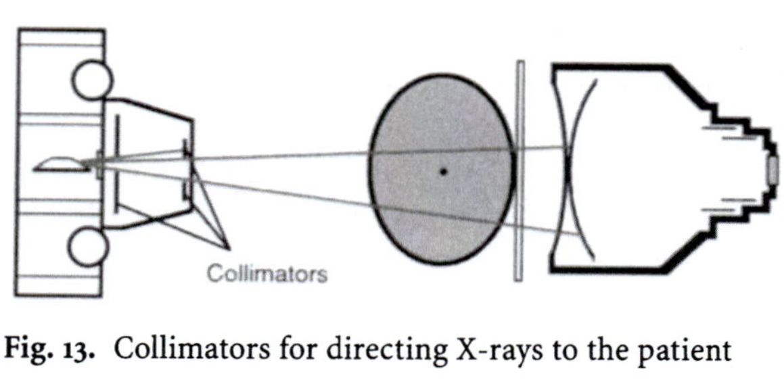

Fig. 13. Collimators for directing X-rays to the patient

Imaging Chain

To detect and produce an image, several components are necessary. The first X-ray systems needed only a film or a film screen combination and a developing machine. Fluoroscopy without an image intensifier is now no longer allowed in several countries. An examination system for angiography uses an image intensifier, which is coupled via an optical system to a video camera, amplifiers for the video signal, video monitors, a digital image processor, and a hard copy unit for films or opaque material. In Germany, digital storage of images during fluoroscopy is required for interventional and pediatric examinations. In cardiology, a 35-mm cine camera is very often coupled to the optical system by a semitransparent mirror. The image passes through several transformation steps before it is presented to the medical user. Depending on the transformation stage, the image is represented as light, electrons, electrical voltage, or digital numbers. Each of these stages has to be optimized to reach the best possible image quality.

Image Intensifier

The image intensifier (Fig. 14) converts the radiation profile in the patient to a bright image at the output window. The present image intensifiers are the result of 20 years of research. Input screens based on caesium iodide (CsI) have been introduced, providing a sensor with both high quantum efficiency and high spatial resolution far superior to the ZnCdS screen used earlier.

The X-ray detector is contained in a metal body with vacuum inside. Behind the input window there is a scintillating screen backed with a photo emitting layer. In the input screen, X-ray quanta generate light, which stimulates the emission of electrons in the photo cathode. These electrons are accelerated in a high electrostatic field (25–35 kV). Charged with high kinetic energy, the electrons hit the output phosphor screen, producing a bright light image at the exit of the image intensifier. The image intensifier works with lower exposure levels than X-ray exposure with a film screen cassette. The contrast of the acquired images is electronically amplified. Image intensifiers are produced in different sizes. Input windows with a diameter of 23 cm (9 in) and 18 cm (7 in are used in cardiology; peripheral and abdominal angiography require larger coverage with an input diameter of up to 38 cm

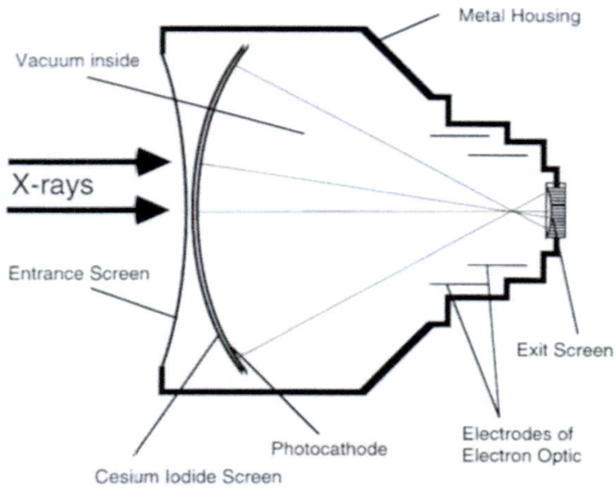

Fig. 14. Image intensifier

(15 in) or 40 cm (16 in). In the latter, a smaller entrance field may be selected electronically. At the output screen of the image intensifier, only this region of interest appears with enhanced brightness. In order to image both large fields (e.g., aortography) and small fields (coronary arteries), the field of view can be changed in two, three, or five steps depending on the type of equipment, e.g., 38 cm, 31 cm, 25 cm, 20 cm and 17 cm. A smaller field means higher spatial resolution at the expense of a higher radiation dose. Since the field size is also reduced, the dose areaproduct, which is a relevant measure for effective patient dose, may remain constant.

To compare the performance of image intensifiers it is important to measure the degree to which the radiation at the entrance is absorbed and transformed to light intensities at the output. The following figures are valid for a 23-cm image intensifier. Other sizes and fields need other reference values. The ratio of luminance to dose rate is called conversion factor or gain. The conversion factor lies between 17 and 46 $(Cd/m^2)/(\mu Gy/s)$. Very important is the DQE, which gives the percentage of the incoming quanta which are actually used to generate the image [26]. DQE is measured as the quotient of the SNR at output and input. DQE for the spatial frequency zero should be greater than 55%.

The ability to visualize objects of different sizes and varying contrast is summarized in the MTF [27, 28]. The modulation at the spatial frequency of 1 lp/mm is called characteristic modulation and should exceed 59%. For low spatial frequencies, i.e., large objects, the fall-off of the modulation factor is measured. This fall-off is also called low frequency drop or veiling glare and can be measured as the contrast ratio [29]. Typical values of image intensifiers are higher than 25:1 or lower than 10% of the MTF. The smallest resolvable object is defined by the spatial resolution, which is normally measured using a test object with lead bars 0.05 mm thick and different groups of line pairs per millimeter. Spatial resolution should exceed 3 lp/mm for the 23-cm field. The geometrical distortions are also known as the pincushion effect. As the geomagnetic field changes, the pathway of the electrons within the image intensifier is altered. Thus distortions change when the image intensifier is moved around the patient. The imaging quality of image intensifiers has been improved dramatically in recent years, providing an image quality sufficient to replace film-screen systems in most exposure situations.

Optical System

The output image of the image intensifier is so bright that it can be split by the optical system for the different viewing subsystems. This is necessary

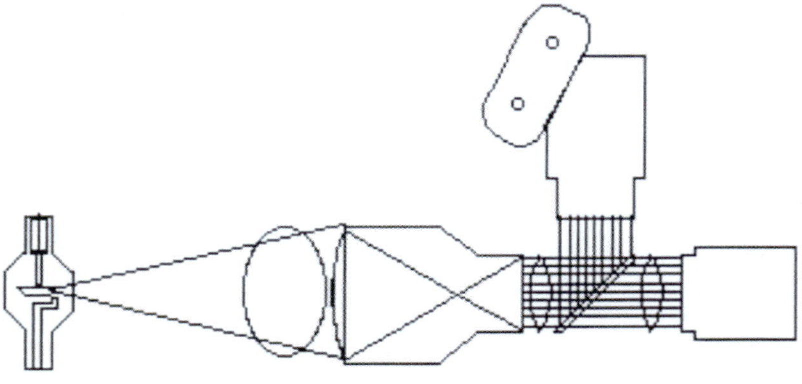

Fig. 15. Optical system connecting image intensifier, video system, and cine system

for displaying images on monitors and recording them on film simultaneously. To connect two subsystems, the image is separated into two copies by a semitransparent mirror. One image is projected to the attached film camera, the other to the video system. A light sensor measures the image brightness for the exposure control. In cardiology, a 35-mm camera is attached to the optical system and receives the bright image of the image intensifier through a semitransparent mirror (Fig. 15). The quality of the optical system is measured as MTF and veiling glare. Optical zooming or overframing may be used for fluoroscopy to acquire a portion of the intensifier output image with improved image quality as long as the video camera limits the resolution.

Future purely digital image systems for interventional medicine may be fitted with simple fiber-optic couplers instead of the tandem optic. This would lessen the MTF and veiling glare degradation.

Video Chain

Both diagnostic and therapeutic catheterization procedures require television fluoroscopy for image transmission and real time viewing at different locations independently of the position of the image intensifier. The video camera is coupled to the optical system. The bright image is projected to the photo-sensitive target of the video tube. This illumination changes the conductivity of the target, which is directly coupled to an electrically conductive layer. This results in a charge distribution on the inner surface of the target. In the vacuum of the tube, an electron beam scans the charge distribution of the image stored on the input target. The resulting variations in the electron current are detected and transformed into the video signal by an amplifier. Video tubes can be distinguished by the composition of their target material. Commonly used types include Plumbicon, Saticon, and Vidicon. In their performance they differ in resolution, dynamic range, time lag, and noise characteristic. In the future, video tubes will be replaced by solid state sensors, so-called charge-coupled devices (CCD). A CCD is basically a silicon chip with a large number of integrated cells, which are sensitive to light. Each cell is isolated from the others and accumulates electrical charge depending on the intensity of the incidental light. In addition, the chip contains read-out amplifiers to convert the amount of charge to a voltage. Because the image cannot be read out in one step, it has to be partitioned in separate lines (video tube) or in lines and columns (CCD) which are read one after the other. There are different patterns scanning the image on the input

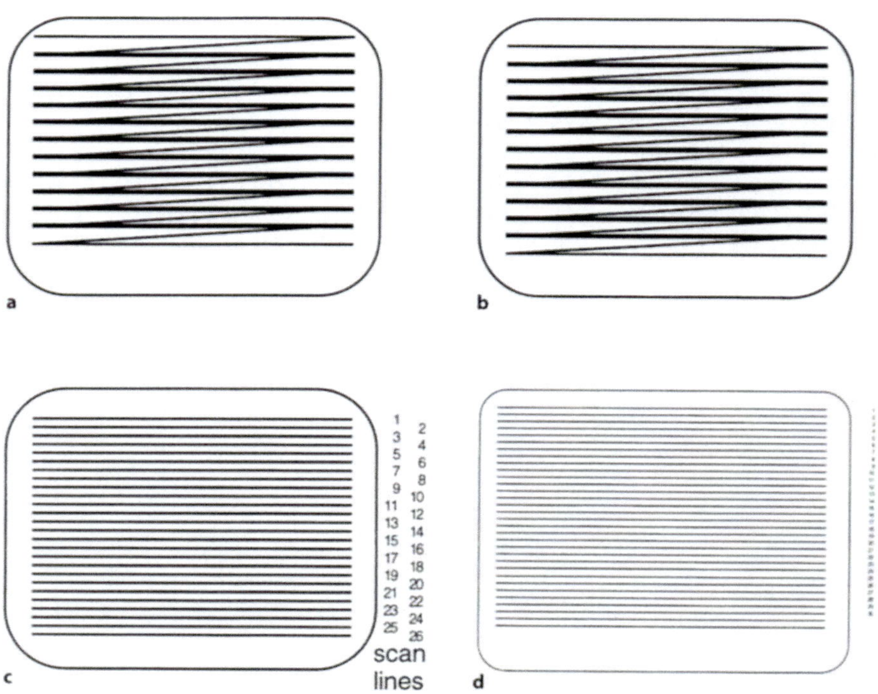

Fig. 16 a – d. Scanning modes of video signals. **a – c** Interlaced mode. **a** First field (1 mol/50 s). **b** Second field (1 mol/50 s). **c** One frame made up of two fields (1/25 s). **d** Progressive mode. One frame progressively scanned in 1/25 s

target of the video sensor (Fig. 16). The time needed to scan an image depends on the scanning speed and the number of lines.

The resulting image consists of an array of video lines. In video standards, all lines of an image together are called the frame. In conventional video practice, interlaced scans are used to avoid flicker. This is realized by separating one frame into two fields, which are shown one after the other in a fast sequence. The first field covers an image by reading out half of the lines. Each line is spaced apart by the width of a line. The second field then reads out the remaining half of the lines, which fall in the space left between the lines of the first field. This interlaced scanning method is appropriate for continuous fluoroscopy. The standard frame rate is 25 frames/s in Europe and 30 frames/s in the United States. The interlaced mode is defined in detail as an international Comité Consultative International des Radiocommunications (CCIR) standard.

To improve temporal and spatial resolution, modern X-ray systems use pulsed exposures with non-interlaced scanning and variable frame rate. Each image is read out line by line in an uninterrupted sequence. This mode of operation is also used by computer displays. For these kinds of video signals there are no standards and more variations exist, mainly characterized by the number of scanned lines, e.g., 625 or 1249 in Europe, and the frame rate. So called multisync displays are able to display video signals of different specifications. In practice, this means that fast moving objects require a rapid sequence of images, i.e., a high frame rate. To show small details, a high number of lines is needed. Both parameters are summarized in the bandwidth of the system, which is a main descriptor of a video system. The bandwidth is defined as the range of electrical frequencies needed to write an image on a video monitor. It can easily be calculated by the multiplication of frame rate, quadratic number of lines and the aspect ratio of the image, e.g.,

$$25\ \text{Hz} \times 625^2 \times (43) \approx 13\ \text{MHz}$$

The units are megahertz or one million cycles per second. Standard video systems have a bandwidth of 5–10 MHz, and high-resolution video chains have a bandwidth greater than 20 MHz. The MTF and the SNR are further parameters describing the performance of a video system [30].

Digitization

All X-ray detectors basically acquire an image as a continuum of signal intensities. In order to use the advantages of digital data processing, images have to be cut into small pieces of information which can be represented as binary digits (bits) ready for storage and processing in a computer. Between maximum and minimum intensity in the image, i.e., its dynamic range, there are only a finite number of possible intensity steps, also called gray values. Each gray value is represented as a digital value (Fig. 17) [31].

The number of possible digital values, i.e., the number of gray levels, is defined by the number of bits. Eight bits are equivalent to 256 gray levels. In

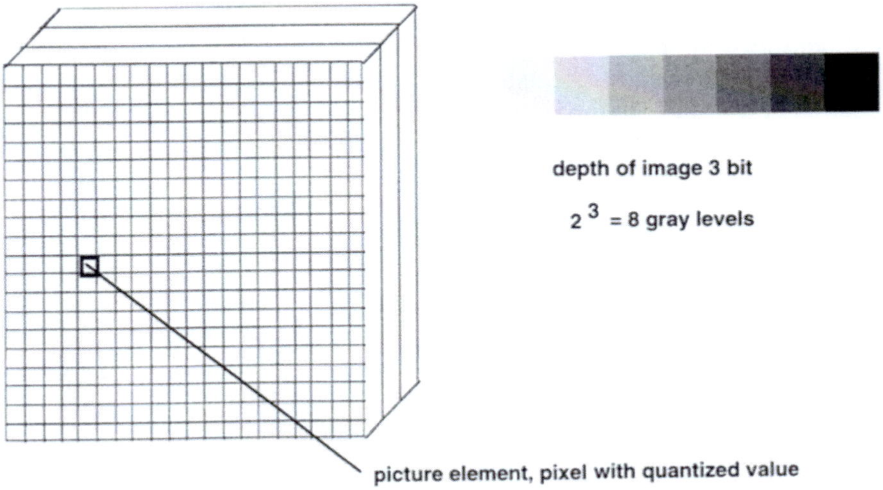

Fig. 17. Example of a digital image matrix with 20 × 20 pixels and 3-bit depth; 2^3=8 gray levels

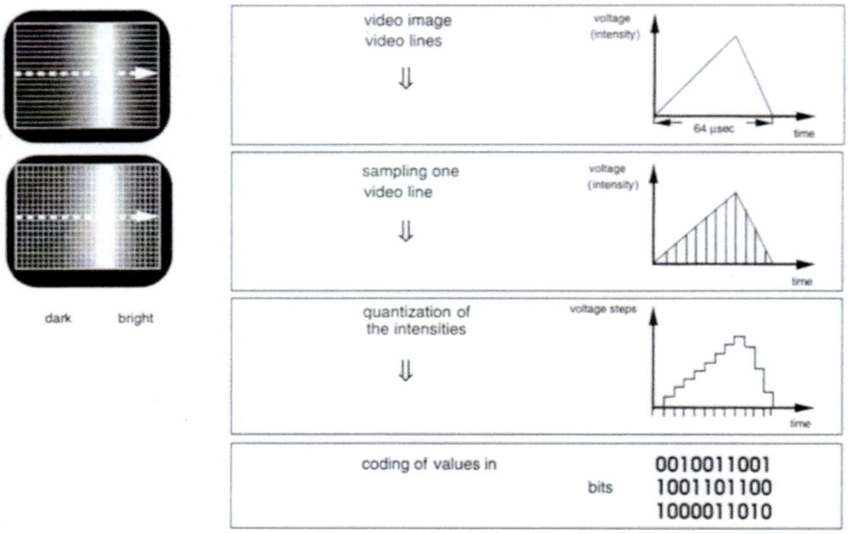

Fig. 18. Digitization of a video image

practice, this means that in an image digitized with 8 bits, each pixel may have a discrete value between 0 and 255. The number of bits alone is not sufficient to describe the contrast rendition of imaging equipment. It has to be related to the range of dose values summarized in the characteristic curve and to the amount of noise in the image.

Converting an image into a finite set of numbers is called digitization (Fig. 18). Two steps are necessary for the transition of an analog to a digital image. First, the image is divided into small picture elements, so-called pixels. In the next step, the mean intensity within the pixel is matched to a discrete intensity value.

Most current angiographic systems use a video camera for scanning the image at the output screen of the image intensifier. This process converts the continuous two-dimensional image into a finite number M_1 of raster lines. This number limits the resolution of the image in the vertical direction. In a second step, these lines are sampled at M_2 evenly spaced points. The image now consists of $M_1 \times M_2$ sample points. It is represented by rows and columns of pixels. If the size of the pixels is much smaller than the smallest detail in the image, there is no loss of information (Shannon's theorem). The pixel size is therefore the main determinant of the spatial resolution, defining which spatial frequencies may be transmitted by the imaging system provided the contrast is sufficient.

If a CCD camera is used, instead of the analog video camera, the scanning process is dropped and a two-dimensional sampling process takes place, as given by the size of the CCD array. The output of the CCD camera is an analog video signal. In any case, the mean intensity within a pixel is converted or "quantized" to a discrete intensity (gray) level. This is performed by the analog-to-digital converter (ADC). In future, the image chain may be replaced by a X-ray converter directly coupled with an array of $M_1 \times M_2$ discrete semiconductor cells. Although promising results have been obtained by different laboratories, these devices have to prove their superiority in routine angiography.

Whereas M_1 and M_2 determine the spatial resolution, the precision with which the intensities are represented is given by N. The size of M_1 and M_2 is given by video standards and the bandwidth of the camera. Typical matrix sizes are 512 × 512 or 1024 × 1024. In angiography with only a few images per second the 1024×1024 matrix is applied, whereas in cardiology with high frame rates the 512×512 matrix is prevalent. The ratio of height-to-width of the pixel, the so-called aspect ratio, is not necessarily 1; however, this is expedient for further steps of image processing and geometric measurements. The number of possible gray levels N depends on the number of bits used to represent the intensity. Using 8 bits, there are $N=2^8=256$ gray levels; for 10 bits, 1024 gray levels are used. For high-precision quantization, the quantization error is reduced, but a larger storage capacity is needed. However, image noise, in particular the quantum mottle, often limits the precision of the gray levels. As a practical compromise quantization step should be smaller than 1.5 times the standard deviation of the noise [32]. Therefore, for cardiac images taken at image exposures of 0.1 – 0.5 μGy, 256 gray levels (8 bits) are sufficient. For DSA, ten bits are needed if an image chain with a linear transmission characteristic is used. In the first DSA systems, the video signal was first logarithmically amplified and then digitized. In this case, analog digital conversion with 8 bits is sufficient. In practice logarithmic processing of an image is needed for DSA to show the path of a vessel undisturbed by overlaying tissues and bones with varying thickness.

Table 1. Spatial resolution (lp/mm) for digital images of different matrix size recorded with different image intensifier fields of view

Field of view		Matrix size			
(cm)	(in.)	256^2	512^2	1024^2	2048^2
14	5.5	0.9	1.8	3.7	7.3
17	6.7	0.8	1.5	3.0	6.0
23	9	0.6	1.1	2.2	4.5
33	13	0.4	0.8	1.6	3.1
41	16	0.3	0.6	1.2	2.5

Tables 1 – 3 show some typical data on digital images. In Table 1, the spatial resolution as limited by the number of pixels is given for matrix sizes M^2 of 256^2 – 2048^2 and for the image intensifier field of view D between 14 cm (zoom) and 41 cm (overview). The resolution in line pairs per millimeter is calculated as $M/2D$, assuming exact framing. The corresponding pixel size at the input screen is D/M. If the resolution due to focal spot blurring is limited to 1.5 lp/mm, a matrix size of 512^2 would be adequate for the 17-cm field of view. For a largest entrance field (33 cm), 1024 pixels are necessary. If the image is sampled with smaller spatial frequencies, aliasing effects appear because the Nyquist theorem is violated. Only for single-shot vascular images with high X-ray dose, small focal spot, and a large field of view may a 2048^2 matrix be necessary [33].

In Table 2 the required memory size is stated for images of different matrix sizes and gray levels, whereby it is assumed that the 10- and 12-bit images are not stored as 16-bit images, as is often done for convenience in digital computers. Fast algorithms are available for lossless compression, and these reduce the required space by a factor of 2 – 3. For angiographic sequences, the capacity required to store one angiographic study in the solid-state memory of the computer is of great practical interest. Therefore, in Table 3, the memory requirement for a cine run of 10 s for 8-bit images and various pulse frequencies is indicated. Provided sufficient digital random access memory (RAM) is available in the workstation, the image sequence can be displayed smoothly as a loop. If only a subset of images need to be displayed, 5 or 20 MByte is sufficient for images of 512^2 or 1024^2 matrix size, respectively. The minimal memory requirement for a single angiographic cine run of 512^2 matrix and a pulse rate of 12.5 fps is 32 MByte. For real-time display of biplane angiograms, this size must be doubled. A cardiac workstation should therefore be equipped with at least 64 MByte. If several series need to be displayed rapidly, e. g., throughout an angioplasty procedure, or when fast biplane calculations need to be performed, the digital imaging system requires considerably more memory or a real-time magnetic disk to store the acquired images.

Table 2. Image storage (MByte) for digital images of different matrix size and gray levels

Gray level		Matrix size			
(bit)	(n)	256^2	512^2	1024^2	2048^2
8	256	0.063	0.25	1.00	4.0
10	1024	0.078	0.31	1.25	5.0
12	4096	0.094	0.38	1.50	6.0

Table 3. Storage capacity (MByte) used per 10 s for digital images of different matrix size recorded with different image sequences

Image sequences		Matrix size			
(bit)	(fps)	256^2	512^2	1024^2	2048^2
8	2	1.3	5.0	20	80
8	8	5.0	20.0	80	320
8	12.5	7.8	31.3	125	500
8	15	9.4	37.5	150	600
8	25	15.6	62.5	250	1000
8	30	18.8	75.0	300	1200

fps, frames per second

Image Storage

For direct online viewing of images with diagnostic quality during catheterization and interventions, a large image memory is required to store all digitally acquired images. The storage capacity is measured in megabytes of memory. One 512 × 512 image needs 0.25 MByte, a 1024×1024 image 1 MByte. Modern systems offer storage capacities of several thousand

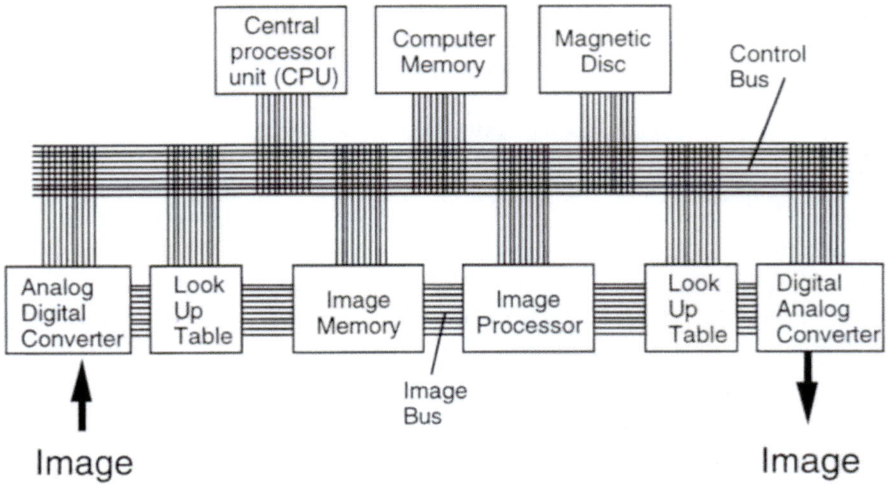

Fig. 19. Block diagram of an image processor

megabytes (gigabytes). Storage and recall in real time have to be supported by the image processor and the digital storage media. The digital storage of images may reduce fluoroscopy time by using stored images for orientation. These stored images are also needed during interventional procedures for the documentation of the procedure and the comparison of images. Digital images are the prerequisite for analytical processing.

Image Processing

The image processor is the core of the digital subsystem (Fig. 19). Via fast transmission lines, so-called busses images are moved between the analog to digital converter, image memory, processor, storage devices, and digital to analog converters.

The availability of images in a digital format gives the opportunity to compensate for degradation during the detection process, to adapt the image presentation to the needs of the observer, and to analyze objects visible in the image. These tasks are called image restoration, image enhancement, and image analysis.

Image Restoration. In projection radiography, an image is degraded due to the geometrical conditions of imaging with X-rays and the imperfections of the X-ray imaging system. The main factors responsible for image degradation are reduction of the image sharpness due to the finite size of the focal spot, the detector electronic imperfections and movements of the object, geometrical distortions, and reduction in contrast due to scattered radiation, quantum and electrical noise, and veiling glare of the detector. Regions with low or high absorption of X-rays may lead to over- or underexposed regions in the image. These effects can be partly compensated by digital image processing automatically performed during the acquisition process.

Image Enhancement. In addition, specific details of the image such as blood vessels are enhanced in their visibility by the enhancement of edges interactively controlled by the user.

The algorithms of image processing can be divided into three groups: (1) changing the intensity value of one pixel at a time independently of other pixels, doing this for all pixels of an image (point operations), (2) changing the intensity value of a pixel in relation to the surrounding pixels (neighborhood operations), and (3) changing the pixel values in respect to preceding and following images in a series.

Point operations are performed using so-called look up tables (LUT). LUT are fast digital memories loaded with a list of intensity values. Each intensity value has an address, which is related to the intensity values of the input image. An LUT may therefore be used to implement transformations of a pixel value between stored intensity values and displayed gray levels. Each pixel value of the input image is used to select an address in the LUT. The value of the pixel is then replaced by the content of the selected address. The stored intensity values cover a range of intensity levels limited by the number of bits of the LUT. Practical examples are enhancement of contrast (Fig. 20) or a logarithmic characteristic curve to compensate for the exponential at-

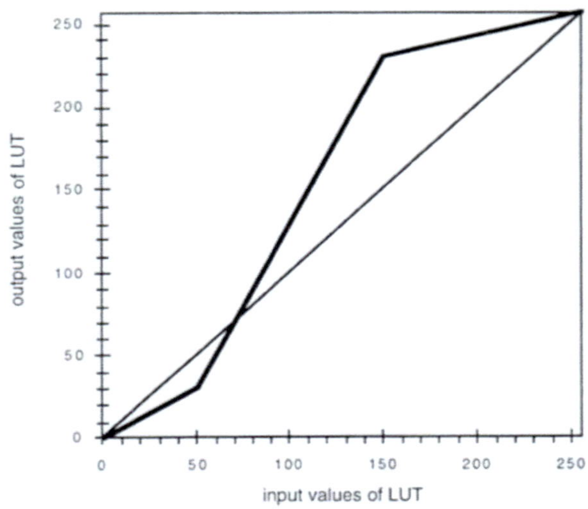

Fig. 20. Contrast enhancement using a look-up table (*LUT*; Window technique). In contrast to the film in the digital image vessels are presented by low intensity values

tenuation of X-rays by the object. The contrast of a vessel in respect to the background is enhanced by lowering the intensity values in the image representing the vessel and raising the values of the background (white compression).

The input values between 50 and 150 are stretched, i.e. the slope is (230 – 30)/(150 – 50)= 2 instead of 1, thus doubling the contrast range. From this example it is obvious that other intensity ranges are compressed. This effect is used for reducing the appearance of those parts of an image which are diagnostically irrelevant. In cardiology, white compression reduces the brightness in the areas with lung tissue surrounding the heart, while the contrast within the heart is enhanced.

Neighborhood operations are accompanied by filters which change the value of the central pixel according to the intensities of the environment. A simple filter of this kind is the smoothing of an image by averaging all pixel values in a region of interest (ROI) and applying this operation to all parts of the whole image. This algorithm is used to reduce noise. Another method is to enlarge the intensity differences within an ROI in the image. These gradient filters are enhancing edges. The size of the ROI defines what size of objects are emphasized. The size of the ROI is also called the kernel size of a filter. Thus these filters are characterized by the kernel size, which is equal to the number of pixels in the ROI; 3×3 and 5×5 kernels are often used. Assuming a pixel size of 0.2 × 0.2 mm, the kernel size is 1 × 1 mm and objects of this size will be enhanced. Small ROI only enhance small objects, and large kernels only enhance large objects.

A median filter reduces noise and single dropouts in the image by replacing each pixel value by the median value of the pixels in its neighborhood.

A favorite method of enhancing structures is unsharp masking (Fig. 21). A blurred copy of an image, the so-called mask, is subtracted from the original image, resulting in an image which contains only edges. By adding these edges to the original image, a sharper image is produced as a result. The big advantage of this method is that it is easy to implement and the amount of edge enhancement can be controlled. This is important, since too much edge enhancement may lead to overshooting intensities at the edges, visible as bright and dark shadows next to edges.

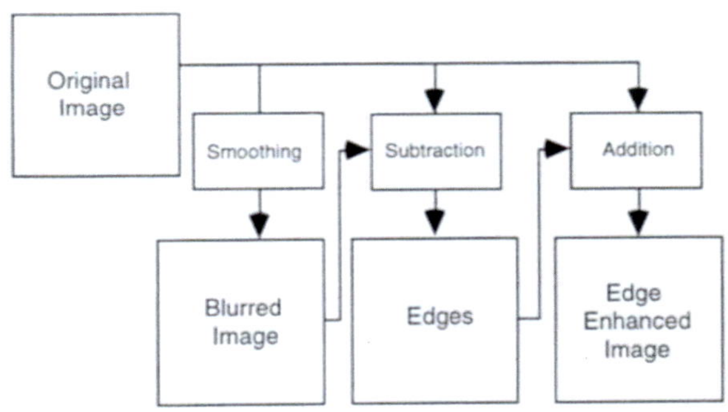

Fig. 21. Principle of unsharp masking. From the original image a blurred version of the same image is subtracted, resulting in an edge image. A fraction of this edge image is then added to the original image

Multiple images can be combined into one by adding or subtracting the intensity values of both images pixel by pixel. Adding two images results in an image with less noise; the SNR is improved by a factor of $\sqrt{2}$. Adding multiple (n) images leads to an improvement by a factor of $\sqrt{n}$. Subtracting two images shows only the differences between the two images. If one image is taken before the arrival of contrast media in a vessel and another with the contrast medium filled vessel, the subtracted image represents only the contrasted vessel. Because of the small signal amplitudes in the subtracted image, subtraction is often completed by electronic contrast enhancement. All overlaying structures are removed, and even small vessels are clearly visualized. The mask image is subtracted from each image taken during filling of the vessel tree. The re-

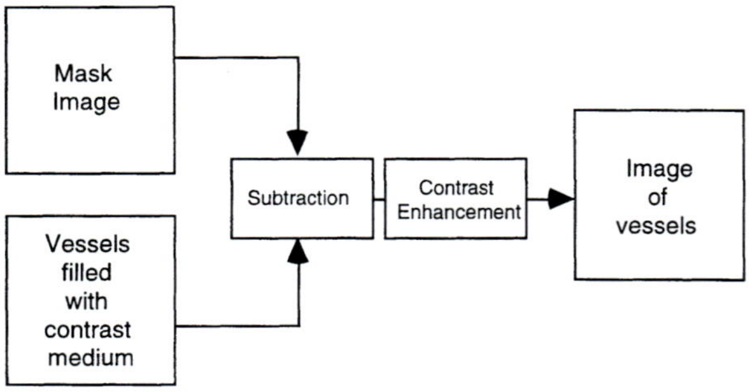

Fig. 22. Principle of digital subtraction angiography. A mask image is subtracted from a series of images taken during a passage of contrast medium. After subtraction the contrast of the images is enhanced

sult is a series of subtracted images. DSA was the first digital method applied in angiography and has now become a standard processing operation (Fig. 22).

By weighted image subtraction, contrast enhancement of the opacified vessels can be achieved without losing the reference to other anatomical structures. DSA fails only in situations where there are movements between the acquisition of the mask image and the images taken during the passage of contrast media. These recordings can be corrected by choosing a new mask image ot of the sequence of images, which is taken closer to the mask image. This mask image can be taken before or after maximum opacification of the vessel. Another method is digitally shifting mask and filling image to get a better fit of both, so-called pixel shift. In the case of rapidly moving vessels, e.g., the coronary arteries, this method cannot be used, however. In this case, the method of choice is unsharp masking separately applied to each image in a series.

When digital image processing was first introduced in the 1970s and early 1980s, the described operations needed substantially longer than the acquisition and only a few images could be stored. Subsequently, the computing speed and memory space were gradually improved. Nowadays, most processing can be done online, i.e., faster than the acquisition, and there is only a short time delay before the resulting image is visible on the monitor. Images are processed directly during the acquisition process and are displayed in the examination room. This mode has mainly replaced film exposures taken with film changers or cine cameras. Films are only used to document the resulting digital images. In principal, during fluoroscopy the same methods as in the exposure mode, such as contrast and edge enhancement and subtraction, can be used online. In addition, there are special fluoroprocessing methods. Noise in the images can be reduced by recursive filtering. This is an algorithm in which the intensities of a series of images are averaged in such a way that the most recent images are given the highest weight. This is done to avoid movement artifacts.

Previously acquired and stored images can be displayed and superimposed onto the live online images, providing a "road map" for orientation during percutaneous interventions and in difficult anatomical areas.

Image Analysis. The numeric representation of an image as a digital matrix permits easy calibration of distances, angles, volumes, and intensities. Objects in the image can be quantitatively analyzed in their size, shape, and orientation. The main practical measurement in angiography is the quantitative assessment of a stenosis, which is particularly important during interventions. The size of the balloon catheter is matched to the directly measured width of the vessel lumen. By measuring the changes in density in a series of images, density-time curves can be obtained to assess the perfusion of tissues.

By combining projections from different angles, three-dimensional representations of a vascular tree can be synthesized.

Standard measurement methods are automated to guarantee fast performance. To allow a high degree of reproducibility, a thorough validation of the algorithms is mandatory.

Image Display

For image display, it is very important to use a flicker-free monitor with high luminance and a high number of scanning lines. This requires a refresh rate of more than 70 images/s, a luminance exceeding 200 cd/m^2 and more than 1000 video lines. Using a high-definition, 1000-line video system, playback is performed using a scan converter independent of the line rate and the pulses per second at acquisition. Display of digital images is more flexible than that of film. The image can be shown without time delay; it can be zoomed and magnified, and the brightness and contrast are set interactively. Various digital filters can be used for edge enhancement. Slow-motion and freeze-frame presentation without flicker or noise bars can be routinely obtained. Therefore, digital systems have become essential in online monitoring of the outcome of interventional procedures and in decision making. To allow simultaneous display of images in the examination room, multiple monitors are needed. At least one monitor for real-time viewing per plane and one or two monitors for the presentation of stored images are needed for comparisons. At the control desk, monitors with a diameter of 38 cm (15 inches) and 50 cm (20 inches) in the examination room are used.

Cine Film Projector

There are two types of projectors available for viewing cine images: (1) the intermittent film advance projector and (2) the rotating prism projector. If image quality is most important, the intermittent projector will do the job best. Moreover, for quietness and convenience, the rotating prism projector may be better. Further important features are high-intensity light source, transport of film forward and reverse at variable speeds, wall projection, zooming mechanism permitting magnified projection, and remote control operation. For the digitization of film images, the adaptation of a video camera using a connection to a video frame grabber of a computer is necessary.

Documentation and Archiving

The classical medium for the documentation of angiograms is film. Film can be easily exchanged between institutions, has a long lifetime, and can be viewed at light boxes or viewing systems all around the hospital. With the advent of digital angiography, the images are primarily stored as digital data in the memory of the image processor. After the examination has been completed, the images are reviewed on the video monitor of the workstation, their contrast and brightness is adjusted, and a set of images is selected for printing on film. Normally, only the relevant images of a run are selected. In the early days of digital angiography, the video signal of the monitor was transferred to a video hard copy unit, also called a video imager. A video imager contains a camera which makes pictures of the video images presented on a built-in monitor. Most video imagers use different lenses to combine multiple images on one film. The film sizes are comparable to the standard sizes used in film-screen radiography. Nowadays, films are printed directly using digital image data. The digital image is transferred to a laser imager. A very fine laser beam is modulated by the stored intensity value of the image matrix. To generate an image, a hard copy film passes in a precise and stable motion past the laser beam. The modulated laser beam moves perpendicular to the direction of the film movement writing the image to the film. Laser imagers produce hard copies of the images with high spatial and contrast resolution in desirable formats. Even now, films are still one of the main storage media. Depending on the national laws and regulations, these documents have to be safely archived for 10–30 years. Several working groups are studying the possibility of monitor reading aimed at a total replacement of film and a storage of images and reports in a digital form on optical disks or optical tapes. Advantages of a digital archive are the reduction in storage space, the automated access to the images, and the possibility of transferring digital images via networks. For the exchange of digital angiographies, the data sets may be duplicated without any loss of information.

Since dynamic processes such as the blood flow in a vessel and the beating heart have to be visualized in angiography, images have to be reviewed in a fast sequence. This is not feasible with films and therefore requires digital storage of images and extra monitors for viewing. Image sequences can be stored as a video signal on video tapes. Because of their limited lifetime, magnetic tapes may only be used as a short-term storage and exchange medium. Video disks may be used as an exchange medium, but standardization is lacking. They are not suitable as an archiving medium, since there is a loss of information. The current best solution is storage of angiographic data on digital optical laser disks.

Angiographic Image Acquisition

Analog Versus Digital Angiography

Although conventional film-based systems are highly advanced and technically sophisticated, they have several fundamental limitations that are becoming increasingly important to three developments:

1. Vascular interventions impose a great demand on real-time X-ray imaging.

2. Digital communication systems are increasingly used in health care, and images should become part of the multimedia database.
3. Due to rapid improvements in the cost-benefit relation in computer technology, advanced digital data processing is being increasingly used. Benefits include speed and flexibility of data access, processing of image series, and application of quantitative techniques for extracting objective data.

However, despite this progress, the conventional system still has certain advantages. Film is a well-standardized medium, easy to review by anyone. Worldwide exchange is easy. Light boxes and cine film viewing stations are available in all hospitals with high homogeneous brightness. It is technically simple to view image sequences in fast-forward and -backward mode. The film has a long guaranteed lifetime. The spatial and temporal resolution of the cine film are also excellent, and it has a large dynamic range.

The advantages of digital radiographic vascular imaging systems can be described as follows:

Availability. Compared to the digital image stored in a computer system, film is not available until several minutes following the procedure, which has important drawbacks when further examinations depend on image-based diagnosis. Later, film may get lost being sent to another physician.

Dose saving. Radiation dose is reduced by the use of pulsed fluoroscopy, last image hold mode, and low frame rate angiography using digital frame gap-filling techniques.

Improved display. By the use of a digital scan converter, real-time display and playback is performed using a high-definition video system and a flicker-free monitor with high scanning line numbers independently of the line rate and the pulses per second at acquisition. Using real-time image processing, the display of small structures can be further improved by edge enhancement filters and digital zoom. Biplane images may be displayed side by side with the same scale for objects within the isocenter of the gantry. During an intervention, a reference scene can be displayed next to or overlaid on live fluoroscopy.

Contrast enhancement. Using proper LUT for white compression or gray-level windowing, image contrast can be adjusted easily. By digital subtraction of a preinjection image, background structures can be removed and the contrast of opacified veins, arteries, or cardiac chambers is amplified. Dynamic subtraction enables the quantity of contrast medium to be reduced. Perfusion of the heart muscle can be visualized by mask mode subtraction and ECG-gated averaging of several images of the capillary phase of a coronary arteriogram.

Image restoration. Due to the nonideal behavior of the image chain, image degradation such as geometrical distortions, scatter radiation and veiling glare, beam hardening, and decrease in contrast ratio affects quantitative measurements. Digital image processing tools are available to restore some of these degradations.

Direct measurements. Diagnostic decisions from angiographic data are primarily based on qualitative, visual analysis of single images or of the passage of a contrast bolus through the beating heart and the arteries. One important stimulus for the development of computerized angiography [17, 18] was the desire to quantify cardiovascular anatomy and function [19]. For example, from geometrical measurements the dimensions of the cardiac chambers and their contraction pattern can be assessed [20, 21]. By measuring the density of contrast-enhanced structures, functional data such as the cardiac ejection fraction or the regurgitation fraction of insufficient valves can be determined [22, 23]. For coronary angiography and for the morphology of peripheral arteriography, localized arterial stenosis must be measured accurately [24]. In a digital environment, all measurements can be performed online provided the corresponding software program is available. Subjective steps such as tracing the edges can be automated, increasing accuracy and decreasing analysis time. Image calibration may not only be performed by calibration balls or grids, but also analytically based on the recorded geometric magnification. Derived data such as the left ventricular volume curve can easily be combined with physiological measurements such as the ventricular pressure. Combined analysis of biplane images or of images of different modalities are promising.

Picture archiving and communication. The storage space for keeping all the screen films and 35-mm cine film rolls from several years is immense. Digital storage saves space and also allows direct access using local or wide-area networks. Copies can be drawn without loss of information. In addition, in a computerized system combination with other data such as physiological data or images of other modalities is easier and faster than using analog storage devices, provided the respective software is available and the digital data exchange protocol is standardized.

Less pollution. Film development and fixation cause pollution due to the release of silver and bromine; this is not the case when the images are stored digitally.

The major impediment to cine film replacement was the missing standard for image exchange. Some laboratories replaced film by analog videotapes or analog optical disks. Others worked with digital tapes or magneto-optical disks. As described below, American and European committees have now accepted a standard for digital imaging and communication in medicine.

Acquisition Modes

To produce optimum-quality X-ray images, a sufficient radiation dose must reach the X-ray detector. During exposure, the dose at the receptor plane is therefore measured and automatically adjusted to a constant level by the X-ray generator. There are three modes of using X-rays in vascular diagnostics: (1) fluoroscopy, (2) cine exposures, and (3) exposure of image series. Fluoroscopy is employed to guide invasive procedures. Typically, continuous radiation at a low dose rate is used. Since attenuation may change quickly, rapid changes in the dose rate are accomplished by adjusting the tube voltage. The images are displayed online on video monitors. Modern systems automatically adjust the radiation in order to optimize image quality while keeping the radiation exposure at a minimum. Here, the continuous radiation is replaced by X-ray pulses of short duration applied for each image required. This mode is called pulsed fluoroscopy (Fig. 23) and provides sharper fluoroscopic images. To avoid any flicker, the images have to be stored in a digital memory and are continuously displayed during exposure gaps (see digital image processor). Depending on the lighting conditions, the human visual system integrates images within about 100–200 ms. It is therefore possible to reduce the radiation dose rate if the frame rate is kept below 10 frames/s and the dose rate can be kept low (0.01 μGy/s).

During fluoroscopy, both tube voltage and current are controlled depending on the attenuation of the patient and the characteristic curve of the equipment (Fig. 24). There are basically three image acquisition strategies: high image quality, low patient dose, and a compromise between the two.

Exposures are employed to visualize and document the diagnostic findings and results of interventions with maximum resolution. The applied methods vary depending on the examined organ. For cardiology, cine exposures with a detector dose of 0.2–1 μGy/frame and high frame rates (12.5–50 images/s) are done to depict fast-moving vessels or the beating heart. Images in series with up to eight images/s and radiation exposures of 0.5–2 μGy are applied to show vessels in other parts of the body with maximum resolution. Since tube voltage is mainly determined by the attenuation of the tissue and the contrasted vessels, the radiation dose is controlled by changing the current and the duration of the exposure.

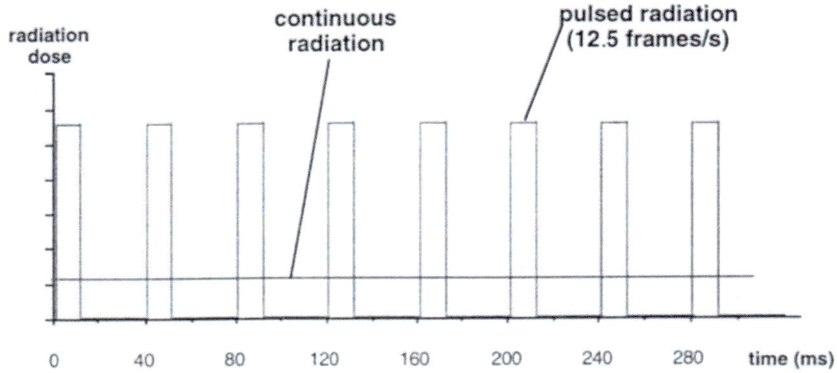

Fig. 23. Principle of pulsed fluoroscopy. Classical fluoroscopy works with continuous radiation, resulting in a low dose per image and blurring of moving objects. Pulsed fluoroscopy uses single short exposures. The images are stored digitally and are displayed until the next exposure occurs. By this method the number of images per second can be reduced, which may lead to less X-ray exposure. Pulsed fluoroscopy results in sharper images

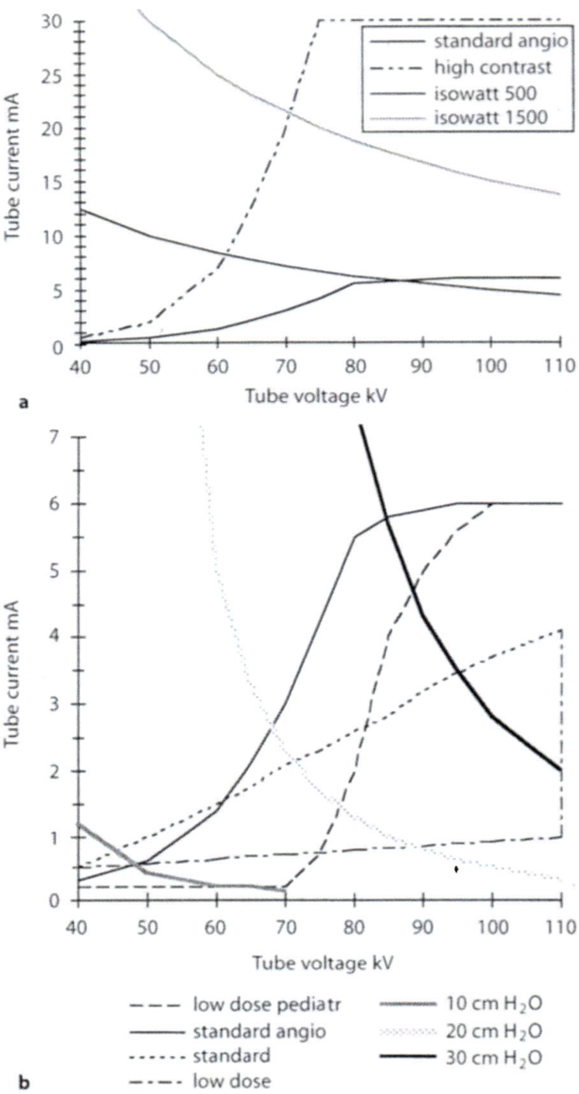

Fig. 24 a, b. Characteristic curves for angiographic fluoroscopy. Tube voltage and current are controlled by the X-ray absorption of the patient. Both parameters are increased until the dose rate at the detector leads to a bright fluoroscopic image. There are several strategies to increase the parameters kV and mA. **a** A typical control curve for angiography and a second one for high-contrast angiography. All control curves are limited by the loadability of the X-ray tube. The isowatt 500 and 1500 curves indicate these limits for different tubes. High dose rates are used in combination with additional beam filtration, i.e., 0.2–0.5 mm Cu to reduce the soft shares of the radiation. **b** Characteristic curves during fluoroscopy for changing the voltage and current of the tube depending on the absorption of the patient. There are different strategies to control voltage and current. For low-dose fluoroscopy the tube voltage is increased, for high-contrast fluoroscopy primarily the current is changed. As a practical example, the absorption curves for 10 cm, 20 cm, and 30 cm H_2O have been included in the diagram. These curves are valid for 0.4 μGy/s at the entrance of the image intensifier and SID=0.9 m

Exposure Control

The proper exposure of an image is guaranteed by measuring the received radiation at the detector. The control system changes the exposure parameters in such a way that an optimum preprogrammed dose value is obtained. During fluoroscopy, the mean brightness level of the image is controlled by changing the three exposure factors, voltage, current, and exposure time (Fig. 25). Each of these parameters has some limitations. Changing the voltage results in a wide dynamic range, but also in much larger changes in dose compared to the other parameters.

Since the contrast of iodine falls with increasing voltages, the contrast of the vessel is also lowered. A range of 60–80 kV for children and 70–90 kV for adults is recommended. Variation in the current is limited to about 800 mA, depending of the type of tube and the size of the focal spot used. The duration of exposure can be varied. In cardiology, times between 5–8 ms for adults and 2–4 ms for children are used. Short duration is employed to avoid motion artifacts of moving vessels. Shorter exposures will degrade the image quality because of time lag in the image intensifier.

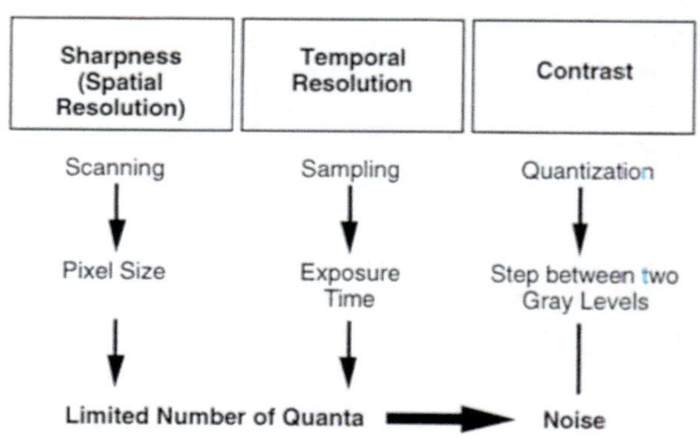

Fig. 25. Image quality may be defined by sharpness, contrast, and temporal resolution. In addition to the basic exposure parameters like voltage, current, and exposure time, digital radiography is limited by pixel size and size of the quantization step. These two parameters are interrelated by the acceptable noise level in the image. Since the number of quanta per pixel is limited, this leads to noise in the image. As a consequence, the size of the quantization step has to be adjusted

Reduction in Scattered Radiation

The best practical method to reduce stray radiation is the proper use of collimators to limit the radiation beam to the exposed area.

A collimator is a radiation-absorbing metal sheet. It is located in the tube housing and should be as close as possible to the anode (see Fig. 13). Circular and rectangular collimators are available. Partially absorbent contoured filters are often used to mask low-absorbing parts in the image, for example bright areas of lung tissue around the heart. Direct radiation to the detector has to be avoided. Proper collimating also minimizes off-focus radiation. This reduces radiation to patient and staff. To further reduce the amount of scattered radiation in the image, radiographic grids are placed between the patient and the image detector, resulting in an increased image contrast. Because of the inherent absorption of the grid, the radiation exposure has to be increased. Focused grids with 40 lines/cm and a factor of 6:1 and 10:1 are used for cine angiography. Carbon fiber grids are recommended because of the low absorption of primary radiation. The performance of the grid depends very much on the characteristics of the X-ray equipment used. Digital imaging systems offer contrast enhancement schemes to compensate for the influence of scatter in the image.

Radiation Safety and Guidelines

Radiation Exposure

Guidelines. Owing to ultrasound techniques and magnetic resonance angiography, it is possible to shorten or even dispense with some vascular X-ray examinations. However, the demand for definite and reliable definition of the cardiac and vascular structures has increased due to the expansion of percutaneous, minimally invasive, and surgical cardiovascular interventions. In addition, in coronary X-ray imaging, for example, the radiation dose has been increased owing to the introduction of interventions. In individual cases, this can lead to a high radiation exposure. In general, with the increasing use of interventional procedures, radiation exposure to patients and staff working in the X-ray room has increased.

Therefore, physicians performing catheterizations should have special training in radiation physics and radiation protection. At this stage, various national guidelines must be considered for each country. The International Commission on Radiological Protection (ICRP) has published important recommendations [34].

Some of the basic relationships and guidelines are presented here: for in-depth information, the reader is referred to the original literature [2, 34, 35]. To assess the radiation energy released in tissue, it is best to measure the ionization of air by a calibrated ionization chamber. By using a transparent ionization chamber fixed at the housing of the X-ray tube, all the radiation sent to the patient is measured to obtain the so-called dose-area product. Since this quantity is independent of the distance from the focal spot, the radiation exposure can be derived when the focus-to-object distance is known.

Units. The amount of electrical charge is measured in coulombs per kilogram of air. The traditional unit of the ionization dose is the roentgen (R); 1 R liberates 2.58×10^{-4} coulomb/kg air, which corresponds to the generation of 2×10^9 pairs of ions in 1 cm^3 air under normal pressure at 0°C.

As X-rays are part of the electromagnetic energy spectrum, the natural units of the radiation energy absorbed per kilogram mass are joules per kilogram. The name of this unit is gray (Gy), and 1 Gy is equal to 1 J/kg. The dose rate is measured as grays per second. For air, water, and tissue, the relation between the ionization dose and the absorbed dose is about 1 R = 8.7 mGy. Due to higher absorption, the conversion factor for muscle is 9.2 and for bone about 36, provided diagnostic X-ray energies are used.

In order to take into account other biologically effective kinds of radiation, e.g., neutrons, the quantity dose equivalent (DE) has been introduced. Its unit is the Sievert (Sv). For diagnostic radiation, the DE of 1 Gy is 1 Sv. Older units are rad and rem (100 rad = 1 Gy, 100 rem=1 Sv).

Another unit is the effective dose equivalent (EDE). This quantity is a weighted average of the organ doses, whereby the weighting factors take into account the estimated radiosensitivity for the genetic or somatic effects of the respective organs. For a total body exposure the EDE equals the DE. The Biological Effects of Ionizing Radiation (BEIR) committee [35] has estimated that the lifetime excess risk of death from radiation-induced cancer is about 8% per 1 Sv EDE. This figure is lower for elderly men and probably twice as high for children and infants.

Image Doses. As discussed above, the image intensifier entrance dose may not be lowered under a certain limit because there is a threshold level of object contrast to noise below which small objects cannot be visualized. For film cassette systems, the minimum dose is determined by their sensitivity. Some typical image doses are listed in Table 4.

Table 4. Typical image doses and dose rates

Acquisition mode	Sensitivity[a] (mGy/D)	Image dose[a] (*D*) (µGy)	Resolution[b] (lp/mm)
Screen-film systems			
High definition	50	20.0	4.0
	100	10.0	3.4
Universal	200	5.0	2.8
High speed	400	2.5	2.4
	800	1.3	2.0
Image intensifier systems[d]			
Fluoroscopy at 50 fps		0.2 – 0.6 µGy/s	1.5
		0.004 – 0.012 µGy/frame	0.5
Cine coronary arteriography,		0.1 – 1.0 µGy/frame	2
single shots, DSA		5 µGy	3

DSA, digital subtraction angiography; fps, frames per second.
[a] Dose required to obtain an optical density of value 1.
[b] Minimum values are given.
[c] Related to a field diameter of 25 cm

The dose at the image intensifier input is set, depending on the application, at about 0.1 µGy (10 µR) per single frame for the cine mode and at 0.5 µGy (50 – 100 µR) for a low image frequency. For intravenous DSA, a higher dose must be used because of the low image contrast. In the case of fluoroscopy, the dose rate may be reduced drastically (down to 0.2 µG/s≈20 µR/s) because the moving image seems to be less noisy than the static one, as the human eye averages the stochastic fluctuations over a duration of about 200 ms. The resolution given in Table 4 is obtained by the features of the cassette system or limited by quantum noise for an object of 30 % image contrast.

Some systems provide the option of high-contrast fluoroscopy. In this mode, the milliampere value is increased by a factor of 3 and the kilovolt value is decreased correspondingly. In consequence, image contrast is improved and radiation exposure is increased considerably. The upper value of the screen dose should be kept below 0.6 µGy/s. High-contrast fluoroscopy should be selected only for a short time, e.g., to improve the visibility of a small device for an intervention.

These figures apply to an image intensifier input screen with a diameter of 23 cm (9 in). For smaller fields of view, a higher image dose must be applied to keep the brightness of the output screen constant. The image dose may be increased in inverse proportion to the reduction in area and/or the diaphragm in front of the television camera is opened correspondingly. Because of the associated high-input dose, the smallest field of view should be used only when highest spatial resolution is necessary.

Balancing System Resolution. According to Rose's criterion stated earlier (Eq. 6), spatial resolution depends on the dose at the image intensifier input screen and on the contrast. Let us assume that the resolution of an object of 10 % contrast recorded with a dose of 0.1 µGy is only 0.5 lp/mm. If the resolution is to be raised to 1.5 lp/mm, one either has to increase the dose tenfold or to increase the contrast threefold (Eq. 7). Higher contrast may be attained by a more selective technique of injection. Another method would be to reduce the X-ray voltage in a suitable way (e.g., from 80 to 75 kV; see Fig. 5).

However, to make optimal use of the information given, one may also choose to adjust any of the other stages of the image chain determining the resolution of the system. This approach is called balancing the system. Apart from the quantum noise, the size of the tube's focus and the size of the digital pixel elements may limit the spatial resolution and must be mutually adjusted.

With a diameter a of the focal spot and a magnification m of the recorded object, the resolution limit is $1/a(m - 1)$. The magnification is calculated as quotient of the source-to-image distance and the source-to-object distance. For example, at a magnification of 1.4 and an effective focal spot of 1.3 mm, the resolution of the system is limited to 1.9 lp/mm. For a spot size of 0.6 × 0.6 mm, focal blurring is usually not critical.

The resolution may be limited by the matrix of digitization, especially for the largest field of view (Table 1). At a screen diameter of 17 cm and 512 lines, it is possible to obtain a resolution of 1.5 lp/mm. We can see that, in general, it is not useful to emit rays at a high dose if digitization with an old 256-matrix system is employed. On the other hand, storing a 1024-matrix system or higher is not justified if all the other components of the imaging system are not equivalent to this high resolution.

In addition, structure mottle (stemming from the graininess of the image intensifier output screen) and electronic noise of the television preamplifier may degrade resolution. In most systems, these components are less important than quantum and digitization noise. In difference images (DSA), structure noise vanishes while quantum noise increases.

Motion blur may also contribute to the total image blur. The motion of the objects during the time of exposures must be small. Otherwise, a blurring of the edges of the shadows occurs for large objects and a loss of contrast for small objects. While in peripheral arteriography with 2 frames/s the exposure time may be 150 ms or even longer, in cardiology it is limited to 2–4 ms for children and to 5–8 ms for adults. For imaging the coronaries, short exposure times must be selected even when only end-diastolic images are obtained at a low frame rate.

Some people using a conventional cine film system believe that noisy images are caused by silver crystals in the emulsion of the cine film. However, cine film material now no longer produces quantum mottle. In high-sensitivity screen films, structure noise of the screens may limit spatial resolution.

Digital images may look noisier than cine films. However, assuming that the same low dose was applied, this is due to utilization of methods for contrast enhancement such as digital edge enhancement or image subtraction. These techniques amplify not only the contrast of the opacified vessels, but make noise more visible as well. The SNR is improved without increasing the dose.

Radiation Protection. Legislation limits radiation doses only to the staff, not to patients. The principle of optimizing the application of radiation is ALARA (i.e., as low as reasonably achievable). Practical application of the ALARA principle must be investigated in all diagnostic applications of radiation. The issue is not reduction in radiation at any price, but optimizing its application. This requirement is combined with the guideline that any medical application of radiation must be performed under an authorized physician and that there is strict surveillance of radiation protection and quality control of appliances.

Measuring patient entry exposure routinely heightens the awareness of the angiographer of the need to use the minimum exposure at all times. Proper dose management requires a clear, real-time display of the utilized dose rate, the total dose per examination, and cumulative fluoroscopy time. If it is not measured, radiation exposure can be estimated from the voltage, current, exposure time, filtration, and geometry of the X-ray source. In any case, all data on image generation, both fixed and variable, should be routinely recorded for review and documentation.

Depending on the image dose rate (Table 4), the size of the patient, and the field of view, the entrance surface dose of the patient from the direct beam of a fluoroscopic X-ray system is typically between 0.01 and 0.05 Gy/min. Less than 1 h of fluoroscopy and several cine angiographic runs may be connected with an interventional radiographic procedure. The total exposure of about 3 Gy can result in skin injury and epilation.

It is logically also in the interest of the staff inside the X-ray room to limit patient exposure, as the scattered radiation spread by the patient is still about 1% of patient exposure. In adult cardiology in particular, radiation exposure of the angiographer and assistant can reach high levels [36]. Most of the staff dose is attributed to scatter from the patient. Compared to fluoroscopy, the scatter rate is high during cine filming, and highest at a high frame rate and with a biplane unit. By doubling the distance to the patient, the angiographer can reduce his or her exposure by a factor of 4. The use of dosimeters is mandatory for anyone working in the laboratory. Instruction on the principles of radiation protection and methods of minimizing patient and staff exposure should be given on a regular basis.

Radiation exposure of the operator depends very much on the position in respect to patient and X-ray tube. Most of the radiation is due to the backscattered radiation from the patient. This is most critical in those situations in which the tube is positioned above the patient. Systems with an image intensifier above the table and a shielded tube under the table are optimal. An X-ray-dense glass shield suspended from the ceiling should be positioned between tube and operator. Leaded drapes should be attached to the patient support. Mobile protective barriers should be considered for the protection of other workers in the laboratory.

Lead aprons protect most of the active bone marrow and the gonads: 0.5 mm lead stops 98% of the scattered beam, and a 0.25-mm lead apron, which is lighter, still stops about 96% and may be used to protect the back. In addition, leaded collars should be worn to protect the thyroid. Eyeglasses with glass equivalent to 0.5 mm lead decrease exposure of the eyes considerably. Ordinary glass lenses have some protective value, but plastic lenses offer virtually no protection.

Lowering Exposure

There are several operator-related methods of lowering radiation exposure. These include controling the optimal X-ray spectrum by selecting the tube voltage and proper X-ray filter, collimating the beam to the area of interest, and keeping the effective time of exposure as short as possible.

X-Ray Spectrum. The highest quantum detection efficiency of the CsI screen of the image intensifier is in the 33- to 55-keV range. Photons below that energy only increase patient dose and should be stopped by a filter. Studies comparing different filter materials led to the conclusion that aluminum, copper, and iron filter are optimal for a broad range of applications [37, 38]. At least 2.5 mm aluminum are routinely used.

Clear visualization of small vessels filled with iodine contrast agents is the primary task in vascular applications. Furthermore, small-sized interventional instruments such as balloons, catheters, and guidewires must be visualized during fluoroscopy. When mean photon energy is increased above 50 keV, both detection efficiency and image contrast become worse, but the dose absorbed by the patient becomes smaller (Fig. 5). Larger objects require higher photon energy. The larger the object thickness, the higher the optimum photon energy and the tube voltage are. A tube with high loadability permits the use of strong filtration, which narrows the X-ray spectrum.

Additional filtration is especially recommended for high absorption, e.g., obese patients or steeply angled projections. The additional filters mainly used are 0.1 to 0.5-mm thick copper sheaths, depending on the heat storage and dissipation rate of the tube [39]. Since these filters also reduce the amount of hard radiation, it is necessary to apply a significantly higher energy to reach an image quality similar to the nonfiltered situation. For thick filters, there is a trade-off between the reduction in patient dose by removing low-energy photons and the degradation of image quality in terms of the SNR. Table 5 presents these relations qualitatively.

Table 5. Change in patient dose and image contrast with change in voltage

Voltage	Radiation	Absorption	Entrance dose	Image contrast
Low	Soft	High	Large	Hard
High	Hard	Low	Small	Soft

Projection. The smallest field of view of the image intensifier may be selected to increase spatial resolution (Table 1). However, the associated increase in the image dose may cause the system for automatic exposure control to set kilovolt values to a high level and to select a large focal spot. Both factors degrade image quality.

Steeply angulated views entail significant increases in the output capacity of the X-ray generator. The long absorption pathway in the patient and the extended source-to-input distance associated with these views may lead to high tube voltages. The inevitable result is an unsatisfactory image quality when large patients are examined.

Collimating. The X-ray beam size must not exceed the visible image dimensions. If possible, the collimator edges should be visible during fluoroscopy. Careful collimating of the beam to the specific area of interest decreases both patient and operator EDE. An important beneficial effect of collimating is the increased image contrast, since scattered radiation is reduced as the irradiated field size decreases. Semitransparent, sickle-shaped filters are useful to avoid saturation effects and to homogenize the image. Exact positioning of collimators and semitransparent filters can be assisted by placing virtual collimators in the last image hold.

Appropriate lead shielding of organs of the patient not examined is mandatory. Protection of the gonads is of particular importance.

Effective Irradiation Time. The simplest way of reducing radiation should not be overlooked, i.e., to only radiate as long as necessary. This is not only a question of operating the unit. A short time of exposure can also be achieved by the help of technical devices. Pulsed fluroscopy is one example. For continuous flicker-free display, digital memory is used for gap-filling.

Another example is the use of image memory integrated within the digital X-ray unit for freezing the last image of a fluoroscopic sequence and showing it as a still image for some time after the end of the fluoroscopy. In order to reduce the quantum noise, this image is usually averaged over the last four to ten frames. For example, to determine the position of the catheters, only a very short exposure is required.

For angiographic series, reduction in the effective time of exposure can also be achieved. In digital angiography, it is possible to choose an image rate that is adapted to the application mode and the medical issue. In cardiology, it is no longer necessary to conduct every examination with 50 or 60 images/s, as was done when conventional video systems were used. Digital X-ray units allow a very flexible technique of shooting, and gap-filling techniques are used for playback. High frame rates may still be necessary for analyzing ventricular function or for capturing a short pass of contrast medium, especially in pediatric cardiology. In some cases, it is enough to record end-diastolic and end-systolic images triggered by the ECG.

Any sequence should be as short as possible. This is supported by an electronically controlled injector triggered by the start of exposure and by high-quality monitors and digital contrast enhancement techniques.

Medical Issue

All the above-mentioned means and relationships should be considered when designing and operating an angiography system. The question of the optimum setting for the individual parameters mainly depends on issues such as patient size, the site of injection of the contrast medium, and, above all, the need to visualize very small structures. For example, in the case of examinations of the heart, the decision concerning optimum settings depends on whether the ventricular morphology, the definition of the great vessels, the coronary artery tree, or a localized stenotic area is to be visualized. Guidelines for standard examinations have been published [40, 41].

To maintain images of consistently high quality, the staff of the catheterization laboratory must understand the capability, function, operation, and limitations of all the components in the imaging chain. The aim is to utilize the methods of keeping patient radiation exposure low, but to still obtain the information which is diagnostically necessary. However, good quality of the image on the one hand and low exposure on the other are not always opposing factors. Automatic exposure control provides an optimal exposure mainly when the lead collimators at the tube are faded in correctly and the patient is positioned in the correct way in terms of the central region of the picture, because the brightness of this region is used to control the exposure. This also helps to obtain good picture quality and low radiation exposure.

It is fundamental that the diagnostic questions and patient-related factors are defined as clearly as possible before radiation is applied and that the required dose per image and the pulse rate are adjusted to meet these demands. To achieve this goal, a clear understanding of the technical aspects of examination is necessary. Thus the question of how to put the ALARA principle into practice arises in every case and must be considered anew whenever a new unit is installed.

Quality Control

Constancy Tests. To ensure optimum performance, the angiographic equipment requires testing after installation using the acceptance test and later repeatedly using the constancy tests. These tests mainly concern the following: input dose levels for the most commonly used imaging modes, stability of brightness and optical density, exposure time, stability of voltage, focal spot size, spatial resolution, contrast resolution, temporal resolution, and subtraction artifacts [42].

Standardized acceptance tests are necessary to assure that the equipment has all the capabilities required and to verify performance of all components. It is also used to establish a reference performance level for future comparison. The acceptable radiation dose levels are set and documented together with typical images of test phantoms.

Constancy tests should be done quarterly or when image quality is degraded and/or essential components have been exchanged. These tests should include characterization of the dynamic range of the system, the spatial and contrast resolution, the automatic exposure control circuit, and the input radiation doses for typical, well-defined conditons. Fluoroscopy and cine exposure values should be monitored every 3 months to verify their acceptability. Automatic adjustment of the beam size should be verified for units with multiple-mode image intensifiers.

All test results should be fully documented. The digital imaging system itself can help to evaluate the images of the constancy test reproducibility, not only for the whole image chain but for each component. Image intensifiers deteriorate at a rate of 5%–7% per year and may need to be replaced in 3–5 years depending on the frequency of examinations. Their conversion factor and contrast ratio values fall gradually below the level of acceptability required to maintain safe exposure levels and high image quality.

In addition, the computer for image processing is part of the system, as are the monitors. Brightness and contrast must be adjusted in a standard fashion using a test picture. There are special standards for acceptance and constancy testing of DSA systems.

For conventional systems, special attention must be paid to the film processor. Problems concerning the film subsystem can significantly degrade image quality. Inadequate control of the processing cycle is one of the most common causes of poor-quality images. Factors affecting quality of photographic processing are time, temperature, and replenishment of developing media and its agitation. Sensitometry is an objective method of measuring density, sensitivity, gross fog, average gradient, and exposure range from the characteristic curve of the film. Normal and abnormal conditions and any trends are detected by plotting the results, measured daily or at least weekly, against time.

Quality Assurance. This is more than just quality control. It is a comprehensive program including training of staff, procedures that guarantee acquisition of high-quality images at reasonably low X-ray exposure, correct interpretation of these images, reliability of quantitative measurements, ergonomic quality of the complete system, and long-term internal and external quality assurance procedures. It must be understood as a dynamic process managed as a feedback loop within each department and between the users and the manufacturers.

Automatic data logging, e.g., of X-ray exposure, during fluoroscopy and cine runs is of considerable help. Complete documentation and adequate screening is very important for any quality assurance. In the catheterization laboratory, the particular areas of activity (e.g., the physiological system, the X-ray equipment, the image processing workstation with all its parts, and the hospital information system) should be regarded as subsystems of one integrated system. The basic guidelines for assessment and quality control are standardized, and complete documentation of each patient examination, including medication, angiograms, measurements, actions, events, and complications is mandatory. Optimum utilization of catheter laboratory technology for interventional procedures is one of the major safeguards for high-quality cardiovascular interventions.

Special Applications

In the preceding paragraphs, general aspects and requirements valid for all kinds of angiographic examinations have been presented. Angiographic systems may be separated into general-purpose systems and specialized systems. In the following, those features which are needed for specific examinations are outlined.

Cardiac/Coronary Applications

For cardiac applications, the equipment has to satisfy special requirements. Multiaxial positioning is needed to allow steeply angulated radiographic views. When the heart is positioned in the rotational center of the gantry, it is projected onto the center of the image intensifier for all angulations. To obtain steep sagittal plane angulation, image intensifiers with diameters larger than 23 cm (9 in) are not recommended. To allow the procedure to be performed from both sides via the femoral or brachial approach, free access to the patient is required. Easy manual positioning and automatic movement to preprogrammed positions by microprocessor control are necessary. Free and fast access to the patient is required in emergencies. The table must be stable to allow emergency treatment, including resuscitation. The table should also be comfortable to allow lengthy procedures, particularly in elderly patients. The advantages of biplane feature in adult cardiology include reliable right ventricular volume determination, the ability to visualize the coronary artery tree from two orthogonal views simultaneously, and easier and faster placement of catheters and devices in interventional procedures.

In cardioangiography of adults, exposures with 25 and 30 images/s or 12.5 and 15 images/s for coronary arteries are necessary in Europe and the United States, respectively. Lower frame rates allow a lower radiation dose rate and should be used whenever the diagnostic situation permits. The different frame rates are due to the different frequencies of the public power supply, i.e., 60 Hz in the United States and 50 Hz in Europe. The image frequency of the video signals is synchronized to these frequencies to avoid hum and other artifacts in the image. Consequently, the pulse rates of fluoroscopy and image series are also in phase with these oscillations.

Quantitative image analysis is an integral part of diagnostic evaluations in cardiology. In addition to quantification of coronary artery stenosis, the ventriculogram is quantitatively analyzed and the electrophysiological and hemodynamic parameters determined. To this end, interactive methods of border definition and automated calculations are available. Ejection fraction and coronary flow reserve are the main quantitative parameters of the ventricular function. To calibrate the software for geometrical measurements, a grid, sphere, or catheter with known size is used. For an object in the center of the X-ray beams, analytical calibration is possible. During interventional procedures, rapid measurements of distances are needed.

Before the advent of digital catheterization laboratories, the 35-mm cine film was the primary storage medium in cardiography. Larger-format spot-film radiography and serial-film radiography are now rarely used in adult cardiac catheterization; however, they are important in examinations of patients with certain congenital heart disorders, e.g., diseases of the aorta, and pulmonary, cerebral, visceral, and peripheral vessels. Typically, the 35-mm camera is attached to the image intensifier. It receives a copy of the image by using a semi-transparent mirror. Special 35-mm projectors are used for display. Despite all the technical developments thus far, the 35-mm film remains the "gold standard" in cardiology. Videotapes (VHS and S-VHS) are widely used as an alternative, inexpensive storage medium. The video image quality is lower than in other storage media and its shelf time is limited.

The weak point of digital heart catheterization laboratories at present remains the storage and archiving of the images as digital data. Videotapes are acceptable only as an intermediate step and means of data transfer. CD-Medical has been designed as a digital storage medium for images and may replace 35-mm cine film as the archiving medium of cardiac image series in the near future. CD-Medical is a digital optical disk similar to an audio CD. It is a specialized CD-ROM and can store over 500 MByte of data, corresponding to 4000 single digital images with a compression of 1:2. In addition, image series for real-time viewing are stored on the same disk with higher compression ratios of 1:7 up to 1:15. To support real-time viewing of image series, a data set with the very high compression ratio of 1:60 may be added to the CD. CD-ROM can be read by all modern computer systems and has made it possible to archive digital cardiograms with diagnostic quality. CD-Medical promises easier handling than cine film. It needs no chemical processing, requires less storage space, and is cheaper. Each CD-Medical disk is designed to hold one patient study. The images are stored as original digital data. To view single images and image series, simple personal computers are needed as viewing stations. The disks can be duplicated without loss of information. American and European committees of National Electrical Manufacturers association (ACR-NEMA and CEN TC251 WG4) have now accepted a standard for digital imaging and communications in medicine (DICOM-3) [43]. Several manufacturers followed the recommendations of the American College of Cardiology [44] and the European Society of Cardiology [45] and offer angiographic systems that employ the standardized recordable CD (CD-R) as an integrated medium [46]. This is a real breakthrough and opens up the way for open digital and uniform communication. The 35-mm film, still used as the main medium for image archiving and exchange of angiograms, can be replaced by the CD-R and used to store all image sequences of one examination.

Pediatric Applications

In cardioangiography of children, biplane systems with a small image intensifier diameter of 23 cm (9 in) and high frame rates, i.e., 25 and 30 or 50 and 60 exposures/s are needed in Europe and the United States, respectively. Subtraction of a mask image has to be available for reviewing acquired ventriculograms and postoperative intravenous angiocardiograms. Special analytical programs are used for the analysis of right ventricular function and vascular malformations. Because of the small dimensions in infants and children, the gonadal dose is relatively high. The higher activity of bone marrow increases the risk of later malignant disease. Due to the long life-span ahead of children, a strict indication for X-ray examination must be given, and radiation protection is of particular importance.

Peripheral Vascular Applications

To visualize the blood flow through peripheral vessels, it is necessary to cover the area from the abdominal projection to the feet without interruption. The long film cassettes that were formerly used have now been substituted by a sequence of films or a set of digitally acquired images. There are three methods allowing uninterrupted peripheral X-ray arteriography: (1) film changer with stepping, (2)

DSA runs per position, and (3) DSA as one run following the contrast bolus, so-called bolus chasing.

In film-based peripheral angiography, a stationary changer of large films (35 × 35 cm) is used. Modern C-arms offer a combination of image intensifier and film changer (30 films, 4 exposures/s), so-called PUCK. During the passage of the contrast medium, the examination table and the patient are moved stepwise from the abdominal position to the feet. At each position an exposure is taken. To adjust for the varying thickness of the object, a stepwise reduction in tube voltage is needed. The timing of the table movement and of each exposure has to be carefully programmed in advance, according to the assumed flow of contrast medium through the vasculature. Handling of the film cassettes is cumbersome, and there is a time delay before the images of the examination are developed and ready for reading on the light box. Even with properly timed and exposed series, vessels below the trifurcation regularly have such low contrast that they are hardly visible. With the advent of digital image storage and image intensifiers with a large field of view to cover the abdomen, it became possible to perform peripheral angiography with electronic image acquisition. During the procedure the images are shown on video monitors, allowing the flow of the contrast medium to be controlled directly. Abdominal angiography requires image intensifiers with large fields of view (38 – 40 cm in diameter) and additional reduction in field size (electronic zoom) for small objects to obtain a spatial resolution comparable with conventional films. For a 38-cm image intensifier, the smaller diameters are 31, 25, 20, and 17 cm. With a 38-cm image intensifier, it is possible to cover the entire length from bifurcation to the feet with five to six overlapping positions. The most commonly used matrix size of the image is 1024×1024. A smaller matrix may be applicable for a small field of view and for the visualization of small contrasts.

To improve visualization of the small vessels with diluted contrast medium, DSA is needed. It requires a pixel depth of 10 bits or 8 bits with analog logarithmic amplification.

There are several methods of performing DSA. The most common method is the stepwise approach with a DSA run at each position, resulting in a complete overview of the whole situation. Timing problems do not exist with this technique, and different flow speeds in the two legs do not present any problem, because image acquisition is continued until the bolus has passed the location. This stepwise DSA requires multiple injections, but each injection may be done with a lower volume than is usual for a complete runoff.

Another method is to acquire the images as one complete runoff with only one injection. With bolus chasing, a continuous table shift is used during the run in order to keep track with the progress of the bolus in the vessels. Exposures are made during the table movement, and an automatic exposure control ensures reduction in tube voltage in relation to object thickness and short exposure times to avoid lack of sharpness due to motion. The bolus chasing technique offers two operating modes, interactive and automatic.

The *interactive mode* is the ideal choice for handling peripheral runoff procedures where the ability to see and control exactly what is happening is of primary importance. The acquisition run is controlled via a hand switch changing the speed of the table top. The operator can follow the contrast bolus, as it is displayed in real time on the monitor. If a second run is made without contrast fluid, the images can be viewed with subtraction. The *automatic mode* is often preferable in situations where large numbers of routine examinations are performed. In the automatic mode, examination parameters are preset by prior measurement of knee arrival time. This procedure requires only minimal contrast medium and X-ray doses. The table movement speed and exposure rate can be set exactly in accordance with the individual patient's anatomy. In both modes, the radiologist is always free to perform additional image acquisition for DSA, if required.

The size of the vessels can be measured manually and is used to calculate the degree of stenosis. Calibration of the measurements is possible with fiducial points. Programs exist for automatical contour detection and subsequent calculation of vessel dimensions and analysis of stenoses.

Neurovascular Applications

Angiography systems for neuroangiography should be optimized for high spatial resolution, e.g., to show small vessels such as the lenticostriate or the anterior spinal artery. Digital fluoroscopy and digital acquisition with 1024×1024 image acquisition, processing, real-time display, storage, and analysis are required for a fast and save examination. The faint contrasts have to be enhanced by digital image processing. The most commonly used exposure method is intra-arterial DSA. The high speed of the blood flow requires image series of 6–12.5 exposures/s. The applied image processing functions are contrast enhancement, noise reduction, edge enhancement, and mask subtraction DSA.

To facilitate the positioning of catheters during fluoroscopy, special functions called road mapping and trace subtraction are used. For road mapping, the actual fluoroscopic image is overlaid with a digitally stored image taken in advance showing the vessel filled with contrast medium. The two images are combined to form one image on the monitor. This gives a better orientation in advancing the catheter. To improve the sharpness of the images, pulsed fluoroscopy is recommended. If the number of exposures can be reduced to less than five frames per s, considerable reduction in dose is possible. To reduce noise in fluoroscopy, multiple images may be continuously averaged. This method can also be used for dose reduction, but it leads to lack of sharpness due to moving objects.

The system has to be easily maneuverable and should allow easy access to the patient, especially during interventions. The main functions have to be controlled near the table, including direct interaction with the images on the monitors in the catheterization laboratory. To shorten the duration of the examination, acquisition programs for setting dose (kV, mA), exposure time, frame speed, focus size, and image processing parameters have to be preprogrammed. The digital images are calibrated and used to quantitatively analyze diameter and stenosis of vessels and perfusion of tissue.

The three-dimensional structure of the cerebral vessels requires multiple projections to cover the part of the vascular tree being studied without distortions. Angulations and rotations of the system therefore have to be performed fast and easily. Biplane systems are used to reduce the duration of the procedure and to reduce contrast medium. A new method of image acquisition is rotational angiography. It adds perspective to the images. During a fast rotation of X-ray tube and image intensifier around the ROI, a series of images is taken in short sequence showing the vessel of interest in different projections. The dynamic display of the image series gives a good impression of the three-dimensional situation. The total range of rotation varies between 90° and 180°. To cover the vessel with good opacification by the bolus of the contrast medium, the rotational speed has to be as high as 30°/s. A frame rate of 8–25 images per s is sufficient. To avoid lack of sharpness due to movements, the duration of the X-ray pulses has to be limited to 8–15 ms. In a second run, mask images not containing contrast material may be acquired. These mask images are subsequently subtracted from the first series with the opaque vessel to improve the contrast of the vessels. Rotational angiography is used for orientation. When the best projection angle is found to show an abnormality, a separate run is made using the conventional technique.

Venography

Direct visualization of the vessels during the peripheral runoff and the dynamic display of the image series give a good impression of the three-dimensional situation. Tiltable tables are needed to allow complete filling of the vessels.

In venography screen film systems are widely used because of their large field of view and insensitivity to direct X-ray exposure. Digital venography requires good positioning of the patient legs using peripheral filters to avoid direct exposure to the image intensifier, which would lead to artifacts due to veiling glare. The advantages of digital venography are dose reduction by use of the image intensifier, direct display of dynamic filling, improved dynamic range, and DSA for contrast enhancement.

Multifunctional Systems

Modern angiographic systems offer such flexibility in specification and operation that they can be configured both for general angiography and special applications such as neuroangiography or cardioangiography. All applications need a powerful X-ray generator and tube, patient support, a stand with a wide range of possible projection and good maneuverability, digital image storage and processing unit with 1 K × 1 K image matrix, and accessories such as displays, viewers, a film processor, and an injector. High image quality and ease of operation are general requirements. Exposure parameters for the different examination types can be stored as presets. In respect to size of the image intensifier, frame speed, and size of image memory, a compromise has to be found. General angiography requires an image intensifier with a large field of view, e.g., with a diameter of 38 cm. This may be an obstacle for some specific projections in neuro- or cardioangiography. If a biplane system is installed, the lateral plane can be moved to a parking position if it is not needed.

System Design and Purchase Selection

At first glance, it seems advantageous to build and buy a universally designed X-ray system for all kinds of cardiovascular imaging. However, there are also obstacles in using these systems.

Facilities for clinical procedures can differ in many technical features. For instance, in cardiology high pulse rates and short pulse times are necessary, whereas image subtraction (DSA) is more important for peripheral angiography. In pediatric cardiology, however, image subtraction is also frequently used to diagnose congenital heart disease. Different applications also require different sizes of the image intensifier and of the spatial resolution. Some applications need a flexible biplane isocentric gantry. Solutions for digital long-term storage may be different for a cardiology department and a radiological facility. Each subdiscipline uses specific software programs for image quantification. Equipment designed to fulfill all the different requirements in a perfect way would be expensive and difficult to operate.

Before a new radiographic imaging system is purchased, the main clinical requirements should be considered. Defining the clinical requirements carefully will help to avoid the mistake of choosing a particular system without first determining the current and future needs. When image quality is of prime importance for a certain type of procedure, specific in-built facilities must be provided. On the other hand, it may be beneficial to the institution to purchase a more general imaging system that will provide acceptable image quality for vascular and cardiac types of examinations, but potentially at the expense of image quality and performance for each application.

The following questions must be asked: How many examinations of each kind are done annually? What are the clinical needs in a few years? How important are interventional facilities? How much money is available?

To obtain the optimum system, understanding the pros and cons of the different options is essential, first to write a purchase specification document and then for proper discussion with the different manufacturers. Hardly any systems provide consistently high quality images for all types of examinations; however, a suitable compromise can be achieved between universal and specific applications. It is important that each user understands the inherent differences between the equipment design of different manufacturers and is aware of how each design decision may affect the overall image quality and performance. During the negotation phase, the buyer and future user is in the strongest position to obtain a state-of-the-art system that fulfills all the requirements for a reasonable price. However, whenever possible, he or she should avoid special case solutions because, as a rule, later updates are rarely possible and servicing may be more difficult.

Conclusion

Although X-ray imaging, the oldest of all medical imaging techniques, was 100 years old in 1995, significant progress in applications and in technical development is still underway. Purely diagnostic vascular radiographic examinations have become less important, whereas new fields of minimally invasive therapy have been added. There is a close relationship between the development of interventional procedures on the one hand and of hardware and software solutions for improved image acquisition, high-quality presentation, and fast analysis techniques on the other hand.

The widespread use of catheter interventions has fostered an ongoing interest in the improvement of on-site image quality and fast quantitative evaluations, providing the operator with important information on the result and allowing decisions to be made on the spot. In addition, digital systems offer the potential for online fusion and combined analysis of biplane projections or of vascular images from other imaging modalities, such as vascular ultrasound.

Imaging with X-rays is basically limited by the physical nature of radiation and the generation of a projectional image. Even with an ideal detector system, the image quality is degraded by quantum noise, scattered radiation, and geometrical distortions.

From the technical point of view, a chain is only as strong as its weakest link. The imaging system is an example of this kind of chain. Its elements are not perfect, and different image degradations limit image quality and quantitative measurements. Promising future developments are related to the detector system, the image processor, the software for image processing, and fast digital storage media. Understanding the principles of the state-of-the-art imaging technology is crucial to proper selection, purchase, and operation of a vascular or cardiac imaging system. Even for a well-designed system, a fully automatic, one-button operation scarcely leads to optimum images at reasonably low exposure rates.

Proper collimation and positioning, proper frame rate and zooming selection, proper preparation and breathing of the patient, and correct bolus injection presuppose basic understanding of the principles of radiography and expertise of trained staff. Consistent operation, easy maneuverability, and reliability of the equipment reduces the risk for the patient and allows fast access in critical situations. Radiation dose for the patient and staff should be kept at the lowest possible level. This is of utmost importance for long interventional procedures and pediatric examinations. Continuous discussion of image quality is necessary to ensure continued optimal imaging, especially for training of new staff in the catheterization laboratory.

Quality control of the radiographic system and quality assurance of the complete examination are becoming increasingly important. Quality assurance of interventional procedures would be supported by complete data logging and integration of all subsystems. Patient name and identification has to be transferred online from the patient data information system of the department, and a complete report must be generated.

Whereas the advantages of real-time digital radiovascular imaging are now obvious, the general introduction of completely filmless equipment was slower than expected in the middle of the 1970s, when the first vascular images were digitized in real time at Wisconsin and Kiel. Requirements for the general use of filmless systems were to assure equal quality of the digital and conventional images and to standardize the digital media for exchange and the format for network communication. The most important incentive for introducing filmless laboratories was to achieve real benefits for the patient and examiner.

The latter requirement has still not been completely fulfilled due to a suboptimal design of presently available systems. The requirement for standardized communication systems is essential for the future development towards filmless systems. We expect that fully digital systems will rapidly spread as soon as the potential benefits relating to openly distributed management systems are fully realized. Workstations form an important part of the strategy behind the communication infrastructure. In contrast to the cine film projector, the medical workstation allows related data of the same patient to be presented immediately in addition to radiographic images. Versatile functions in image processing can be added, such as online pressure volume analysis or image fusion or quantitative pre- and postoperative comparisons.

The best solutions for cost-effective digital archiving systems depend on the application and environment. The pros and cons of a centralized archive versus distributed access systems must be examined. A general rule is to keep local data local and to start on a small scale. A link to the hospital information using the tools of the world wide web may be helpful in the local or global environment for clinical exchange of information.

Driven by changing medical issues and requirements, exciting new developments are therefore continuing to take place even in the oldest method of vascular imaging. Continued vigorous scientific and engineering efforts will be necessary to determine the ultimate role of digital vascular radiography in assessing both the morphological and functional aspects of the circulation.

References

1. Löster W (1982) Physik der Röntgenstrahlung. In: Stieve FE (ed) Strahlenschutzkurs für Ärzte. Hoffmann, Berlin
2. Krestel E (1990) Imaging systems for medical diagnostics. Publicis MCD, Munich
3. Hay GA (1982) Traditional x-ray imaging. In: Wells PNT (ed) Scientific basis of medical imaging. Churchill Livingstone, Edinburgh, pp 1–53
4. Rosenbusch G, Oudkerk M, Ammann E (1995) Radiology in medical diagnostics. Evolution of X-ray applications 1895–1995. Blackwell Science, Oxford
5. Rose A (1973) Vision: human and electronic. Plenum, New York
6. Fujita H, Morishita J, Meda K, et al (1989) Resolution properties of a computed radiographic system. Medical imaging III. SPIE 1090: 263–275
7. Dainty JC, Shaw R (1974) Image science. Academic, New York
8. Giger ML, Doi K (1984) Investigation of basic imaging properties in digital radiography. 1. Modular transfer function. Med Phys 11: 287–295
9. Fujita H, Doi K, Giger M (1985) Investigation of basic imaging properties in digital radiography. 6. MTFs of II-TV digital imaging systems. Med Phys 12: 713–720
10. Roerig H, Nudelmann S, Fisher HD, Frost MM, Capp MC (1981) Photoelectric imaging for radiology. IEEE Trans Nucl Sci NS-28(1): 190–204
11. Barnes GT (1982) Radiographic mottle: A comprehensive theory. Med Phys 9: 656–667
12. Giger ML, Doi K (1984) Investigation of basic imaging properties in digital radiography. 2. Noise Wiener spectrum. Med Phys 11: 797–805
13. Giger ML, Doi K, Fujita H (1986) Investigation of basic imaging properties in digital radiography. 7. Noise Wiener spectra of II-TV digital imaging systems. Med Phys 13: 131–138.

14. Metz CE, Wagner RF, Doi K, Brown DG, Nishikawa RM, Myers KJ (1995) Toward consensus on quantitative assessment of medical imaging systems. Med Phys 22(7): 1057-1061
15. Fu TY, Roehrig H (1984) Noise power spectrum, MTF and DQE of photoelectronic radiographic systems. Application of optical instrumentation in medicine XII. SPIE 454: 377-386
16. Rupp S (1991) Digitale Radiographie. Optimierung der Bildqualität durch Bildbearbeitung. Reihe 10 (161). VDI, Düsseldorf
17. Kruger RA, Mistretta CA, Houk TL, Riederer SJ, Shaw CG, Goodsitt MM, Crummy AB, Zwiebel W, Lancester JC, Rowe GG, Flemming D (1979) Computerized fluoroscopy in real time for non-invasive visualization of the cardiovascular system. Radiology 130: 49-57
18. Brennecke, R, Brown TK, Bürsch JH, Heintzen PH (1976) Digital processing of angiocardiographic image series using a minicomputer. Computers in cardiology. IEEE Computer Society, Long Beach, pp 255-260
19. Heintzen, PH, Brennecke R, Bürsch JH, Lange PE, Malerczyk V, Moldenhauer K, Onnasch DGW (1975) Automated video-angiocardiographic image analysis. Comput Mag 8: 55-64
20. Lange PE, Onnasch DGW, Farr F, Malerczyk V, Heintzen PH (1978) Analysis of left and right ventricular size and shape, as determined from human casts. Eur J Cardiol 8: 431-501
21. Sheehan FH (1991) Cardiac angiography. In: Markus ML, Schelbert HR, Skorton DJ, Wolf GL (eds) Cardiac imaging. Saunders, Philadelphia, pp 109-148
22. Bürsch JH, Heintzen PH, Simon R (1974) Videodensitometric studies by a new method of quantitating the amount of contrast medium. Eur J Cardiol 1: 437-446
23. Onnasch DGW, Jarrens U, Heintzen PH (1991) Determination of cardiac ejection and valvular regurgitant fraction by on-line digital densitometry - methodology, validation, and application. Int J Cardiac Imaging 7: 113-124
24. Reiber JHC, Serruys PW (1991) Quantitative coronary angiography. In: Markus ML, Schelbert HR, Skorton DJ, Wolf GL (eds) Cardiac imaging. Saunders, Philadelphia, pp 211-280
25. Jötten G (1979) Röntgentechnik. In: Lichtlen PR (ed) Koronarangiographie. Perimed, Erlangen, pp 21-52 (Beiträge zur Kardiologie, vol 11)
26. Hillen W, Eckenbach W, Quadflieg P, Zaengel T (1991) Signal-to-noise ratio performance in cesium iodide x-ray fluorescent screens. SPIE Med Imaging V, Image Üjys 1443: 120-131
27. Beekmans AAG (1982) Image quality aspects of x-ray image intensifiers. Medicamundi 27: 25-29
28. CIE IEC 1262-2 (1994) Medical electrical equipment: characteristics of electrooptical x-ray image intensifiers. Part 2: Determination of conversion factor. Part 6: Determination of contrast ratio and veiling glare index. International Electrotechnical Commission Central Office, Geneva
29. Seibert JA, Nalcioglu O, Roeck W (1984) Characterization of the veiling glare PSF in image intensified fluoroscopy. Med Phys 11: 172
30. Spekowius G, Boerner H, Eckenbach W, Quadflieg P, Laurenssen GJ (1995) Simulation of the imaging performance of x-ray image intensifier/TV camera chains. Proc Int Soc Optical Eng SPIE 2432: 12-23 (Medical Imaging 95)
31. Balter S (1993) Fundamental properties of digital images. Radio Graph 13: 129-141
32. Verhoeven L (1991) Design considerations of digital fluoroscopy/fluorographic equipment. AAPM Summer School
33. Fujita H, Giger ML, Doi K (1988) Investigation of basic imaging properties in digital radiography. 12. Effect of matrix configuration on spatial resolution. Med Phys 15: 384-390
34. International Commission on Radiological Protection (ICRP) Recommendations of the International Commission on Radiological Protection (ICRP publication 69). Pergamon, Oxford
35. National Academy of Science Committee on the Biological Effects of Ionizing Radiation (1990) Health effects of exposure to low levels of ionizing radiation (BEIR V). National Academic, Washington DC
36. Johnson LW, Moore RJ, Balter S (1992) Review of radiation safety in cardiac catheterization laboratory. Cathet Cardiovasc Diagn 25: 186-194
37. Sandborg M, Carlson C, Carlson GA (1994) Shaping x-ray spectra with filters in x-ray diagnostics. Med Biol Eng Comp 32: 384-90
38. Nagel HD (1989) Comparison of performance characteristics of conventional and K-edge filters in general diagnostic radiology. Phys Med Biol 34: 1269-1287
39. den Boer A (1994) Reduction of radiation exposure while maintaining high-quality fluoroscopic images during interventional cardiology using novel x-ray tube technology with extra beam filtering. Circulation 89: 2710-2714
40. Pepine CJ, Allen HD, Bashore TM et al (1991) ACC/AHA Guidelines for cardiac cathetrization and cardiac catheterization laboratories. J Am Coll Cardiol 18: 1149-1182; Circulation 84: 2214-2247
41. Leitlinien der Bundesärztekammer zur Qualitätssicherung in der Röntgendiagnostik (1995) Dtsch Arztebl 92(34/35): C-1515-1527
42. Cowen AR (1991) Digital x-ray measurements. Sci Technol 2: 691-707
43. Parisot C (1995) The DICOM standard. A breakthrough for digital information exchange in cardiology. Int J Cardiac Imaging 11 [Suppl 3]: 171-177
44. Nissen SE, Pepine CJ, Bashore TM et al (1994) Cardiac angiography without cinefilm: erecting a "tower of Babel" in the cardiac catheterization laboratory. JACC 24: 834-837
45. Simon R, Brennecke R, Hess O, Meier B, Reiber JHC, Zeelenberg C (1994) Recommendations for digital imaging in angiocardiography. Eur Heart J 15: 1332-1334
46. Digital Imaging and Communications in Medicine (DICOM) - Part 12 (1995) Media Formats and Physical Media, Annex F: CD-R Medium, NEMA Standards Publication PS 3.12 (Draft)

X-ray Contrast Agents

W. Krause

Introduction

In contrast to ultrasonography (color Doppler) and magnetic resonance angiography (MRA), which are both possible without the use of contrast agents, radiography (angiography, digital substraction angiography, computed tomography) needs contrast enhancement of the vessel lumen to visualize blood vessels. As early as 1895, shortly after W.C. Röntgen's discovery of X-rays, it became evident that contrast could be increased by using elements with high atomic numbers such as barium, bismuth, and lead [1]. Iodine and bromine were also discovered as suitable contrast-giving elements. Sodium and lithium iodide and strontium bromide were the first water-soluble contrast media [2]. Iodine was identified as especially suitable and has therefore been used exclusively as the X-ray absorbing atom in water-soluble contrast agents until the present day. The blood concentration of iodine necessary for adequate contrast enhancement has to be greater than 1 mg/ml in computed tomography (CT) and 10–100 mg/ml in projection radiography, depending on vessel diameter and location and radiological technique. Accordingly, the doses which have to be administered in cardiovascular radiography are the highest used in any field of medicine.

The first contrast agent, sodium iodide, proved, however, very toxic. Subsequent research was therefore directed towards designing organically bound iodine compounds that masked the halogen ion, making it "biologically invisible" to the body. The first urographic contrast medium with one organic iodine atom per molecule was Uroselectan, which became available in 1929 [3]. The introduction of a second iodine atom led to Uroselectan-B, the first angiographic contrast agent [4]. Modern substances based exclusively on the triiodobenzene ring system were synthesized in the early 1960s [4–6]. The features of an ideal contrast agent include the following characteristics: a high density differencee relative to surrounding tissue, biological inertness, low viscosity, rapid and complete excretion, and a low price.

All presently available iodinated contrast agents contain either three (monomers) or six (dimers) iodine atoms per molecule. The first characteristic, high density, has therefore been fulfilled. Biological inertness mostly depends on electrical charge, osmolality, and hydrophilicity. Further, as yet unknown parameters are summarized under the term "chemotoxicity." Another physicochemical feature, viscosity, is also determined by the chemical structure of the molecule and by the components of the preparation. The price of contrast media has become one of the main issues after the introduction of nonionic substances which in Europe are three to five times and in the USA five to ten times more expensive than the conventional ionic agents.

Extensive research efforts have been directed to further decrease biological interaction and to make compounds available which are isotonic to blood and have a low viscosity. The synthesis of low-price contrast agents, however, has so far not been successful.

Contrast agents for vascular injection are identical to substance used for urography or CT, so practically all of the following data are applicable to both areas of indication.

Chemistry

The underlying principle of all presently available contrast agents is the symmetric coupling of three iodine atoms to a benzene ring. The three remaining positions are used for "hydrophilic shielding" in order to improve both solubility and tolerance. The first widely used derivative based on these "classical" ionic structures was diatrizoate, which was introduced in 1953 and still remains in clinical use. Other more recent ionic compounds include iothalamate (Conray), ioxithalamate (Telebrix), iodamide (Uromiro), ioglicate (Rayvist) and metrizoate (Isopaque). All these compounds can be collectively referred to as "high-osmolality" contrast media (HOCM). Of the ionic monomers, at present, only diatrizoate in the form of either pure sodium or meglumine salts or mixtures thereof, retained some clinical importance.

The next significant step was the synthesis of the first nonionic compound, metrizamide (Amipaque), in 1969 [7]. The drawback of this substance, however, was its chemical instability, requiring its distribution in a freeze-dried form and reconstitution before use. The first ready-to-use nonionic contrast medium was iopamidol (Isovue, Niopam, Solutrast) followed by iohexol (Omnipaque), iopromide (Ultravist), ioversol (Optiray), iopentol (Imagopaque), iomeprol (Iomeron), and iobitridol (Xenetix). All these compounds are "low-osmolality" contrast agents (LOCM). Another LOCM with a different type of structure is ioxaglate (Hexabrix). This is a dimeric substance with one remaining carboxyl group. It might therefore be classified as an ionic LOCM. The most recently introduced compounds are the nonionic dimers iotrolan (Isovist) and iodixanol (Visipaque), which are isotonic to blood and therefore are called ICM ("isotonic contrast media"). Representative structures of one compound from each class are shown in Fig. 1.

The chemical stability of the contrast media is sufficiently high to achieve shelf lives of up to 5 years. The long shelf life is due either to the stability of the compounds themselves or to added preservatives. These include buffering systems to maintain a defined pH value and chelating agents to mask trace levels of metals such as iron which might initiate deiodination. Stability is monitored by measuring pH and free iodide and amine groups. Another possibility of degradation includes intramolecular rearrangement, which is observed in certain contrast agents.

Physical Chemistry

Classification criteria for contrast agents are water solubility, electrical charge, osmolality, viscosity, and hydrophilicity.

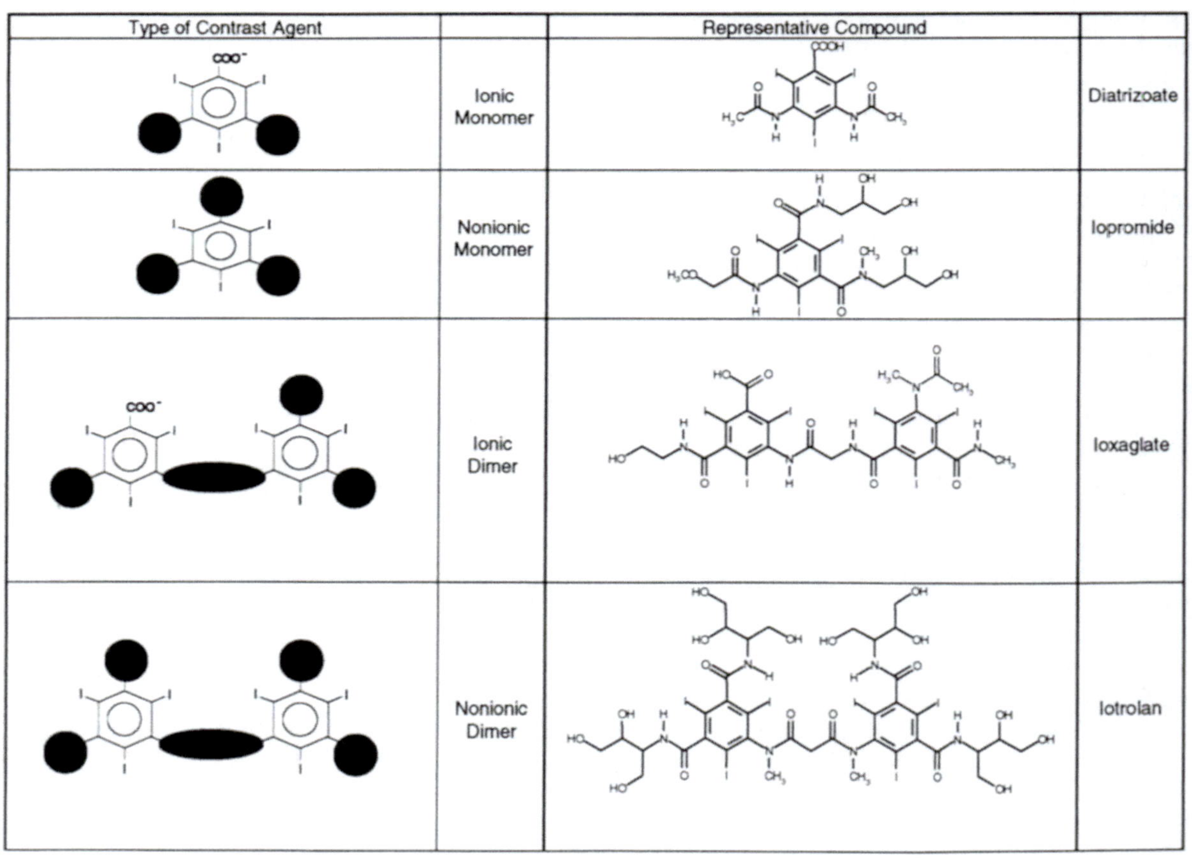

Fig. 1. Types of contrast agent and representative chemical structures

High *water solubility* of a contrast agent is a basic requirement. The highest available concentrations are 320 mg iodine/ml for ionic and nonionic dimers and 370–400 mg iodine/ml for nonionic monomers. The limiting factor for dimers is, however, not insufficient solubility, but high viscosity.

Negative electrical charge of a carboxyl group is an exclusive characteristic of ionic contrast agents (HOCM and ionic LOCM) and has been identified as one of the major factors contributing to undesired biological activity. Ionic contrast agents are salts of iodine-containing anions and of sodium or meglumine cations. The latter do not contribute to the absorption of X-rays. They do, however, influence interactions with biological systems such as proteins or enzymes and are responsible for hemodynamic side effects. The iodine-containing anions bind circulating calcium cations [8], thereby producing hypocalcemia, which may lead to bradycardia, alterations in T-wave configuration, and ventricular fibrillation [9, 10]. To avoid these side effects, the modern compounds are electrically neutral.

Osmolality (mosmol/kg) is influenced by the molar concentration of the contrast agent, by association/dissociation effects, and by hydration. At concentrations of 300 mg iodine/ml , HOCM are characterized by osmolalities in the range of 1500 mosmol/kg, low-osmolarlity nonionic monomeric substances by 500–800 mosmol/kg [11]. This is still considerably higher than the value of blood (300 mosmol/kg). Isotonicity at clinically relevant concentrations (300 mg iodine/ml) has only been achieved for nonionic dimers such as iotrolan and iodixanol. Osmolality-related adverse effects include hemodynamic effects such as depression of myocardial contractile performance associated with a decrease in *dP/dt*, increase in left ventricular end-diastolic pressure, and subsequent decrease in blood pressure [12–16]. Bradycardia [17], increase in pulmonary resistance, pain, endothelial damage, blood-drain barrier disturbance, thrombosis, and thrombophlebitis have also been reported.

Viscosity (mPa) is influenced by the temperature of the solution, the size and shape of the molecule, and by intermolecular interactions. Increasing the temperature sharply decreases viscosity. Often contrast media are therefore warmed up to 37°C before injection. For ionic compounds there is a clear dependence of viscosity on the counterions used. Sodium salts have lower values than meglumine salts. Viscosity directly affects the handling of the solution, higher viscosities limiting the injection rate. In angiography, where narrow catheters and high injection rates are used, a lower viscosity is preferable. The viscosities of commercially available contrast media range from 4.5 to 8.5 mPa at concentrations of 300 mg iodine/ml and 27°C.

Hydrophilicity is responsible for sufficient and – on the gross scale – for biological tolerance of the compound. Hydrophilicity is determined by measuring the partition between a lipophilic organic phase such as *n*-butanol or *n*-octanol and an aqueous buffer. The most hydrophilic contrast agent is the nonionic dimer iotrolan ($p = 0.005$), which is more than ten times as hydrophilic as nonionic monomers.

Pharmacokinetics

The pharmacokinetics of all iodinated extracellular contrast agents are practically identical [18, 19]. Following rapid intravenous injection there is a biphasic decline in blood levels characterized by half-lives of 3–10 min for the first phase and 1–2 h for the second. The first phase is attributable to distribution within the vascular system and diffusion from the intravascular space into the extracellular tissue, and the second phase corresponds to renal elimination.

The *distribution* of the contrast agents within the body is determined by their extremely high hydrophilicity. As a consequence, protein binding is low (<5%) and membranes are not permeated to any significant extent. These compounds are therefore not able to pass the blood-brain barrier, they are not excreted into breast milk, and they are not absorbed after oral administration in significant amounts. Their volume of distribution is practically identical to that of the extracellular space volume (0.25 kg).

Due to their highly hydrophilic character, *biotransformation* is not necessary and, indeed, never has been described for any angiographic contrast agent. Deiodination is not normally observed to any significant extent, but may be sufficient to cause hyperthyroidism in susceptible patients. Furthermore, a certain amount of free iodide probably is due to degradation of the contrast agent within the preparation [20]. Iodide levels in formulations are typically below 10 µg/ml; in a total dose of 100 ml of contrast medium, up to 1 mg of free iodide is administered. This amount does not comprise the function of an intact thyroid gland. In patients with latent hyperthyrosis prophylactic treatment with perchlorate and thiamozolies mandatory (see below).

Elimination of contrast agents proceeds rapidly and mainly via the kidneys (>95% of dose). Glomerular filtration is the predominant mechanism. Active tubular excretion has been observed for ionic monomeric contrast agents and tubular reabsorption for nonionic compounds or ionic dimers [21]. These processes, however, comprise only very small proportions of the injected dose. As a consequence, the total clearance of the contrast agents is practically identical to the individual glomerular filtration rate (GFR). The elimination of iodine or the decline in CT enhancement has therefore been used to determine GFR in patients [22, 23]. Impaired renal function will prolong the half-life of contrast agents up to 10 h or more. Extrarenal (biliary) excretion is increased in these patients, up to 20% of the dose as compared to less than 5% in normal subjects. Due to excellent tolerance of the nonionic contrast agents, their use might even be considered in dialysis patients [24, 25]. In renal risk patients doses have to be minimized (<2 ml/kg) and the following measures taken: discontinuation or dose reduction of potentially nephrotoxic concurrent medication (nonsteroidal antirheumatics, aminoglycosides, hydroxyethyl starch infusions), sufficient hydration (500–1500 ml physiological saline), premedication with diuretics (furosemide, 20 mg i.v.) – which, however, is not universally accepted – and continuous dopamine infusion (3–4 μg/min). If renal function deteriorates, mannitol infusion (up to

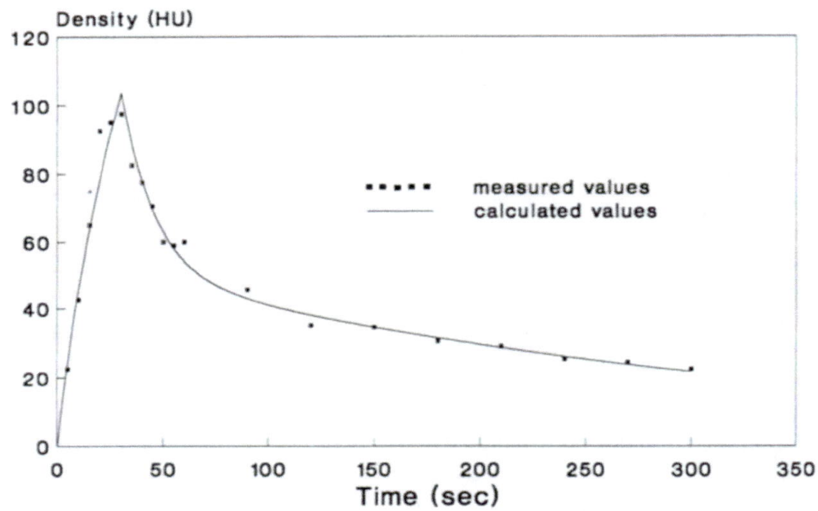

Fig. 2. Enhancement of the aorta after intravenous injection of a conventional contrast medium (diatrizoate 306) at a dose of 300 mg iodine/kg body weight and a rate of 2 ml/s. Measured values were taken from the literature [110] and the curve was calculated by computer-fitting using the programm Topfit [111]

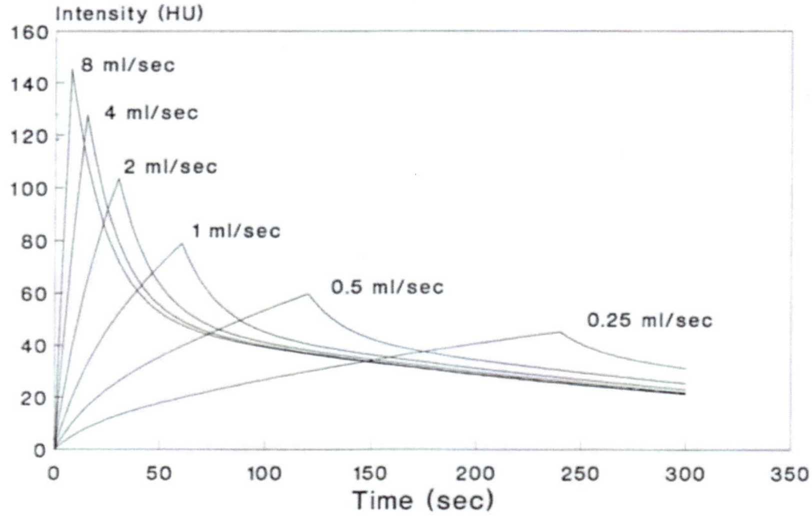

Fig. 3. Effect of the intravenous injection rate on the enhancement of the aorta. The curves were obtained by computer simulation using the data from Fig. 2

25 g over/3 h), then dopamine and furosemide as above should be given, and if necessary hemodialysis [26]. It has been shown that contrast agents are easily dialyzable (55 ml/min at a blood flow of 200 ml/min) and are effectively removed from the body by hemodialysis.

Half-lives, total clearance, and routes of elimination at the dosages used in clinical practice are independent of the amount injected (Figs. 2, 3).

Indications for Use of Contrast Media

In this section the use of contrast agents for a number of different angiographic indications will be briefly reviewed.

The need for *cerebral angiography* has been declining since the introduction of noninvasive techniques such as CT angiography (CTA), MRA, and Doppler ultrasonography. Remaining angiographic indications include arteriosclerosis, arteritis, aneurysms, and arteriovenous malformations. Thedoses used in conventional angiography are 8–10 ml

Table 1. Reported adverse reactions to contrast media used in angiographic procedures

Reference	Contrast medium	No. of patients	Results
Cardiac procedures			
Davis et al. [94]	HOCM	7553	Myocardial infarction 0.25 %, stroke 0.03 %
Johnson et al. [30]	>82 % HOCM	222553[a]	Death 0.10 %, myocardial infarction 0.06 %, stroke 0.07 %
Hirshfeld et al. [42]	HOCM	4630	Minor reactions 14 %, major reactions 1.3 %
Davidson et al. [59]	LOCM	8517	Ventr. tachycardia/fibrillation 0.1 %, bradycardia 0.2 %, thrombotic events 0.18 %, prolonged angina 0.3 %
Wisneski et al. [44]	LOCM	60	Ioxaglate 43 %, iopamidol 7 %
Klinke et al. [45]	LOCM	150	with ioxaglate more effects than with iopamidol
Barrett et al. [46]	HOCM vs LOCM	1490	LOCM significantly superior to HOCM
Steinberg et al. [112]	Iohexol vs diatrizoate	1955	LOCM significantly superior to HOCM in regard to mild, moderate, and overall reactions; no difference for minor and severe reactions
Cohen et al. [113]	Iohexol vs diatrizoate	1390	3.7 times higher chance of side effects with diatrizoate
Percutaneous transluminal coronary angioplasty			
Gasperetti et al. [114]	Iopamidol vs diatrizoate	184	Thrombosis: iopamidol 18 %, diatrizoate 4 %
Lembo et al. [115]	Iopamidol vs diatrizoate	913	Major effects: iopamidol 10.8 %, diatrizoate 10 % Thrombus: iopamidol 7.2 %, diatrizoate 3.2 %
Esplugas et al. [116]	Iohexol vs diatrizoate	100	Major effects: iohexol 8 %, diatrizoate 4 % Thrombus: iohexol 22 %, diatrizoate 2 %
Piessens et al. [117]	Iohexol vs ioxaglate	500	Major effects: iohexol 3.2 %, ioxaglate 2.8 % Thrombus: iohexol 7.2 %, ioxaglate 3.2 %
Cerebral procedures			
Cronquist [118]	HOCM vs LOCM	973	LOCM slightly superior to HOCM
Skalpe [27]	Iohexol vs metrizoate	1509	LOCM not significantly superior to HOCM
Sumie and Kateyama [119]	Iotrolan vs iopamidol	168	Significantly less heat sensation with iotrolan
Bien [65]	Iotrolan vs iohexol, iopromide	373	Significantly better contrast and less heat sensation with iotrolan
Visceral procedures			
Enge [120]	Iohexol vs ioxaglate	841	Minimal and mild side effects: iohexol <2 %, ioxaglate >8 %
Peripheral procedures			
Hori [121]	Iotrolan vs iopamidol	160	Significantly less heat sensation with iotrolan
Gmeinwieser and Wenzel-Hora [122]	Iotrolan vs iopamidol, iohexol, iopromide	541	Minor events iotrolan 2.3 %, LOCM 4.6 %; significantly less pain with iotrolan

[a] No. of procedures.
HOCM, High-osmolality contrast medium; LOCM, low-osmolality contrast medium.

(300 mg iodine/ml) in the carotid arteries, 6 ml (300 mg iodine/ml) in the vertebral artery, and 60 ml (350 – 370 mg iodine/ml) in the aortic arch [27].

Usually, complications (see Table 1), which are reported by 1% – 2% of the patients and may include hemiparesis, dysarthria, disturbances of vision, and unconsciousness, are induced primarily by the invasiveness of the technique and not by the contrast media. The underlying mechanism is probably embolism provoked by the catheter. The use of thin catheters, frequent flushing with heparinized saline, and a careful catheterization technique will reduce the incidence of these side effects. Additional measures are the prophylactic intake of aspirin 1 – 2 h to the examination and the use of nonionic contrast agents [28].

The indications for *spinal angiography* are vascular malformations, dural arteriovenous fistula, and preoperative assessment of scoliosis and tumors. Digital subtraction angiography (DSA) is the method of choice. Individual segmental arteries are visualized via a transfemoral catheter with 1 – 2 ml contrast medium (200 mg iodine/ml for DAS and 300 mg iodine/ml for cut-film technique), arteriovenous malformations with 5 ml, and the vertebral artery with 4 – 5 ml. A total dose of 300 ml (300 mg iodine/ml) should not be exceeded. If there are symptoms of spinal irritation, any further injection of contrast medium should be avoided. Complications include those induced by the method itself (primarily injury of the vessel wall) and those provoked by the contrast medium, distinction between the two being often difficult. For spinal angiography the use of nonionic contrast agents is strongly recommended [28].

In *angiography of the peripheral and visceral vessels* the advantage of intra-arterial DSA is the smaller amounts of contrast medium required compared to cut-film changers; its disadvantage is the slightly lower spatial resolution. Intravenous DSA gives poorer contrast and more overlap with other body structures. It should only be used when direct access is not possible. The indications for angiography of the peripheral and visceral vessels are stenoses, occlusions, and interventional procedures. In conventional aortography up to 100 ml contrast medium (300 – 370 mg iodine/ml) are used and approximately half that volume is required for an intra-arterial DSA study. Injections are typically performed with an automatic injector. Visualization of the arteries of the arm by conventional or DAS technique usually requires 10 – 20 ml (300 mg iodine/ml); for arteriography of the hand 5 – 10 ml is needed. For intravenous DSA of the peripheral vessels the dose has to be increased to 40 ml and the injection rate should be 16 – 20 ml/s when administered into a central vein. A total volume of 300 ml contrast medium should not be exceeded. The contrast medium requirements for selective areriography of the visceral vasculature vary widely depending on the vascular territory in question and the physician's technique.

Cardioangiography is required for quite a number of indications including diseases of the myocardium, pericardium, cardiac valves, and the aorta. Coronary arteriography typically requires from three to five injections on the left and right side of 6 – 10 ml each (320 – 370 mg iodine/ml). The overall doses should not exceed 4 – 5 ml/kg, although some authors use total doses even up to 7 ml/kg [29]. Data from the Society for Cardiac Angiography and Interventions Registry [30] show that on average approximately 130 ml is required for conventional cardioangiography and 200 ml for percutaneous transluminal coronary angioplasty.

Abdominal angiography ist employed to study vascular anatomy preoperatively, to search for hypervascularized tumors or metastases, and during embolization procedures. Typically, 300 mg iodine/ml is used for conventional angiography and 100 – 150 mg iodine/ml for intra-arterial DSA. Doses in standard techniques vary from 5 – 10 ml for transhepatic portography to 30 ml for arteries of the celiac trunk. for intra-arterial DSA, the volumes do not exceed 20 ml (superior mesenteric artery) [31].

Renal arteries can be investigated by intravenous DSA using 35 – 40 ml contrast medium (300 mg iodine/ml) at a flow rate of 20 ml/s. Intraarterial DSA is indicated whenever intravenous DSA gives suboptimal results or during interventional procedures. In nonselective arteriography, on average 25 ml (300 mg iodine/ml) is injected into the abdominal artery at a flow rate of 15 – 20 ml/s. Typically, 20 ml is injected at 8 ml/s in selective angiography. For plain film techniques the volumes have to be increased to 35 – 40 ml.

Venous disorders are examined by *phlebography*, either using conventional techniques or DSA. The volume of contrast medium is adjusted to according to the indication; it is usually 0.7 ml/kg per extremity. For DSA of the pelvic veins 30 ml contrast medium (300 mg iodine/ml) is followed by 30 ml saline. The injection rate is 3 – 5 ml/s [32].

Ionic contrast media have been in use for angiographic indications for more than 30 years. In cardioangiography the mixed sodium/meglumine salt of diatrizoate (Urografin) has been shown to be better tolerated than the pure sodium or meglumine salt. Increasingly high doses and rapid injection rates in patients with multiple disease, however, may result in undesirable side effects. To reduce the adverse reactions associated with the use of ionic contrast agents, nonionic substances are recommended. As would be expected from the abovementioned characteristics, nonionic LOCM are well tolerated and safely applicable. Guidelines for the use of LOCM have been issued by several authorities. Further progress could be achieved by introducing the nonionic dimers. Due to their isotonicity the heat sensation during injection is significantly reduced and cardiac as well as hemodynamic adverse reactions are minimized. However, large-scale clinical trials demonstrating the superiority of nonionic dimers have not yet been reported.

A summary of recommended concentrations and volumes for angiographic indications is presented in Table 2. General handling and storage advice is given in Table 3.

Table 2. Concentration and dose recommendations for different applications of contrast medium administration

Technique	Concentration (mg iodine/ml)	Dose (ml)
Arteriography Abdominal	300	5–50
Aorta	300–370	10–50
Cardiac	370	40–60
Cerebral	300	4–12
Coronary	370	4–8
DSA, i.a.	75–300	6–60
DSA, i.v.	300–370	50–150[a]
Extremities	300	10–70
Phlebography	150–300	20–50

[a] Multiple injections of 20–50 ml

Table 3. Recommendations for the handling and storage of contrast media

Storage	At room temperature in the dark *Not* in the refrigerator
Shelf life	2–5 years (see expiration date)
Handling before use	Take from the dark immediately before use Use only clear solutions Crystals may be solubilized by warming up to 80°C If solution will not become clear, discard Viscous preparation may be injected at 37°
Handling after opening	Use within 4 h, under no circumstances use after 12 h Do not pour out of container Do not resterilize

Side effects of Contrast Media

The mechanisms of contrast media-induced adverse reaction can be divided into two categories: first, the easily understood side effects provoked by nonisotonicity and, second, the less well comprehended range of so-called "biological interactions." These interactions of contrast agents with biological macromolecules are considered to be the first step in the direction of molecule-specific toxicity. Molecular binding is mediated by ionic charge, hydrogen bondage and hydrophobic interaction between less hydrophilic parts of the contrast agent molecule and the macromolecules. To avoid these interactions, nonionic molecules, alkylated nitrogens, and hydrophilic substituents with a sufficient number of hydroxyl groups have been introduced. Due to their relative biological inertness, the contrast agents are the best tolerated pharmacologic compounds available for use in medicine. High doses of iodine of up to 1.5 g/kg body weight, equivalent to more than 100 g iodine or 200 g per dose of substance, can be safety administered.

The incidence of side effects is extraordinarily low. They may be classified according to severity (mild, moderate, severe, fatal), target organ (kidneys, heart, skin, etc.), dependence on dose (dose-dependent, dose-independent), and time of appearance (early and late). Minor side effects include nausea, vomiting, urticaria, pruritus, pain at the injection site, and transient arrhythmia. Moderate adverse reactions are severe vomiting, extensive urticaria, headache, bronchospasm, and edema (face or larynx). Severe reactions are syncope, convulsion, schock, hypotension, cardiac arrest, and pulmonary edema. The mortality associated with intravenously injected contrast agents appears to be less than 1 per 165 000 patients [33]. It seems to be higher with intra-arterial or intracardiac injection, probably because the patients requiring these procedures are more sick. A summary of the side effects reported for HOCM and LOCM and their possible mechanisms is given in Table 4.

Electrophysiological effects are mainly observed after intracoronary or intracardiac injection of contrast media and include sinus bradycardia, arteriovenous conduction disturbances, QT prolongation, and ST segment and T wave changes [12–17, 34, 35]. Most side effects are osmolality-related and are therefore reported especially for high-osmolar compounds [9, 10]. The ionic character of HOCM results in binding of calcium. As a consequence, ventricular fibrillation is observed in approximately 1 out of 200 cardiac angiographic procedures [36].

Table 4. Effects of contrast agents in different regions of the body

System	Effect	Mechanism
Cardiovascular	Vasodilatation	Osmolality
	Bradycardia	Osmolality
	Contractility ↓	Charge (calcium binding)
	Disturbance of microcirculation	Osmolality, viscosity (?)
Peripheral	Pain	Osmolality
	Vascular injury:	
	Cell shrinkage	Osmolality, chemotoxicity
	Opening of tight junctions	Osmolality, chemotoxicity
	Blood pressure ↓	Osmolality
	Vascular tone ↓	Osmolality
	Blood volume ↑	Osmolality
	Hematocrit ↓	Osmolality
	Plasma electrolytes ↓	Charge, osmolality
	Erythrocytes: deformation	Osmolality, charge
	Leukocytes:	Charge, osmolality, chemotoxicity
	Histamine release	Chemotoxicity
	Phagocytosis ↓	Charge, chemotoxicity
	Lymphocytes: "allergoid" reaction	Osmolality, charge
	Platelets: inhibition of aggregation	
	Arachidonic acid:	Osmolality
	Metabolism ↑	Osmolality
	Inactivation ↓	Osmolality
	Blood coagulation time ↑	Osmolality, chemotoxicity
	Blood pH ↓	Osmolality, chemotoxicity
	Complement system: activity ↓	Osmolality, chemotoxicity
	Enzyme systems: activity ↓	
Neural	Blood-brain barrier: damage	Osmolality, chemotoxicity
	Epileptogenicity	Charge, osmolality
	Sedative effects	Osmolality, chemotoxicity
	Neural deficits	Charge, osmolality
	EEG changes	Charge, osmolality
Renal	Glomerular permeability ↑	Charge, osmolality
	Tubular vacuolization	?
Local	Tissue damage	Charge, osmolality
General (allergoid)	Nausea	Chemotoxicity
	Vomiting	Chemotoxicity
	"Allergoid" reactions	Chemotoxicity

Hemodynamic effects of contrast media include myocardial depression followed by a decrease in blood pressure and in *dP/dt* and an increase in left ventricular end-diastolic pressure [14, 37–40]. This may provoke or exacerbate myocardial ischemia especially in patients with preexisting stenosis or heart failure. Nonionic low-osmolality substances have been shown to be less likely to produce ischemia [13–15]. Another, osmolality-related and therefore dose-dependent characteristic of HOCM is vasodilatation and the sensation of warmth or even pain. For low-osmolality or isotonic agents this effect is reduced or not observed [41]. Hirshfeld reports 14% of patients with minor reactions and 1.3% with major effects, mainly changes in arterial pressure and pulmonary vascular congestion, after HOCM in a series of 4630 cardiac angiographic procedures [42]. Interestingly, 5.4% of the procedures had to be shortened because of concern about adverse effects and 0.7% due to actual reactions. In a similar study in 8517 patients using LOCM [43] the incidence of ventricular tachycardia/fibrillation was 0.1%, bradycardia 0.2%, thrombotic events 0.18%, and prolonged angina 0.3%. Direct comparisons of contrast agents have not very often been performed. There is, however, clear evidence that nonionic compounds are better tolerated than ionic ones including the low-osmolar ionic agent ioxaglate [44–46]. The new nonionic dimers, iotrolan and iodixanol, seem to be superior to the monomers due to their isotonicity as demonstrated in animal experiments [47] and in human trials [48]. Before their broader use, concern was widespread that their relatively higher viscosity would affect blood flow especially in the microcirculation. However, in experimental studies no effects of isotonic dimers such as iotrolan on microcirculation have been documented in the rat mediastinum, intesine, or heart [49–52].

The *hemostatic system* is primarily influenced by ionic contrast media (HOCM and LOCM) due to their anticoagulant and antiplatelet activities [53–60] and resulting antithrombotic effects, which are less prominent with nonionic compounds. To avoid side effects, prolonged contact between blood and contrast medium should be avoided and heparin (5 IU/ml) should be added to the preparation. Apart from contrast agents, however, thrombogenicity during angiography can be influenced by numerous additonal factors such as the length of the procedure, the length of time the catheter remains in the vascular system, the severity of vascular disease, the operator's concomitant use of heparin, the intensity of catheter flushing, the type of catheter material, and the operator's skill, Although this is not generally accepted, the last issue probably has the greatest impact not only on thromboembolic risk but also on procedural safety. During coronary interventions, the risk of thrombosis is increased due to intimal disruption. The data regarding dependence of the frequency of thromboembolic events during PTCA on the type of contrast agents are equivocal. It appears likely that, compared to the above-mentioned factors in the procedure, the choice of the particular contrast agent is of negligible significance.

Neurologic effects of contrast agents are primarily due to interactions with the blood-brain barrier, manifested by EEG changes and, rarely mild, fully reversible neurologic functional disturbances. The blood-brain barrier is particularly susceptable to the agents with a high osmotic pressure. Accordingly, low-osmolarlity or isotonic contrast agents exhibit only minimal effects, as demonstrated in animal experiments [61, 62]. In addition to changes in blood-brain barrier permeability, changes in the cerebral blood flow have been reported in the literature. While some authors reported cerebral vasodilatation [63], others observed vasoconstriction [64]. These differences remain physiologically unexplained and may be due to difficulties in measuring cerebral blood flow accurately in a given experimental preparation. Multiple comparative studies performed over the last 30 years have shown that the overall procedure risk of transient neurologic deficits in cerebral angiography is 0.5%–5.5% and that of permanent neurologic deficits is 0%–1% of all cases [65]. The introduction of DSA and the use of LOCM has considerably reduced the overall risk. The increased use of nonionic dimers is expected to reduce this risk even further.

The spectrum of *renal adverse reactions* ranges from mild and transient changes in laboratory parameters to the requirement for hemodialysis. It has been estimated that approximately 12% of all hospital-acquired episodes of renal failure have been caused by contrast medium administration [66]. The incidence of contrast medium-induced nephropathy is uncertain; estimates range from 0%–10% [67–69] up to 30% [70–72]. LOCM are less likely to induce permanent nephropathy [73, 74]. Risk factors for the development of contrast-induced nephropathy include pre-existing renal insufficiency, insulin-dependent diabetes mellitus, and dehydration [75]. Recent data indicate that multiple myeloma by itself is not a risk factor, but rather that other factors associated with this disease, such as azotemia, dehydration, and albuminura, constitute a higher risk. The clinical signs of renal nephropathy induced by contrast media are well described. Serum creatinine increases within 24 h and reaches peak values at 3 days, accompanied by oliguria. Within 10 days polyuria develops and creatinine values normalize. Mild forms may remain undetected. Symtomatic patients should be carefully monitored and some may require dialysis. In rare cases, irreversible nephronal change may result in a requirement for chronic hemodialysis. Although several theories have been advanced to explain the acute contrast agent-related suppression of glomerular filtration rate, a multifactorial pathogenesis is now widely accepted [76]. both glomerular (hemodynamic) and tubular components are involved. Renal blood flow changes in a biphasic manner: an initial steep increase is followed by a more prolonged decrease. These fluctuations are higher the "nearer" the injection site is to the kidney (renal arteries > intra-arterial > intravenous). Prophylactic measures include adequate hydration and discontinuation of comedication with biguanides and other drugs affecting renal clearance. As mediators of the altered glomerular hemodynamics norepinephrine, the renin-angiotensin system, prostaglandins, calcium [77], adenosine and, recently, nitric oxide [78] have been considered. Damage to the tubular system induced by contrast media has been associated with changes in urinary enzyme excretion, e.g., *N*-acetyl-β-glucoseaminidase [79–81]. The new nonionic dimers seem to be better tolerated than the monomers [82]. A meta-analysis of 14 controlled, double-blind, comparative studies showed that iotrolan has had less influence on renal function than iohexol, iopamidol, or iopromide [83].

In addition to the above-mentioned side effects, there is the general class of *"allergy-like" reactions* with an overall incidence of 1%–2%. This class can be subdivided on the basis of severity into two groups, the mild and dose-depenfent reactions due to release of mediators which cannot be inhibited by corticosteroids, and the more severe, dose-independent, pre-existing allergy or priming factors related reactions which respond to corticosteroids. Allergy-like symptoms include urticaria, bronchospasm and laryngospasm, edema, hypotension, and, rarely, hypotensive shock. The incidence of severe reactions is approximately 0.1% and mortality is less than 1 in 10000 patients. None of the proposed explanations for "allergy-like" reactions, such as histamine release, antibody formation, complement activation, and changes in leukotriene formation, has been universally accepted. Psychological factors such as stress and anxiety may play an important role in triggering "allergy-like" reactions. Since a clearly defined cause has not been found, the question of pretesting and pretreatment of patients without a history of allergic reactions is controversial [84, 85]. A careful inquiry, however, into known allergies or previous effects is mandatory. Additional risk factors include renal and cardiac insufficiency, diabetes, and advanced age. General prophylaxis consists of administration of corticosteroids (cf. Chap. 7) and atropine. Concomitant treatment with antihistaminics (H_1 and H_2) proved useful in high-risk patients [86, 87]. LOCM are reported to cause a lower incidence of "allergy-like" reactions than HOCM [46, 88].

The debate about the superiority of nonionic contrast media over ionic agents has for a long time been undecided. Numerous clinical data available now, however, clearly show that the incidence of side effects is decreased by a factor of 3–10 when nonionic instead of ionic contrast media are used. The types of adverse reactions seem to be identical for both groups. For HOCM side effects range from 0.5% to 24% of all cases, whereas for nonionic contrast media 0.7% to 3% has been reported [33, 89–104]. The incidence of fatal reactions with LOCM is probably lower than with HOCM, although this has not been unequivocally proven due to the low incidence of this event (1 out of 10 000–100 000 cases).

To assist physicians in choosing whether and when to use nonionic LOCM, guidelines have been issued by several authorities. The American College of Cardiology recommends using nonionic contrast agents in "selected patients at high risk for hemodynamic complications (including congestive heart failure, severe aortic stenosis, cardiogenic shock, and left main coronary artery disease) during cardiac catheterization and in patients with a history of allergic reaction to contrast medium" [105]. In general, the ACC recommends that the physician should determine the choice of contrast agent in consultation with the patient. The American Society of Cardiovascular and Interventional Radiology proposes the use of low-osmolality compounds [106] for painful examinations and patients with marked anxiety, for patients with hemodynamic instability or limited cardiac reserve, and for persons with an inability to tolerate a marked osmotic load, children and elderly patients, patients with hyperosmolar states (dehydration), renal failure, prior reactions, and a strongly allergic diathesis or asthma. The Royal Australian College of Radiologists Guidelines recommend [107] that "high risk patients, asthmatic subjects and patients over 50 years" should only receive nonionic contrast media. Low-risk patients should have corticosteroid pretreatment (methylprednisolone, 32 mg 12 h and 2 h before injection). If pretreatment cannot be arranged or if the study is urgent, then the use of nonionic contrast agents is recommended. In Central Europe, Scandinavia, and Japan the use of HOCM has practically been discontinued and LOCM are used exclusively.

In summary, HOCM and LOCM seem to cause the same type of side effects but severity is clearly different. High-osmolality ionic compounds have a 3–10 times higher risk of provoking adverse reactions than low-osmolality nonionic agents. For the new nonionic dimers, extensive clinical comparisons with nonionic monomers are not yet available.

Prevention/Premedication and Treatment of Side Effects

The incidence of adverse reactions is markedly less when nonionic LOCM are used instead of ionic HOCM (diatrizoate) or LOCM (ioxaglate). However, even with nonionic compounds side effects cannot be ruled out.

Patients with an *allergic history* should be pretreated with corticosteroids (methylprednisolone 32 mg p.o. 12 h and 2 h before study) and antihistaminics (demetindenmaleate 0.1 mg/kg i.v. plus cimetidine 5 mg/kg i.v.).

In patients with *hyperthyroidism* the use of iodinated contrast media should be avoided. If they are used, prophylatic treatments with perchlorate (400 mg t.i.d.) and thiamozole (20 mg b.i.d.) or carbimazole (10 mg t.i.d.) from 4 days before to 3 weeks after study is mandatory.

Pheochromocytoma patients should be pretreated for approximately 2 weeks with individual doses of α-blocking agents to avoid a hypertensive crisis or sudden hypotension. Medical treatment of allergic, thyroid-related, and hypotensive emergencies has been described in the literature [108].

In *sickle-cell anemia* the deformation of erythrocytes due to osmotic overload is less marked with LOCM than with HOCM. Deformed and rigid erythrocytes are unable to pass through narrow capillaries, resulting in stasis and, possibly, ischemic tissue damage. Intra-arterial contrast media injections are to be performed only when absolutely indicated. Special caution with both groups of contrast media is mandatory, and where possible isotonic LOCM should be used.

In patients with *impaired renal function* (renal insufficiency, diabetes mellitus, cardiac insufficiency, myeloma, advanced age, etc.) the use of contrast medium is restricted and special precautions are mandatory. Serum creatinine values should be measured before and after contrast medium administration, the doses must be minimized (2< ml/kg) and nephrotoxic medication (nonsteroidal antirheumatics, aminoglycosides, hydroxyethyl starch, etc.) has to be discontinued. Further prophylactic measures include adequate hydration during the entire peri-interventional period, the – not generally accepted – administration of diuretics (furosemide 20 mg and more i.v.), the administration of dopamine (continuous infusion, 3–4 µg/kg min), and the avoidance of repeated contrast medium administrations within days. If renal function deteriorates, the infusion of mannitol (25 g/3 h) and dopamine/furosemide as needed is recommended. Ultimatively, hemodialysis may be required.

Risk evaluation is also mandatory in *pregnancy*, when the use of X-rays should be omitted whenever possible. During *breast feeding* the use of contrast agents is allowed, since contrast media are not excreted into the milk and they are not absorbed in the gastrointestinal tract in any significant amounts.

Although contrast media-induced side effects are very rare, especially when nonionic low-osmo-

Table 5. Treatment of contrast media adverse reactions (according to Siegle [108])

Adverse reaction	Treatment	
	Mild reaction	Severe reaction
Heat, nausea, vomiting	Fresh air, oxygen (2–6 l/min)	Valium (5–10 mg i.v.)
Urticaria	None	diphenyhydramine (50 mg p.o. or i.m. or 25–50 mg i.v.) or hydroxyzine (25 mg p.o. or i.m.) Cimetidine (300 mg p.4o. or i.v.) or ranitidine (50 mg i.v.) Epinephrine (1:1000 0.3 ml s.c. or 1:10 000 1 ml i.v. over 3–5 min)
Angioedema	Local cooling; epinephrine (1:1000; 0.3 ml s.c.); oxygen (2–6 l/min); diphenhydramine (50 mg i.m.); cimetidine (300 mg p.o. or i.v.)	
Bronchospasm	Epinephrine (1:1000; 0.3 ml s.c. or 1:10 000 1 ml i.v. over 3–5 min at 10 µg/min) Oxygen (2–6 l/min) Albuterol or metaproterenol (2 breaths)	Aminophylline (250 mg i.v.) Intubation *If prolonged, add:* Hydrocortisone (250 mg i.v.) Diphenhydramine (50 mg i.m.) Cimetidine (300 mg i.v.) *If necessary, add:* Morphine (5 mg i.v.)
Hypotension with bradycardia	Trendelenberg position I.v. fluids (saline or lactated Ringer's solution)	Atropine (0.75 mg i.v.) *If ineffective:* Dopamine (5–10 µgg/kg/min i.v.)
Hypotension with tachycardia	Trendelenberg position I.v. fluids *If no response but remaining mild:* Epinephrine (1:1000; 0.3 ml s.c.)	I.v. fluids Epinephrine (1:1000 0.3 ml s.c.) Oxygen (2–6 l/min) Intubation *If persistent:* Dopamine (5–10 µg/kg min i.v.)
Pulmonary edema	Oxygen (2–6 l/min) Raise head and upper body Furosemide (40 mg i.v.)	*If unconscious:* Intubation *If agitated:* Morphine (10–15 mg i.v.) Epinephrine (1:1000 0.3 ml s.c.)

lar compounds are used, the physician and staff must be aware of potential side effects and must know how to treat them. The availbility of well-trained staff and treatments for the management of side effects is mandatory. Table 5 gives a summary of how to treat adverse reactions to contrast media effectively [108].

Future Developments

The four basic characteristics of the ideal contrast agent for angiographic indications are nonionicity, isotonicity, hydrophilicity, and low viscosity. During the past 20 years safe and well-tolerated angiographic contrast media have been developed. Modern nonionic monomeric substances exhibit low osmolalities and low viscosities. The nonionic dimers are isotonic to blood and extremely hydrophilic and are therefore particularly suited for angiography and interventions. Their only drawback is their relatively high viscosity, which limits concentrations to 320 mg iodine/ml. For cardiac/coronary applications, higher concentrations, in the range of 350–400 mg iodine/ml, are, however, preferable, and the combination of isotonicity and low viscosity would represent further significant progress.

Other possible future developments are related to improvements in X-ray angiography technology. Monochromatic X-rays, for example, would be useful to operate at an energy characteristic of iodine (K-edge). This could both considerably increase patient safety, by reducing radiation, and improve image quality, by increasing spatial and temporal image resolution. Using synchrotron radiation, the usefulness of monochromatic radiation in cardioangiography has been demonstrated [109].

A further line of research is directed towards compounds which do not extravasate. These substances are either particles with a diameter smaller than 5 μm or polymers with molecular weights greater than 40 000. For this purpose, polymers based on dextran or other backbones have been synthesized. These molecules are too big to pass through the endothelial gaps into the extravascular space. The problem still to solve, however, is the improvement of tolerance and the retention of these compounds in the body. Compounds which do not leave the vascular system would above all have the advantage of clearer delineation of fine vascular structures and prolongation of the residence time within hyper- or hypovascularized tumors, allowing more precise visualization. It remains to be seen whether any of these compounds will become clinically applicable in the future.

References

1. Haschek E, Lindenthal TO (1896) Ein Beitrag zur praktischen Verwertung der Photographie nach Röntgen. Wien Klin Wochenschr 9: 63–64
2. Osborne ED, Sutherland CG, Scholl AF, Rowntree LG (1923) Roentgenography of urinary tract during excretion of sodium iodide. JAMA 80: 368–373
3. Binz A, Rath A, von Lichtenberg A (1931) The chemistry of Uroselectan. Z Urol 25: 297–301
4. Wallingford VH (1953) The development of organic iodide compounds compounds as X-ray contrast media. J Am Pharm Assoc Sci Ed 42: 721–728
5. Langecker H, Harwart A, Junkmann K (1954) 3,5-Diacetylamino-2,4,6-triiodbenzoesäure als Röntgenkontrastmittel. Nauny Schmiedebergs Arch Exp Pathol 222: 584–590
6. Hoppe JO, Larsen HA, Coulston FJ (1956) Observation on the toxicity of a new urographic contrast medium, sodium 3,5-diacetamno-2,4,6-triiodobenzoate (Hypaque sodium). J Pharmacol Exp Ther 116: 394–403
7. Almén T (1969) Contrast agent design. Some aspects on the synthesis of water-soluble agents of low osmolality. J Theor Biol 24: 216–226
8. Morris TW, Sahler LG, Fischer HW (1982) Calcium binding by radiopaque media. Invest Radiol 17: 501–505
9. Piao ZE, Murdock DK, Hwang MH, Raymond RM, Scanlon PJ (1988) Contrast media induced ventricular fibrillation: a comparison of Hypaque-76, Hexabrix and Omnipaque. Invest Radiol 23: 466–470
10. Missri J, Jeresaty RM (1990) Ventricular fibrillation during coronary angiography: reduced incidence with nonionic contrast media. Cathet Cardiovasc Diagn 19: 4–7
11. Krause W, Miklautz H, Kollenkirchen U, Heimann G (1993) Physicochemical parameters of X-ray contrast media. Invest Radiol 29: 72–80
12. Higgins CB (1985) Cardiotolerance of iohexol, a survey of experimental evidence. Invest Radiol 20: 565–569
13. Bettmann MA, Bourdillon PD, Bary WH, Brush KA, Levin DC (1984) Contrast agents for cardiac angiography: effects of a nonionic agent vs. a standard agent. Radiology 153: 583–587
14. Gertz KW, Wisneski JA, Chiu D, Akin JR, Hu C (1985) Clinical superiority of a new nonionic contrast agent (iopamidol) for cardiac angiography. J Am Coll Cardiol 5: 250–258
15. Gerber KH, Higgins CB, Yuh YS, Koziol JA (1982) Regional myocardial hemodynamic and metabolic effects of ionic and nonionic contrast media in normal and ischemic stetes. Circulation 65: 1307–1314
16. Bashore TM, Davidson CJ, Mark DB (1988) Iopamidol use in the cardiac catheterization laboratory: a retrospective analysis of 3313 patients. CARDIO 5: 4–10
17. Thomson KR, Evill CA, Fritzsche J, Benness GT (1980) Comparison of iopamidol, ioxaglate and diatrizoate during coronary arteriography in dogs. Invest Radiol 15: 234–241
18. Hartwig P, Mützel W, Taenzer V (1989) Pharmacokinetics of iohexol, iopamidol, iopromide, and iosimide

compared with meglumine diatrizoate. In: Taenzer V, Wende S (eds) Recent developments in nonionic contrast media. Thieme, Stuttgart, pp 220-223
19. Feldman S, Hayman A, Hulse M (1984) Pharmacokinetics of low- and high-dose intravenous diatrizoate contrast media administration. Invest Radiol 19: 54
20. Wang YCJ (1980) Deiodination kinetics of water-soluble radiopaques. J Pharm Sci 69: 671-675
21. Zurth C (1984) Mechanism of renal excretion of various X-ray contrast materials in rabbits. Invest Radiol 19: 110
22. Almén T, Bergquist D, Frennby B, Hellsten S, Lilja B, Nyman U, Sterner G, Tornquist C (1991) Use of urographic contrast media to determine glomerular filtration rate of each kidney with computed tomography and scintigraphy. Invest Radiol 26: S72-S74
23. Effersoe H, Rosenkilde R, Groth S (1990) Measurement of renal function with iohexol or a comparison of iohexol, ^{99m}Tc-DTPA, and ^{51}Cr-EDTA clearance. Invest Radiol 25: 778-782
24. Corradi A, Menta R, Cambi V (1990) Pharmacokinetics of iopamidol in adults with renal failure. Arzneimittelforschung 40: 830-832
25. Waaler A, Svaland M, Fauchald P (1990) Elimination of iohexol, a low osmolar nonionic contrast medium, by hemodialysis in patients with chronic renal failure. Nephron 56: 81-85
26. Scherbach JE, Kollath J, Riemann HE (1991) Unerwünschte Kontrastmittelwirkungen an der Niere. In: Peters PE, Zeitler E (eds) Röntgenkontrastmittel - Nebenwirkungen, Prophylaxe, Therapie. Springer, Berlin Heidelberg New York, pp 65-69
27. Skalpe IO (1993) Clinical use of iodinated media for the visualization of vessels, organs and organ systems. In: Dawson P, Clauss W (eds) Contrast media in practice. Springer, Berlin Heidelberg New York, pp 119-121
28. Latchaw RE (1993) The use of nonionic contrast agents in neuroangiography. A review of the literature and recommendations for clinical use. Invest Radiol 28: S55-S59
29. Romaniuk P (1993) Angiography and thoracic aortography. In: Dawson P, Clauss W (eds) Contrast media in practice. Springer, Berlin Heidelberg New York, pp 144-161
30. Johnson LW, Lozner EC, Johnson S (1989) Coronary areriography 1984-1987: a report of the registry of the Society for Cardiac Angiography and Intervention. Cathet Cardiovasc Diagn 17: 5-10
31. Rödl W (1993) Angiographic procedures for the liver, spleen, pancreas and portal venous system. In: Dawson P, Clauss W (eds) Contrast media in practice. Springer, Berlin Heidelberg New York, pp 161-169
32. Hagen B (1993) Phlebography. In: Dawson P, Clauss W (eds) Contrast media in practice. Springer, Berlin Heidelberg New York, pp 133-138
33. Katayama H, Yamaguchi K, Kozuka T, Takashima T, Seez P, Matsuura K (1990) Adverse reactions to ionic and nonionic and nonionic contrast media: a report from the Japanese Committee on the safety of contrast media. Radiology 175: 621
34. Hirshfeld JW Jr, Laskey W, Martin JL, Groh WC, Untereker W, Wolf GL (1983) Hemodynamic changes included by cardiac angiography with ioxaglate: comparison with diatrizoate. Am J Cardiol 2: 954-957
35. Feldman RL, Jalowiec DA, Hill JA, Lambert CR (1988) Contrast-media related complications during cardiac catheterization using Hexabrix or Renografin in high risk patients. Am J Cardiol 61: 1334-1337
36. Johnson LW, Lozner EC, Johnson S (1989) Coronary arteriography 1984-1987: a report of the Registry of the Society for Cardiac Angiography and Intervention. I. Results and complications. Cathet Cardiovasc Diagn 17: 5-10
37. Friesinger GC, Schaffer J, Criley JM, Gaertner RA, Ross RS (1965) Hemodynamic consequences of the injection of radiopaque material. Circulation 31: 730-740
38. Vine DL, Hegg TD, Dodge HT, Stewart DK, Frimer M (1977) Immediate effect of contrast medium injection on left ventricular volumes and ejection fraction. Circulation 56: 379-384
39. Bettmann MA (1982) Angiographic contrast agents: conventional and new media compared. AJR 139: 787-794
40. Cohan RH, Dunnick NR (1987) Intravascular contrast media: adverse reactions. AJR 149: 665
41. Hagen B, Klink G (1983) Contrast media and pain: hypotheses on the genesis of pain occurring on intra-arterial administration of contrast media. In: Taenzer V, Zeitler E (eds) Contrast media in urography, angiography and computerized tomography, Thieme, Stuttgart, pp 50-56
42. Hirshfeld J, Kussmaul K, Diabattiste P (1990) Safety of cardiac angiography with conventional ionic contrast agents. Am J Cardiol 66: 355-361
43. Davidson C, Mark D, Pieper K (1990) Thrombotic and cardiovascular complications related to nonionic contrast media during cardia catheterization: analysis of 8517 patients. Am J Cardiol 65: 1481-1484
44. Wisneski JA, Gertz KW, Dahigren M, Muslin A (1989) Comparison of low-osmolality ionic (ioxaglate) versus nonionic (iopamidol) contrast media in cardiac angiography. Am J Cardiol 63: 489-495
45. Klinke WP, Grace M, Miller R, Naqvi SZ, Roth D, Roy L (1989) A multicenter randomized trial of ionic (ioxaglate) and nonionic (iopamidol) low-osmolality contrast agents in cardiac angiography. Clin Cardiol 12: 689-696
46. Barrett BJ, Parfrey PS, Vavasour HM (1992) A comparison of nonlonic, low-osmolality radiocontrast agents with ionic, high-osmolality agents during cardiac catheterization. N Engl J Med 326: 431-436
47. Muschick P, Wehrmann D, Schuhmann-Giampieri G, Krause W (1994) Cardiac and haemodynamic tolerability of different X-ray contrast media in the anaesthetized rat. Cardiovasc Intervent Radiol 17 Suppl 2: S125
48. Morris TW (1993) The physiologic effects of nonionic contrast media on the heart. Invest Radiol 28: S44-S46
49. Klopp R, Niemer W, Schippel W (191) Kontrastmittelwirkungen auf die Fliessbedingungen der Mikrozirkulation (tierexperimentelle Studie). In: Peters PE, Zeitler E (eds) Röntgenkonstrastmittel: Nebenwirkungen, Prophylaxe, Therapie. Springer, Berlin Heidelberg New York, pp 52-64
50. Klopp R, Niemer W, Schippel W, Münster W, (1992) Veränderungen der intestinalen und myocardialen Mikrozirkulation nach Applikation verschiedener Rontgenkontrastmittel. In: Richter K (ed) Digitale und interventionelle Radiologie bei Herz- und Gefäßerkrankungen. Blackwell, Berlin pp 192-196

51. Strickland NH, Rampling MW, Dawson P, Martin G (1992) Contrast-media induced effects on blood rheology and their importance in angiography. Clin Radiol 45: 240-242
52. Klopp R, Niemer W, Schippel W, Krause W (1994) Changes in the microcirculation of the intact rat heart after iodinated and Gd-containing contrast agents. Cardiovasc Interven Radiol 17 Suppl 2: S123
53. Stommorken H, Skalpe IO, Testart MC (1986) Effect of various contrast media on coagulation, fibrinolysis, and platelet function: an in vitro and in vivo study. Invest Radiol 21: 348-154
54. Robertson HJF (1987) Blood clot formation in angiographic syringes containing nonionic contrast media. Radiology 163: 621-622
55. Gabriel DA, Jones MR, Reece NS (1991) Platelet and fibrin modification by radiographic contast media. Circ Res 68: 881-887
56. Dawson P, Hewitt P, Mackie IJ (1986) Contrast, coagulation, and fibrinolysis. Invest Radiol 21: 248-252
57. Grollman JH Jr, Liu CK, Astone RA, Lurie MD (1988) Thromboembolic complications in coronary angiography associated with the use of nonionic contrast medium. Cathet Cardiovasc Diagn 14: 159-164
58. Au PK (1991) Nonionic contast media and intracatheter clot formation during use of a perfusion balloon catheter. Cathet Cardiovasc Diagn 22: 235-236
59. Davidson CJ, Mark DB, Pieper KS (1990) Thrombotic and cardiovascular complications related to nonionic contrast media during cardiac catheterization: analysis of 8517 patients. Am J Cardiol 65: 1481-1484
60. Hwang MH, En Piano A, Murdock DK (1989) The potential risk of thrombosis during coronary angiography using nonionic contrast media. Cathet Cardiovasc Diagn 16: 209-213
61. Krause W (1994) Preclinical characterization of iopromide. Invest Radiol 29 Supl 1: S21-S32
62. Wilson AJ, Evill CA, Sage MR (1991) Effects of nonionic contrast media on the blood-brain barrier. Osmolality versus chemotoxicity. Invest Radiol 26: 1091-1094
63. Nakstad PH (1989) The reaction of cerebral arteries to non-ionic contrast media during cerebral angiography. Neuroradiology 31: 247-249
64. Du Boulay GH, Wallis A (1986) Cerebral arterial constriction due to contrast media. Acta Radiol Suppl (Stockh) 369: 518-520
65. Bien S (1995) Iotrolan, a non-ionic dimeric contrast agent in cerebral angiography. Eur Radiol 5: S45-S48
66. Hou SH, Bushinski DA, Wish JB, Cohan JJ, Harrington JT (1983) Hospital-acquired renal insufficiency: a prospective study. Am J Med 74: 243-248
67. Byrd L, Sherman RL (1979) Radiocontrast-induced acute renal failure. A clinical and pathophysiologic review. Medicine (Baltimore) 58: 270-279
68. Diaz-Buxo JA, Wagoner RD, Hattery RR, Palumbo PJ (1975) Acute renal failure after excretory urography in diabetic patients. Ann Intem Med 83: 155-158
69. Port KF, Wagoner RD, Fulter RE (1974) Acute renal failure after angiography. Am J Radiol 121: 544-550
70. Mason RA, Arbeit LA, Givon F (1985) Renal dysfunction after arteriography. JAMA 253: 1001-1004
71. D'Elia JA, Glenson RE, Arday W, Malarick C, Godfrey K, Warran J (1982) Nephrotoxicity from angiographic contrast material. A prospective study. Am J Med 72: 719-725
72. Temel JL, Marcer R, Onaindia JM, Serano A, Quereda C, Ortuno J (1981) Renal function impairment caused by intravenous urography. Arch Intem Med 72: 719-725
73. Taliercio CP, Vlietstra RE, Ilstrup DM (1991) A randomized comparison of the nephrotoxicity of iopamidol and diatrizoate in high risk patients undergoing cardiac angiography. J Am Coll Cardiol 17: 384-90
74. Hill JA, Winniford M, Van Fossen DR (1991) Nephrotoxicity following cardiac angiography: a randomized double-blind multicenter trial of ionic and nonionic contrast media in 1194 patients. Circulation 84 Suppl 2: 333
75. Rich MW, Crecelius CA (1990) Incidence, risk factors, and clinical course of acute renal insufficiency after cardiac catheterization in patients 70 years of age or older: a prospective study. Arch Intern Med 150: 1237-1242
76. Porter GA (1993) Effects of contrast agents on renal function. Invest Radiol 28: S1-S5
77. Deray G, Martinez F, Cacoub P, Baumelou B, Baumelou A, Jacobs C (1990) A role for adenosine, calcium, and ischemia in radiocontrast-induced intrarenal vasoconstriction. Am J Nephrol 10: 316-322
78. Lasser EC, Lamkin GE (1994) Is there a role for nitric oxide in contrast material toxicity? Invest Radiol 29 Suppl 29: S102-104
79. Talner LB, Rushman HN, Cael MN (1972) The effect of renal artery injections of contrast material on urinary enzyme excretion. Invest Radiol 7: 311-322
80. Thomsen HS, Golman K, Hemmingsen L, Larsen HA, Skaarup P, Svendson O (1993) Contrast media-induced nephropathy: animal experiments. Front Eur Radiol 9: 83-108
81. Parvez Z, Rhamamursky S, Patel NB, Moncada R (1990) Enzyme markers of contrast media-induced renal failure. Invest Radiol 25: S133-134
82. Berns JS, Rudnick MR (1992) Radiocontrast media associated nephrotoxicity. Kidney 24: 1-5
83. Clauß W, Dinger J, Meißner C (1995) Renai tolerance of iotrolan 280 in European clinical studies. Eur Radiol 5: S79-S84
84. Fischer HW, Doust VL (1971) An evaluation of pretesting in the problem of serious and fatal reactions to excretory urography. Radiology 103: 497
85. Leonello PP, Frewin DB, Russell WJ, Gilligan JE, Jolley PT (1980) Adverse reactions to radiographic contrast media administered by the intravascular route. Aust Radiol 24: 311
86. Lasser EC, Lang J, Sovak M, Kolb W, Lyon S, Hamlin E (1977) Steroids: theoretical and experimental basis for utilization in prevention of contrast media reactions. Radiology 125: 1
87. Greenberger PA (1987) Clinical studies on the pretreatment of high risk patients submitted to contrast media procedures. In: Parvez Z (ed) Contrast media. CRC Press, Boca Raton, p 165
88. Gertz KW, Wisneski JA, Miller R (1992) Adverse reactions of low osmolality contrast media during cardiac angiography: a prospective randomized multicenter study. J Am Coll Cardiol 19: 899-906
89. Pendergrass HP, Tondreau RL, Pendergrass KP, Ritchie DJ, Hildreth EA, Askovitz Sl (1958) Reactions associated with intravenous urography. Historical and statistical prview. Radiology 71: 1
90. Coleman WP, Ochsner SF, Watson BE (1964) Allergic

reactions in 10 000 consecutive intravenous urographies. South Med J 57: 1401
91. Toniolo G, Buia L (1966) Risultati di una inchiesta nazionale sugli incidenti mortali da inizione di mezzi di contrasto organo-iodati. Radiol Med 2: 625
92. Wolfromm R, Dehouve A, Degand F, Wattez E, Lange R, Crehalet A (1966) Les accidents graves per injection intraveineuse de substances iodees pour urographie. J Radiol Electrol 47: 346
93. Witten DM, Hirsch FD, Hartman GW (1973) Acute reactions to urographic contrast medium. AJR 119: 832
94. Davies P, Roberts MB, Roylance J (1975) Acute reactions to urographic contrast media. Br Med J 2: 434
95. Shehadi WH, Toniolo G (1980) Adverse reactions to contrast media. Radiology 137: 299
96. Ansell G, Tweedie MCK, West CR, Evans P, Couch L (1980) The current status of reactions to intravenous contrast media. Invest Radiol 15: S32
97. Hobbs BB (1981) Adverse reactions to intravenous contrast agents in Ontario 1975-1989. J Can Assoc Radiol 32: 8
98. Pinet A, Lyonnet D, Maillet P, Groleau JM (1982) Adverse reactions to intravenous contrast media in urography - results of national survey. In: Amiel (ed) Contrast media in radiology. Brikhäuser, Basel, p 14
99. Michel JR (1982) Prevention of shocks induced by intravenous urography. In: Amiel (ed) Contrast media in radiology. Birkhäuser, Basel, p 11
100. Hartman GW, Hattery R, Witten DM (1982) Mortality during excretory urography: Mayo Clinic experience. AJR 139: 919
101. Schrott KM, Behrends B, Clauß W, Kaufmann M, Lehnert J (1986) Iohexol in der Ausscheidungsurographie. Fortschr Med 104: 153
102. Lasser EC, Berry CC, Talner LB (1987) Pretreatment with corticosteroids to alleviate reactions to intravenous contrast material: a randomized multi-institutional study. N Engl J Med 317: 845
103. Palmer FJ (1988) The RACR survey of intravenous contrast media reactions - final report. Aust Radiol 32: 426
104. Wolf GL, Arenson RL, Cross AP (1989) A prospective trial of ionic vs nonionic contrast agents in routine clinical practice: comparison of adverse effects. AJR 152: 939
105. Ritchie JL, Nissen SE, Douglas JS et al (1993) Use of nonionic or low osmolar contrast agents in cardiovascular procedures. J Am Coll Cardiol 21: 269-273
106. Bettmann MA (1989) Guidelines for use of low-osmolality contrast agents. Radiology 172: 901-903
107. Benness GT (1988) Guidelines revisited. Australas Radiol 32: 424-425
108. Siegle RL (1992) Contrast reactions, treatment and risk management. Refresher course #317, RSNA '92. Radiology 185: 57
109. Dix WR (1995) Intravenous coronary angiography with synchrotron radiation. Prog Biophys Mol Biol 63: 159-191
110. Clausen C, Lochner B (1983) Dynamische Computertomographie. Springer, Berlin Heidelberg New York, p 39
111. Heinzel G, Woloszczak R, Thomann P (1993) Topfit 2.0 Pharmacokinetic and pharamcodynamic data analysis system for the PC. Fischer, Stuttgart
112. Steinberg KP, Moore RD, Powe NR (1992) Safety and cost effectiveness of high-osmolality as compared with low-osmolality contrast material in patients undergging cardiac catheterization, N Engl J Med 326: 425-430
113. Cohen MB, van Fossen DB, Murphy MH, Halpern E (1992) Adverse events following cardiac angiography: a randomized double-blind multicentre trial of ionic and nonionic contrast media. Cathet Cardio Vasc Diagn 26: 74
114. Gasperetti CM, Feldmann MO, Burwell LR (1991) Influence of contrast media on thrombus formation during coronary angioplasty. J Am Coll Cardiol 173: 443-450
115. Lembo NJ, King SB, Roubin GS, Black AJ, Douglas JS (1991) Effects of nonionic versus ionic contrast media on complications of percutaneous transluminal coronary angioplasty. Am J Cardiol 67: 1040-1050
116. Esplugas E, Esquier A, Jara F (1991) Risk of thrombosis during coronary angioplasty with low osmolar contrast media. Am J Cardiol 68: 1020-1024
117. Piessens JH, Stammen F, Vrolix MC (1993) Effects of an ionic versus a nonionic low osmolar contrast agent on the thrombotic complications of coronary angioplasty. Cathet Cardiovasc Diagn 28: 99-105
118. Cronquist S (1982) Iohexol in cerebral angiography. Survey and present state. Acta Radiol Suppl 366: 135-139
119. Sumie H, Kateyama H (1993) Iotrolan in cerebral angiography: a Japanese phase III multicenter comparative study with iopamidol. Eur Radiol 5: S39-S44
120. Enge IP (1993) Safety of nonionic agents in visceral angiography. Invest Radiol 28: 539-542
121. Hori S (1995) A Japanese phase II multicenter comparison of iotrolan 280 with iopamidol 33 in peripheral arteriography. Eur Radiol 5: S24-S29
122. Gmeinwieser JK, Wenzel-Hora BI (1995) Peripheral and pendle angiography with iotrolan 280 versus nonionic monomers: results of the European clinical phase II and II trials. Eur Radiol A 530-S38

Magnetic Resonance Angiography

M. Lipton and G. Karczmar

Introduction

Arteriography has a long history, dating back 100 years. The first recorded angiogram was performed only 3 months after Roentgen's discovery of X-rays by injecting sodium iodide solution into the artery of an amputated human limb. Since that time remarkable developments in X-ray technology, improved contrast media and most recently in digital imaging have resulted in excellent, safe procedures. Furthermore, interventional radiology techniques, e.g., balloon angioplasty, have also become an extension of arteriography and venography. Despite the rapid advances in new techniques, angiography is still regarded as the gold standard for displaying and diagnosing disease of the cardiovascular system.

Given this history together with the prevalence and availability of digital X-ray imaging, it is logical to question the value of developing magnetic resonance angiography (MRA). The answer lies in the expectation that MRA will provide even more capability than conventional X-ray angiography. MRA procedures, furthermore, can be totally noninvasive, since contrast media is not essential for most applications. Vessel patency, especially distal to severe stenoses or even total occlusions, may be demonstrated by MRA. Allergic reactions to iodine are avoided. Patients with severe renal disease and high creatinine levels in whom conventional angiography is contraindicated can be safely studied. Additionally, MRA has the potential for displaying both veins and arteries, obtaining three-dimensional displays, and measuring blood flow velocity. MRA techniques are still being developed, refined, and improved. Furthermore, the remarkable flexibility of MR technology in terms of magnet design, field strength, pulse sequences, postprocessing, and, more recently, developments in interventional MR procedures is indeed exciting.

Several techniques have now become established for obtaining clinical MRA of particular anatomical areas. The choice of technique is important, since it should be tailored to answer the clinical question. Some discussion is warranted in regard to obtaining useful and consistently diagnostic MRA studies. There is a fundamental advantage if an experienced angiographer can work closely with the MR technologist performing the study, and also with a physicist conversant with MRA methods. The capability and limitations of the equipment and the preparation of well-designed protocols is critical. Optimizing technique by examining normal volunteers is a good preliminary step, which in our experience is well advised before offering a clinical service to clinicians in any given anatomical area.

An understanding of MRA requires some familiarity with basic MR imaging methods. Therefore, this chapter will provide a brief introduction to the physical basis of MR imaging. Subsequently, the physics of several common MR angiographic methods will be reviewed, and examples of state-of-the-art clinical MRA will be illustrated and discussed.

The Nuclear Magnetic Resonance Signal

Polarization of Atomic Nuclei

Magnetic resonance (frequently referred to as nuclear magnetic resonance) signals are detected from atomic nuclei which possess angular momentum. According to the classical analogy, these nuclei behave like tiny bar magnets when placed in a magnetic field, producing detectable magnetic polarization. The magnetic moment does not parallel the external field (i.e., the applied field) but instead precesses around it. The precession frequency is determined by the strength of the nuclear magnetic moment (or the gyromagnetic ratio, *g*) and the strength of the applicd field (*B*), and is given by the Larmor equation:

$$\omega = \gamma B$$

The applied field is commonly measured in gauss (G), the gyromagnetic ratio in hertz (Hz) per gauss, and the Larmor frequency, ω, is commonly expressed in Hertz. The nucleus which is detected for conventional medical imaging purposes is the nucleus of the water proton. The energy which causes the nuclear magnetic moments to align with the field is very tiny – on the order of one millionth of the thermal energy at room temperature. Therefore the tendency of nuclei to align against the applied field is very weak. Out of two million water proton nuclei at room temperature in a 2-tesla magnet, the net polarization is on the order of one nucleus. This small polarization means that MR signals are very weak. They can only be detected when the number of nuclei studied is very large. For example, water protons in the human body are present in a concentration of roughly 80 molar. A large volume of water molecules produces a signal strength on the order of millivolts in a well-tuned detector coil.

Excitation and Detection of the MR Signal

At equilibrium nuclear magnetic moments generate a net polarization along an applied field. The field produced by the nuclear moments adds to the main field and causes a slight change in field strength (on the order of one part per million) which is very difficult to detect. The net nuclear polarization can only be detected with a reasonable signal-to-noise ratio if it is perturbed from its equilibrium position. This is done by applying a small radiofrequency (RF) magnetic field (generally on the order of between 1 and 10 G) at right angles to the large static field. This small field affects only those nuclei which are precessing about the static field at close to the frequency of the RF field. These nuclei are said to be at the "resonant" frequency. For example, in a 2-tesla (20000-G) field, protons precess at a frequency of 85 MHz. Therefore, they can only be excited by an RF energy at a frequency of 85 MHz.

Figure 1 illustrates schematically the excitation and detection process. The RF field rotates nuclear polarization away from the applied field (i.e., the *z*-axis) and leaves the polarization in the *xy* plane. The excitation normally requires very short RF pulses with durations of tens to hundreds of microseconds. When the RF field is turned off, nuclear polarization is left in the *xy* plane, where it continues to precess at its Larmor frequency. The precession of nuclear magnetism induces alternating current in an inductor tuned to the resonance frequency. This current is amplified and detected using equipment similar to a radio receiver. The signal is Fourier transformed so that the resonance frequency can be determined.

The MR signal from water in the human body typically lasts on the order of 10–100 ms. There are two primary mechanisms by which signal is lost in vivo. (a) Immediately after the excitation pulse, the nuclear magnetic moments are in phase in the *xy* plane and the maximum signal is detected. Howe-

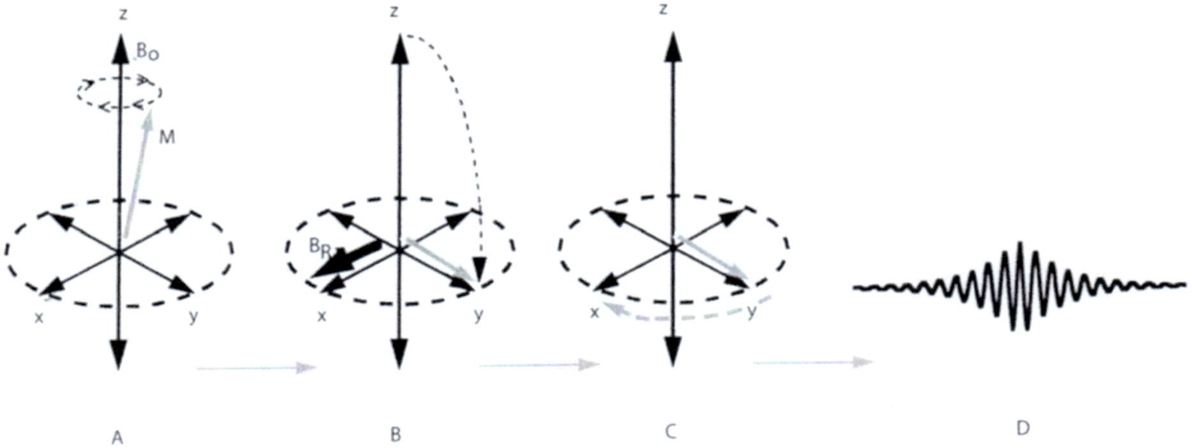

Fig. 1 A–D. Process of the excitation and detection of MR signals. **A** A radiofrequency field (B_{RF}) is applied along the *x* axis. In the laboratory frame, the RF field is much smaller than the B_0. Although the RF affects nuclear precession, the effect is small compared to precession about B_0 and is not shown in the figure. In the rotating frame, B_{RF} is the only magnetic field and magnetizatin which is on resonance precesses around it into the transverse (*xy*) plane. **C** B_{RF} is turned off and magnetization is left in the transverse plane where it precesses about B_0, inducing **D** a current in the detector coil

ver, the many tiny nuclear magnetic moments which make up the net nuclear polarization do not precess at exactly the same frequency, and loss of phase coherence decreases the signal that is detected. (b) Nuclear magnetic moments gradually leave the *xy* plane and realign along the applied field (the *z* axis). These two types of relaxation are called T_2 (or T_2*) and T_1 relaxation respectively.

A series of consecutive excitation pulses must be separated by a period of time during which magnetization returns from the transverse plane to the *z* axis. This is referred to as T_1 or longitudinal relaxation and is discussed below. If the time between excitation pulses is much less than the characteristic longitudinal relaxation time, T_1, then there is very little recovery of *z* magnetization and after a few excitations there is very little *z* polarization which can be rotated into the transverse plane – i.e., the magnetization is saturated. Under these conditions, the relatively small amount of signal which is detected is strongly dependent on the value of T_1.

Basic Principles of Imaging

An understanding of the basic principles of MR imaging is necessary to an understanding of MR angiography. Therefore, MR imaging methods are briefly reviewed here. A number of excellent textbooks provide a comprehensive introduction [see 1–3] The use of magnetic resonance to form images was pioneered by Lauterbur [4], Damadian and Mansfield [6]. Following this early work, the Fourier methods which are now most commonly used for imaging were introduced by Kumar et al. [7]. Subsequently, a wide variety of alternative "non-Fourier" imaging methods have been developed [see 8]. The present discussion will focus on Fourier imaging methods.

Effects of a Magnetic Field Gradient on Signals from Objects

The frequency of MR signals is sensitive to the local field experienced by the nuclei (see above). Although this frequency is primarily determined by the strength of the field of the main solenoid, small deviations, on the order of 100 parts per million, can occur because of gradients in the applied field. This sensitivity to magnetic field inhomogeneities is the property which is used to produce MR images.

Consider the MR signals from water in a test tube. In a perfectly uniform magnetic field, the water protons give rise to a single sharp resonance (Fig. 2a). However, if a linear magnetic field gradient is applied along the long axis of the test tube, the value of the magnetic field at various points along the gradient is offset from the value of the main field. If the gradient is symmetrical about the center of the magnet (the offset is zero at the center), the size of the offset is the product of the distance from the magnet center and the gradient amplitude. The *offset field* causes water protons at different locations along the gradient to precess at slightly different frequencies, determined by the distance from the magnet center. This causes dephasing of nuclear magnetic moments in the *xy* plane. The Fourier transform of the decay of the water signal in the *xy* plane as a function of time is a profile of the proton density in the test tube. If we know how large the magnetic field gradient is (i.e., in G/cm), then we can determine how long the test tube is, based on the width of the profile. For example, if the applied magnetic field gradient is 1 G/cm, or about 4250 Hz/cm for protons (the gyromagnetic ratio for protons is 4250 Hz/G), a 5-cm-long test tube will give a signal with a bandwidth of approximately 21250 Hz (Fig. 2b). The amplitude of

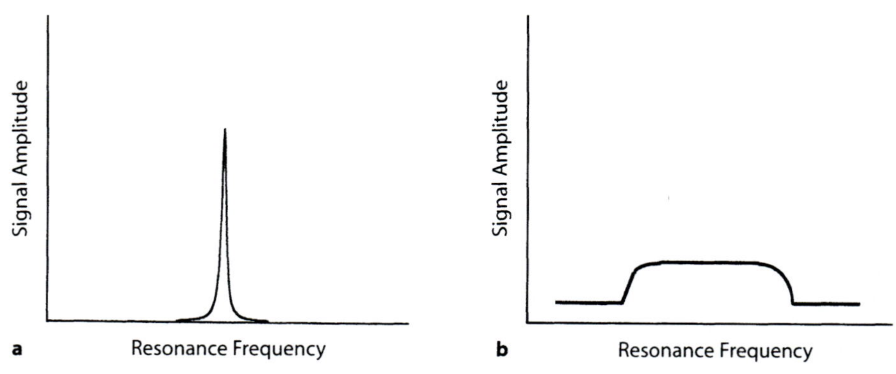

Fig. 2a. Lorentzian line shape obtained in a uniform field. **b** signal from test tube with a gradient along the long axis

the Fourier transformed signal is proportional to the amount of water at each position along the gradient (i. e., the volume of the cross-section of the test tube at each position). Note that one end of the profile is rather sharp, reflecting the flat surface of the water at the top of the test tube, while the other end is rounded, reflecting the rounded bottom of the test tube. The accuracy of the profile depends on the linearity of the gradient.

Of course, application of a linear gradient across an object provides only a one-dimensional image of an object,which is of limited utility. A number of tools have been developed which make it possible to obtain much more useful MR images. The following sections describe these tools and discuss how, in combination, they are used to obtain high-resolution three-dimensional images of objects. Water protons which are used for conventional medical imaging are present in high enough concentrations and have long enough T_2*s to allow very high resolution imaging in vivo. Therefore, the following sections emphasize imaging of tissue water protons. However, MR imaging methods can also be applied to signals from other nuclei.

Gradient Echoes

The "gradient echo" plays a vital role in virtually every imaging technique, and as discussed below, is essential to "phase-sensitive" MR angiography methods. Immediately after nuclear magnetic moments are rotated from the *z* axis to the *xy* plane all the moments are aligned (that is, they are phase-coherent), and therefore the net polarization is at a maximum. This means that the amplitude of the detected signal is at a maximum. Application of a static field gradient causes magnetic moments at different positions in the gradient to precess at slightly different frequencies. As a result, the spins dephase over time, and the net polarization decreases. However, if the gradient is reversed, the dephasing caused by the gradient is also reversed and signal returns to approximately the maximum value (somewhat reduced by T_1, T_2, and T_2^* relaxation). This recovery of signal is called an "echo" or, more specifically, a "gradient echo," since the dephasing and rephasing is caused by application of gradients in the main magnetic field. Note that, when magnetization is not in the same position along the gradient during the first half of the echo as it is during the second half, complete refocusing does not occur because the absolute value of the precession frequency is not constant. The effect of a gradient echo on signal from flowing blood is the basis of a large class of angiographic methods. These methods are discussed below.

Selective Excitation

The RF energy which is used to excite MR signals has a relatively narrow bandwidth. For signals on resonance, in the rotating frame the exciting RF field is the *only* magnetic field. The effective field is coincident with the RF field. Nuclear magnetic moments which precess at the proper frequency rotate or precess around this field into the *xy* plane, where they produce a signal. However, nuclei which are not on resonance are not strongly affected by the RF field. In the presence of a magnetic field gradient, resonance frequency varies along the gradient, so that only nuclei within a relatively thin slice of tissue are at the resonance frequency of an RF excitation pulse. Therefore, when a magnetic field gradient (referred to as the "slice-selection gradient") is applied during the excitation pulse, magnetization within a narrow slice of tissue can be rotated into the transverse plane – that is, spatially selective excitation can be achieved. Note that in the pulse sequence shown in Fig. 3, a small negative lobe follows the slice-selective gradient. This "slice-rephasing gradient" reverses dephasing of magnetization which occurs due to the influence of the "slice-selection gradient" so that a coherent MR signal can be detected.

A "block pulse" is an RF excitation pulse which turns on instantaneously, delivers constant power for the duration of the pulse, and then turns off instantaneously. Because the sharp edges of this pulse have high-frequency components, the excitation profile of the pulse is not square. Therefore, the pulse does not excite a slice with sharp edges and spatial resolution is degraded. Spatial resolution can be improved if RF pulses with rounded edges are used. Gaussian pulses and sinc-shaped pulses excite slices with fairly sharp edges.

Since spatially selective excitation is designed to excite very well defined slices, only magnetization in the selected slice is perturbed from its equilibrium state along the *z* axis. Therefore, immediately after magnetization in one slice is selectively excited and detected, magnetization in a second slice can be excited and detected. As will be discussed, a number of separate excitations and detections (typically between 64 and 256) are required to

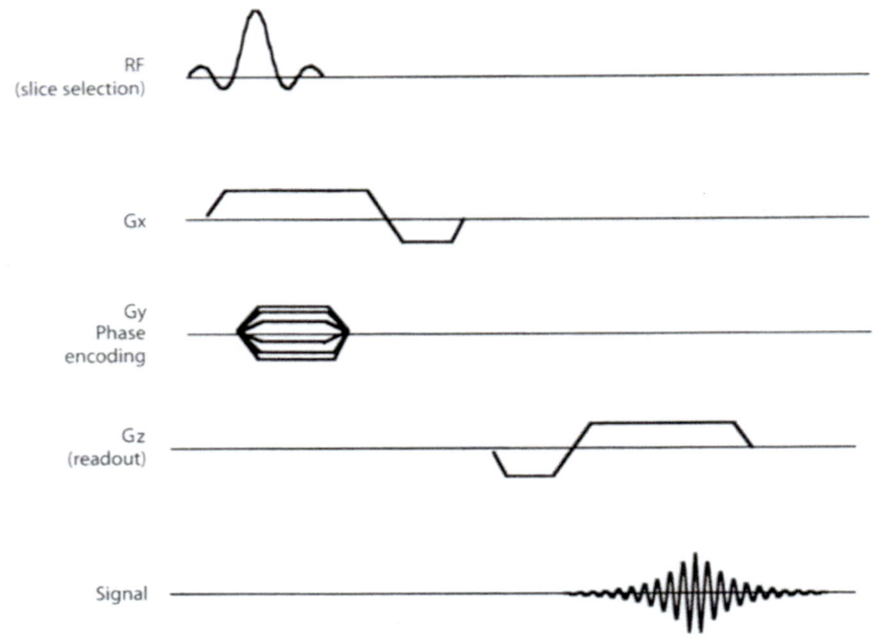

Fig. 3. A pulse sequence used to detect signal in the presence of a readout gradient, including slice-selective excitation (Gx), phase encoding gradients (*Gy*), a dephasing gradient, and a rephasing gradient for readout (*Gz*). In the presence of a readout gradient, signal is initially small because of the dephasing gradient, reaches a peak as phase accumulation is reversed by the readout gradient, and then decays again

form an image. These steps can be performed in parallel for a number of slices until all the data required for a two-dimensional image of each slice is acquired. In practice, up to 16 slices are excited in a typical clinical imaging study. This results in a tremendous savings in imaging time.

Observe Gradients

The preceding section explains how selective excitation provides spatial resolution in one direction by exciting a single well defined slice through the object of interest. This slice must then be imaged in two dimensions. Resolution in one dimension can be obtained by detecting signal in the presence of an observe gradient. As explained above, the Fourier transform of signals detected in the presence of a linear gradient provides a one-dimensional image along the direction of the gradient. The observe gradient is turned on following the excitation pulse, and is applied along one axis in the plane of the selected slice (Fig. 3). A negative dephasing gradient must precede the observe gradient. The dephasing gradient causes signal to decay rapidly as nuclear magnetic moments at different positions in the gradient precess at different frequencies, and phase coherence is lost. When the gradient is reversed and the observe gradient is applied, the dephasing is reversed and the signal increases until a gradient echo is formed. At the peak of the echo all of the polarization in the *xy* plane is roughly in phase. After the maximum is reached, signal begins to decay again under the influence of the observe gradient. The entire echo is detected and digitized, including the initial increase in signal which occurs when the gradient is turned on, and the subsequent decrease. The Fourier transform of the echo profile as a function of time gives a profile of the object along the direction of the gradient. Any motion along the gradient during formation of the echo will produce blurring of the profile.

It is not always necessary to detect an entire gradient echo as shown in Fig. 3. In cases where rapid imaging is required, slightly more than half the echo can be detected to, reducing the signal acquisition time by a factor of almost two. The penalty for this decreased run time is a decrease in signal-to-noise ratio, since only half of the available signal is detected. In addition, phase artifacts can occur when an asymmetrical signal is detected, and reconstruction of the "partial echo" requires measurement or estimation of the phase of the MR signal [9]. Despite this inconvenience, the increased speed of partial echo detection is sometimes required for imaging of flowing blood in large vessels, which is sometimes moving so rapidly that it leaves the field of view before it can be detected.

Phase Encoding

Slice-selective excitation and observe gradients provide spatial resolution along two orthogonal axes. Phase encoding can be used in combination with these two techniques to provide resolution along a third orthogonal axis. Alternatively, phase encoding alone can provide two- or three-dimensional spatial resolution. The phase encoding method takes advantage of the fact that MR spectrometers are phase-sensitive detectors. Following excitation, the x and y components of transverse magnetization are detected independently, and are proportional to the cosine and sine respectively of the phase (i.e., the angle) of the magnetization vector in the xy plane. Thus the phase of the detected signal relative to a reference phase can be determined with great accuracy and precision.

Following slice-selective excitation, all nuclear magnetic moments are in phase in the xy plane. A "phase encoding gradient" is applied for several milliseconds immediately following the excitation pulse. While the gradient is turned on, each nucleus experiences an offset field which is determined by the position of the nucleus along the gradient. The precession rate of the nuclear magnetic moment is either increased or decreased (relative to the rate of precession in the main field) by this offset field. For example, if the phase encoding gradient has an amplitude of 1 G/cm, a nucleus 1 mm from the center of the magnet along the direction of the gradient, after rotation into the xy plane by an RF excitation pulse, will precess at a frequency approximately 425 Hz faster than a nucleus at the center of the magnet (where the offset field due to the gradient is zero). Let us arbitrarily assign a nuclear magnetic moment at the center of the magnet a phase of zero in the xy plane. Even though this magnetic moment is actually precessing about the main field at a high frequency, in the rotating frame (i.e., frame which rotates at the Larmor frequency) there is no precession, and the phase of the magnetization in the xy plane remains at zero. If the gradient is applied for 1 ms, the nuclear magnetic moment 1 mm from the magnet center will arrive at a phase of 150° (while the nuclear magnetic moment at the magnet center remains at a phase of 0°). If the size of the gradient is doubled the phase of the signal detected at 1 mm from the magnet center will be 300°. The increment in phase of the MR signal as a function of phase encoding gradient strength can be measured to determine the position of the nuclear magnetic moment along the gradient. If the gradient is applied for 1 ms, magnetization which accumulates 360° of phase (i.e., one cycle) for each increment of 2.38 G/cm in the applied gradient is 1 mm from the center of the magnet.

In a conventional phase encoding experiment a series of MR signals is acquired following application of phase encoding gradients which are incremented through a series of amplitudes. As a result, the phases of MR signals change as a function of the distance of nuclei from the magnet center and the size of the phase encoding gradient. The position of magnetization can be determined from the Fourier transform of the signals with respect to phase encoding gradient size. The resulting spectrum represents the change in precession frequencies of the nuclei in the selected slice due to the applied phase encoding gradient. A single nuclear magnetic moment would give rise to a single line in the spectrum. A large sample would give a broad spectrum containing a variety of frequency components which is equivalent to a one-dimensional image or profile along the direction of the gradient. Phase encoding gradients can be applied along one, two, or three axes to give one-, two-, or three-dimensional spatial resolution.

Alternative Methods for Sampling "k-Space"

MR imaging is based on detection of the spatially dependent change in phase of magnetization due to the application of magnetic field gradients. This sampling of the shape and density of the object is referred to as "k-space" or "reciprocal space" sampling. Phase changes which are measured in k-space are translated into recognizable images by Fourier transformation. In conventional "spin warp" imaging k-space is sampled row by row along a rectangular grid, as illustrated in Fig. 4a. The example in the figure shows phase encoding along the y axis, with the "observe" or "readout" gradient along x. A row of k-space with a constant y value is selected by applying a phase encoding gradient. Then, all of the x values in that row are measured in rapid succession during the readout gradient echo – that is, the phase of magnetization is measured as a function of time during application of the readout gradient. A separate acquisition is required to measure each row of k-space.

Echo Planar Imaging

However, much more rapid imaging methods are available. These methods rely on rapid gradient

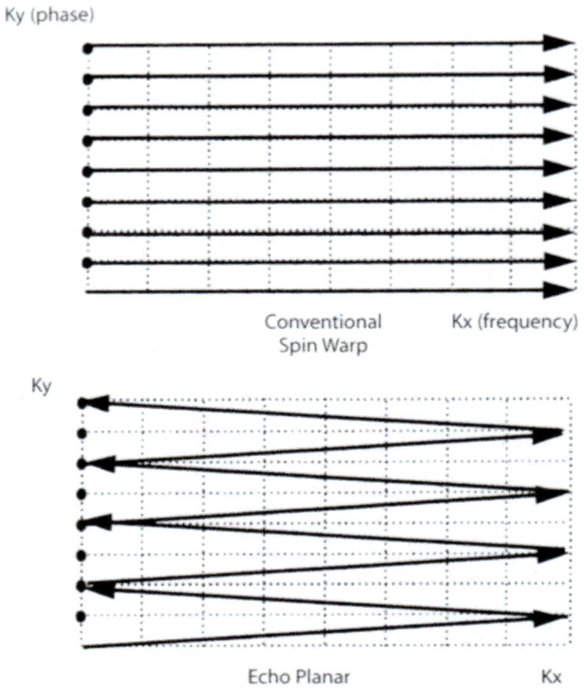

Fig. 4. Trajectories through k-space for conventional spin warp experiment (*top*) and echo planar experiment. In the spin warp experiment, a phase encoding gradient along *y* selects a row of k-space and the readout gradient samples the selected row in a single acquisition. The number of acquisitions required to form an image is equal to the number of rows of k-space that must be sampled. In the echo planar experiment (*bottom*) a gradient along the *x* axis samples the rows of k-space, while at the same time a smaller gradient produces motion along the *y* axis of k-space, so that the net effect is that k-space is traversed along a series of diagonal vectors

switching to sample more than one row of k-space following each excitation. Mansfield and coworkers introduced the first such method [10], which is referred to as echo planar imaging. A simplified version of echo planar imaging is shown in Fig. 5; this schematic is meant to illustrate the important principles of the method, and is not a complete representation of the technique. Immediately after rotation of magnetization into the transverse plane, an oscillating gradient is applied to sample rows of k-space (along *x*), while at the same time a lower amplitude gradient, sometimes referred to as a broadening gradient, moves the detection process along *y*. The net effect is that k-space is sampled along a series of diagonals. This process is repeated until all of k-space has been sampled. In this way, an entire image can be collected following a single slice-selective excitation pulse.

The factor which limits echo planar imaging is T_2* relaxation. Immediately following excitation, the transverse polarization begins to decay due, for example, to local magnetic field inhomogeneity (which is not due to the applied imaging gradients).

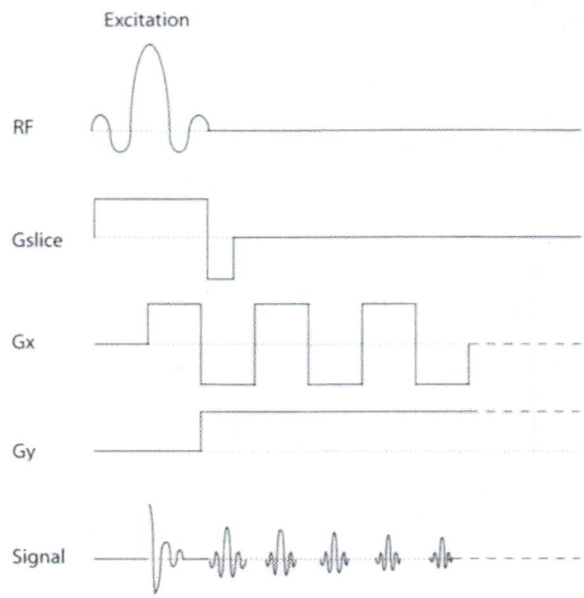

Fig. 5. Echo planar pulse sequence. RF in the presence of a gradient (*Gslice*), (i.e. along the "z" direction), selectively excites signal from a single slice. A gradient along the "x" direction (*Gx*) samples rows of k-space while the "broadening gradient" (*Gy*) moves the k-space trajectory along the "y" direction. An echo is detected for each diagonal through k-space

The time constant for this decay is generally on the order of 40 ms in a voxel with a 1-mm (the gradients across larger voxels are larger and therefore the decay is more rapid). The entire echo planar sequence must be completed before this decay becomes appreciable. Otherwise, much of k-space will not be sampled with an adequate signal-to-noise ratio. The need for very fast imaging requires that applied gradients are large and gradient switching is rapid. This requirement can be met with state-of-the art clinical imaging systems. As a result, echo planar imaging sequences can be applied in as little as 60 ms [11] to obtain spatial resolution of 1–2 mm in plane. This approach is particularly valuable for angiography in organs and tissues which are rapidly moving. For example, echo planar imaging is frequently used for coronary angiography.

Spiral k-Space Sampling

Spiral k-space sampling is under many conditions a more efficient way to obtain k-space information. The edges of k-space, which tend to contribute motion artifacts and reduce signal-to-noise ratio, are avoided with little expense in terms of image resolution [12]. The spiral trajectory can be sampled in a single shot so that the technique is analagous to echo planar imaging. This technique has been particularly useful for cardiac imaging [12].

Relaxation

For clinical purposes MR provides an image of water protons in the body. However, an image of proton density would contain little information. Outside of bone and fat, there is very little variation in water density throughout the body. But in fact, MR images generally provide better contrast for soft tissue than other imaging methods. This is because of the effect of nuclear spin relaxation on image intensity. Polarization in the transverse plane is lost in two ways, as described below.

Longitudinal Relaxation

Transverse polarization can return to its equilibrium position along the *z* axis, but to do so it must exchange an amount of energy equal to the Larmor energy with its surroundings. This is referred to as longitudinal or T_1 relaxation. There are a number of important pathways for T_1 relaxation in vivo. An important relaxation mechanism is the magnetic interaction of neighboring water protons, i.e., water protons on the same water molecule or on neighboring water molecules. Each proton produces a magnetic field which affects neighboring protons. The strength of the interaction depends on the distance between the protons and also the speed with which the magnetic dipoles move relative to each other, due primarily to rotational and translational motion and to exchange of protons between water molecules. The strength of the interaction changes when water molecules are associated with macromolecules (i.e., due to noncovalent binding) so that the speed of motion of the proton magnetic dipoles is reduced. Magnetic interactions between water protons and rapidly relaxing protons on proteins and other large structures are also important, and form the basis for "magnetization transfer imaging". Water protons can be relaxed by paramagnetic substances (i.e., molecules which contain unpaired electrons) such as oxygen or deoxyhemoglobin, or injected contrast agents.

"T_1-weighted images" are images in which T_1 is an important factor in controlling image intensity. Such images can be produced in many ways. One common method is to keep the time between successive excitations much shorter than T_1. After each 90° excitation pulse, very little *z* polarization remains, since all of the magnetization has been rotated into the *xy* plane, where polarization rapidly lost due to transverse relaxation (see below) and the dephasing effects of phase encoding and readout gradients. A second excitation pulse applied very soon after the first pulse will generate very little signal, since there is very little *z* polarization available to rotate into the transverse plane. Thus, when the delay between successive excitations is relatively short, the amount of signal generated depends on how much longitudinal polarization is recovered during this delay period. This recovery is the rate at which polarization returns to its equilibrium position along the *z* axis following saturation, or T_1. In tissues with a short T_1, polarization returns to the *z* axis rapidly after each excitation, and these tissues appear brighter in T_1-weighted images than tissues with a long T_1. For example, fat appears bright in T_1-weighted images because it has a short T_1, while edema appears dark because a high wet-to-dry weight ratio results in a long T_1. Heavily T_1-weighted images play an important role in MR angiography. This is because very strong T_1-weighting can be used to completely suppress signals from stationary magnetization in a slice, while magnetization in flowing blood which enters the slice rapidly is not saturated and thus produces a very large signal which can be used to estimate rates of blood flow and track blood vessels. This method, referred to as the "time of flight" method, is discussed in detail below.

Transverse Relaxation

Following excitation, the large ensemble of nuclear magnetic moments within each image voxel precess at slightly different frequencies, due to small variations in the local field which each nucleus experiences. These variations are caused by variations in local magnetic susceptiblity due to anatomic or physiologic heterogeneity. For example, a large concentration of deoxyhemoglobin in capillaries creates gradients in the magnetic field near the capillaries. These gradients lead to loss of phase coherence of the net transverse polarization, and therefore loss of signal. This process is referred to as T_2* relaxation. In "T_2*-weighted images", image pixels with large magnetic susceptibility gradients appear dark (e.g., regions near deoxygenated veins and capillaries), while image pixels where the magnetic field is homogeneous (e.g., edematous areas) appear bright.

Following the excitation pulse and subsequent loss of coherence in the transverse plane, coherence can be recovered by applying a "180° pulse" or "spin echo pulse." This RF pulse effectively reverses phase accumulation due to differences in resonance frequency so that at the end of the "echo evolution time" an echo is detected – that is, a maximum in the MR signal due to partial recovery of polarization in the transverse plane. The extent to which polarization is recovered following a spin echo pulse depends on T_2 relaxation. Although T_2 relaxation can occur by the same mechanism as T_1 relaxation (see above), T_2 relaxation in vivo is due primarily to diffusion of water molecules through magnetic susceptibility gradients. A special case of this is diffusion of water molecules along the direction of the applied gradient. In the more general case, water molecules diffuse through magnetic field gradients caused by variations in local magnetic susceptibility. Magnetic interactions between "coupled" protons (i.e., due to covalent bonds) also produce T_2 relaxaton. "T_2-weighted images" are images in which T_2 is an important factor in controlling image intensity. Such images can be produced using a spin echo pulse sequence with a long echo evolution time. In this case, tissues with a long T_2, such as edematous areas, appear bright while tissues with short T_2, such as liver (which contains high concentrations of free radicals), appear dark.

MR Instrumentation

This section will provide a brief introduction to the instrumentation required for MR imaging. A more complete discussion can be found in introductory textbooks [1–3].

Magnet

The largest and most expensive part of the MR imaging device is the magnet which is used to provide the polarization of anatomic nuclei. The technical specifications for these magnets are extraordinary. Standard imaging procedures require magnetic fields which are extremely homogeneous, i.e., less than 5 parts per million variation over a 50-cm diameter spherical volume. In addition, the field must be extremely stable with drift rates of less than 1 part per million per week. These requirements are routinely met by a variety of magnet designs. In general, these magnets are large enough to accommodate an entire adult human body, although smaller magnets which are specialized for imaging of extrempties or the head have also been developed. Magnets used clinically range in field strength from 0.1 tesla to 1.5 tesla. In addition, a small number of 4-tesla magnets are being tested for clinical use at the National Institutes of Health, the University of Minnesota, and several other laboratories [e.g., 13, 14]. Higher field strength is generally believed to provide higher signal-to-noise ratio and spatial resolution. However, due to the large fringe fields, high-field magnets are more difficult and expensive to site. They generally require extremely heavy iron shields (on the order of 60 tons), which reduce the fringe field but take up space and require expensive support beams. In addition, imaging at high fields poses technical difficulties – for example, detection and excitation coil tuning and stability is problematic.

Electromagnets (i.e., current flowing through resistive coils) and permanent magnets can be used to provide lower magnetic field strengths (under 0.5 tesla). These magnets are relatively inexpensive and easy to maintain. However, superconducting magnets are universally used at higher field strengths. Superconducting technology makes it possible to produce extremely high magnetic fields with a stability of better than a part per million. Superconducting magnets require a significant investment in maintenance; they require regular charging with liquid nitrogen and liquid helium. Occasionally they must be "ramped down" (that is, the current is removed from the solenoid) for service and this can be a very expensive operation.

The recent advent of actively shielded magnets has considerably reduced siting costs. In this design, an additional solenoid is placed outside of the solenoid which generates the field used for imaging. The outside solenoid is configured so that it cancels the fringe field produced by the inside solenoid. This reduces the need for heavy iron shields and increases the stability of the internal magnetic field.

Gradient Coils

The coils which produce magnetic field gradients used for imaging and angiographic studies are also a technical tour-de-force. They must provide highly linear gradients across large fields of view (about 50-cm diameter spherical volumes). If the gradients are not linear, images become distorted. In order to perform state-of-the-imaging experiments the gradients must have rapid rise times on the order of 200 ms to gradients of 5 G/cm. A problem which impedes the performance of rapidly switched gradient coils is that the changing magnetic fields they produce penetrate conductive materials which are used to construct the magnet. This induces eddy currents which decrease the speed with which gradients can be switched and produces time-dependent gradients in the magnet bore which can create severe artifacts in MR images. In recent years eddy currents have been greatly reduced by the use of self-shielded gradient coils. These coils include active outer shields which are designed to cancel magnetic flux lines which the gradient coils produce beyond the bore of the magnet. Self-shielded gradient coils have greatly increased the feasibility of echo planar imaging and the accuracy of a variety of angiographic measurements which require large gradients and fast switching.

Signal Excitation and Detection

Excitation and detection of MR signals is shown schematically in Fig. 6. A high power RF amplifier produces an RF signal which is coupled into a resonator inside the bore of the magnet which is placed around the target tissue. This high-power pulse rotates magnetization into the transverse plane so that it can be detected as discussed above. In the simplest case the same RF resonator (or "coil") is used for both excitation and detection, but in many cases a large-volume coil is used to produce a homogeneous RF field for excitation while a more sensitive local coil is used to detect signal. In the case of imaging experiments a pulsed magnetic field gradient is usually turned on during detection of the signal. The detected signal is then sent to a preamplifier. The preamplifier must have a very good noise figure (1.8–2.5 dB is common), and must be protected from the high power excitation pulse by passive or active diode networks. Following the initial preamplification the signal is mixed down to audio frequency and amplified further. Finally it is digitized and Fourier transformed. The timing of all of these events is controlled by a computer typically referred to as a pulse programmer. Timing is critical since errors of even a tenth of a part per million can cause amplitude and phase distortions. It is the phase coherence of the entire excitation, detection, and amplification process which makes a variety of phase-sensitive angiographic methods possible as discussed below.

Digital Processing and Display

Since its inception, MR imaging has been heavily dependent on digital data acquisiton control, processing, and display. Timing of each event in MR pulse sequences requires nanosecond precision, and a number of hardware devices, including RF amplifiers, gradient amplifiers, and digitizers, are under the control of a central computer. In general, the

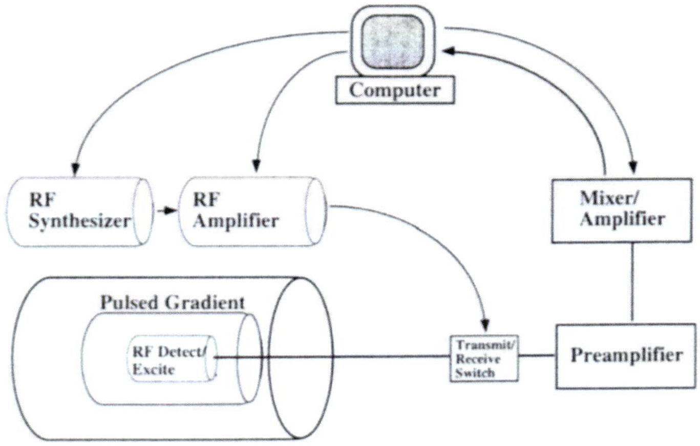

Fig. 6. An MR imaging system. The magnet produces magnetic polarization. Pulsed gradients are used to produce images by labeling each point in the magnet with a specific frequency. RF signals produced by a synthesizer are amplified and then sent to a tuned circuit (RF detection/excitation coil), where they produce a magnetic field which rotates magnetization into the transverse plane. Signal is then detected, amplified, mixed down to audio frequencies, and digitized

computer must be able to control acquisition of MR data while at the same time processing and displaying data which has already been acquired. Several aspects of angiographic studies make high-speed computers especially important for data processing. Angiographic studies which are based on the use of contrast agents require acquisition of a large number of images in a short period of time (0.5 – 10.0 s/image). A series of high-resolution, large field-of-view images can casily generate 100 megabytes of data. Angiographic studies may also require processing and display of large three-dimensional data with views from any desired direction. Currently, a great deal of effort is devoted to development of MR "fluoroscopy". This means that high-speed MR images are acquired continuously during a surgical procedure. Images must be reconstructed and displayed in real time to provide a useful picture for the physician. As a result of these requirements, modern MR scanners are usually operated by computers with central processing units operating at 200 MHz or faster, 64 megabytes of random access memory, and many gigabytes of hard disk space. The instrument control computers are generally connected to off-line workstations which allow further data analysis, viewing, and storage.

Noninvasive Angiographie Methods

CT and X-ray angiography require injection of contrast agents which provide a high signal-to-noise ratio but pose some risk and cause some discomfort. Although MR studies can also be performed with contrast, there is a class of MR methods which do not require injection of exogeneous tracer molecules. These methods rely on magnetic tagging of water molecules, and fall into two general classes, *Bolus tagging* or *time-of-flight* and *phase-sensitive* methods. In both cases, patterns are encoded in the phase or amplitude of water proton magnetization. When water molecules move, the magnetic label moves with them. The motion or decay of these patterns as a function of time can be analyzed to determine the velocity of flow of water molecules. MRA is based on the use of these methods to measure coherent blood flow (i. e., blood flow with relatively constant velocity and direction) in large vessels.

Bolus Tagging or Time-of-Flight

In an early implementation of MR angiography, blood flow was measured in the human forearm [11]. A brief discussion of this work will illustrate some basic principles of angiography. A simplified version of the experiment is illustrated in Fig. 7. A surface coil can be placed over the artery and used to saturate magnetization flowing past the coil. The saturated nuclei become "MR-invisible" since there is no net z polarization which can be detected. A second coil can be placed upstream from the first coil and used to detect signals from blood flowing through the artery. A decrease in the signal from the blood is detected when saturated nuclei reach the second coil. Saturating pulses from coil 1 are delivered at precisely timed intervals, and the time between saturating pulses and appearance of saturated nuclei at coil 2 is measured. The rate of blood flow is calculated on the basis of the distance between the two coils and the time required for saturated nuclei to reach the second coil. The magnetic label, i. e., saturation of the nuclei at a certain position, lasts on the order of several T_1s. Therefore, dynamic processes which occur within one T_1, can be accurately measured using this method.

A more recent generalization of this method which provides much greater flexibility and spatial resolution is to selectively saturate a slice of tissue upstream from the slice which is to be imaged. This is done by repeatedly exciting the upstream slice using 90° slice-selective excitation with a delay between excitation pulses which is much shorter than T_1. This means that the magnetization in the slice which is selectively saturated contains very little longitudinal polarization and produces a very low signal in MR images. Flowing blood from the saturated slice will still be partially saturated when it moves downstream into the slice which is imaged. Therefore the flowing blood will appear dark in the imaged slice. In fact the degree of saturation depends on the time required for blood to flow from lhe saturated slice to the imaged slice (i. e., the "time-of-flight") as well as T_1. Therefore the degree of saturation of the blood signal is a measure of the velocity of blood flow.

2D Time-of-Flight

The "2D time-of-flight" method is currently the most widely used MR angiographic method [15 – 22]. This method is based on the principle that

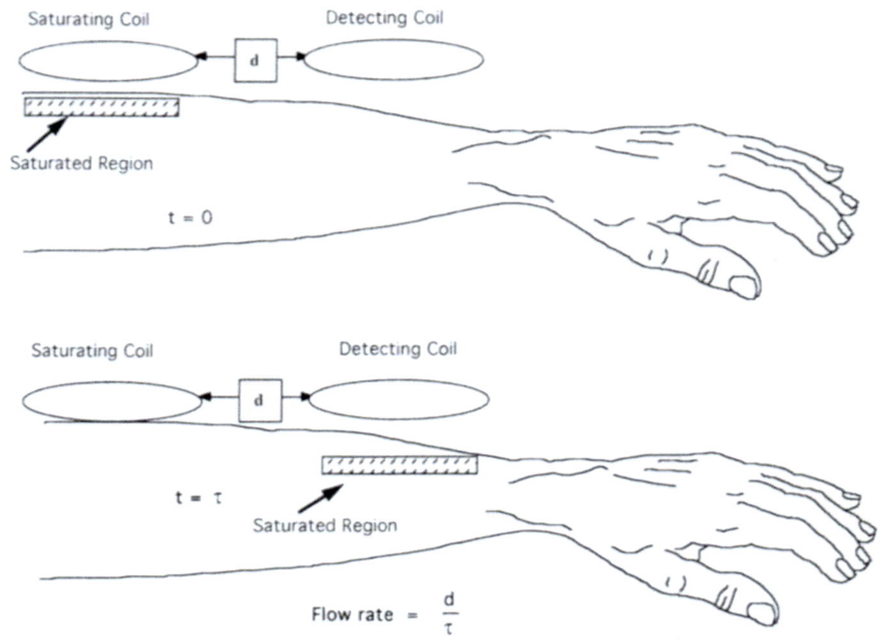

Fig. 7. Illustration of the Singer bolus tracking experiment. A surface coil is placed over the artery and used to saturate magnetization as it flows by. A second coil detects the flowing magnetization

when water proton nuclei within a thin slice are excited using selective excitation as discussed above the signals from the slice can be saturated if the delay between successive excitation pulses is very short compared to T_1. As a result, very little signal comes from static magnetization in the selected slice. However, magnetization which flows into the slice rapidly in blood is not saturated by repeated excitations and appears much brighter than static magnetization in two-dimensional images of the slice. Therefore, large arteries and veins can be easily identified. The optimal contrast between blood vessels and tissue is obtained when the slice which is excited and imaged is perpendicular to the direction of flow since in this way the speed with which blood flows through the slice is maximized. The minimum velocity of blood flow which can be detected is on the order of $\Delta z/TR$ where Δz is the thickness of the selectively excited slice and TR is the time between excitation pulses; that is, blood must flow through the excited slice during the time between excitations so that most of the blood present in the slice at any given time is relatively unsaturated. Typically, a series of transverse slices through tissue containing larger blood vessels is imaged to provide a series of cross-sectional views of the arteries, which are then analyzed using a maximum intensity projection (MIP) algorithm [22, 23] which provides a view of the entire vessel.

A number of variables must be optimized to obtain good contrast between flowing blood and static material:

Pulse length: Low-angle excitation pulses (30° or less) may provide improved signal-to-noise ratio for blood that flows through the slice relatively slowly, but may inadequately suppress (i.e., saturate) signals from static material.

TR: A shorter TR provides improved suppression of signal from static material but may also decrease signal from blood if the flow velocity is low.

Slice thickness: A thinner slice is more sensitive to slower-flowing blood, since $\Delta z/TR$ is small. In addition, a thinner slice minimizes loss of signal due to turbulence. However, the signal-to-noise ratio generally requires that slices be 2 mm thick or greater.

Image resolution: Smaller pixels sizes provide better delineation of the contours of arteries and veins, and also reduce problems due to turbulence. However, signal-to-noise ratio considerations place a lower limit of approximately 1 mm on in-plane spatial resolution.

Gradient strength: In order to image flowing blood, the phase and frequency of the blood magnetization must be accurately determined during application of phase encoding and readout gradients. High-resolution images require that the integral of the applied gradients (duration x amplitude) be large. To obtain approximately 1 mm in-pla-

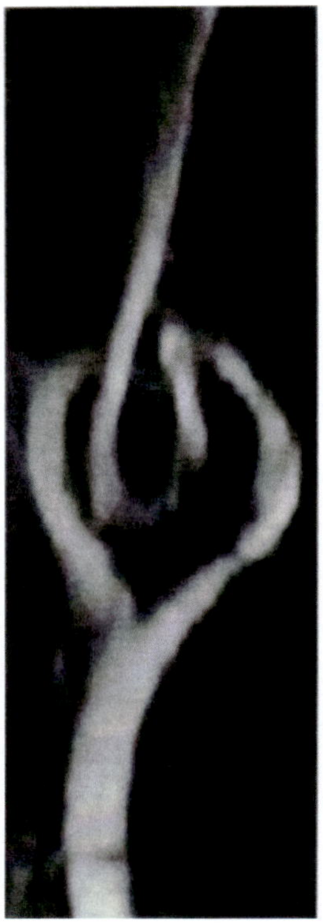

Fig. 8. This is a 2D time-of-flight image of the carotid region obtained at the University of Chicago, on a GE 1.5-tesla Signa system using a spoiled GRASS sequence with a TR of 41 ms and a TE of 8.7 ms. Image matrix size was 256 x 128. Sixty slices were obtained in approximately 10 min and combined using a maximum intensity projection (MIP) algorithm. Voxel size in the MIPs was approximately 0.6 x 1.2 x 1 mm. The tortuous internal carotid artery was difficult to display in conventional projections, but is well demonstrated using this edited MIP

ne spatial resolution, either large-amplitude gradients (5–10 G/cm) must be applied for short periods of time (200–500 μs) or lower-amplitude gradients (0.5–1 G/cm) must be applied for longer periods of time (2–5 ms). If the motion of the blood along these gradients is significant, large motion artifacts result and the image quality is inadequate. Therefore higher-amplitude gradient pulses must be applied for short time periods to image rapidly flowing blood. On the other hand, it is advantageous to use lower-amplitude readout gradients when the velocity of blood allows, since in the absence of significant T_2* losses this can significantly improve signal-to-noise ratio [24].

A number of techniques have been developed to improved visualization of arteries. One is selective saturation of slices downstream from the arterial section which is to be imaged. This saturates venous blood which enters the slice and thus differentiates between arterial and venous signals [25]. Improved suppression of tissue signals can be achieved using magnetization transfer methods. An RF field applied far off-resonance saturates broad signals due to protons bound to macromolecular structures, notably proteins [26, 27]. Due to coupling between protons in the aqueous phase and these bound protons, saturation of the broad resonance results in transfer of saturation to the narrow water resonance and thus greatly decreases image intensity (up to 50%). Since magnetization transfer effects are relatively weak in blood but strong in most tissue [28], this procedure results in significant reduction in the signal from stationary material relative to signal from blood and thus increases the relative brightness of the arteries.

Figure 8 is a high-resolution image of the carotid region obtained using the 2D time-of-flight method. The image was reconstructed using an MIP algorithm from images of 128 transverse slices acquired sequentially. This examination is one of the most popular applications of 2D time-of-flight.

3D Time-of-Flight

In the case of very rapidly flowing blood, three-dimensional imaging methods can be used rather than the multiple slice methods used for 2D time-of-flight images [29–31]. This means that a relatively thick slice is selectively excited and phase encoding is used to provide additional spatial resolution along the slice direction. Phase encoding is also used in the second dimension, and a readout gradient is used along the third dimension to provide high-resolution three-dimensional images of the selectively excited slice. This approach can provide better spatial definition along the slice direction than the two-dimensional method. However, only very rapid blood flow is imaged effectively, since blood must traverse the thick slice which is excited in a time which is short compared to T_1.

Figure 9a shows a large cerebral arteriovenous malformation imaged using the 3D time-of-flight approach at the University of Chicago using a Signa 1.5-tesla system. Areas with high flow rates are well depicted, while slower flowing blood in large venous structures is not well visualized. For comparison, Fig. 9b shows an image of the same patient obtained using phase contrast angiography (see p. 127). The phase-sensitive method shows slow-flowing blood more clearly.

Advantages and Disadvantages of Time-of-Flight Methods

Time-of-flight methods are currently the most widely used MR angiographic methods. This is primarily because they are extremely straightforward. De-

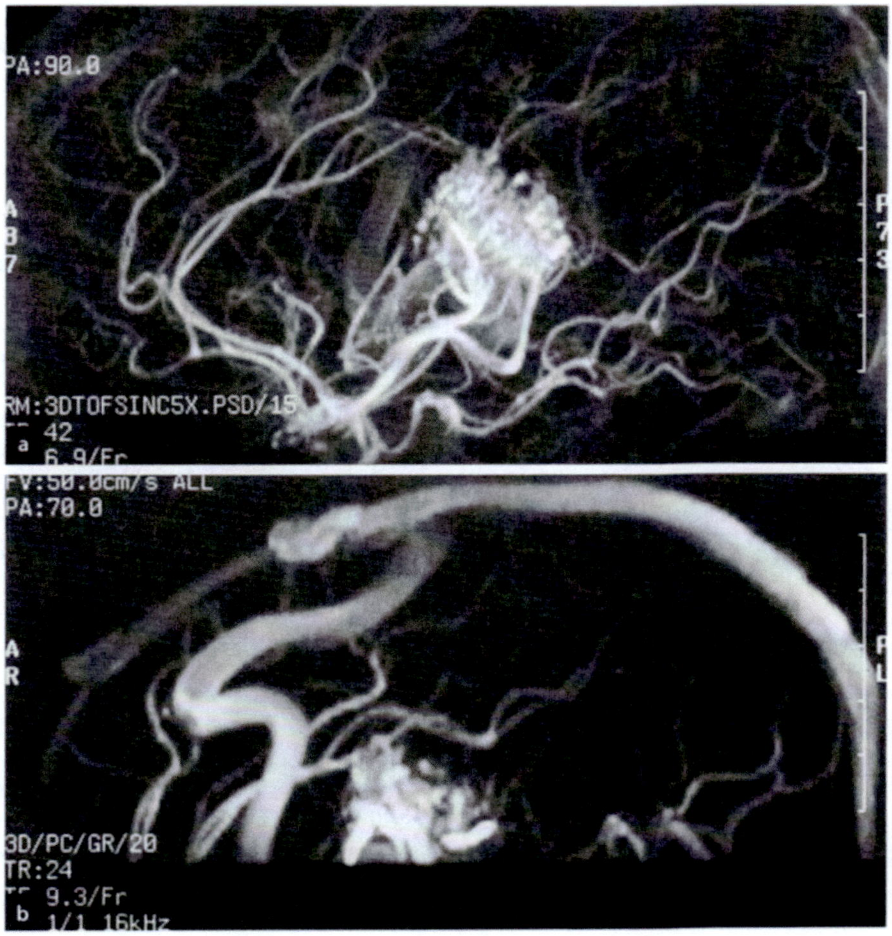

Fig. 9 a. A large cerebral arteriovenous malformation is demonstrated by means of a 3D time-of-flight study performed at the University of Chicago using a Signa 1.5-tesla system with a TR of 42 ms and a TE of 6.9 ms. Imaging time was 10 min and the matrix was 256 x 192 x 60. Voxel size was 0.6 x 0.9 x 0.8 mm. Areas with high flow rates are well depicted, while slower-flowing blood in large venous structures is typically less sensitive to 3D time-of-flight techniques. **b** Same patient, 3D phase contrast study with a TR of 42 ms and a TE of 6.9 ms. The image was acquired in approximately 10 min. Voxel size was 0.6 x 1.2 x 1 mm. Slow-flowing blood in the veins draining the malformation is elegantly depicted

spite the many variations of the technique mentioned above, a usable image of a large vessel which contains rapidly flowing blood can be obtained simply by selecting a relatively narrow slice and imaging with a short TR. Time-of-flight methods are less sensitive than phase-sensitive methods to motion artifacts and artifacts due to turbulence. This makes them particularly useful for studies of the abdominal cavity, where they are becoming competitive with conventional angiography [32]. On the other hand, accurate quantitation of blood flow velocity and direction is more difficult with time-of-flight methods than with phase-sensitive methods. In addition, improvements in hardware, particularly the development of fast self-shielded gradients, will tend to favor phase-sensitive methods.

Phase-Sensitive Methods

In recent years, the popularity of phase-sensitive methods has increased [33–38]. These methods take advantage of the fact that the frequency of precession of transverse magnetization changes as it moves along a magnetic field gradient. To understand this, we compare the effect of a gradient echo on stationary and flowing magnetization. Following rotation into the transverse plane by an excitation pulse, stationary magnetization precesses at a relatively constant rate. If a static field gradient pulse (a dephasing gradient) is applied, the frequency at which the magnetization precesses will change while the gradient is on by an amount ($\Delta\omega_a$) based on the position of the magnetization along the gradient. This will result in a net accumulation of phase relative to the phase the magnetization would acquire in the absence of a gradient. After a time t, a refocusing gradient is applied. For stationary magnetization, the change in precession frequency in the presence of the refocusing gradient ($\Delta\omega_b$) is the negative of the change in the precession frequency during the initial dephasing gradient. Therefore, the accumulation of phase during the refocusing gradient exactly reverses the loss of phase during the dephasing gradient, and the net phase at the end of the gradient echo is "0", i.e., a gradient echo is formed. However, if magnetization moves during the period between gradients, the position in the dephasing gradient is not the same as the position in the refocusing gradient, and $\Delta\omega_a$ is no longer the negative of $\Delta\omega_b$. In this case:

$$\Delta\omega_a - \Delta\omega_b = \gamma G_I{}^* (x_a - x_b) \quad (2)$$

where γ is the gyromagnetic ratio (Hz/G), G_I the area of the gradient waveform, x_a is the position of magnetization during the dephasing gradient and x_b is the position of magnetization during the refocusing gradient. Therefore the net phase accumulation at the end of the gradient echo is

$$\text{phase} = (\Delta\omega_a - \Delta\omega_b) \text{ x } t \quad (3)$$

This simplified analysis assumes that a very large gradient is applied for a very short period of time, so that there is very little motion of blood with respect to the gradient during the time the gradient is applied; most of the motion is assumed to occur during the echo evolution period *t*. With this assumption, the velocity of flow can be calculated from the change in phase:

$$\text{velocity} = \Delta \text{ phase}/(t \text{ x } \gamma \text{ x } G_I \quad (4)$$

Since the phase of transverse magnetization is measured, only motion which occurs on the order of the constant for decay of transverse magnetization, i.e., $T_2{}^*$, is detected. However, this period, on the order of 25–50 ms, is long enough for the motion of blood in major vessels to be easily detected when gradients of 0.5 G/cm or higher are used. For example, with a gradient strength of 1 G/cm applied for 5 ms, a gradient echo evolution period of 25 ms, and blood flow velocity along the gradient of 1 cm/s, a gradient echo would result in a change of phase of approximately 180°; this change can easily be detected. This method is designed to detect blood which flows at constant velocity. In some vessels, such as the aorta, more complicated methods [39, 40] must be used to account for both velocity and constant or increasing acceleration.

The evolution period and gradient strength used for the gradient echo must be carefully selected. If flow is so rapid that the change in phase of signals from blood is greater than 180°, the velocity of blood flow can be dramatically underestimated. For example, a change in phase of 450° may be misinterpreted as a change of 90°, leading to an estimate of the flow rate which is 20% of the true value. This is a typical problem for discrete sampling methods. In order to determine the true rate at which the phase of magnetization is advanced by flow, the phase must be allowed to advance no more than 180° in one sampling period, i.e., during the evolution time of the gradient echo. One way to make accurate measurements is to perform Fourier analysis of flow velocity. To do this, a series of gradient echoes are acquired, gradient amplitudes are incremented in steps jand the change in the phase of magnetization caused by each gradient echo is measured. The change in phase is plotted against gradient strength, and the Fourier transform gives a "spectrum" of blood flow velocities. The highest rate of blood flow which can be measured using this method is the flow rate which advances the phase of magnetization by 180° for each increment in gradient strength. More rapid flow rates will be undersampled and therefore underestimated. Although the Fourier analysis provides accurate measurements across a range of blood flow velocities, it is not often used because of the time requirement. When combined with a standard imaging experiment, each of a number of velocity encoding gradient echoes must be combined with the series of phase-encoding steps (typically 64–128 steps) which are used to form the image.

The phase-sensitive method measures *only* the rate of blood flow along the gradient. Gradients which form the gradient echo can be applied along any three orthogonal directions to determine the direction of blood flow. This procedure is time consuming, since a separate image must be obtained to determine the rate of flow in each direction. A more practical alternative is to apply velocity encoding gradients along the direction of the vessels which are under investigation; this can be determined from high-resolution reference images.

High-quality phase contrast images can be obtained in which *only* signals from blood flowing at a selected velocity appear. This procedure is illustrated in Fig. 10. First an image is obtained in which no velocity encoding gradients are applied. Next, an image is obtained in which velocity encoding gradients are adjusted so that magnetization in flowing blood which is to be imaged undergoes a 180° phase shift due to its motion through the gradient. The first complex data set is then subtracted from the second to obtain an image in which only flowing blood appears. Alternatively, the two data sets can be added to obtain an image in which only signals from stationary tissue appear, and signals from flowing blood are greatly attenuated. Note that this procedure selects only one velocity component in blood which is flowing along one direction. Only magnetization flowing along the applied gradient at a speed such that a 180° phase shift occurs during the gradient echo will appear in the difference image; other velocity components will be significantly attentuated. However, it is possible to obtain a series of images which emphasize blood flowing at different velocities in three orthogonal directions.

An example of a phase-sensitive image of a large cerebral arteriovenous malformation is shown in Fig. 9 b. Slower flowing blood is more clearly visualized in the phase-sensitive image than in the analogous 3D time-of-flight study (Fig. 9 a). This is particularly important for the examination of large venous structures.

In addition to their important practical applications, phase shifts due to flow through applied gradients can pose problems. An important artifact occurs because flow velocity in blood vessels is not uniform. The phase accumulation experienced by different velocity components will be different, and this leads to phase dispersion, which decreases the signal-to-noise ratio of MR images. This artifact can be minimized by reducing the effective evolution time of gradient echoes and the duration and amplitude of gradients which are applied for velocity encoding purposes. This will reduce the amount of phase dispersion which occurs, but at the same time reduces sensitivity to slowly flowing components. Another method for reducing the effects of turbulence is to reduce voxel size. This decreases the amount of phase dispersion which can occur in each voxel, i. e., decreases linewidth, at the expense of a reduced signal-to-noise ratio.

It is important to note that velocity-dependent phase shifts are caused not only by "velocity encoding" gradients, but by other applied gradients as well. For example, slice selection gradients can cause phase shifts and other artifacts [41]. One reason for this is that the frequency of moving magnetization changes during the selective excitation

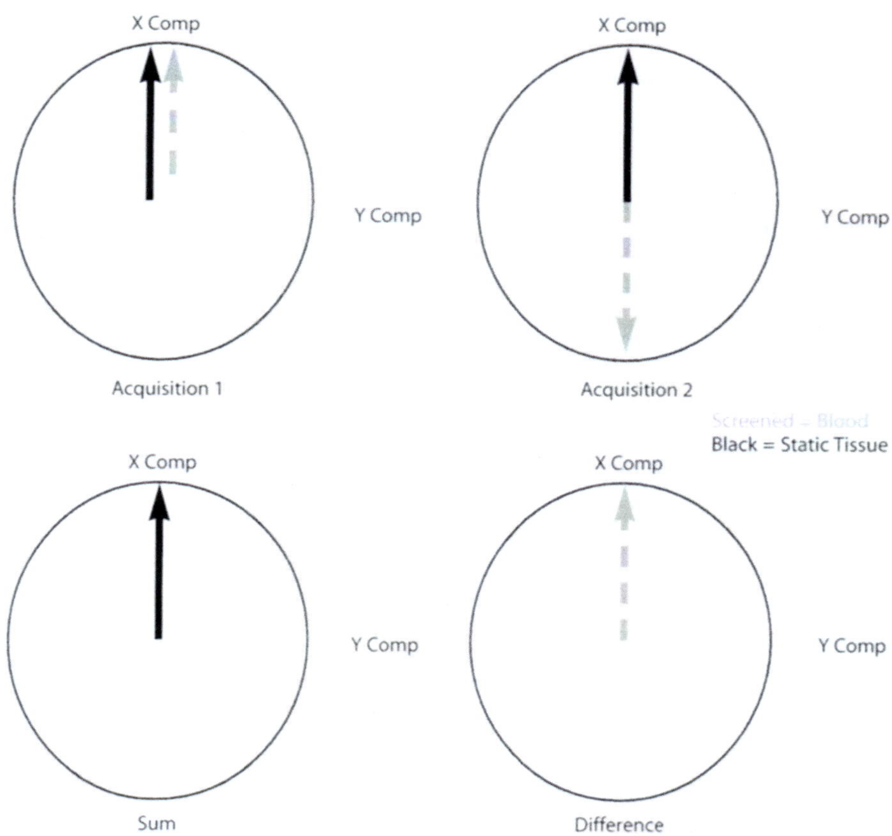

Fig. 10. Detection of a selected velocity component. First an image is obtained in which no velocity encoding gradients are applied. Next, an image is obtained in which velocity encoding gradients are adjusted so that magnetization in flowing blood which is to be imaged undergoes a 180° phase shift due to its motion through the gradient. The first complex data set is then subtracted from the second to obtain an image in which only flowing blood appears. Alternatively, the two data sets can be added to obtain an image in which only signals from stationary tissue appear, and signals from flowing blood are greatly attenuated

pulse. In the extreme case, magnetization which was not initially in the selected slice enters the slice during the excitation pulse, but does not experience the full effect of the pulse. In this ease, the transverse phase and amplitude is distorted. In addition, the position of magnetization along the slice selection gradient may be different during the excitation pulse and during the refocusing pulse, leading to undesirable phase shifts. The same thing can occur along the direction of the readout gradient. Due to nonuniform flow, velocity-dependent phase shifts can result in loss of signals and artifacts. In some cases, "flow compensation gradients" are added in the slice selection and readout directions to minimize these effects.

Phase-sensitive angiography has a number of practical advantages. Vessels are clearly distinguished from surrounding tissue based on changes in phase of magnetization due to blood flow. Therefore, vessel morphology can be studied with high resolution in three dimensions. By varying the amplitude and direction of velocity encoding gradients, rates of blood flow can be measured with high precision and the direction of blood flow can be accurately determined. An important application of this technique is detection of stenosis. Stenosis causes turbulence so that blood flows at a range of different velocities and in different directions. As a result, the gradient echo does not generate magnetization with a single phase which is characteristic of the velocity of flow. Rather, magnetization arrives at a range of phases, and this lack of phase coherence results in dramatic attenuation of the echo. Thus stenosis or other turbulence-creating malformations appear as areas of phase cancellation – that is, dark areas.

An important weakness of phase-sensitive MR angiographic methods is sensitivity to motion artifacts. If a large gradient is placed across the sample to provide sensitivity to blood flow, then any motion of the sample along the direction of the gradient produces a phase shift. Thus breathing movements or other involuntary motions have a significant effect on the appearance of the images. A second disadvantage is that each measurement detects only a narrow range of blood flow velocities along a single direction. This range is determined by the amplitude and duration of the velocity encoding gradients which are applied. Velocity components which are slower than those selected or along a different direction than that of the applied gradient will not produce detectable changes in the images. Components at a greater velocity than those selected will be "folded back" – that is, their velocity will appear to be much lower than it actually is. In order to properly analyze all velocity components in all directions, a large number of independent examinations must be performed and the time required becomes exorbitant.

Studies of heart function are an important area for application of this method. The heart is a difficult target, since mechanical motion of the heart can affect the apparent rate of flow of blood and can also cause image artifacts which make quantitative interpretation difficult. A number of approaches have been developed to minimize motion artifacts:

Cardiac gating: Excitation and detection can be triggered at a chosen phase of the cardiac cycle, generally determined from EKG monitoring during MR studies. In addition to reducing artifacts, cardiac gating also allows measurement of blood flow at different phases of the cardiac cycle. This procedure is referred to as "cine MR" and produces very high quality images which can be used to assess cardiac function [42, 43].

Fast imaging: Artifacts can also be reduced by using rapid imaging methods such as echo planar imaging, which reduce the amount of heart motion which occurs during acquisition of images.

Retrospective gating: A conventional MR image typically requires 128–256 phase encoding steps. For retrospective gating, a much larger number of phase encoding steps are performed at random points in the cardiac cycle. Information obtained concomitantly from a motion detector either a mechanical detector or a pulse sequence [44] is later used to group the phase encoding steps according to the point in the cardiac cycle at which data were acquired. A series of images can then be produced which show the heart at various phases in the cycle. An important goal of current research is to develop MR angiographic methods which provide high-quality, clinically useful images of coronary arteries [45, 46]. This is very difficult because of the small size and complicated curvature of the coronaries. However, a great deal of progress has been made in this area. If these methods come into clinical practice they may prove superior to conventional methods because they are completely noninvasive and provide completely three-dimensional images of the arterial tree.

Contrast Agents for Angiography

Early in the development of MR imaging it was hoped that MR would provide such strong intrinsic contrast that contrast agents would not be needed. However, it was soon discovered [47–49] that a variety of substances could dramatically improve contrast in MR images. Generally, contrast agents are paramagnetic substances which have very large magnetic moments. Magnetic interactions between the unpaired electrons of contrast agents and water protons in living tissue cause T_1, T_2, and T_2* relaxation which leads to changes in signal intensity. The change in signal amplitude will depend on the distribution of the contrast agent. For example, gadolinium-albumin-DTPA is generally an intravascular contrast agent which increases signal from blood relative to surrounding tissue, and can be used to evaluate vascular function Gadolinium-DTPA is rapidly extracted from the vasculature but provides intravascular contrast during the first pass of the contrast bolus.

Currently, gadolinium-containing substances are the only FDA-approved contrast agents. Concentrations of gadolinium-DTPA as low as 200 μM can be detected with high spatial resolution. However, following an intravenous bolus injection, concentrations of contrast in blood vessels during the first pass often reach 50 mM. In large vessels such as the aorta, this causes a large decrease in the T_1 of blood, so that the vessel appears much brighter in T_1-weighted images, i.e., images in which the repetition time is minimized (Fig. 11). In smaller vessels and/or when a gradient echo imaging sequence with a long TE is used, changes in T_2* are detected [48, 49]. Large concentrations of contrast agents trapped in blood vessels during the first pass of contrast produce significant changes in, local magnetic susceptibility (due to the high magnetic susceptibility of the contrast agent) [49–51]. This causes large time-dependent magnetic field gradients and hence dephasing of transverse polarization in the vicinity of the blood vessels. As a result, there is significant loss of signal as the contrast bolus passes through arteries and arterioles [50, 51]. This type of contrast is particularly important in the kidneys, where the filtering process produces high concentrations and a heterogeneous distribution of contrast agent and thus large magnetic field gradients. This may account for some of the dark areas visible in the kidneys in Fig. 11.

Changes in T_1, and T_2* in and around major vessels are most pronounced during the first pass of gadolinium-DTPA when the bolus is concentrated, i.e., before it passes through the capillary system where it is dispersed and extractecl into the extravascular space. Rapid gradient echo imaging of the bolus of contrast as it moves down major vessels can be used to estimate the speed at which the bolus moves and therefore rate of blood flow. In addition, cross-sectional views of the contrast bolus as it propagates through the arterial system can provide excellent views of stenoses and other malformations. Use of contrast agents provides extremely high signal-to-noise ratio because their effects on both T_1 and T_2* can produce changes of 50 % or more in MR signals. Therefore the signal-to-noise ratio of difference images which show the change in signal produced by the contrast bolus is almost as high as the signal-to-noise ratio of conventional MR imaging. T_1-weighted images can often be analyzed to determine the concentration of contrast in the blood vessels, on the basis of the change in T_1, produced by the contrast agent. In addition, T_1 contrast clearly delineates the boundaries of vessels. T_2* contrast can also be used to determine contrast concentration [48, 49] but is somewhat less quantitative than T_1 contrast. The T_2* effects spread beyond the blood vessel containing contrast and thus it may be difficult to identify vessel boundaries accurately [49–51]. This problem is compounded because changes in T_2*-weighted image intensity caused by contrast depend strongly on the size and orientation of the blood vessels in each image voxel.

Conclusion

MRA was first developed for studies of the head and neck. The carotid bifurcation is the most common site of extracranial atherosclerotic disease threatening the blood supply to the brain. MRA is growing in popularity in this area, and in many centers it is becoming a routine procedure. It should however, be regarded at the present time as a useful screening technique only, not a diagnostic examination. This is because MRA has limitations, including overestimation of the degree of stenosis due to turbulent bloodflow, with resultant signal loss. It yields insufficient information concerning the arterial wall – the presence, severity, and nature of both atherosclerotic plaques and the arterial lumen itself. Small ulcerations are commonly missed and occasionally large ones may be hidden. Subintimal hemorrhage and hematomas can also be overlooked even by the most experienced. An important complementary techni-

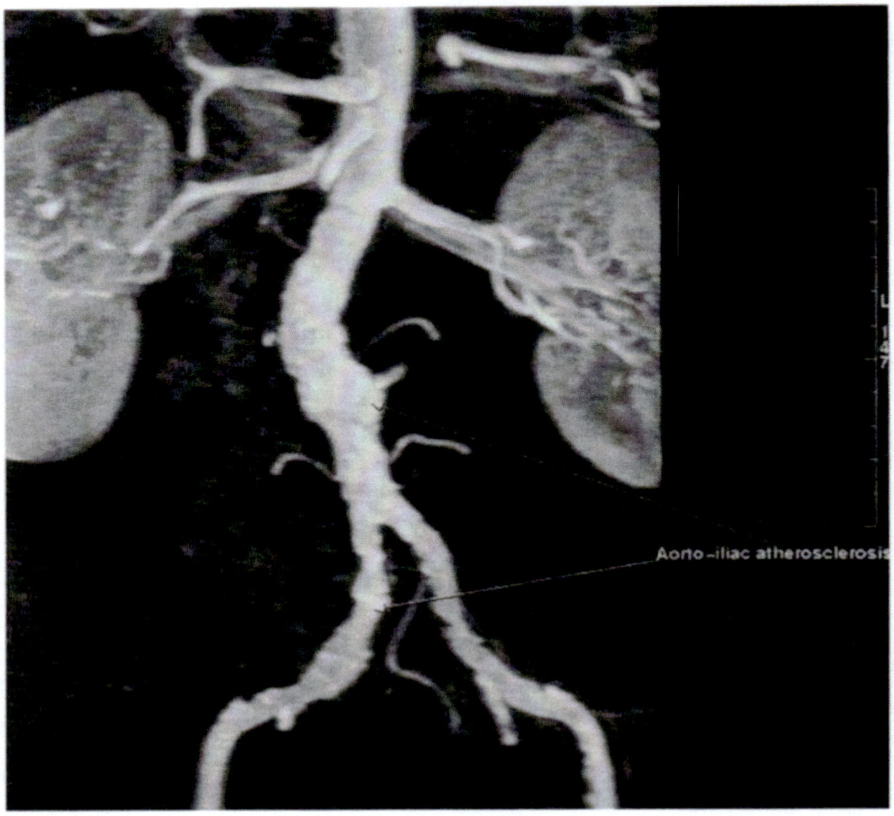

Fig. 11. Gadoloinium contrast-enhanced image of the abdominal aorta and its branches using a Spectris Injector (Medrad Corporation, Pittsburgh, Pennsylvania), demonstrate normal renal and visceral vessels but marked atherosclerosis of the iliac arteries (*arrows*) using fast T_1-weighted images. Twenty-eight slices were obtained during breath holding following contrast injection. Pulse sequence was 3D fast gradient echo with TR 7.1 ms and TE 2 ms. In-plane resolution was 1.2 x 2.5 mm

que is spin echo imaging which allows the wall and blood vessel lumen to be evaluated. Time-of-flight imaging in 2D and 3D is to some extent machine-dependent, but most scanners can adequately show the extracranial as well as the intracranial vasculature. When blood flow is extremely slow, phase contrast imaging may be required to demonstrate the "string sign" involving high-grade stenoses. Such patients may be incorrectly thought to have a total occlusion unless the distal vessel is seen.

Intracranial vessels are studied to identify arterial stenoses, arteriovenous malformations, aneurysms and tumors. In the future, newer MR techniques may reduce signal loss, leading to improved contrast and spatial resolution. The recent commercially available echo planar techniques with subsecond scanning may provide diagnostic studies more compar able to digital subtraction selective angiography. The expectations for MRA, therefore, are great. Measurements of blood flow in vessels and possibly regional tissue perfusion are other exciting possibilities. The use of contrast-enhancing paramagnetic agents requires further validation in this context.

In addition to screening, MRA is valuable for post-treatment follow-up. MRA of the renal arteries, pelvis and lower extremities is believed by many to be still in its infancy, but its potential is great. Practical considerations include situations in which the blood supply is so reduced that conventional arteriography is either very difficult or inadequate; patients with a severe allergy to iodine and those with high creatinine levels due to renal failure are also very suitable candidates for MRA. Many of these patients suffer from diabetes mellitus and have extensive small-vessel disease. Surgeons expect the radiologist to demonstrate very small peripheral vessels, such as those in the feet, in great detail, and this is challenging for MRA. Furthermore, in patients with acute embolic obstruction, thrombolytic therapy needs to be instituted urgently. MRA can detect such emboli, but takes additional time and thus delays the implementation of catheter-delivered intraarterial thrombolysis therapy. Similar arguments could be made for patients requiring other types of vascular interventional therapy. At present, MRA cost-effective but in general less readily available than conventional angiography. Convincing outcome analysis studies are lacking, and are very difficult to perform [52].

Thoracic studies are challenging because of motion artifact and the number and complexity of vascular structures in the chest. Screening for venous and arterial congenital cardiac and other anomalies as well as acquired disease is possible, and more centers are gaining experience with these procedures. Numerous publications have described the value of MRA techniques in the thorax [45, 46, 53–56]. Most cardiac imaging techniques require some form of EKG gating [56], although high-speed gradient echo imaging and, more recently, echo planar imaging is changing the outlook of cardiovascular MR applications. The general concensus is that no one MR technique is adequate for studying the thoracic vasculature. This is why radiologists need to tailor their studies to the clinical problem, and why a team approach including a physicist working together with physicians and technologists is required for the best studies. Further refinements, experience, and, most importantly, the forces driving health care reform and regulation will determine which studies will be reimbursed, when they should be performed, and with what priority. Screening and diagnosis of vascular disease comprises a major component of health care, and competing technologies including nuclear medicine, ultrasonography, (transthoracic, transesophegeal, and intravascular), interventional studies, and MRA must be considered in terms of cost and efficacy. It is imperative that both the technical factors and the clinical needs are understood by everyone involved in this exciting field, since the welfare of the patient is the real objective, not the technology.

References

1. Fukushima E, Roeder SBW (1981) Experimental pulse NMR. Addison-Wesley, New York
2. Gillies RJ (1994) NMR in physiology and biomedicine. Academic, New York
3. Cho ZH, Jones P, Singh M (1993) Foundations of medical imaging. Wiley, New York
4. Lauterbur PC (1973) Image formation by induced local interactions: examples employing nuclear magnetic resonance. Nature 242: 190–191
5. Damadian R, Goldsmith M, Minkoff L (1977) Fonar image of the live human body. Physiol Chem Phys Med NMR 9: 97–105
6. Mansfield PC, Grannell PK (1973) NMR "diffraction" in solids? J Phys C Solid State Phys 6: L422–L426
7. Kumar A, Welti D, Ernst RR (1975) NMR Fourier zeugmatography. J Magn Reson 18: 69–83
8. Cao Y, Levin DN (1992) MR imaging with spatially variable resolution. J Magn Reson Imaging 2: 701–709
9. Foo TK, Shellock FG, Hayes CE, Schenk JF, Slayman BE (1992) High-resolution MR imaging of the wrist and eye with short TR, short TE, and partial-echo acquisition. Radiology 183: 277–281
10. Stehling MK, Turner R, Mansfield P (1991) Echo-planar imaging: magnetic resonance imaging in a fraction of a second. Science 4: 43–50
11. Singer JR (1960) Flow rates using nuclear or electron paramagnetic resonance techniques with applications to biological and chemical processes. J Appl Phys 31: 125
12. Meyer CH, Hu BS, Nishimura DC, Macovski A (1992) Fast spiral coronary artery imaging. Magn Reson Med 28: 202–213
13. Ugurbil K, Garwood M, Ellermann J, Hendrich K, Hinke R, Hu X, Kim SG, Menon R, Merkle H, Ogawa S et al (1993) Imaging at high magnetic fields: initial experiences at 4 T. Magn Reson Q 9: 259–277
14. Duewell SH, Ceckler TL, Ong K, Wen H, Jaffer FA, Chesnick SA, Balaban RS (1995) Musculoskeletal MR imaging at 4 T and at 1.5 T: comparison of relaxation times and image contrast. Radiology 196: 551–555
15. Miyazaki T, Yamashita Y, Shinzato J, Kojima A, Takahashi M (1995) Two-dimensional time-of-flight magnetic resonance angiography in the coronal plane for abdominal disease: its usefulness and comparison with conventional angiography. Br J Radiol 68: 351–357
16. Caputo GR, Higgins CB (1992) Magnetic resonance angiography and measurement of blood flow in the peripheral vessels. Invest Radiol 27 Suppl 2: S97–S102
17. Caputo GR, Masui T, Gooding GA, Chang JM, Higgins CB (1992) Popliteal and tibioperoneal arteries: feasibility of "two-dimensional time-of-flight MR angiography and phase velocity mapping. Radiology 182: 387–392
18. Servois V, Laissy JP, Feger C, Sibert A, Delahousse M, Baleynaud S, Mery JP, Menu Y (1994) Two-dimensional time-of-flight magnetic resonance angiography of renal arteries without maximum intensity projection: a prospective comparison with angiography in 21 patients screened for renovascular hypertension. Cardiovasc Intervent Radiol 17: 138–142
19. Tkach JA, Ruggieri PM, Ross JS, Modic MT, Dillinger JJ, Masaryk TJ (1993) Pulse sequence strategies for vascular contrast in time-of-flight carotid MR angiography. J Magn Reson Imaging 3: 811–820
20. Masui T, Caputo GR, Bowersox JC, Higgins CB (1995) Assessment of popliteal arterial occlusive disease with 2D time-of-flight. J Comput Assist Tomogr 19: 339–454
21. Anderson CM, Lee RE (1995) Magnetic resonance angiography: time-of-flight Techniques. Syllabus for the Categorical Course on Cardiovascular Imaging, Sept 9–10. American College of Cardiology
22. Chen H, Hale J (1995) An algorithm for MR angiography image enhancement. Magn Reson Med 33: 534–540
23. Shapiro LB, Tien RD, Golding SJ, Totterman SM (1994) Preliminary results of a modified surface rendering technique in the display of magnetic resonance angiography images. Magn Reson Imaging 12: 461–468
24. Sigal R, Bittoun J, Jolivet O, Behnam N, Suminski M, Zannoli G, Francke JP (1995) High resolution T_1 weighted magnetic resonance imaging of the deep brain structures using a reduced bandwidth. Br J Radiol 68: 261–265
25. Miyazaki M, Kojima F, Ichinose N, Onozato Y, Igarashi H (1994) A novel saturation transfer contrast method for 3D time-of-flight magnetic resonance angiography:

a slice-selective off-resonance sine pulse (SORS) technique. Magn Reson Med 32: 52-59 Published erratum appears in Magn Reson Med 32: 671
26. Zhou D, Bryant RG (1994). Magnetization transfer, cross-relaxation, and chemical exchange in rotationally immobilized protein gels. Magn Reson Med 32: 725-732
27. Balaban RS, Ceckler TL (1992). Magnetization transfer contrast in magnetic resonance imaging. Magn Reson Q 8: 116-137
28. Dousset V, Franconi JM, Degreze P, Balderrama J, Lexa F, Caille JM (1994) Use of magnetisation transfer contrast to improve cerebral 3D MR angiography. Neuroradiology 36: 188-192
29. Talagala SL, Jungreis CA, Kanal E, Meyers SP, Foo TK, Rubin R, Applegate GR (1995) Fast three-dimensional time-of-flight MR angiography of the intra-cranial vasculature. J Magn Reson Imaging 5: 317-323
30. Lin W, Haacke EM, Tkach JA (1994) Three-dimensional time-of-flight MR angiography with variable TE (VARIETE) for fat signal reduction. Magn Reson Med 32: 678-683
31. Horikoshi T, Fukamachi A, Nishi H, Fukasawa I (1994) Detection of intracranial aneurysms by three-dimensional time-of-flight magnetic resonance angiography. Neuroradiology 36: 203-207
32. Ecklund KE, Hartnell GG, Hughes LA, Stokes KR, Finn JP, Longmaid HE (1994) MR angiography as the sole method for evaluating abdominal aortic aneurysms: correlation with conventional techniques and surgery. Radiology 192: 345-350
33. Wedeen VJ, Rosen BR, Brady TJ (1987) Magnetic resonance angiography. Magn Reson Annu 3: 113-178
34. Moran PR, Moran RA, Karstaedt N (1985) Verification and evaluation of internal flow and motion. True magnetic resonance imaging by the phase gradient modulation method. Radiology 154: 433-441
35. Dumoulin CL, Yucel E, Vock P, Souza SP, Terrier F, Steinberg FL, Wegmuller H (1990) Two- and three-dimensional phase contrast MR angiography of the abdomen. J Comput Assist Tomogr 14: 779-784
36. Hamilton CA, Moran PR, Santago P II, Rajala SA (1994) Effects of intravoxel velocity distributions on the accuracy of the phase-mapping method in phase-contrast MR angiography. J Magn Reson Imaging 4: 752-755
37. Ikawa F, Sumida M, Uozumi T, Kuwabara S, Kiya K, Kurisu K, Arita K, Satoh H (1994) Comparison of three-dimensional phase-contrast magnetic resonance angiography with three-dimensional time-of-flight magnetic resonance angiography in cerebral aneurysms. Surg Neurol 42: 287-292
38. Vock P, Terrier F, Wegmuller H, Mahler F, Gertsch P, Souza SP, Dumoulin CL (1991) Magnetic resonance angiography of abdominal vessels: early experience using the three-dimensional phase-contrast technique. Br J Radiol 64: 10-16
39. Edelman R, Rubin JB, Buxton RB (1990) Flow. In: Edelman R, Hesselink JR (eds) Clinical magnetic resonance imaging. Saunder, Philadelphia, pp 109-183
40. Van Tyen R, Saloner D, Jou LD, Berger S (1994) MR imaging of flow through tortuous vessels: a numerical simulation. Magn Reson Med 31: 184-195
41. Young IR, Bydder GM, Payne JA (1986) Flow measurement by the development of phase differences during slice formation in MR imaging. Magn Reson Med 3: 175-179
42. Hundley WG, Clarke GD, Landau C, Lange RA, Willard JE, Hillis LD, Peshock RM (1995) Noninvasive determination of infarct artery patency by eine magnetic resonance angiography (see comments). Circulation 91: 1347-1353
43. Hartiala JJ, Foster E, Fujita N, Mostbeck GH, Caputo GR, Fazio GP, Winslow T, Higgins CB (1994) Evaluation of left atrial contribution to left ventricular filling in aortic stenosie by velocity-encoded eine MRI. Am Heart J 127: 593-600
44. Sachs TS, Meyer CH, Hu BS, Kohli J, Nishimura DG, Macovski A (1994) Realtime motion detection in spiral MRI using navigators. Magn Reson Med 32: 639-645
45. Duerinckx AJ, Urman MK, Atkinson DJ et al (1994) Optimal imaging planes for coronary MR angiography. J Magn Reson Imaging 4(P): 123
46. Dinsmore RE (1995) Noninvasive coronary arteriography - here at last? Circulation 91:1607-1608
47. Mendonca-Dias MH, Gaggelli E, Lauterbur PC (1983) Paramagnetic contrast agents in nuclear magnetic resonance medical imaging. Semin Nucl Med 13: 364-376
48. Young IR, Bailes DR, Burl M, et al (1982) Initial clinical evaluation of a whole body nuclear magnetic resonance tomograph. J Comput Assist Tomogr 6: 1-18
49. Rosen BR, Belliveau JW, Aronen HJ, Kennedy D, Buchbinder BR, Fischman A, Gruber M, Glas J, Weisskoff RM, Cohen MS et al (1991) Susceptibility contrast imaging of cerebral blood volume: human experience. Magn Reson Med 22: 293-299
50. Villringer A, Rosen BR, Belliveau JW, Ackerman JL, Lauffer RB, Buxto, RB, Chao YS, Wedeen VJ, Brady TJ (1988) Dynamic imaging with lanthanide chelates in normal brain: contrast due to magnetic susceptibility effects. Magn Reson Med 6: 164-174
51. Zhong J, Gore JC (1991) On the relative importance of paramagnetic relaxation and diffusion-mediated susceptibility losses in tissues. Magn Reson Med 22: 197-203
52. Lipton MJ, Metz CE, Ranahan LA (1996) Outcome and benefit analysis in MRI. Encyclopedia of nuclear magnetic resonance. Wiley, London, pp 3419-3424
53. Debatin JF, Leung DA, Wildermuth S, Holtz D., McKinnon GC (1995) Advances in vascular echoplanar imaging. Cardiovasc, Intervent Radiol 18: 277-287
54. Hartnell GG (1993) MR angiography of the thoracic aorta. MRI Clin 1: 315-326
55. Potchen EJ, Haacke EM, Siebert JE, Gottschalk A (eds) (1993) Magnetic resonance angiography: concepts and applications. Mosby, St Louis
56. Lanzer P, Botvinick EH, Schiller NB, Crooks LE, Arakawa M, Kaufman L, Davis PL, Herfkens R, Lipton MJ, Higgins CB (1984) Cardiac imaging using gated magnetic resonance. Radiology 150: 121-127

Computed Tomographic Angiography

J.E. Wilting and F.W. Zonneveld

Introduction

Angiography is the gold standard for the imaging of vessels, while computed tomography (CT) is useful for imaging of bone and soft tissue. The term "computed tomographic angiography" (CTA) encompasses all methods that use CT to image vascular structures with the help of contrast agents. This chapter concentrates on CTA performed with intravenous injections. A stack of cross-sectional images is generated, providing information on the vascular structures and their relation to the surrounding anatomy. Since there is no superimposition of vessels, the real 3D geometry can be derived from the data set, which is particularly important for visualization of convoluted and curved vascular trajectories. After injection of a contrast bolus, data acquisition must be complete within a limited time frame, as the concentration of the contrast agents in the blood pool decreases over time. This time frame is influenced by injection techniques and individual patient physiology.

The limits of CTA are largely determined by the technical properties of the CT scanner. This chapter

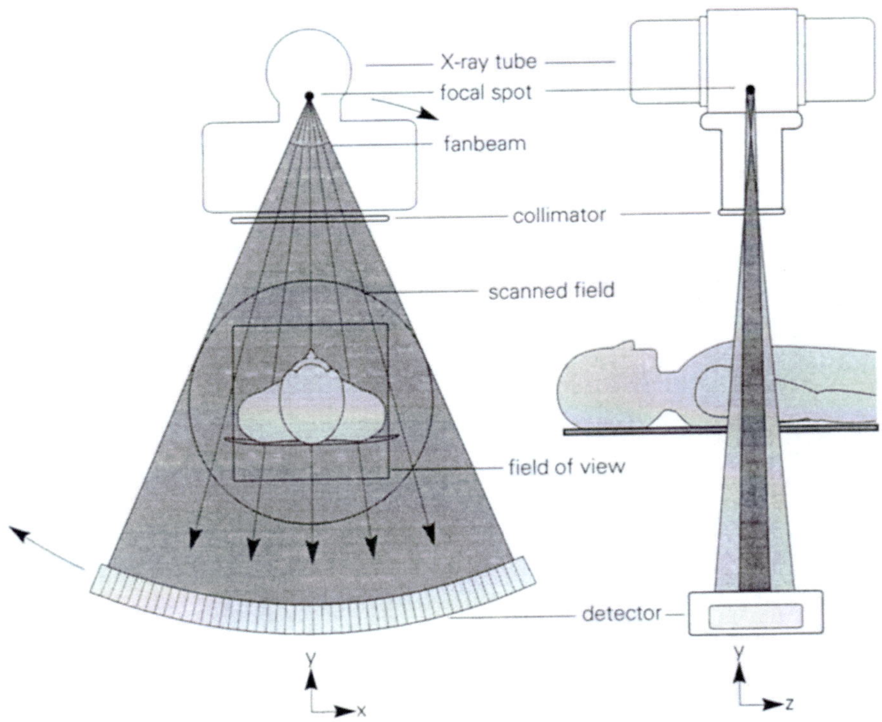

Fig. 1. Basic CT geometry (figure not to scale). Schematic view in the *xy*-plane (*left*) and the *yz*-plane (*right*). The *X-ray tube* rotates with the *detector* array around the patient. The patient is positioned within the scanned field, that is, the area in which sufficient data can be acquired to reconstruct an image. The emission in the imaging plane is fan-shaped and is denoted *fanbeam*. The detector measures the attenuation of X-rays by the patient in one direction at a time. By rotating the tube and the detector array, these measurements are acquired in all directions. A set of measurements by the detector array acquired at a certain position of tube and detector array is denoted a *view*. A full rotation has to be made to gather enough views for one reconstruction, showing the local attenuation coefficients in every voxel of scanned volume. The area that is reconstructed is determined by the *field of view* (FOV), which can be chosen anywhere within the scanned field. The *collimator* determines the slice thickness. The width of the *focal spot*, the aperture width of the detector elements, and the number of views determine the axial spatial resolution. The imaging plane can be angulated around the *x*-axis, allowing a tilt from approximately -30° to +30° for the optimal scan plane in the volume of interest. However, in spiral scans, tilting is usually not applied. The table supporting the patient can be moved in the *z*-direction to allow different scanning positions

will therefore start with an introduction of the principles and instrumentation of spiral CT. Contrast injection and optimal timing, major issues in vascular applications, are discussed next. Several ways of dealing with the large amount of images generated are described in the section on viewing and postprocessing. Next, with an awareness of effect of choices in acquisition and postprocessing, we discuss various applications and protocols. The chapter concludes with an overview of the advantages, shortcomings, pitfalls, and future of CTA.

Principles and Instrumentation of Spiral CT

To ensure optimal diagnostic procedures in any anatomical region in the individual patient, a detailed understanding of the technology and working principles of CT scanners is needed. The basic geometry of CT is shown in Fig. 1. Figure 2 shows an example of a spiral CT scanner.

All CT scanners consist of a yoke, with an X-ray tube on one side and a detector array on the other, that rotates around the patient. The user can select voltage (e.g., 100–140 kV) and current (e.g., 10–300 mA) to determine the quality and quantity of the X-ray emitted. The X-rays emitted by the tube are attenuated by the patient. The output of the detectors is digitized and recorded by a computer. By calibrating the scanner without a patient, it is possible to compare the attenuated with the nonattenuated X-ray intensities, and thus calculate the attenuation in the patient.

The attenuation information is fed into a reconstruction algorithm that takes the detector readings recorded in the various projections and calculates an image matrix of linear attenuation coefficients μ (cm^{-1}). This algorithm is based on smearing the profiles back over the direction in which they were acquired. Since blurring is inherent in this process, the profiles are filtered with a sharp filter before being backprojected, to compensate for this blurring effect. Therefore, this reconstruction algorithm is denoted "filtered back projection".

The attenuation coefficients are transformed into Hounsfield units (HU), named after the inventor of CT, Sir Godfrey Newbold Hounsfield. This scale is such that, by definition, air has the value of -1000 HU and water 0 HU. This is achieved by defining:

$$\text{CT number}_{\text{tissue}} = 1000\,\frac{\mu_{\text{tissue}} - \mu_{\text{water}}}{\mu_{\text{water}}}$$

The attenuation value of blood is around 55 HU. Since liver, muscle, and cerebral tissue have attenuation values of the same order of magnitude, contrast agents are employed to differentiate the structures of interest from surrounding tissue.

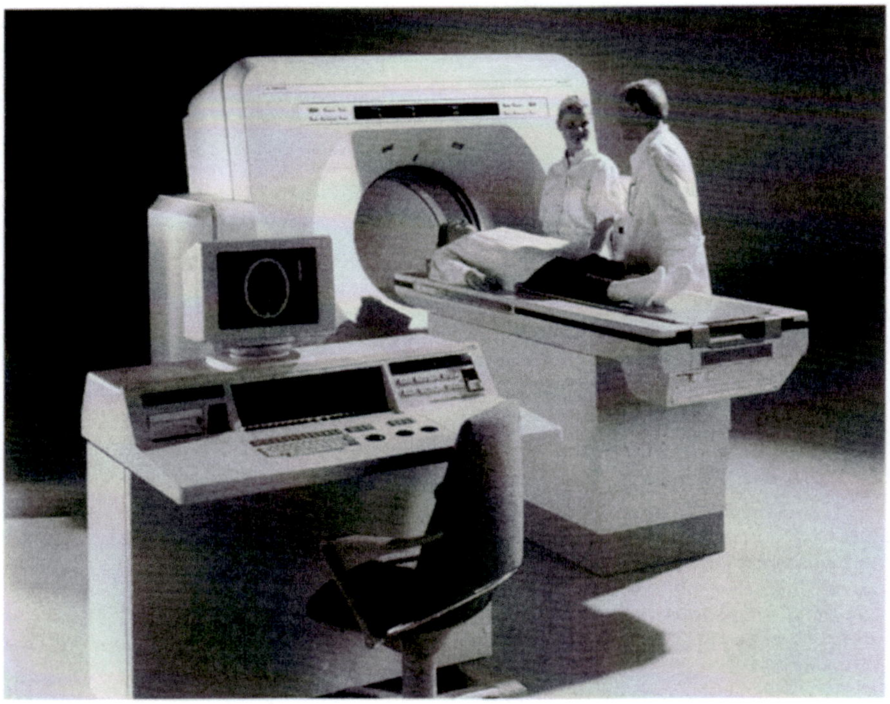

Fig. 2. Tomoscan AV Expander Plus, Philips Medical Systems Nederland bv, Best, the Netherlands. CT scanner with slip ring, allowing data acquisition of 100 rotations in 100 s, very suitable for computed tomographie angiography (CTA). A patient is lying on the CT table and can be moved into the gantry. The gantry contains a yoke on which the X-ray tube and detector array are mounted. In the foreground are the operator's console for the examination and the monitor for the image display

For visualization, the Hounsfield values must be translated into shades of gray. Since the human eye can discriminate only a limited number of gray levels, choices have to be made about the range of Hounsfield values to be allocated to the available gray levels. This is referred to as the "windowing technique". The user chooses a window level (WL) denoting the Hounsfield unit attached to the mean gray level, and a window width (WW) denoting the range of Hounsfield units that are imaged within the gray scale.

A wide range of literature is available for further study of the principles underlying CT [1–4].

In conventional CT, the combination of tube and detectors rotates through 360°, after which the table, with the patient, moves to the next slice position. This technique is referred to as "slice-to-slice imaging" or "conventional CT." Due to the cable limits on conventional scanner, clockwise and counterclockwise rotations alternate, resulting in an interscan delay of about 4 s. With the advent of slipring scanners, however, with their sliding contacts for power supply and usually optical or other wireless connections for data transport, continuous rotation has become possible, the patient being moved slowly through the gantry aperture during the rotation. For reconstruction, each slice is made up from the data acquired in one rotation. Both the X-ray and the detector array describe a helix around the patient, and therefore this technique is denoted "spiral" or "helical CT." In spiral CT data are acquired without an interscan delay, achieving up to 100 rotations of 1 s or less each, which allows imaging of the vascular structure within the period of optimal contrast enhancement.

To ensure a sufficient radiation dose for diagnostic image quality, tube technology is crucial in the design of a CT scanner. Instead of the maximum allowable tube current per rotation, which is important in conventional CT, the important issue is now maximum allowable current that can be sustained for the full duration of the scan. New tube technology, using spiral-groove bearings, allows the tube to dissipate its heat through conduction in addition to radiation, resulting in a much higher cooling rate [5, 6]. Heat capacity has been increased as well. These two factors help to allow more scanner rotations at a higher tube current. The latter is especially important for thin slices. More information on the technique of spiral CT can be found in the literature [7–11].

Factors Affecting Image Quality

This section discusses the CT-related factors that influence the quality of the images acquired. Two basic beam geometries influence the sharpness of the image: one is the geometry in the scan plane, which determines the axial spatial resolution; the other is the geometry perpendicular to the scan plane, which determines the longitudinal resolution. Resolution cannot be regarded separately from other parameters of image quality discussed in this same section. New parameters introduced by spiral scanning are discussed in the next section.

Axial Resolution

The spatial resolution in the scan plane is determined by the composite distance between tube, center of rotation, and detector array, the width of the focal spot, and the aperture width of the detector channels. While tube and detector array rotate around the patient, a number of projections, or views, are recorded.

The spatial resolution of a CT scanner is always measured at the center of rotation, the isocenter. The intensity distribution of an image of a single infinitesimal point is denoted the point spread function (PSF). The width of this PSF is a measure of the spatial resolution. In practice, however, it is measured using a thin stainless steel wire of finite thickness in a phantom. In a CT image this wire is not reconstructed as a true point, but as a blurred dot. A profile drawn through this dot shows the gradual transition of the attenuation value from the surrounding tissue to a maximum Hounsfield value in the center of the wire. The width of the PSF is usually given by measurement of the profile at a level halfway between the Hounsfield value of the surrounding tissue and the maximum. This measurement is referred to as the "full-width-at-half-maximum" (FWHM).

A different way to express spatial resolution is to measure the number of line pairs per centimeter that can be imaged. This is measured by scanning a high-contrast grid. Blurring causes a decrease in contrast of the imaged line pairs. For standard body scanning, most scanners have a resolution at which 50% of the contrast is left at about 4–5 line pairs per centimeter. With the use of sharper filters (high-resolution filters) this can increase to 11 line pairs per centimeter [12].

Partial Volume Averaging

Although axial spatial resolution is defined independently of slice thickness, the latter may have an adverse effect on sharpness in the appearance of the image. The reason for this is that averaging of details across the slice thickness has a blurring effect on the image, and it can also be the source of artifacts. This effect is referred to as "partial volume averaging." If there is much variation in structure in the longitudinal direction, e.g., as in a stenotic artery, the blur may complicate the assessment of such a stenosis.

The size of the reconstructed area, the field of view (FOV), and the number of pixels determine how large a tissue volume is represented by one pixel. The larger the volume represented by one pixel, the greater the partial volume averaging will be.

Longitudinal Resolution

The longitudinal resolution is influenced by the slice thickness and the slice index. For tiny structures that are parallel to the scan plane, such as the circle of Willis, a slice thickness of 1–2 mm is used, whereas for larger structures running perpendicular to the scan plane a slice thickness of up to 10 mm is applied. The slice thickness is determined by the height of the focal spot and the width of the slice thickness collimator, which is between the patient and the tube. For slice-to-slice imaging, the slice sensitivity profile (SSP) generally coincides with the dose distribution in the longitudinal direction, at the axis of rotation. Ideally, the shape of the SSP is that of a plateau with steep slopes. The collimator is adjusted such that the FWHM of the SSP equals the desired slice thickness. To achieve the thinnest possible profiles, postpatient collimation is sometimes used to reduce the effective slice thickness. However, this only results in narrowing the SSP; it does not reduce patient radiation.

The slice index determines the distance between the isocenter of two adjacent slices. Scanning with overlapping slices, i.e., with a slice index smaller than the slice thickness, improves the longitudinal resolution, but also increases patient dose. A small detail that just fits within the SSP is depicted more clearly than a detail that is captured partly by one slice and partly by the next. This illustrates how the location of the center of the SSP with respect to a detail is important. Longitudinal resolution is of special importance for reformatted and postprocessed images that make use of a stack of contiguous or overlapping slices.

Noise

The most important factor that degrades the image is quantum noise. Its origin lies in the statistical fluctuations of the detected X-ray photons. The signal can be expressed relative to the noise in the signal-to-noise ratio (SNR). The more signal is measured – that is, the more X-ray radiation is measured in the detectors – the more this fluctuation is averaged out. This implies that for minimal disturbance due to noise in a pixel, the size of the pixel, the patient dose per slice, and the slice thickness must be maximal. Thicker and denser objects attenuate the X-rays more, thus reducing the amount that can be measured by the detectors and increasing the appearance of noise in an image. Less efficient detector systems increase noise for the same reason. Smooth convolution filters average measurements and therefore reduce image noise. Acquisition parameters to reduce noise are: slice thickness (increased), tube voltage (kV), scan time, and tube current (mA).

Partial Volume Averaging, Resolution, and Noise

To minimize the partial volume effect, thin slices are required. However, this means a decrease of the SNR, thus degrading the image quality. The SNR can be increased again by increasing tube current, which in turn is limited by the tube technology. Thicker slices can be used on the one hand to speed up data acquisition and thus reduce artifacts due to patient motion, and on the other hand to improve the SNR. Therefore a compromise is needed between slice thickness and image quality, which is tuned to the contrast of the relevant image details [13].

The filtering of the profiles that takes place before the backprojection can make use of different convolution filters to optimize image quality. In areas with detailed structures where high resolution is important, e.g., the lung parenchyma, the high-frequency signals in the profiles are important and are therefore enhanced (edge enhancement). The noise increases accordingly. However, since contrasts are high (approximately 1000 HU), a wide window is used to study the images, and therefore the noise is hardly visible. In areas where discrimination of low contrast is very important, e.g., the liver and the brain, noise can be very disturbing and can be suppressed using a smoothing convolution filter. The result is a smoothed image where only relatively large structures, with little contrast with their surroundings are clearly depicted. For imaging vascular structures, moderate filters are used.

Spiral Acquisition

In slice-to-slice imaging too much time is lost in bringing the table from one imaging position to the next. If the acquisition takes too long, the contrast bolus dilutes, the contrast is excreted by the kidneys, and the best enhancement conditions may be missed. This problem is overcome with spiral CT, where the patient moves while the X-rays are being emitted and the rotation is continuing. This greatly reduces examination time, which is of especial importance in CTA.

Another advantage of spiral acquisition is that, with appropriate choice of parameters, longitudinal resolution can be improved without increasing the patient's radiation dose. To reconstruct images from spiral acquisition, interpolation is needed.

Interpolation Methods

We will now describe how flat slices can be reconstructed from raw data with a helical geometry. The raw data collected during subsequent scanner revolutions must be interpolated prior to reconstruction, such that the resulting "measurements" can be treated as if acquired in a single flat plane. Then the filtered backprojection can be used again to reconstruct the image, as in a conventional scan. The two interpolation methods used most often differ mainly in terms of effective slice thickness, i.e., the FWHM of the SSP. The older method is an interpolation between two adjacent full spiral rotations (Fig. 3a). The raw data acquired in these two consecutive scan rotations are interpolated pairwise to a data set, as if acquired in one plane of rotation. Then the filtered backprojection reconstruction method can be applied. This technique is generally referred to as the "360° reconstruction algorithm," since measurements that are a full rotation away are used to project the data on the reconstruction plane. Since two rotations are used to reconstruct one image, the FWHM of the effective slice thickness increases by approximately 30% [14–16].

To avoid this increase of slice thickness, the 180© algorithm was developed (Fig. 3b). Whereas in the 360© algorithm the two measurements that are used to calculate an interpolation are always recorded in the same direction, in the 180© algorithm the two measurements are in opposite directions. Given the geometry of the scanner, these two measurements are always within the rotation angle range of 180° $\pm$ γ from one antoher, with γ being the fan angle. Measurements taken close to the reconstructed plane are used without interpolation. Measurements at the beginning and end of one rotation are discarded since they are acquired at a location too far away from the plane of reconstruction. Instead, the opposite measurements, lying in the scan plane, are used again. Although this 180° algorithm gives an increase in noise of about 8%, it has the advantage that the effective slice thickness increases only minimally in comparison to slice-to-slice imaging. The disadvantage of this method is that, especially in regions with sharp transitions in the direction perpendicular to the scan plane, streaking artifacts may occur due to inconsistent data [14]. This inconsistency is due to the fact that consecutive views measure attenuation not only in consecutive directions, but in consecutive z-locations as well. Furthermore, along cone-shaped or inclined surfaces of a contrasting density, artifacts such as a crescent-shaped band of intermediate density may be seen. This artifact is referred to as a "spiral" artifact. Others sometimes refer to it as a "stairstep" artifact. However, the term "stairstep artifact" is generally used to refer to the discontinuity of structures lying obliquely to the direction of movement of the patient, although this effect is not strictly an artifact, but is inherent in the CT imaging principle [17].

Table Increment

The larger the table increment per rotation, the larger the scanned volume per reconstructed slice. This affects the SSP in the sense that it is widened: the dose per slice at the center diminishes somewhat and spreads out over a larger range in the longitudinal direction, causing an increase in effective slice thickness, independent of the collimated slice thickness. The table speed is usually chosen to correspond to the slice thickness divides by the rotation time.

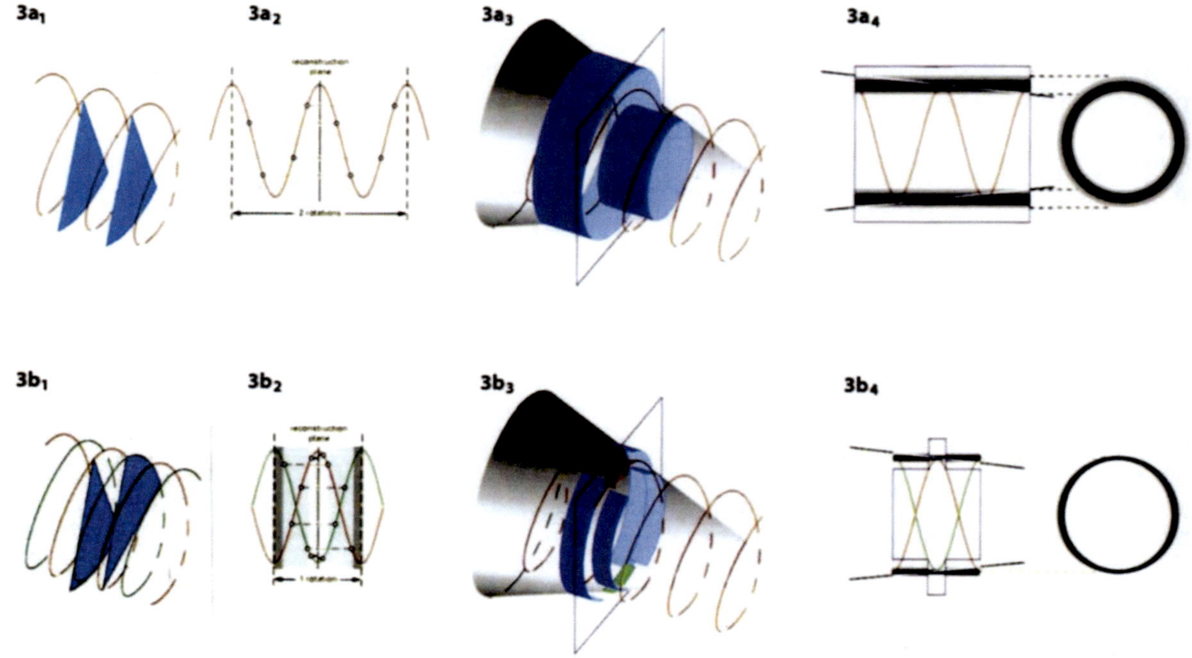

Fig. 3a, b. Differences in interpolation algorithms and their effects on image sharpness. **a** relates to the 360° interpolation algorithm, **b** to the 180° interpolation algorithm. In both parts, the *red line* shows the tube position with respect to the table position, the *blue fan* shows the fanbeam with, at the top, the focal spot and the detector array opposite to it. The figures are not to scale and are only meant to give the reader an understanding of how the interpolation algorithsm work.

a_1 shows the fanbeams in two locations, one rotation apart. The two views acquired at these locations are used for a reconstruction anywhere in between the two, using a weighted average of the two measurements with the same detector. **a_2** shows the projection of the tube position in the *yz*-plane with respect to the plane of reconstruction. Two full rotations are needed to reconstruct one image. Every view gets a weighing factor inversely proportional to the *z*-distance to the image plane. **a_3** demonstrates the data acquisition of a spiral CT of a cone. Data acquisition starts at a location where the cone is wide and ends where the diameter declines substanially. The *blue zones* show the diameters of the start and end of the acquisition. The first and the last view are the ones that are most distal to the reconstruction plane. Since these views are given only low weighing factors, their contribution is minimal. Views proximal to the reconstruction plane are given high weighing factors. The effect for the axial image of the cone is shown in **a_4** the surface of the cone is heavily blurred.

b_1 shows two fanbeams, the second after the tube has rotated 180° plus the fan angle. In each of the views acquired after rotation between 180° minus fan angle to 180° plus fan angle, exactly one measurement can be found which is acquired parallel but opposite to a measurement in the first view. For each detector in the detector array, the curve belonging to the tube position as shown in the *red spiral* can be shown as a "pseudospiral." As an example, the curve of the middle detector is drawn in *green*, showing where the parallel measurements are taken from for interpolation. With this interpolation method only one rotation is used for a reconstruction. **b_2** Now that only one rotation is used for reconstruction, it is not always advantageous to use both measurements in the same way. The *dark gray areas* denote the regions where the first and last views in one rotation are acquired relatively far away from the plane of reconstruction. Therefore, the measurements of the pseudospiral are used to obtain a data set suitable for reconstruction. Near the reconstruction plane, the *white area*, the measurements in the pseudospiral are too far away and are hardly used for interpolation. Thus measurements in the dark gray areas contribute little to the data set for reconstruction, whereas those in the white areas are accounted for more heavily. Averaging takes place in the area in between these regions. **b_3** shows the effect on a spiral scan of a cone. Again the *blue zones* show the areas that contribute to the blur. Near the reconstructed plane, the *red band* shows the area almost without interpolation. The *green band* shows the measurements of the pseudospiral used almost without interpolation. **b_4** Here we see that, since there was little interpolation in the red and green zones, the blurring on those positions is minimal. At a greater distance from that position there is blurring to half the extent of the blurring in the 360° interpolation algorithm. Note that the image of the cone is not rotationally symmetric; the location of the blurred part of the cone will rotate if more reconstructions are made at different locations. Note that drawings are not to scale and are only intended to give the reader an understanding of how the interpolation algorithms work. Details on angles and weighing factors can be found in the literature [14]

Pitch

In radiological literature the dimensionless ratio between table increment per rotation and slice thickness is referred to as the "pitch". Generally, a pitch of 1 is applied. To extend the length of the spiral scan the pitch can be increased to 2, allowing double the volume to be scanned with the same tube heating and total radiation dose to the patient. The skin dose, defined as the maximum absorbed dose per kilogram body tissue near the skin of a patient, is reduced in this way. However, this is achieved at the cost of decreased lingitudinal resolution due to more partial volume averaging, and, more importantly, of worse spiral artifacts. Some radiologists allow a pitch of up to 1.5. However, the effects on the axial images is negative: with increased pitch the patient moves more during the acquisition and the resulting streaking artifacts are comparable to those induced by patient motion.

Reconstruction Index

The reconstruction index has a similar function to the slice index in conventional scanning, but rather than denoting the center-to-center distance between two adjacent rotations, it is that between two adjacent reconstructions. Since the acqusition is a continuous spiral, any position on the lingitudinal axis can be chosen as the center lication of a reconstructed slice. This means that the localization of the SSP with respect to any detail can always be optimized. This is especially important for very localized lesions such as vascular stenoses. With two reconstructions per rotation a higher longitudinal resolution is achieved than in contiguous slice-to-slice scanning with the same slice thickness [18-20]. For vascular applications two to three reconstructed images per rotation are advantageous; more reconstructions will give little improvement, but increase computing time. Note that these extra reconstructions are acquired without increasing patient radiation dose.

Spiral CT Data Acquisition for Vascular Applications

The attenuation value of blood is mainly determined by the protein content of the blood cells. Blood from healthy individuals with normal hematocrit and hemoglobin levels has a CT numer of 55 ± 5 HU. When blood coagulates, hemoconcentration due to retraction of fibrin occurs with a corresponding increase in hematocrit levels, and thus an increase in CT density. In a later stage, degradation of fibrin and blodd cells, together with the subsequent absorption of albuminous substances, leads to a reduction in attenuation value of some tens of Hounsfield units [21]. The contrast between blood and the surrounding soft tissue, e.g., liver, muscle, cerebral tissue, is little. To increase this contrast, iodine-containing contrast agents can be injected.

Although there are some applications where intra-arterial catheters are used, e.g., CT arteriography, one of the strengths of CTA is that arteries can be imaged with contrast that is administered intravenously. To guarantee optimal acquisition we need to address several issues. Any contrast medium bolus in the vascular structure starts to dilute immediately after injection, until it is homogeneously spread out in the blood pool. In conventional CT, the acquisition time frame is primarily determined by the rate of excretion of the contrast agent by the kidneys. The introduction of spiral CT now allows imaging in the bolus phase of contrast injection, thus showing optimal contrast enhancement of arteries directly after administration of the contrast agent. This bolus is formed by injection of a large volume at high rate.

Injection of contrast media

CTA employs standard contrast agents utilized in X-ray angiographic studies. Since any adverse reaction to contrast agent may induce patient motion, an thus artifacts, nonionic agents should be used. In order to obtain a homogeneous contrast bolus, an automatic injector should be used [22]. Agents with iodine concentrations of up to 370 mg iodine per milliliter (I/ml) are used. In general, for vascular applications, up to 170 ml contrast agent with 300 mg I/ml are recommended, at injection rates of 3-5 ml/s [23 -25]. The total volume of contrast agent depends on the volume to be imaged, but should not exceed 2 ml/kg body weight. The time needed for acqusition determines the length of the bolus needed and therefore the injection rate.

Delay Times

More than for any other CT application, timing is critical in CTA (see Fig. 4). Numerous parameters affect the timing and profile of the vessel enhancement. These factors may include the patient's size, age, weight, cardiac output, metabolic status, and degree of hydration. Although there ist consensus that scanning during the optimal time window, i.e., the period of the maximum vessel contrast enhancement, is important, there is no general agreement on how to achieve this.

After administration in the antecubital vein the delay in appearance of the contrast agent in the arteries of interest is always variable. Once arrived in the arterial system, the contrast agent is quickly diluted and both venous and parenchymal opacification begins. Therefore it is important to estimate this delay and to perform the acquisition during the time of maximum arterial enhancement. The appropriate delay time, i.e., the time that elapses between the start of the contrast injection and the beginning of the scan, must be estimated for each individual patient. A number of approaches have been recommended:

1. Fixed delay after the start of the contrast injection. The delay is empirically determined per application, depending on injection rate, quality of contrast agent, and the volume to be imaged. Sometimes differences are made by age category. This method is quick and simple, but since the time to peak enhancement varies among patients, it is not always the best method.
2. (Semi)automatic enhancement recognition. A series of multiple low-dose scans is performed until an arbitrary threshold of enhancement in a region of interest is achieved. Then a transition is made to a routine scan series. This method assumes similar levels of enhancement for different patients; variations mean that some patients never reach the chosen threshold and are therefore scanned too late, while others have much higher enhancement levels and are scanned too early.
3. "Time to peak" in a test bolus. With this method, an enhancement curve in a region of interest is made in each individual patient after injection of a small test bolus (up to 20 ml at an injection rate of 3–5 ml/s). The time to peak, sometimes with an additional delay time to compensate for the duration of the injection, is taken as the delay time. Van Hoe et al. [26] showed that the time to peak of a test bolus correlates well with a minimum enhancement of 50 HU, but the correlation with the time to maximum enhancement was not studied. This method is most time-consuming, and assumes similar patterns of enhancement independent of the amount of contrast agent [24, 25].

Although, enhancement may sometimes be more accurate with the latter two methods, in radiological practice most physicians use empirically determined fixed delay times.

Patient Preparation and Instruction

Since acquisition time per reconstructed image is around 1 s, CTA is highly susceptible to motion. Therefore, the patient is instructed to avoid any voluntary motion during scanning. This will reduce motion artifacts and may prevent omission of parts of the structures. Ideally all studies should be done in a single breathhold. After hyperventilation most patients can hold their breath for 40 s, some for even 50 s. This time frame can be used for for longitudinal coverage, or for increased resolution in the longitudinal direction. Some radiologists prefer to use multiple spirals to allow intermediate patient breathing.

For cranial an carotid vessels, the patient should be immobilized as much as possible and be instructed not to swallow during the scan. Unlike other abdominal studies with CT, bowel clearance an opacification is not needed for CTA of the abdominal arteries.

Quantification of Vessel Diameters

Images of the blood vessels, like those of other structures, are influenced by the finite resolution of the CT, which can be described as blurring of the images with the PSF in the axial direction and the SSP in the longitudinal direction. This blurring causes the borders between adjacent tissues with different attenuation coefficients to be imaged as if the transition were gradual. The threshold value for determining the borderline of the two structures should be taken as the mean of the Hounsfield values of the two adjacent tissues using the FWHM method. Using this technique, vessels of at least twice the width of the SSP and PSF can be measured accurately in the respective directions. This means that vessels parallel to the scan plane with a diameter of 4 mm can be accurately measured using a 2 mm slice thickness. The FWHM of the PSF for abdominal applications generally is 1.2 mm [12], so vessels with diameters larger than 2.4 mm can be measured accurately. Stenotic parts with smaller diameters can be overestimated, and thus the degree of stenosis will be underestimated. When structures of higher densities are present, such as atherosclerotic calcifications, the opposite may occur. Measurements of diameters should be assessed perpendicular to the vascular axis. This eliminates the significant errors which can be introduced when an oblique segment of a vessel is measured in the axial plane. Multiplanar reformations can be used to achieve optimal measurements (see Fig. 5 and section on viewing and postprocessing, below).

Parameter Choice

In the section on principles and instrumentation, the effects of various parameters on image quality were discussed. Now we will describe how to arrive at a general protocol depending on diagnostic objectives, system limits, an biological limits, especially in regard to the radiation dose delivered to the patient.

First the minimal volume that has to be imaged must be determined. Next, the maximal allowable slice thickness to discriminate diagnostically relevant structures should be selected; selecting thinner slices than are clinically relevant increases the patient dose unnecessarily. Then the other parameters can be set.

In principle, the ideal tube voltage and current are the same as in slice-to-slice imaging. With 140 kV instead of 120 kV the tube output will increase by 40% with minimal degradation of the contrast. This should be used for regions of high attenuation such as the shoulders and hips. The current setting is in general chosen to be the maximum allowable tube current for the number of rotations planned, in order to minimize disturbance from noise. Compared to conventional scanning, the tube current is limited by the heat capacity and cooling rate over a longer time period. Further, the rotation time for CTA is most often chosen as 1 s. Due to these factors, the radiation generated per rotation is less than that in conventional scanning, and the SNR is impaired. This means that the images are relatively noisy and hence adge-enhancement filters cannot be used. However, too much smoothing will blur the structures, so the reconstruction filter is adjusted to optimize the balance between SNR and the spatial resolution. The scan direction should be chosen to be the same as that of the blood flow in order to "ride the wave." However, close to the injection site the contrast is only minimally diluted, causing more attenuation than can be handled by the scanner calibration. This may cause artifacts, in which case the opposite acquisition direction is recommended. The aim of this reversed acquisition is that the part close to the injection is imaged after the injection has stopped and the concentration of contrast is reduced.

The limited number of rotations can be dealt with by using either multiple spirals or pitches larger than 1. The advantage of multiple spirals is that the patient is allowed to breath in between scans, but the loss of contrast enhancement may be unacceptable, or may require an extra contrast injection. Increasing the pitch may result in artifacts, as described above. In order to reduce the volume that is mapped on each pixel, the FOV should be chosen such that it includes only the area of interest.

Viewing and Postprocessing

The reconstructed axial slices can be studied at different window settings and photographed on film, as with conventional CT. These axial slices contain all available information that is acquired with the CTA. The main advantages of CTA compared to conventional angiography, e.g., acquiring information not only of the lumen but of plaques, the vessel wall, and surrounding tissues as well, are best appreciated on these images (Fig. 4a). The main purpose of viewing and postprocessing facilities is to help extract the topographic morphology in a quick and easy way. Although radiologists will have a 3D impression of the geometry after viewing consecutive 2D slices, various methods can be used to augment this process of 3D awareness. They are either based on temporal clues, offering different images in time, on static aspects such as different cutting planes or shading, or on a combination of these.

Data Preserving Techniques

The following display techniques offer the physician different ways to study the entire dataset acquired with CTA.

Cine Display

The entire stack of images can be displayed in an interactive cine or movie mode. Tracking through the vascular structures in the craniocaudal direction of the data set allows the 3D structure of the vessels to

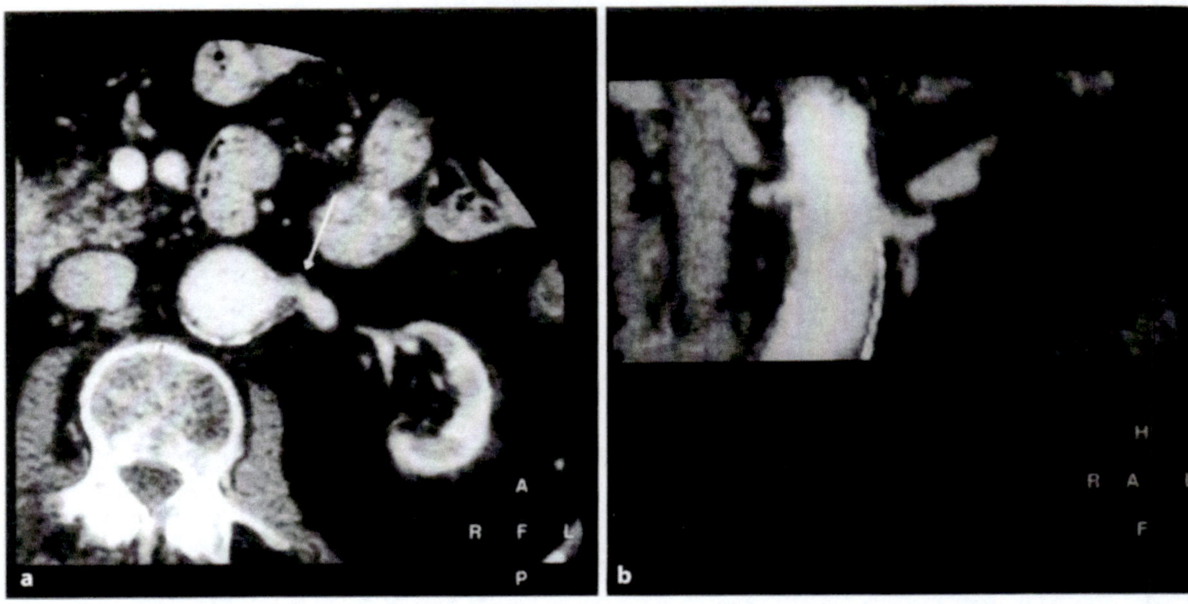

Fig. 4a, b CTA of the renal arteries showing exactly how to left renal artery originate from the aorta. a On the axial scan the left renal artery shows an ostial stenosis *(arrow)* and mural thrombus on the dorsal wall of the aorta. **b** Oblique multi planar reformation (MPR) of the aorta through the renal arteries. Maximum contrast is achieved just above the renal arteries. Scanning could have started a few seconds later. *A*, anterior; *P*, posterior; *H*, head; *F*, feet; *R*, right; *L*, left

be appreciated. In this way, the vessels of interest can be followed through the stack of images in order to study the morphology. No information is lost. Displaying the axial images in a short time frame gives a 3D impression.

Multiplanar Reformatting

The stack of axial slices can be reformated into orthogonal or oblique planes or any other desired plane, denoted "multiplanar reformations" (MPR). Since spatial resolution in the longitudinal direction in the MPR is usually inferior to in-plane resolution in axial slices, the reformatted images will appear degraded. The data set is still of high quality, but instead of high resolution in the plane that is imaged, small steps can be made to adjacent planes, allowing optimal location of the reformatted plane. Figure 4b shows an oblique MPR of the aorta with the origins of the renal arteries.

To facilitate optimal MPR, vessel tracking algorithms can be of use. Vessel tracking is a segmentation technique in which the center of a vessel is traced through a data set (Fig. 5). Visualization of the vascular structure is then achieved by reconstructing a curved MPR parallel or a flat MPR perpendicular to the axis determined by the vessel tracking algorithm. The latter can then be used for assessing the degree of stenosis.

Data Reduction Techniques

Various methods have been developed for creating topographic images of vascular trees by data reduciton. In general they are referred to as 3D reconstruction techniques. The relevant data for assessment of the vascular structure are extracted from the original data set an presented to the user. In contrast to conventional angiography, these methods allow the vascular trees to be viewed from any desired direction in a 3D space.

Maximum Intensity Projections

To provide images and data comparable to those of conventional angiography, maximum intensity projections (MIP) can be made. First a viewing point is defined. From this point, imaginary rays are cast through the data set onto an image plane. The Hounsfield value of the volume element or voxel with the highest density along each ray is preserved and mapped onto the MIP image. Since only the structures with the highest Hounsfield value are depicted, structures of high attenuation that are not

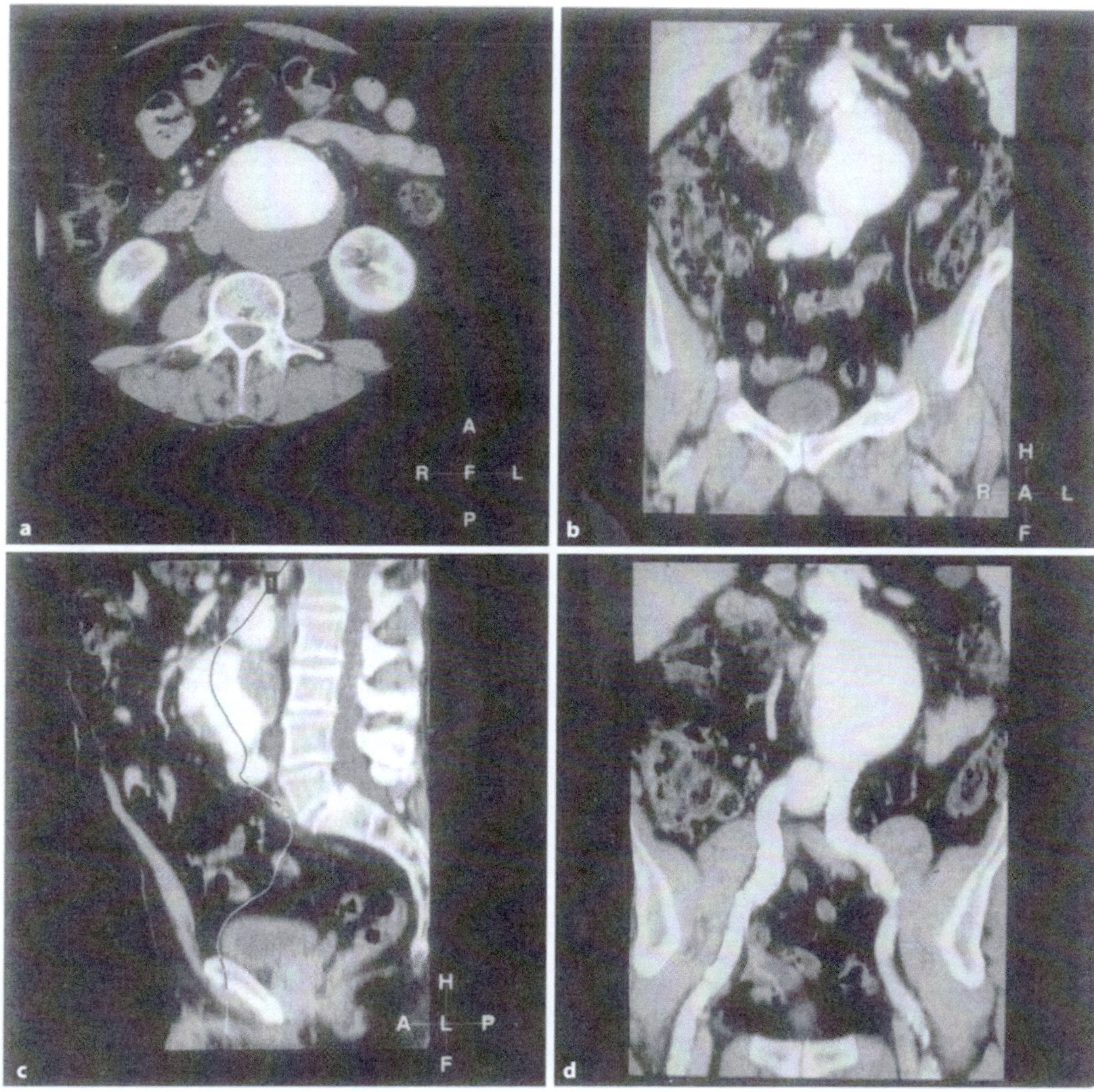

Fig. 5 a–d. CTA of the abdominal aorta. By determining the middle of a vessel in two orthogonal planes (**a, b**), the vessel axis can be followed. The trajectory defined in this way is shown as projected onto the sagittal plane (**c**). A curved MPR can then show the vessel as if located in a stretched coronal plane (**d**). These images visualize the total extent of the aneurysms and they can be used for length measurements, as required for stent design. Reconstructions perpendicular to this vessel axis can be used for determining the diameter of the lumen and the thrombus. Note that, since the axis of the vessel is stretched, the surronding tissue is displayed in a deformed fashion

of interest, e.g., bone, should be excluded from the data set. This exclusion process is called the editing of the dataset. To omit the editing procedure, a slab MIP can be taken. In this method only a part of the volume is used for the projection. The slab and editing functions should be used to reduce the volume of interest, which will speed up the MIP while increasing its quality (Fig. 6). In itself, every MIP image is a 2D projection of a astructure. A spatial effect is achieved by presenting a series of MIP images, each rotated over a small angle, in a cine loop. To introduce more depth into the static MIP images, the so-called "closest vessel projection" was developed, by which vessels that are in front of others are still dis-

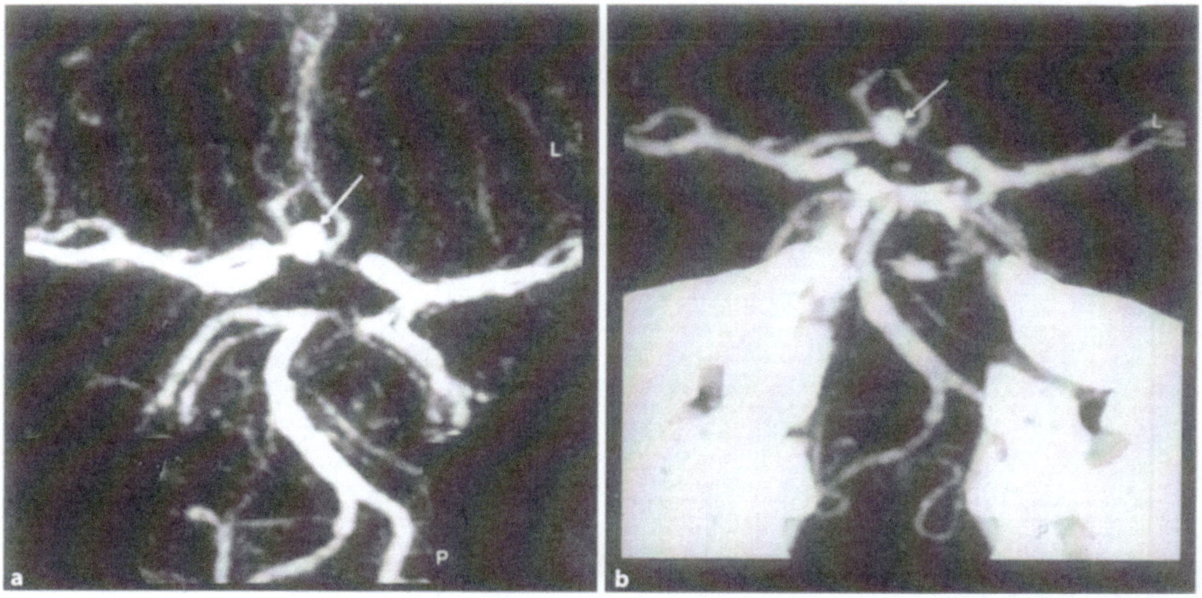

Fig. 6 a, b. CTA of the circle of Willis. **a** Edited maximum intensity projection (MIP) of the circle of Willis, showing an aneurysm of the anterior communicating artery (*arrow*). All bony structures have been removed by editing. **b** Slab MIP of the same data set representing a 2-cm-thick slab. By using a smaller volume for postprocessing no editing is needed. Since in a small volume fewer irrelevant structures contribute to the MIP, the quality of the image improves

played even if the vessels behind have higher densities. The remaining problem is that small vessels still look too transparent. This can be overcome by the use of surface or volume rendering. More information on MIP can be found in the literature [27].

Surface Rendering

Surface rendering algorithms serve the same purpose as MIP. In this procedure the vascular structure is defined as the structure within two selected Hounsfield values. Structures that have attenuation values in the same range, but do not belong to the vascular tree, are edited away by the user. This segmentation process may be facilitated by the use of vessel trace algorithms. Again a vantage point is selected, but this time from each imaginary ray the first voxel with a Hounsfield value within the selected range is marked. In this way the surface description of the vascular tree is extracted. Rendering is done by the use of virtual light sources, using shaded surface display (SSD) [28]. One view is sufficient to give the 3D impression, but a cine loop can help. The disadvantage of this technique is that both thresholding and editing are very user-dependent. The sizes of the structures depend heavily on the threshold settings used for the surface extraction. This means that stenosis can apparently be "caused" and "cured" by choosing different thresholds and editing (Fig. 7). Further, the rendered image only shows a surface: the different attenuation values for calcifications, plaque, and other structures are lost and therefore discrimination between these structures and the vessel lumen is no longer possible.

Volume Rendering

This technique probably most closely resembles conventional angiography, but has the advantage that the viewpoints are not restricted to those of the acquisition. Again a viewpoint is selected and imaginary rays are sent through the data set (ray tracing). This time, however, all voxels are accounted for. The weighing factor for the various Hounsfield values determine the appearance of the projection. Voxels partly belonging to different tissues can be given an intermediate weighing factor. This avoids some of the problems of surface rendering. Another advantage of volume rendering is that the tissue opacity is selctable [29]. A disadvantage is that the image can remain transparent, which adversely affects the depth perception cues.

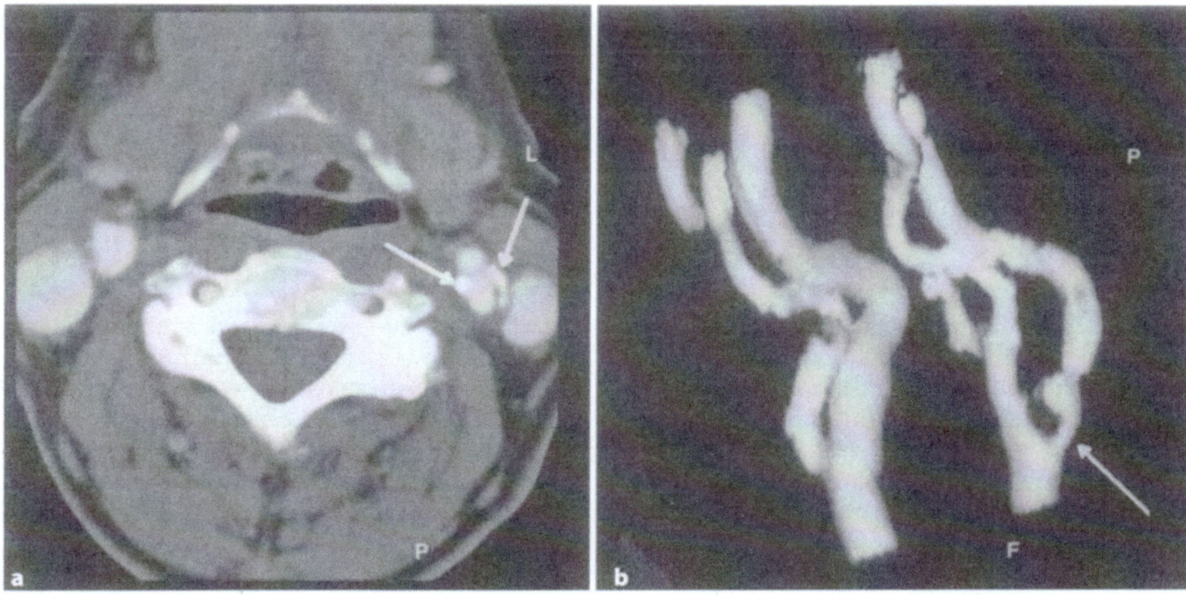

Fig. 7 a. b. CTA of the carotid arteries. **a** Calcification (*arrows*) around the bifurcation of the left carotid artery. **b** Shaded surface display of the carotid arteries. Lumen diameters are influenced by removal of calcified plaques (*arrow*) and by the selected thershold. Axial slices should be studied to establish the degree of the more distal stenosis in the internal carotid artery.

MIP and surface an volume rendering can be helpful for gaining a quick overview of the patiens's vasculature. Of the three, the MIP is the most user-independent, quick and available and is therefore the most frequently used. However, to obtain exact information, the axial or flat MPR images should be studied. For example, if calcified atherosclerotic plaques are present in a concentric or near-concentric fashion, the degree of stenosis is often difficult to determine from the MIPs [30].

Clinical Applications and Protocols

In this section we will discuss the kind of pathology that can be imaged using CTA, and the considerations for specific parameter choices. For further diagnostic issues and clinical results, the reader is referred to the literature [31–35].

Atherosclerotic Disease

Atherosclerotic disease induces degenerative changes in the intima and media of the arterial wall with calcium deposition in sclerotic plaques. The artery loses its elasticity and the lumen can be narrowed. Blood clots easily on the plaque, further reducing the lumen of the vessel.

The degree of stenosis greatly influences patient management and it is therefore important to use optimal techniques to determine its severity. CTA provides sufficient contrast to differentiate between calcification in the wall of the atherosclerotic vessel and intraluminal contrast [36]. However, in practice the limited resolution impairs exact spatial discrimination.
Atherosclerosis may occur in any artery. Here we will highlight those vascular territories where we can show some of the specific advantages and limitations of CTA that are already known.

Carotid Arteries

The carotid arteries typically run perpendicular to the scan plane. In general, structures with tissue interfaces perpendicular to the scan plane have the advantage that partial volume effects are minimal or absent. Therefore, one might expect that the use of thick slices in carotid artery imaging would result in good quality investigations. However, in the internal carotid artery, at the carotid bifurcation, stenoses may be very severe but focal. In such cases, thick slices will cause a blurring of the stenoses, which will appear to be less severe but longer. Other reasons for using thin slices are the often convoluted or kinked arteries, or the horizontal course of the internal carotid artery at the bifurcation. The expected geometry of the vasculature therefore indicates the use of thin slices. The increased noise, however, limits the use of slices thinner than 2 mm. To allow sufficient *z*-axis coverage, a compromise is found using a slice thickness of 2–3 mm.

Renal Arteries

Atherosclerosis of the renal arteries may cause stenoses and thus reduce blood flow to the kidneys. Although this ist not the most common cause of high blood pressure, accounting for less than 5% of patients with systemic hypertension, CTA is capable of detecting and grading renal artery stenosis and therefore assisting patient management. Prior to vascular intervention the form and location of the stenosis can be visualized. Thus, it is possible to differentiate between stenoses at the origin and in the trunk (see Fig. 4a) [36a], which is important for deciding on the appropriate surgical or endovascular treatment [37]. In addition, for preinterventional conventional angiograms, the optimum projections to visualize the renal arteries can be determined by measuring the angle at which they originate from the aorta in axial slices.

Acquisition starts with an abdominal scan (slice thickness 10 mm) without contrast to visualize both kidneys. A test bolus is used to determine the delay time between start of injection and start of acquisition. Then a volume acquisition is planned containing both renal arteries. The slice thickness of 3 mm is mainly determined by the minimum thickness that still has acceptable noise levels. More on accuracy of CTA for renal artery stenoses can be found in the literature [24].

Peripheral Vasculature

Atherosclerosis in the peripheral vasculature often spans long segments in the pelvis and the lower limbs. Since CTA is limited as to permissible slice thickness and the number of rotations, the volume that can be imaged imposes limits on the length of imageable vascular territory. However, once the region of interest has been defined, as is the case for example, in iliac artery stenting and assessment of postprocedural complications, CTA is a good tool for avaluation [38, 39]. To cover enough volume, a slice thickness of 5 mm and more is chosen as long as the image quality permits.

Aneurysms, Dissections, and Ruptures

Aneurysms represent focal widenings of the artery. These aneurysms tend to grow, get filled with blood clots, and dissect. Some areas are specifically of interest for CTA.

Circle of Willis

The circle of Willis is typically oriented parallel to the scan plane. The vessels are narrow, so that thin slices are needed in order to avoid partial volume effects. Examinations are generally aimed at detecting aneurysms. Aneurysms in this region tend to be relatively large compared to the vascular structure itself, making spatial resolution not a serious limiting factor. Based on a CTA study, the size, orientation, location, and involvement of other vessels can be defined and treatments planned. CTA is well suited to depict anatomy and pathology of the circle of Willis [40] (Fig. 6).

Thoracic and Abdominal Aorta

For large vascular structures such as the thoracic and abdominal aorta, visualization of large volumes is required, which can be achieved using 10-mm-thick slices. However, if aneurysms or dissections are present, it is important to identify branching arteries, which requires the use of thinner slices. As a compromise, slice thicknesses varying from 5 to 10 mm are used. In patients with aortic dissections where the false lumen is not thrombosed, CTA is capable of clearly visualizing the intimal flap separating the true end the false lumen, as well as documenting the relationship of the branching vessels to each lumen [23, 41]. If an endoprothesis is to be implanted, distance measurements in a 3D space using a vessel-traced MPR are important to determine precisely the length and diameter of the required implant [42].

Thrombosis and Embolism

Blood clot formation and peripheral embolization are frequently complications of an underlying pathology. CTA shows particular promise in precise and reliable definition of the extent of thrombi.

Pulmonary Embolism

The pulmonary arterial tree is complex. Careful differentiation between vascular structure and adjacent tissues such as intersegmental lymph nodes, along with integration of physiologic data, is needed to explain asymmetry in pulmonary arterial opacification. CTA appears to be useful to depict proximal pulmonary embolism, to evaluate suspected chronic thromboembolic pulmonary hypertension, and to monitor patients with documented central emboli [43]. Central pulmonary emboli are better seen with CTA than with conventional angiography because there is no superimposition of other structures. However, horizontal vessels in the middle lobe and lingula may be poorly visualized because of volume averaging, requiring a careful balance between the size of the imaged volume and spatial resolution. This results in the choice of a 5-mm slice thickness. In addition, peripheral portions of the upper and lower lobe may be inadequately scanned, possibly due to insufficient time delay between contrast initiation and data acquisition. CTA signs of emboli are partial or complete filling defects, "railway track" sign and mural defects [44].

Other Vascular Applications

Vascular pathology is not the only reason for imaging the vasculature. The visualization of the morphology of the vascular tree can also be used as a road map for surgical treatment. Information on the integrity of the vasculature is important for the assessment of transplant candidates.

Liver Vessels

Although the main goals of liver imaging are screening, quantification, and characterization of liver lesions, the location of lesions with respect to important vascular structures such as the portal and the intrahepatic vessels is also clinically important [45]. 3D display of intrahepatic vascular structures, together with tumor(s) and liver surface, offers the possibility of perceiving complex individual morphology in a coherent fashion. In this way specific resections can be planned in detail, and potentially hazardous phases of the operation can be avoided or anticipated, thus reducing complications. However, such examinations are time-consuming.

Transplant Candidates

CTA can be used to study the integrity, morphology, and patency of the hepatic and renal arterial anatomy in transplant donor candidates [46]. The presence of accessory renal arteries or prehilar renal arterial branching can be identified [47].

Imaging Protocols

The protocols given in Table 1 are usesd in The University Hospital, Utrecht, in the Netherlands, and have been developed in cooperation with neuro- and vascular surgeons. Instead of fixed delay times, as indicated in the table, delay can also be determined using test boli. The protocols are designed to provide optimum image quality, i.e., maximum resolution and contrast along with a low noise level. Protocols are, of course, dependent on the equipment used, and the examples given in Table 1 are therefore intended to be used only as a guideline.

Image Acquisition

The matrix is set to 512^2 and the pitch to 1. Parameters are set following the protocols listed in Table 1. In all protocols a power injector is used. For thoracic and abdominal studies, the breathing technique should be rehearsed with the patient. For most applications in adults, the total amount of contrast agent is 150 ml of contrast with 300 mg I/ml, e.g., Ultravist 300, in the injector, of which 140 ml is injected at a rate of 3 ml/s. If lower injection rates are used with the same total amount, the bolus length increases, allowing longer imaging times. To build up the bolus, the first 4 ml is injected at a maximum rate of 4 ml/s.

A scanogram or survey image is made to determine the start position of the spiral acquisition. If the scanogram does not provide enough information, a low-resolution scan with relatively thick slices and possibly a pitch of 2 can be used to identify the location of the vascular structures of interest. This can be done with less than half the normal radiation, in order to reduce patient dose [48].

Instead of fixed delay times, a test bolus can always be used to determine the best delay time for the individual patient. First, a position is determined where the enhancement during acquisition should be optimal. Then the injection protocol, e.g., starting with 2 ml at a rate of 2 ml/s, followed by

Table 1. CTA Protocols for a CT scanner that allows up to 70 rotations.

	Abdominal aorta[a]	Aorta	Thoracic aorta	Abdominal aorta, post-operative, endoprosthesis	Carotid arteries	Circle of Willis[b]	Pulmonary artery	Renal arteries
Start position	Celiac trunk	Aortic arch	Diaphragm	Celiac trunk	Lower level of C6	Orbitomeatal line	Diaphragm	Superior mesenteric artery
Scan direction	Craniocaudal	Craniocaudal	Craniocaudal	Craniocaudal	Craniocaudal	Craniocaudal	Craniocaudal	Craniocaudal
No. of rotations	50	50	50	50	50	50	50	50
Slice thickness (mm)	5	10	5	5	2–3	1–1.5	5	2–3
Reconstruktion index (mm)	2	5	2	2	2	1	2	1
Voltage (kV)	140	140	140	140	120	140	120	140
Current (mA)	225	225	225	225	250	125	250	250
Field of view (mm)	250	250	250	250	160	160	Full screen	250
Filter	Smooth abdominal	Smooth abdominal	Smooth abdominal	Smooth abdominal	Standard head	Standard head	Standard abdomen	Smooth abdominal
Delay (s)	30	30	30	30	25	25	20	[c]
Injection rate (ml/s)	3	3	3	3	2.5	4.5	2.5	3

[a] If the number of scans is limited, a second spiral scan can be made as soon as possible after the first scan with slice thickness 10 mm and reconstruction index 5 mm, down to below the ischium.
[b] angulation parallel to the plane from the upper orbital edge to just below the foramen magnum.
[c] Determined by test bolus.

13 ml at 3 ml/s, can be started. After a delay of 12 s an axial slice is made every 4$s, at low current to reduce patient dose. The time from the start of injection until the time at which the image with the maximum enhancement is acquired is taken as the delay time. Extra seconds can be added to the delay time to compensate for the longer injection time needed for the total amount of contrast.

Data Documentation

CTA produces a large number of images. If more reconstructions are made per rotation, the extra reconstructions can be used for viewing and postprocessing. Since cine display is an important viewing tool for CTA, the best way to store the images is in a digital format, e.g., on optical disks. If filming is required, film costs can be reduced by filming only one image per rotation. Another option is to use postprocessed image like MIPs or SSDs to show the overall vasculature and to print the axial images of the diseased area only.

Value of CTA

For exact figures regarding the sensitivity and specificity of CTA compared with other diagnostic procedures, the reader is referred to the articles mentioned in the previous section. In this section only selected comments on advantages, disadvantages, and some possible pitfalls of CTA will be made.

Advantages of CTA

Some important advantages of CTA have already been mentioned: its ability to obtain real 3D visualization of the vasculature, which can be presented in any way desired using the viewing and postprocessing functions, as well as direct correlation of the vascular structure and the surrounding tissues. This can be achieved after just one injection of contrast agent, with one acquisition that can be acquired in less than 1 min. Another advantage over conventional angiography is the minimal invasiveness, reducing morbidity and mortality. Both these issues make CTA a patient-friendly and cost-effective tool in the work-up of patients with vascular disease. The radiation dose to the patient is reduced, and radiation exposure of the staff is eliminated.

Compared to sonographic techniques, CTA offers the advantage of being user-independent and not restricted to areas without bone or air. Compared to magnetic resonance angiography (MRA), image data acquisition in CTA is generally faster. In addition, CTA does not suffer from the flow-related artifacts observed in MRA [26, 49].

Shortcomings of CTA

The most important disadvantages of CTA compared to conventional angiography are the lower spatial resolution and the greater susceptibility to motion. These factors limit the clinical use of CTA. Further, CTA does not offer possibilities for intervention.

Compared to ultrasound and MRA, the need for radiation and contrast agents is the most obvious disadvantage of CTA. Besides the common CT artifacts [50], artifacts generated by very high attenuation values within the subclavian and brachiocephalic veins may occur during or immediately after injection. Furthermore, the plane with optimal resolution is relatively fixed, i.e., the axial plane. Images in planes other than axial must be reconstructed by reformating the data.

In CTA imaging of intracranial vessels, surrounding calcifications may partly obscure aneurysms in postprocessed images, whereas this is not a problem in MRA [49].

If the venous system is filled as well, segmentation can be complicated. Furthermore, differentiation of the lumen from calcified plaque, and of the vascular structures from bone, especially in the skull base for examination of the circle of Willis, may be very laborious and time-consuming. The various postprocessing algorithms that are available are usually time-consuming and not always practical in a clinical setting.

Pitfalls of CTA

The most important pitfall in CT in general, and in CTA specifically, is the effect of partial volume averaging and limited spatial resolution. All structures are blurred to some extent and this must be accounted for in evaluating CTA studies. The gradual transition from one structure to the adjacent tissue means that the choice of window level and with always influences the appearance of where the vessel wall is located. This effect is most apparent in surface renderings, where the user is forced to choose a threshold. Choosing higher thresholds will show displays with reduced vessel diameters, as explained above in the section on quantification of vessel diameters (p. 142).

Table speed and slice thickness influence the appearance of stenoses. Increasing the number of reconstructions does not change this, but will increase the chance of optimal visualization by optimal localization of the slice with respect to the structure.

Filling defects may occur, simulating occlusions. Especially in complex structures, like the bronchovascular tree, it can be difficult to obtain optimal simultaneous filling of both the central and peripheral part. Further, insufficient contrast enhancement may cause intimal flaps to be missed [51].

Pulsation artifacts may very closely mimic the appearance of an aortic dissection [52–55]. These artifacts occur because the scan duration of 1 s closely approximates the duration of a single cardiac cycle. Within this cycle the aorta moves over a distance of a few millimeters in the scan plane. On close inspection the artifact appears as if the aorta is depicted twice in slightly different positions. With slower scanning, this movement will cause a blurring effect in the depiction of the vessel wall.

An understanding of the physics of CT together with a knowledge of the anatomical characteristics of the morphology and physiology of the area to be investigated, can allow most pitfalls to be avoided.

Future Prospects

With improvements in tube technology, it will be possible to acquire even higher quality images with thinner slices. At that point, the limits of the system will no longer remain the determining factors of paramter choice, but rather the scanning parameters will be determined by the acceptable radiation dose for the total examination.

The development of blood pool agents that will provide optimal enhancement of the vasculature for a much longer period of time will eliminate the problem of choosing exactly the right delay between contrast injection and acquisition. However, differentiation between venous and arterial structures by their enhancement patterns is then lost; venous filling may impair discrimination between an artery and its accompanying vein.

Since patient motion is another important image-degrading parameter, acquisition will always have to be fast and therefore blood pool agents may not be as beneficial as they seem to be at first sight.

CTA may emerge as a tool to screen before angiography or may replace angiography altogether in cases of trauma or other emergencies. CTA will gain in value for posttreatment evaluation of vascular implants. Its spatial resolution will allways be limited compared to that of conventional angiography, but it will be valued for the real 3D information it provides, its ease of use and its cost-effectiveness.

References

1. Newton TH, Potts DG (eds) 1981 Radiology of the skull and brain. Technical aspects of computed tomography. Mosby, St Louis
2. Swindell W, Webb S (1992) X-ray transmission computed tomography. In. Webb S(ed) The physics of medical imaging. IOP, London, pp 98-127
3. Zonneveld FW (1983) Computed tomography. Philips Medical Systems, Best, the Netherlands
4. Zonnveveld FW (1987) Principles of computed tomography. In. Zonneveld FW (ed) Computed tomography ot the temporal bone and orbit, techniques of direct multiplanar, high-resolution CT and correlative cryosectional anatomy. Urban and Schwarzenberg, Munich, pp 1-24
5. Schreiber P (1990) Heat management in X-ray tubes. Medicamundi 35: 49-56
6. Behling R (1990) The MRC 200: a new high-output X-ray tube. Medicamundi 35: 57-64
7. Zeman RK, Brink JA, Costello P, Davros WJ, Richmond BJ, Silverman PM, Vieco PT (eds) Helical/spiral CT; a practical approach. McGraw-Hill, New York
8. Fishman EK, Jeffrey RB (eds) (1995) Spiral CT: principles, techniques and clinical application. Raven, New York
9. Kalender WA (1994) Technical foundations of spiral CT. Semin Ultrasound CT MRI 15(2): 81-89
10. Napel SA (1995) Basic prinicples of spiral CT. In: Fishman EK, Jeffrey RB (eds) Spiral CT: principles, techniques and clinical applications. Raven, New York, pp 1-9
11. Brink JA, Heiken JP, Wang G, McEnery EW, Schlueter FJ, Vannier MW (1994) Helical CT: principles and technical considerations. Radiographics 14: 887-893
12. Davros WJ, Zemann RK (1995) Comparison of helical/spiral CT scanners. In: Zeman RK, Brink JA, Costello P, Davors WJ, Richmond WJ, Silverman PM, Vieco PT (eds) Helical/spiral CT, a practical approach. McGraw-Hill, New York, pp 299-324
13. Zonneveld FW, Vijerberg GP (1984) The relationship between slice thickness and image quality in CT. Medicamundi 29(3): 104-117
14. Crawford CR, King KF (1990) Computed tomography scanning with simultaneous patient translation. Med Phys 17: 967-982
15. Kalender WA, Polacin A (1991) Physical performance characteristics of CT scanning. Med Phys 18: 910-915
16. Polacin A, Kalender WA (1994) Measurement of slice sensitivity profiles in spiral CT. Med Phys 21: 133-140
17. Vieco PT (1995) Head, neck and spine. In. Zeman RK, Brink JA, Costello P, Davros WJ, Richmond BJ, Silverman PM, Vieco PT (eds) Helical/spiral CT; a practical approach. McGraw-Hill, New York, pp 27-104
18. Wang G, Vannier MW (1994) Longitudinal resolution in volumetric x-ray computerized tomography - analytical comparison between conventional and helical computerized tomography. Med Phys 21: 429-433
19. Steenbek JCM, ter Haar rRomeny BM, van Leeuwen MS (1993) Comparison of resolution in longitudinal direction. In: Lemke HU, Rhodes ML, Jaffe CC, Felix R (eds) Computer assisted radiology - Computergesttzte Radiologie. Springer, Berlin Heidelberg New York, pp 489-494
20. Kalender WA, Polacin A, Sues C (1994) J Comput Assist Tomogr 18: 167-176 A comparison of conventional and spiral CT: an experimental study on the detection of spherical lesions.
21. Wegener OH (ed) (1992) Whole body computed tomography. Blackwell, Boston, p 87
22. First German consensus conference on spiral CT. Insert in European Radiology (2), April 1996
23. Rubin GD, Walker PJ, Dake MD, Napel S, Jeffrey RB, McDonnell CH, Mitchel RS, Miller CM (1993) Three-dimensional spiral computed tomographic angiography: an alternative imaging modality for the abdominal aorta and ist branches. J Vasc Surg 18: 656-665
24. Rubin GD, Dake MD, Napel S, Jeffrey RB, McDonnell CH, Sommer FG, Wexler L, Williams DM (1994) Spiral CT of renal artery stenosis: comparisions of three-dimensional rendering techniques. Radiology 190: 181-189
25. Galanski M, Prokop M, Chavan A, Schaefer CM, Jandeleit K, Nischelsky JE (1993) Renal arterial stenoses: spiral CT angiography. Radiology 189: 185-192
26. Van Hoe L, Marchal G, Baert AL, Gryspeerdt S, Mertens L (1995) Determination of scan delay time in spiral CT-angiography: utility of a test bolus injection. J Comput Assist Tomogr 19: 216-220
27. Napel SA (1995) Principles and techniques of 3D spiral CT angiography. In: Fishman EK, Jeffrey RB (eds) Spiral CT: principles, techniques and clinical applications. Raven, New York, pp 167-182
28. Tiede U, Hoehne KH, Bomans M, Pommert A, Riemer M, Wiebecke G (1990) Surface rendering, investigation of medical 3D-rendering algortihms. IEEE Comput Graphics Appl 10(2): 41-53
29. Drebin RA, Carpenter L, Hanrahan P (1988) Volume rendering. Comput Graphics 22: 65-74
30. Marks MP, Napels S, Jordan JE, Enzmann DR (1993) Diagnosis of carotid artery disease: preliminary experience with maximum-intensity-projection spiral CT angiography. AJR 160: 1267-1271
31. Van Leeuwen MS, Polman LJ, Noordzij J. Velthuis B (1994) Computed tomography angiorgraphy. In: Lanzer P, Resch J (eds) Vascular diagnostics. Springer, Berlin Heidelberg, New York, pp 443-462
32. Rubin DR, Dake MD, Napel SA, McDonnell CH, Jeffrey RB (1993) Three-dimensional spiral CT angiography of the abdomen; initial clinical experience. Radiology 186: 147-152

33. Rubin GD (1994) Three-dimensional helical CT angiography. Radiographics 14: 905-912
34. Rubin GD, Dake MD, Semba CP (1995) Current status of three-dimensional spiral CT scanning for imaging the vasculature. Radiol Clin North Am 33(1): 51-70
35. Zeman RK (1995) Vascular system and three-dimensional CT angiography. In: Zeman RK, Brink JA, Costello P, Davros WJ, Richmond BJ, Silverman PM, Vieco PT (eds) Helical/spiral CT; a practical approach. McGraw-Hill, New York, pp 265-285
36. Cumming MJ, Morrow IM (1994) Carotid artery stenosis: a prospective comparison of CT angiography and conventional angiograpy. AJR 163: 517-523
36a. Kaatee R, Beek FJA, Verschuyl EJ, van der Ven PJG, Beutler JJ, van Schaik JPJ, Mali WPTM (1996) Atherosclerotic renal artery stenosis: ostial or truncal? Radiology 199: 637-640
37. Marks MP, Katz DA (1995) Spiral CT angiography of the cerebrovascular circulation. In: Fishman EK, Jeffrey RB (eds) Spiral CT: principles, techniques and clinical applications. Raven, New York, pp 197-208
38. Rubin GD, Jeffrey RB (1995) 3D spiral CT angiography of the abdomen and thorax. In: Fishman EK, Jeffrey RB (eds) Spiral CT: principles, techniques and clinical application. Raven, New York, pp 183-195
39. Freund M. Palmié S, Hutzelmann A, Heller M (1995) Doppel-spiral-CT-Angiographie. Fortschr Rongenstr 163(2): 177-180
40. Katz DA, Marks MP, Napel SA, Bracci PM, Roberts SL (1995) Circle of Willis: evaluation with spiral CT angiography, MR angiography, and conventional angiography. Radiology 195: 445-449
41. Zeman RK, Berman PM, Silverman PM, Davros WJ, Cooper C, Kladakis AO, Gomes MN (1995) Diagnosis of aortic dissection: value of helical CT with multiplanar reformation and three-dimensional rendering. AJR 164: 1375-1480
42. Eikelboom BC, Balm R (1994) Endovascular prosthesis implantation: clinical integration of imaging modalities and image processing. Philips Medical Systems, Best, The Netherlands (no. 522 982 48151 1994-11)
43. Remy-Jardin M, Remy J, Wattinne L, Giraud F (1992) Central pulmonary thromboembolism: diagnosis with spiral volumetric CT with the single-breath-hold technique - comparison with pulmonary angiography. Radiology 185: 381-387
44. Costello P (1995) Thorax. In: Zeman RK, Brink JA, Costello P, Davros WJ, Richmond WJ, Silverman PM, Vieco PT (eds) Helical/spiral CT, a practical approach. McGraw-Hill, New York, pp 265-285
45. Van Leeuwen MS (1994) Triphasic spiral CT if the liver and three-dimensional liver imaging. Thesis, University of Utrecht
46. Winter TC III, Freency PC, Nghiem HV, Hommeyer SC, Barr D, Croghan AM, Coldwell DM, Althaus SJ, Mack LA (1995) Hepatic arterial anantomy in transplantation candidates: evaluation with three-dimensional CT arteriography. Radiology 195: 363-370
47. Rubin GD, Alfrey EJ, Dake MD, Semba CP, Sommer FG Kuo PC, Dafoe DC, Waskerwitz JA, Bloch DA, Jeffrey RB (1995) Assessment of living renal donors with spiral CT. Radiology 195: 457-462
48. Rubin GD, Silverman SG (1995) Helical (spiral) CT of the retroperitoneum. Radiol Clin North Am 33: 903-923
49. Schwarz RB, Tice HM, Hooten SM, Hsu L, Stieg PE (1994) Evaluation of cerebral aneurysms with helical CT: correlation with conventional angiography and MR angiography. Radiology 192: 717-722
50. Joseph PM (1981) Artifacts in computed tomography. In: Newton TH, Potts DG (eds) Radiology of the skull and brain, technical aspects of computed tomography. Mosby, St Louis, pp 3956-3992
51. Godwin JD, Breiman RS, Speckmann JM (1982) Problems and pitfalls in the evalutaion of thoracic aortic dissection by computed tomography. J Comput Assist Tomogr 6: 750-756
52. Burns MA, Molina PL, Gutierrez FR, Sagel SS (1991) Motion artifact simulating aortic dissection on CT. AJR 157: 465-467
53. Duvernoy O, Coulden R, Ytterberg C (1995) Aortic motion: a potential pitfall in CT imaging of dissection in the ascending aorta. J Comput Assist Tomogr 19: 569-572
54. Mukherji SK (1992) Motion artifact simulating aortic dissection on CT. AJR 159: 674
55. Posniak HV, Olson MC, Demos TC (1993) Aortic motion artifact simulating dissection on CT scans: elimination with reconstructive segmented images. AJR 161: 557-558

Part I: Diagnostics of Vascular Diseases: State-of-the-Art

Section III: Laboratory Vascular Methods

Assessment of Hemostasis

R.E. Roller, C. Korninger, and B.R. Binder

Physiology of the Hemostatic System

Primary Hemostasis

Contact of platelets with subendothelial collagen induces platelet adhesion, a reaction mediated by von Willebrand factor. Adhesion is followed by platelet conformation change and release of substances such as serotonin, platelet factor-4 (PF-4), β-thromboglobulin, and factor Va. ADP release induces platelet activation, exposure of fibrinogen receptors and thus aggregation. The final product of the primary platelet activation is the platelet ("white") clot, which is stabilized and stregthened by the fibrin clot.

Fibrin Clot Formation

The final product of activation of the coagulation cascade is the formation of the macromolecule fibrin from fibrinogen by limited proteolysis liberating fibrinopeptides (FPA) and (FPB).

Coagulation factors are glycoproteins, either zymogens, which act as enzymes after activation (serine proteases II, VII, IX, XII), or cofactors (V, VIII). With the exception of von Willebrand factor they are all synthesized in the liver, and several are vitamin K dependent (II, VII, IX, X, protein C, protein S). Plasma concentrations and half-lives are given in Tables 1 and 2.

Coagulation is initiated by contact with subendothelial structures (intrinsic system) or by liberation of tissue thromboplastin from injured cellular structures (extrinsic system). The cascade-type coagulation process occurs primarily on surfaces (subendothelium, activated platelets) and thus in loco (Fig. 1 a, b). It is important to note that the so-called intrinsic activating system and the extrinsic one have a common pathway from activated factor X on and are regulated at several levels. Factor XIIa can activate factor VII, thereby leading to incrased

Table 1. Plasma concentrations and half-lives of coagulation factors I–XIII

Coagulation factor	Name	Type	Plasma concentration (mg/dl)	Molecular weight (kDa)	Half-life times (h)
I	Fibrinogen	Substrate	300	340	100–120
II	Prothrombin	Serine protease	3	72	50–60
V	Proaccelerin	Cofactor	3	50	35
VII	Proconvertin	Serine protease	0.1	48	5–6
VIII	Anthihemophilic factor, globulin A	Cofactor	1	2000	6–14
IX	Anthihemophilic factor, globulin B	Serine protease	0.3	80	18–30
X	Stuart Prower factor	Serine protease	0.8	56	40–60
XI	Plasma thrombo-plastin antecedant (PTA)	Serine protease	0.6	160	48–60
XII	Hageman factor	Serine protease/pro-enzyme	3	80	52–70
XIII	Fibrin-stabilizing factor	Transglutaminase	0.8	320	72–96

Table 2. Plasma concentrations and half-lives of other hemostatic factors

	Type of factor	Plasma concentration (μg/ml)	Molecular weight (kDa)	Half-life times (h)
Protein C	Proenzyme/serine protease	4	62	6
Protein S	Cofactor	10 (free form)	69	–
Antithrombin III	Serine protease inhibitor	290	62	61–92
C1-INH	Serine protease inhibitor	240	105	–
Heparin cofactor II	serpin	9	65	–
Plasminogen	Proenzyme/serine protease	20.000	90	0.08 (Lys) 2.2 (Glu)
tPA	Serine protease	0.04	72	0.08
scuPA	Proenzyme/serine protease	0.1	53	0.08
PAI-1	Serine protease inhibitor	0.05	57	–
Protein C inhibitor	Serine protease inhibitor	4	57	–
α_2Antiplasmin	Serine protease inhibitor	70	67	60

C1-INH, C1 inhibitor; t-PA, tissue-type plasminogen activator; scuPA, single-chair urokinase; PAI, plasminogen activator inhibitor.

levels of circulating VIIa, which upon exposure to tissue factor immediately triggers fibrin formation. Furthermore and most importantly, factor VIIa also activates factor IX, thereby generating a loop of activation (Josso loop Xa → VIIa → IXa → Xa), finally bypassing inhibition of the tissue factor pathway by tissue factor pathway inhibitor (TFPI; see below); this explains the bleeding seen in factor VIII deficiency upon injuries. Only when enough factor Xa is generated to activate factor II to thrombin a positive feedback loop is initiated in which factor IIa activates factors VIII and V to factors VIIIa and Va. Only these cofactors in their activated form are capable of sustaining the coagulation cascade at a high enough level to finally lead to fibrin formation.

In addition to induction of the extrinsic coagulation cascade by injury-mediated tissue factor exposure, tissue factor expression on the surface of endothelial cells (EC) can also initiate coagulation;

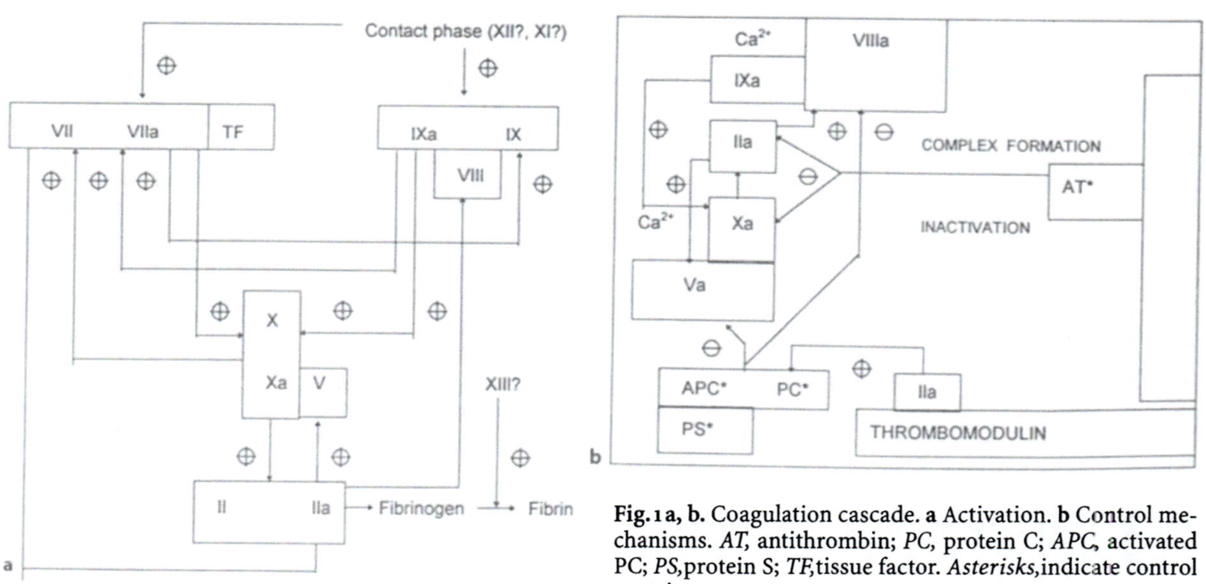

Fig. 1 a, b. Coagulation cascade. **a** Activation. **b** Control mechanisms. *AT,* antithrombin; *PC,* protein C; *APC,* activated PC; *PS,* protein S; *TF,* tissue factor. *Asterisks,* indicate control proteins

this process is a highly regulated one. Tissue factor is upregulated on the surface of EC in response to mediators of inflammation such as tumor necrosis factor-α (TNF-α) or lipopolysaccharide (LPS) itself. Both TNF-α and LPS trigger a cascade of cellular events which are at least partially mediated via activation of the nuclear factor (NF)-κB pathway, leading not only to upregulation of tissue factor, but also to increased expression of plasminogen activator inhibitor-1 (PAI-1), adhesion molecules, and inflammatory cytokines, e. g., interleukin (IL) -1, -6, and -8. The overall response is generation of disseminated intravascular coagulation (DIC) rather than local fibrin clot formation.

Activated coagulation factors are neutralized in plasma with high efficiency by inhibitor systems. The antithrombin III-heparan sulfate heparin system inhibits coagulation factors XIIa, XIa, Xa, IXa, and IIa, preferentially in the fluid phase. Of major importance is the fact that factor Xa bound to factor Va is protected against inhibition by antithrombin (AT)-III, whereas fluid-phase Xa is immediately inhibited by AT-III, thus limiting the coagulation cascade to surfaces exposing factor Va, such as activated platelet. However, AT-III bound to heparin is capable of overcoming the factor Va effect. The protein C-thrombomodulin-protein S system inactivates factors Va and VIIIa, thereby terminating the coagulation cascade, especially at the site of intact endothelium exposing thrombomodulin. TFPI neutralizes factor VIIa and tissue factor, switching off the extrinsic system after an initiated trigger stage.

Fibrinolytic System

The fibrinolytic enzyme plasmin is formed from its zymogen plasminogen (plasma concentration, 20 μg/dl) by two plasminogen activators. Tissue-type plasminogen activator (tPA) released from endothelial cells seems to be mainly responsible for dissolution of fibrin clots; its enzyme activity is regulated by the presence of fibrin and by its major inhibitor, PAI-1, which are both synthesized by the liver and EC and contained in platelets. However, PAI-1 is mainly found in its latent form.

The second plasminogen activator, urokinase plasminogen activator (u-PA), is synthesized by several cells in its inactive precursor form, prourokinase (single-chain urokinase, scuPA), and seems to be responsible for extravascular proteolysis and activation; its activity is regulated by local binding to its high-affinity receptor, a glycosyl-phosphatidylinasitol (GPI)-anchored surface protein. In addition, extravascular proteolysis is also regulated by availability of surface plasminogen-binding sites. Additional factors in the regulation of fibrinolysis are α-antiplasmin, which can become cross linked to fibrin, contributing to the higher resistance of cross-linked fibrin towards fibrinolysis [1]. Plasmin formation is generally regulated by the exposure of lysin residues (especially *N*-terminal ones) to the kringle structures contained in plasminogen and other proteins (tPA, uPA, prekallikrein, apolipoprotein (a), hepatocyte growth factor). Enzyme binding of native Glu-plasminogen includes a conformational change mimicking the Lys form of plasminogen, which is more readily activated than the Glu form.

Analytical Methods in Hemostasis

Primary Hemostasis

Bleeding Time

Bleeding time is a global method for evaluating primary hemostasis; interactions between platelets, von Willebrand factor, and endothelium are assessed. Bleeding time is primarily prolonged in conditions in which the platelet count is reduced and in qualitative platelet disorders. All bleeding time methods are difficult to standardize and are thus problematic to interpret.

Duke's Technique
A puncture approximately 4 mm deep is made at the fingertip while the capillaries are under increased pressure (40 mm Hg) due to an inflated blood-pressure cuff on the upper arm. This method has little practical merit, since false-negative (below 50 000 platelets per μl) and false-positive results can be expected [2].

Incision Methods
These methods as described by Borchgrevink [3] (commercial Simplate and Template kits are available; Simplate Organon, The Netherlands) are more reliable than Duke's technique. Prolongation can be expected in thrombocytopenia (linear correlation between bleeding time and a platelet count of 10 000 – 100 000 per μl), in thrombocytopathies, in von Willebrand disease, in rare vascular bleeding syndromes, and under the influence of anti-aggregating drugs (e.g., acetyl salicylic acid).

Platelet Count

Platelet count is routinely performed in electronic particle counting machines, using blood anticoagulated by addition of ethylenediaminetetraacetate (EDTA). An erroneously low platelet count may be reported in the presence of large platelets (by a "gate" excluding these cells) or in pseudothrombocytopenia [4] (an artifact frequently encountered in vitro and with no clinical relevance; in vitro platelet aggregation is induced by EDTA). If results are doubtful, a blood smear can be inspected (method described by Fonio) or platelet counting in the Bürker-Trk chamber (method of Brecher and Cronkite [5]) can be performed.

Platelet Function Tests

The principle underlying *platelet aggregation tests* is the increase in photometrically measured light transmission of platelet-rich plasma when aggregated by addition of substances such as ADP [6], epinephrine, thrombin, or collagen. In Bernard-Soulier syndrome (a genetic defect of glycoprotein Ib, which is responsible for von Willebrand factor binding) and in von Willebrands's disease, aggregation with ristocetin is typically reduced, but is normal with ADP, epinephrine, and collagen. In Glanzmann's thrombasthenia (a genetic defect of the glycoprotein receptor IIb/IIIa, an integrin responsible for fibrinogen binding), aggregation with ristocetin is normal, but is abnormal with ADP, epinephrine, and collagen. In uremia and after ingestion of acetyl salicylic acid, aggregation with epinephrine and collagen is reduced. (For further rading on platelet function tests, see [7].)

Tests such as *platelet adhesion* [8] (reduced in von Willebrand's disease), *retraction* (abnormal in thrombasthenia), and *platelet spreading* (abnormal in disorders of thrombopoiesis) are performed under selected clinical conditions.

Blood Coagulation Tests

Global Tests

Global tests are charcterized by low sensitivity and are thus of limited clinical value.

In the whole-blood clotting time (Lee-White) procedure, the clotting time of whole blood is measured immediately after venipuncture in glass tubes at 37°C. The normal value ranges from 6 to 12 min. The whole-blood clotting time is prolonged in severe blood coagulation disorders (intrinsic system, extrinsic system, or end phase of coagulation) and in the presence of heparin, as is the recalcification time (the clotting time of citrated blood following addition of calcium chloride).

The activated clotting time (ACT) is measured by drawing blood into "activating" substances such as celite or glass beads. Normal values largely depend on the techniques used and range from 90 to 145 s. Thus the time range is more practical than in the previously mentioned tests and the test precision is higher (coefficient of variation, 5%). The test can be used for bedside screening and is commonly employed in dialysis units and during catheter interventions. ACT is prolonged mainly in disorders of the intrinsic blood coagulation pathway and in the presence of heparin (sensitivity, 0.1 heparin/ml).

Group Tests

Prothrombin Time

This test, also known as the thromboplastin time or Quick test [9], is based upon recalcification of citrated blood or plasma in the presence of tissue thromboplastin by measuring the fibrin formation. The result of the test mainly reflects the activity of the extrinsic pathway, including coagulation factors II, V, VII, and X, and, to a lesser extent, of fibrinogen (factor I). Heparin as used in clinical regimens does not affect prothrombin time (PT) measurements. In Europe, it is common to express the results of the PT test as a percentage of the normal value by comparing the result (in seconds) with a calibration curve obtained by dilution of normal blood or plasma (the so-called Quick value). In the Anglo-American literature, the results of the PT test are given in seconds, together with the value of the normal control. Alternatively, a prothrombin ratio (the ratio of the patient's PT to normal PT) may be given.

The result is largely influenced by the source and quality of the thromboplastin preparation used. In order to optimize comparability of various PT results, the international normalized ratio (INR) [10], also recommended by the World Health Organisation (WHO), has been proposed and is now increasingly used. It is calculated by potentiating the ratio (R) obtained by the international sensitivity index (ISI) of the thromboplastin used given by the manufacturer:

$$\mathrm{INR} = \mathrm{R}^{\mathrm{ISI}}$$

The method is described in detail in a publication by Kirkwood [11] and allows comparison of thromboplastin preparations of different origin and sensitivity. The INR should generally be used for control of anticoagulant therapy and guarantees comparable results (even with different thromboplastins), given a ratio range of 1.5 – 5.

The PT is prolonged in conditions associated with the reduction of one or more of the coagulation factors II, V, VII, and X (as well as in conditions with severely reduced fibrinogen): i.e., rare hereditary or acquired deficiencies of factors II, V, VII, and X; liver disease (since the factors are produced by the liver); vitamin K deficiency (since factors II, VII, and X are vitamin K dependent), as is seen in newborn babies; diseases with lowered absorption of vitamin K (sprue); total parenteral nutrition; during treatment with cephalosporins; and during treatment with oral anticoagulant drugs. Furthermore, the PT is prolonged in the presence of high levels of heparin and fibrin (fibrinogen) degradation products.

Some PT methods (Normotest, Thrombotest, Immuno, Austria); have been modified by addition of factor V and fibrinogen and thus reflect the activity of vitamin K-dependent coagulation factors II, VII, and X. These tests are therefore sensitive markers of vitamin K deficiency and can be used to monitor liver function or oral anticoagulant therapy.

The therapeutic range for oral anticoagulants differs according to the thromboplastin used and can be obtained from the instructions generally provided by the manufacturers. For most PT reagents, "mild" treatment should be aimed at in patients with a PT of 20% – 25%, and "intensive" treatment for those with a PT of 15% – 20%. In terms of the INR, mild treatment is indicated in patients with an INR of 2 – 3, and intensive treatment in those with an INR of 3 – 4.5. The individual range for a given patient is chosen according to the parti cular diagnosis.

Activated Partial Thromboplastin Time

This is the classic group test for evaluating the intrinsic system of blood coagulation. In principle, it is a recalcification time of citrated plasme low in platelets, whereby prior to recalcification a lipid extract and a negatively charged material are added [12]. Results and sensitivity depend on the lipid fraction (partial thromboplastin) and the activator used. A reference value must be supplied together with the results. Activated partial thromboplastin time (aPTT) values are prolonged when one or more of the following coagulation factors are reduced: V, VIII, XII, prekallikrein (PKK), and high molecular weight kininogen (HMWK). aPTT values are also prolonged in more severe cases of reduction in coagulation factor II (prothrombin) and I (fibrinogen) and in the presence of coagulation inhibitors, such as heparin, or circulating anticoagulants, such as lupus anticoagulants.

The sensitivity for certain abnormal conditions varies between test systems. Some aPTT reagents are especially sensitive for reduction; coagulation factors VIII and IX (hemophilia), some for heparin, and others for circulating anticoagulants (e.g., lupus inhibitors). For the detection of acquired and hereditary defects of coagulation factors, aPTT is primarily used to monitor heparin therapy; in addition to thrombin time, aPTT is a further standard test used to monitor conventional (unfractionated) heparin treatment. In patients on continuous intravenous heparin infusion, an increase in aPTT of two to five times the initial value is used as a guideline.

Thrombin Time

The thrombin time can be used to assess the end phase of coagulation. A small amount of thrombin is added to citrated plasma and the time necessary for formation of a clot is determined. The thrombin time depends on the amount of clottable fibrinogen present and on the inhibitors of the reaction. Thus a prolonged thrombin time occurs in hypo- or dysfibrinogenemia, in the presence of (unfractionate) heparin, and in the presence of substances that interfere with fibrin polymerization (high levels of fibrin and fibrinogen degradation products and paraproteins).

Heparin sensitivity of the thrombin time largely depends upon the amount of thrombin present in the test system. With low doses of thrombin (final concentration, 1 IU/ml), a normal value of 20 – 24 s is obtained, together with a high heparin sensitivity. For the purposes of monitoring treatment with unfractionate heparin, higher concentrations are used (final concentration, 2 IU/ml; normal value, 12 – 17 s) [13].

Reptilase Time and Thrombin Coagulase Time

In this test, reptilase or thrombin coagulase are used to clot fibrinogen. Since these two enzymes are not inhibited by the AT-III-heparin system, the results of the respective tests reflect clottable fibrinogen and interfering substances (such as fibrinogen degradation products and paraproteins), but are not influenced by the presence of heparin. By comparing thrombin time with either reptilase time or thrombin coagulase time, it is therefore possible to distinguish between the effect of heparin and other abnormalities of the end phase of coagulation. Reference values for all tests mentioned are given in Table 3.

Table 3. Reference values for blood coagulation tests

Test system	Reference range
Bleeding time (Duke)	120–240 s
Coagulation time (Lee-White)	<9 min
Thrombin time	10–24 s
Thrombin- coagulase time	<23 s
Reptilase time	<20 s
Thromboplastin time	10–15 s
	70%–125%
Activated thromboplastin time	<45 s

Determination of Single Blood Coagulation Factors

Blood coagulation disorders can more precisely be defined by determination of single coagulation factors. The test systems may be either clotting, amidolytic, or immunologic methods.

The most frequently used single coagulation factor assay involves the determination of fibrinogen by the Clauss method [14]. This method is easy to perform and results are adequately precise (coefficient of variance, 10%). After addition of a high concentration of thrombin to diluted citrated plasma, the measured coagulation time depends (almost exclusively) on the amount of clottable fibrinogen present. Fibrinogen values may, however, be underestimated in hyperfibrinolysis and thrombolytic therapy. Another reliable method has been described by Ratnow and Menzie [15]; this method has excellent precision, but is time consuming.

Low fibrinogen values are present in hereditary deficiencies, disorders of synthesis (liver cirrhosis), and fibrinogen consumption (DIC) and may also be due to volume expansion (polytransfusion). High fibrinogen levels can be found in various diseases, because fibrinogen is an acute phase protein. This coagulation test can thus also be used as a marker for inflammation.

Other single factor assays are performed by testing ability of the patients plasma to correct the clotting time (PT or aPTT system) of a plasma deficient in one specific coagulation factor. This is achieved by using either congenitally deficient plasmas or plasmas in which a specific coagulation factor has been depleted. By testing for factor V activity, for example, it is possible to distinguish between vitamin K deficiency (normal factor V activity) and liver dysfunction (low factor V).

By using immunologic methods it is possible to distinguish between coagulation factor deficiencies (low activity, low antigen) and dysfunctional coagulation factors (low activity, normal or higher antigen).

Determination of blood coagulation factors may be of interest in cardiovascular medicine, since an association between elevated levels of certain blood coagulation factors (finbrinogen or factor VII) with mortality from cardiovascular diseases has been described [16].

Markers for Activation of the Hemostatic System

The ethanol gelation test (EGT [17]) is a method used to demonstrate soluble fibrinogen, fibrin monomer complexes present as a result of thrombin generation. At fibrinogen levels of between 50 and 400 mg/dl, it is, however, a useful test in the diagnosis of disseminated intravascular coagulation.

Intravascular generation of thrombin can be demonstrated indirectly by measuring thrombin, AT-III complexes (TAT) [18], usually by the enzyme-linked immunosorbent assay (ELISA) technique.

Further evidence of thrombin activation is the presence of FPA [19] and FPB, commonly determined by radioimmunoassay [20].

At the level of thrombin generation, the presence of factor Xa is revealed by the occurrence of prothrombin fragment-1,2 (PTF-1,2).

Coagulation Factor Inhibitors

Antithrombin III

To assess antithrombin III (AT-III) enzymatic and immunologic methods are available.

In enzymatic methods, principally thrombin or factor Xa is added to plasma (in the presence or absence of heparin). After a defined incubation time, residual (not AT-III inhibited) enzyme is determined either using a clotting assay method [21] or by chromogenic substrate. The result is commonly expressed as percentage of normal. Immunologic methods either use radioimmunodiffusion, two-dimensional immunoelectrophoresis (Laurell), radioimmunoassys, or ELISA.

Reduction of AT-III occurs in hereditary deficiencies (type I, II, or III) or in acquired disease states, i.e., disorders of synthesis (liver disease) loss (nephrotic syndrome) and consumption (DIC).

Protein C, Protein S, and Activated Protein C Resistance

For protein C, both enzyme kinetic (clotting assays and amidolytic methods) and immunologic methods are available [22, 23]. Under physiological conditions, 60 % – 70 % of protein S is bound to C4b-binding protein, and the remaining 30 % – 40 % of "free" protein S may be measured by enzyme kinetic methods. Activated protein C (APC) resistance [24] can be determined using a modified aPTT coagulation test or by demonstration of a point mutation in the factor V gene (e.g., by polymerase chain reaction, PCR; Table 4).

Table 4. Refernces values for coagulation factor inhibitors

Factor	Reference range
Antithrombin III (AT-III)	75 % – 125 %
Protein C activity	70 % – 140 %
Protein S (total)	70 % – 140 %
Protein S (free form)	>55 %
APC resistance ratio	>2.0 – 2.2

APC, activated protein C

Fibrinolysis Tests

Various test systems have been developed to assess function and capacity of the fibrinolytic system. Systems that enzymatically or immunologically measure individual components of the fibrinolytic system such as tPA, uPA, PAI-1, plasminogen, and α_2-antiplasmin are available. Free plasmin activity is rarely present in blood. After inhibitor depletion by euglobulin fractionation or dilution, however, the plasmin activity generated can be measured by its effect on fibrin. The presence of plasmin-α_2-antiplasmin complexes (PAP) and of fibrin (fibrinogen) degradation products, especially of d-dimer, indicates the presence of plasmin activity in the circulation. In vivo, fibrinolytic activity is generated after release of t-PA from the vessel walls in response to various stimuli. The vessel wall's capacity to release tPA can be tested by venous occlusion or infusion of certain drugs. In the venous occlusion test, a sphygmomanometer cuff is placed on the upper arm and inflated to a pressure midway between systolic and diastolic blood pressure for 5 – 20 min. In the 1-deamino-*D*-Arg-8 vasopressin (DDAVP) test, 0.4 µg vasopressin analogue/kg body weight is infused prior to testing.

Global Tests

After euglobulin precipitation from activated diluted plasma (at low pH), the time to lysis of a fibrin clot produced by addition of thrombin (euglobulin clot lysis time, ECLT [31]) or the lytic area on a standard fibrin plate is measured (fibrin plate method [25]). Using these global tests, both spontaneous fibrinolytic activity and stimulated activity (fibrinolytic capacity after tPA release induced by venous occlusion or DDAVP) can be measured.

The results of the ECLT or the fibrin plate assay reflect a number of variables and are thus difficult to interpret. Shortening of the ECLT is seen during thrombolytic therapy and in hyperfibrinolytic states (e.g., during disseminated intravascular coagulation). Low fibrinolytic activity after stimulation (low fibrinolytic capacity) is a common finding in young survivors of myocardial infarction.

Analysis of Single Fibrinolytic Proteins

Enzymatic and/or immunologic methods [26] are available for all components of the fibrinolytic system. Plasminogen and PAI-1 assays are commonly used in the analysis of patients with thrombosis (since high PAI-1 levels may be associated with thrombophilia and/or vascular disease). α_2-Antiplasmin deficiency is a rare cause of hemorrhagic diathesis.

Fibrin (Fibrinogen) Degeneration Products

Fibrinogen degradation products occur as a consequence of plasmin activity and therefore reflect activation of the fibrinolytic system. Classically, these products are determined by the hemagglutination inhibition test [27]. By this method, mainly fibrinogen degeneration products X and Y, and to a lesser extent D are determined. High levels of these products are found during thrombolytic therapy and in primary or secondary hyperfibrinolysis (due to DIC). The presence of the fragment *D*-dimer is direct evidence for the digestion (and thus presence) of fibrin. For determination of d-dimer, a specific monoclonal antibody is used either in an ELISA or in a latex agglutination test that is easy to perform without special laboratory equipment [32]. Elevated levels may not only be found in states of hyperfibrinolysis, but also in many situations associated with fibrin formation, such as venous thrombosis and pulmonary embolism [28].

As mentioned in the previous section, high levels of fibrinogen degeneration products are associated with a prolonged thrombin, reptilase, and thrombin coagulase time.

Disorders of Hemostasis

Disorders of Platelets

Thrombocytopenia

Reductions in platelet count can be found in various clinical situations.

Disorders of Syntheses
These are seen in rare congenital diseases (Fanconi-anemia, Wiskott-Aldrich syndrome) and may be the consequence of acquired bone marrow dysfunction (e.g., due to leukemia, cytostatic therapy, vitamin B_{12} deficiency).

Enhanced Peripheral Platelet Destruction
This may be due to immunologic mechanisms as in idiopathic thrombocytopenia (ITP), in systemic lupus erythematodes (SLE), in post-transfusion purpura, in thrombotic thrombocytopenic purpura (TTP), and in hemolytic-uremic syndrome (HUS). Nonimmune mechanisms include mechanical destruction (artificial heart valves), increased turnover (disseminated intravascular coagulation), loss (massive bleeding and transfusion with blood low in platelets) and sequestration (splenomegaly). In various clinical settings, a combination of causes is responsible for thrombocytopenia.

Thrombocytopenia is commonly defined as "severe" with platelet counts below 50 000 per μl and "mild" between 100 000 and 150 000 per μl. There is a rough correlation between clinical bleeding tendency and platelet count, with marked individual differences according to the cause of thrombocytopenia and the age of the patient. Spontaneous bleeding is common with values below 20 000 per μl.

Thrombopathy

Thrombopathies are rare disorders characterized by normal or reduced platelet count and disturbed platelet function. In Bernard-Soulier syndrome, platelet adhesion, in thrombasthenia Glanzmann aggregation, and in storage pool disease the platelet release reaction is reduced. Hereditary thrombopathies are characterized by spontaneous skin and mucosal bleeding and by post-traumatic and post-operative bleeding.

Acquired platelet function disorders are much more common and can be due to underlying diseases such as uremia, paraproteinemia, or leukemia. Various drugs can inhibit platelet function, such as dextran and some antibiotics. The most important platelet-inhibiting drugs are acetyl salicylic acid which irreversibly inhibits platelet cyclooxygenase, and nonsteroidal anti inflammatory drugs (NSAID).

Blood Coagulation Disorders

Hereditary Deficiencies

Bleeding
Isolated coagulation factor deficiencies can be severe (coagulation factor activity below 1%), moderate (1%–5%), or mild (>5%). Even severe deficiencies of prekallikrein, HMWK or factor XII are not associated with bleeding tendencies; in factor XI deficiency, bleeding tendency is mild, whereas it is severe in deficiencies of coagulation factors I, II, V, VII, VIII (hemophilia A), IX (hemophilia B), and XIII. The pattern of inheritance is either recessive (no clinical symptoms with one diseased allele) or sex linked in hemophilia; in factor I deficiency it is autosomal.

Typical bleeding manifestations of hemophilia are spontaneous joint and muscle bleeding, hematoma, postoperative and post-traumatic bleeding, and impaired wound healing.

Patients with von Willebrand's syndrome are deficient in coagulation factor VIII due to increased turnover of factor VIII because of deficient binding to vWF, and also in vWF, which mediates platelet adhesion to subendothelium. Von Willebrand's disease has an autosomal dominant or recessive pattern of inheritance; it is more common than hemophilia A and is characterized by both platelet-type and coagulation-type bleeding.

Hereditary Deficiency of Coagulation Factors Causing Thrombosis

Protein C deficiency is a well-known risk factor for thrombophilia is protein C deficiency, which causes deep vein thrombosis (DVT) and is seen in 5%–8% of DVT patients. Two types of protein C deficiencies are known so far. In the more prevalent one (type I), protein C antigen and activity are reduced in parallel. In type II only low protein C functional activity is found. The genetic defects in these disorders have been well defined and include nonsense and missense mutations and some chromosomal deletions. Homozygous protein C deficiency is very rare (1:200 000 – 1:400 000) and is associated with severe thrombosis even in neonates. These babies suffer from necrotic skin lesions caused by thromboembolic occlusion of skin capillaries, DIC, and brain and eye damage. In such cases, treatment with protein C concentrates may be lifesaving. Furthermore, protein C deficiency is sometimes associated with warfarin-induced skin necrosis, which develops early during anticoagulant treatment. This clinical phenomenon is due to the very short half-life ($t_{1/2,}$ 8 h) of protein C compared to other vitamin K-dependent coagulation factors, which leads to an imbalance between pro- and anticoagulant factors.

The classical type of *protein S deficiency* is associated with a reduction in plasma levels of total protein S antigen of approximately 50% and a higher reduction in free protein S antigen and its functional activity. Another type of deficiency has been described in which total protein S antigen levels are in the normal range, but levels of free protein S and its functional activity are disproportionally reduced to less than 40% of normal. In general, it should be borne in mind that total protein S levels are significantly lower and more variable in females and that deficiency of protein S by more than 50% the normal values results in a statistically significant increase in the risk of thromboembolic events. Protein S deficiency is found in 5%–8% of DVT patients.

Two major types of *AT-III deficiencies* have been described. The classical (type I) deficiency state is a result of reduced synthesis of the functionally normal protease inhibitor, whereas in type II deficiency patients have a protease inhibitor with a discrete molecular defect, causing loss of functional activity at normal antigen levels. The prevalence of AT-III deficiency in the general population is 0.2%–0.4%, and it is important to note, that the majority of AT-III-deficient patients identified during screening analysis never exhibit clinical manifestation of a thromboembolic event [29]; however, AT-III deficiency is found in 5%– 8% of patients with DVT.

A novel mechanism for thrombophilia was recently discovered. It is characterized by an inherited resistance of factor V to the anticoagulant action of activated protein C *(APC resistance)*. In more than 90% of patients, it is caused by a single point mutation of the factor V gene. It is highly prevalent in the general population (3%–5%) and in its heterozygous form afflicts affected people with a lifelong hypercoagulable state and a five- to tenfold increase in the risk of thrombosis [30]. This defect is thought to be responsible for 25% of cases of DVT.

Acquired Disorders

Vitamin K Deficiency

This is characterized by a coagulation-type bleeding tendency, and the key abnormality is the prolonged PT. It is commonly the result of oral anticoagulant treatment, but may be found in newborn babies, in patients with malabsorption conditions, and in those receiving total parenteral nutrition (especially during concomitant treatment with cephalosporins). Purely alimentary deficiency states are rare, since vitamin K is not only present in nutrients (vegetables), but is also synthesized by bacteria. Treatment with vitamin K (preferably by infusion, not injection, since anaphylactic reactions are common) usually normalizes blood coagulation within 24h. In an emergency, prothrombin complex concentrates may be used.

Liver Disease

Hepatocellular disease may cause a serious coagulation defect, the severity of which is proportional to the extent of liver damage. The complex disorder is caused by decreased synthesis of coagulation factors and inhibitors, synthesis of abnormal coagulation factors, altered clearance function for activated coagulation factors and components of the fibrinolytic system, such as tPA, and thrombocytopenia. The main finding is the prolonged PT. In more severe cases, fibrinogen levels are reduced and thrombocytopenia is common in cirrhosis. Dysfibringenemia is evidenced by a prolonged thrombin and reptilase time. Due to the complex nature of the hemostatic defect, complete correction is impossible. In an emergency, substitution with fresh frozen plasma, prothrombin complex concentrates (together with AT-III concentrates), and platelet transfusion are effective.

Disseminated Intravascular Coagulation
This disorder results from intravascular activation of the coagulation system, leading to macro- and microthrombosis on the one hand and coagulation factor and platelet depletion with bleeding tendency on the other (consumption coagulopathy). DIC can occur in a number of different clinical situations, such as septicemia, shock, malignancy, and obstetric disorders. Its course may be chronic (as in giant hemangiomas) or acute (as in amniotic fluid embolism). The main clinical feature may be macro- and microthrombosis (acquired respiratory distress syndrome, renal failure) or bleeding. Therapeutic strategies are complex and are still a matter of dispute; they should include inhibition of thrombin formation in addition to treatment of the underlying clinical disorder.

Acquired Coagulation Factor Inhibitors
Occurrence of neutralizing antibodies to a blood coagulation factor is a rare event. Clinically, the resulting coagulation disorders resemble congenital deficiencies of the respective factor.

Antibodies that interfere with the formation of activation complexes, so-called lupus anticoagulants, are much more common. They occur in patients with autoimmune disorders or viral infections, patients receiving drugs, pregnant women, and individuals with no underlying disease. The main feature is the prolonged partial thromboplastin time, and the diagnosis can be established by mixing experiments with normal plasma. Lupus anticoagulants are not associated with any bleeding tendency, but with an increased risk of venous or arterial thrombosis [34] and miscarriage [33]; 60% of lupus anticoagulants are associated with anticardiolipin antibodies.

Hemostasiological Monitoring in Cardiovascular Medicine

Screening of Hemostasis and Monitoring of Treatment

Surgical Procedures and Arteriography

In the absence of a personal or familial bleeding history, the following three laboratory tests are sufficient prior to surgical interventions: PT, aPTT, and platelet caunt. Should one or more of these tests be abnormal, the intervention should be postponed until the cause is disclosed. It must be kept in mind that several rare bleeding disorders cannot be diagnosed by the above-mentioned tests, i. e., rare platelet function disorders, mild coagulation factor deficiencies such as subhemophilia A und B, variants of von Willebrands disease, factor XIII deficiency and α_2-antiplasmin deficiency.

In the case of pathological coagulation tests (or platelet counts), the importance of the therapeutic or diagnostic intervention must be balanced against the risk of bleeding.

It must be kept in mind that acetyl salicylic acid enhances the risk of bleeding in patients, expecially in those receiving heparin prophylaxis.

Heparin Treatment

The European Consensus Conference, held in November 1991 in London, formulated a classification for thromboembolic risk assessment in medical and surgical patients [40]. Suggestions for thromboprophylaxis with unfractionated heparin (UH) and low molecular weight heparin (LMWH) are given. Primary prophylaxis aims at avoiding thromboembolic complications in patients at risk (e.g., after surgery, prolonged bed rest). It is achieved by subcutaneous injection of a fixed dose of heparin, e.g., 5000 units UH, or LMWH, twice or three times daily, usually once daily. In the case of primary prophylaxis, it is not necessary to monitor treatment by means of coagulation tests. It is, however, advisable to test platelet counts regularly, due to a possible heparin-associated thrombocytopenia (HAT). In the case of blood coagulation abnomalities, the thromboembolic risk has to be weighed against the risk of bleeding in deciding whether to perform primary prophylaxis or not.

Secondary thromboprophylaxis with heparin aims at avoiding thrombus extension and reducing the risk of thromboembolism. With UH, after an initial bolus (5000 IU), doses of 20 000–40 000 U per day are adminstered, either by continuous intravenous infusion or by subcutaneous injection (every 6–12 h). Treatment is adequate if the thrombin time is prolonged to twice or three times its initial value (care must be taken to use thrombin time methods with normal values of 12–17 s) or the aPTT is prolonged to 1.5 times to twice its initial value (care must be taken to use sufficiently sensitive aPTT reagents).

Secondary prophylaxis with LMWH is performed by subcutaneous injection of 200 IU/kg per day, as a single dose or in a split dosage regimen. Monitoring is not necessary due to the superior bioavailability of LMWH. Recent meta analysis of UH versus LMWH in the treatment of acute DVT [35] suggested a superior efficacy of LMWH. It is now considered to be safe to treat acute DVT on an outpatient basis.

Oral Anticoagulants

Oral anticoagulant therapy is monitored by PT, PT ratio, or INR. Intensive treatment (INR, 3–4.5) is advisable in arterial thromboembolism and in patients with artificial heart valves, mild treatment (INR, 2–3) in venous thromboembolism, atrial fibrillation, and dilated cardiomyopathy. The duration of oral anticoagulation depends on the indication and patient-specific factors. In patients with artificial heart valves and with cardiogenic arterioembolism, lifelong anticoagulation is indicated. After a first episode of DVT, 3-month anticoagulation treatment is considered to be sufficient. In recurrent venous thromboembolism and in patients with coagulation inhibitor deficiencies (after a thrombotic episode), lifelong anticoagulation may be advisable.

Fibrinolytic Therapy

For thrombolytic therapy in myocardial infarction and massive pulmonary embolism, standardized treatment regimens with streptokinase (SK) and recombinant tissue plaminogen activator (rtPA) are available. Dosage is not modified according to blood coagulation tests. Early heparinization (thrombin time or aPTT control) is generally used in an attempt to avoid early reocclusion. Recently, bedside tPA test sticks have become available to determine tPA blood levels.

Conventional long-term (days) fibrinolytic therapy is commonly performed in patients with arterial or venous thrombosis; urokinase can also be used. In long-term treatment, the effects of fibrinolytic therapy are monitored mainly by determination of fibrinogen (plasmin activity), thrombin time, and aPTT, which reflects the concentration of fibrin (fibrinogen) degradation products. Generally, the dosage is reduced at fibrinogen values below 100 mg/dl; additional heparin is adminstered to achieve thrombin times above twice the normal value.

Venous Thromboembolism

Determination of *D*-dimer levels (qualitative and semiquantitative Latex tests are available) has been recommended for diagnoses of venous thromboembolism and pulmonary embolism. PAP levels correlate significantly with changes in of *D*-dimer levels in patients with DVT. The *D*-dimer test can be of clinical value, provided its limites sensitivity and specificity is kept in mind. False-positive results are found in various disease states (postoperatively, post-traumatically, in septicemia, and in tumours); false-negative results occur in (even recent) isolated calf vein thrombosis, in thrombosis of more than 1 week duration, and in pulmonary embolism. Determination of PAP levels seems to be more sensitive.

Thrombophilia

In patients who have experienced venous thromboembolism (especially in young patients and in patients with spontaneous DVT), thrombophilia screening should be performed. The test result can serve as a criterion for determining the duration of oral anticoagulation, especially when inherited disorders of the coagulation inhibitors protein C, protein S, AT-III, and APC resistance are present in the individual patient. Thrombophilia screening should include tests for AT-III, protein C, protein S. APC resistance (factor V deficiency), lupus anticoagulant, platelet count, levels of fibrinogen, plasminogen, and homocysteine, and fibrinolysis defects, although the latter are not common (determination of tPA and PAI-1 levels). The incidence of AT-III, protein C and protein S deficiencies in the normal population is 1/400, 1/200 000, and 1/16 000, respectively. In patients who have had DVT, the incidence of these deficiencies is 3% (AT-III) 5%–8% (protein C), and 5%–8% (protein S), respectively. APC resistance is present in 5% of the normal population and in 25% of patients with DVT. Hyperhomocysteinemia [36] is an independent risk factor for venous and arterial thrombosis, present in 10% of patients with thrombosis.

Arterial Occlusive Disease

Large clinical studies [37] have demonstrated an alteration in the fibrinolytic and hemostatic system [38] in a statistically significant percentage of patients suffering from arterial occlusive disease. Elevation of fibrinogen, t-PA (and PAI-1), vWF, and protein C inhibitor (PCI) levels not only indicates the state of disease, but may also be used as a prognostic marker for the clinical outcome of patients undergoing interventions [39].

References

1. Binder BR (1995) Physiology and pathophysiology of the fibrinolytic system. Fibrinolysis 9 [Suppl 1]:3.
2. Duke WW (1910) The relation of blood platelets to hemorrhargic disease. Description of a method for determining the bleeding time and report of three cases of hemorrhargic disease relieved by transfusion. JAMA 55: 1185
3. Borchgrevink CF, Waaler BA (1958) The secondary bleeding time. A new method for the differentiation of hemorrhargic diseases. Acta Med Scand 162: 362
4. Vetsch W, Pugin P, Perrin L, Kraemer R, Krafft T, Miescher PA (1978) Pseudothrombocytopenia. Schweiz Med Wochenschr 108: 1595
5. Brecher G, Cronkite EP (1950) Morphology and enumeration of human blood platelets. J Appl Physiol 3: 365
6. Born GVR (1962) Aggregation of blood platelets by adenosine diphosphate and its reversal. Nature 194: 927
7. Bloom AL, Forbes CD, Thomas DP, Tuddenham EGD (1994) Hemostasis and thrombosis, 3ed edn. Churchill Livingstone, Edinburgh
8. Niessner H (1972) Messung der Plttchenadhesivitt mit einer modifizierten Form der Hellem-II Methodik unter besonderer Bercksichtigung des v. Willebrand Jrgens Syndroms. Thromb Diath. Haemorrh 27: 343
9. Quick AJ (1942) Hemorrhargic diseases and the physiology of hemostasis. Charles, Springfield
10. Biggs R, Denson KWE (1967) Standardization of the one stage prothrombin time for the control of anticoagulant therapy. Br J Haematol 1: 84–88
11. Kirkwood TBL (1983) Calibration of reference thromboplastins and standardisation of the prothrombin time ratio. Thromb Haemost 49: 238–244
12. Proctor RR, Rapaport SI (1961) The partial thromboplastin time with kaolin. A simple screening test for first stage plasma clotting factor deficiencies Am J Clin Pathol 36: 212
13. Brill-Edwards P, Ginsberg JS, Johnston M, Hirsh J (1993) Establishing a therapeutic range for heparin therapy. Ann Intern Med 119: 104
14. Clauss A (1957) Gerinnungsphysiologische Schnellmethode zur Bestimmung des Fibrinogens. Acta Haematol (Basel) 17: 237
15. Ratnoff OD, Menzie C (1951) A new method for the determination of fibrinogen in small samples of plasma. J Lab Clin Med 37: 3160
16. Meade TW, North WRS, Chagrabarti RR, Stirling Y, Haines AP, Thompson SG (1980) Haemostatic function and cardiovascular death: early results of a prospective study. Lancet 1: 1050
17. Godal HC, Abildgaard U (1966) Gelation of soluble fibrin in plasma by ethanol. Scand J Haematol 3: 342
18. Elgue G, Pasche B, Blombach M, Olsson P (1990) The use of a commercial ELISA for assay of thrombin-antithrombin complexes in purified systems. Thromb Haemost 63: 435
19. Butt RW, deBoer AC, Turpie AG (1984) Evaluation of a commercial kit for the radioimmunoassay of fibrinopeptide A. J Immunoassay 5: 245
20. Bruhn HD, Conard J, Mannucci M, Monteguado J, Pelzer H, Reverter JC, Samama M, Tripodi A, Wagner C (1992) Multicentric evaluation of a new assay for prothrombin fragment 1+2 determination. Thromb Haemost 68: 413
21. Egeberg O (1965) Inherited antithrombin deficiency causing thrombophilia. Thromb Diath. Haemorrh 13: 516
22. Guglielmone HA, Vides MA (1992) A novel functional assay of protein C in human plasma and its comparison with amidolytic and anticoagulant assays. Thromb Haemost 67: 46
23. D'Angelo SV, Tombesi S, Marcovina S, Albertini A, Della-Valle P, D'Angelo A (1992) Monoclonal antibody based anzyme-linked immunosorbent assays (ELISA) for the measurement of vitamin K-dependent proteins: the effect of antibody immunoreacitvity on plasmaproteins antigen determinations. Throm Haemost 67: 631
24. Dahlbck B, Carlsson M, Svensson PF (1993) Familial thrombophilia due to a previously unrecongnized mechanism characterized by poor anticoagulant response to activated protein C: prediction of a cofactor to activated protein C. Proc Natl Acad Sci USA 90: 1004–1008
28. Schmidt U, Enderson BL, Chen JP Maull KI (1992) D-Dimer levels correlate with pathologic thrombosis in traume patients, J Trauma 33: 312
29. Bauer KA (1995) Management of patients with hereditary defects predisposing for thrombosis including pregnant women. Thromb Haemost 74(1): 94
30. Koster T, Rosendaal FR, deRonde F, Briet E, Vandenbroucke JP, Bertina RM (1993) Venous thrombosis due to poor response to activated protein C: Leiden thrombophilia study. Lancet 342: 1503
31. Fearnly GR (1964) Measurement of spontaneous fibrinolytic activity. J Clin Pathol 17: 307
25. Astrup T, Mllertz S (1952) The fibrin plate method for estimating fibrinolytic activity. Arch Biochem Biophys 40: 346
26. Wojta J, Turcu L, Wagner OF, Korninger C, Binder BR (1987) Evaluation of febrinolytic capacity by a combined assay system for tissue type plaminogen activator antigen and function using monoclonal anti-tissue-type plasminogen activator antibodies. J Lab Clin Med 109(6): 665
27. Merskey C. Lalezari P, Johnson AJ (1969) A rapid, simple, sensitive method for measuring fibrinolytic split products in human serum. Proc Soc Exp Biol Med 131: 871
32. Dale S, Gogstadt GO, Brostad F, Godal HC, Holtlund J, Mork E, Brandsnes O, Borch SM (1994) Comparison of three D-dimer assays for the diagnosis of DVT: ELISA, latex and immunofiltration assay (Nycocard D-Dimer). Thromb Haemost 71: 270
33. Out HJ, Bruinse HW, Christiuens GC, vanVliet M, de-Groot PG, Nieuwenhuis HK, Derksen RH (1992) A prospective, controlled multicenter study on the obstetric risk of pregnant women with antiphospholipid antibodies. Am J Obstet Gynecol 167: 26

34. Ginsberg JS, Wells PS, Brill-Edwards P, Donovan D, Moffatt K, Johnston M, Stevens P, Hirsh J (1995) Antiphospholipid antibodies and venous thromboembolism. Blood 86: 3685
35. Leizorovicz AJP, Simmoneau G, Decousus H, Boissel JP (1994) Comparison of efficacy and safety of low molecular weight heparins and unfractioned heparin in initial treatment of deep vein thromboses: a meta-analysis. BMJ 309(6950): 299
36. denHejer M, Koster T, Blom HJ, Bos GMJ, Briet E, Reitsma PH, Vandenbroucke JP, Rosendaal FR (1996) Hyperhomocysteinemia as a risk factor for deep venous thrombosis. NEJM 334: 759
37. Haverkate F, Thompson SG, Duckert F (1995) Haemostasis factors in angina pectoris; relation to gender, age and acute phase reaction. Results of the ECAT Angina Pectoris study group. Thromb Haemost 73: 561
38. Merlini PA, Bauer KA, Oltrona L, Ardissino D, Cattaneo M, Belli C, Mannucci PM, Rosenberg RD (1994) Persistent activation of coagulation mechanism in unstable angina and myocardial infarction. Circulation 90: 61
39. Huber K, Binder BR (1992) Plasminogen activator inhibitor-1 plasma levels and coronary restenosis. Circulation 85:1279
40. Nikolaides AN (1994) Combined methods. In: Bergquist D, Comerota A, Nikolaides A, Scurr J (eds) Prevention of venous thromboembolism. Heal-Orion, London, pp 225–234

Assessment of Lipoproteins

H. Wieland

Introduction

Disorders of lipid metabolism (dyslipidemias) are very common. They are of major clinical importance because they contribute to the development of premature atheroseclerosis. The disorders of lipid metabolism become manifest as frank hyperlipidemia or as unfavorable concentrations of specific lipoproteins or the presence of abnormal lipoproteins not leading to explicit hyperlipemia.

Diagnosis of hyperlipidemia by lipoprotein quantitation is often triggered by a turbid serum sample or by an abnormal total serum lipid concentration.

Laboratory investigation a dyslipidemia is based primarily on the determination of the concentrations of lipids and lipoproteins. The major breakthroughs in this field have been achieved since the mid-1950s, when it became possible to fractionate the lipids of the plasma into different density classes using preparative ultracentrifugation [143]. This led to the concept of different density classes consisting of complexes of lipids with proteins, the so-called lipoproteins. These particles contain all the relevant lipids and, in addition, special proteins (apolipoproteins) which can be quantified and analyzed by chemical and immunological methods.

The ultracentrifugation of lipoproteins was followed by their differentiation using staining with an ordinary protein electrophoresis on paper. This technique allowed for the first time the large-scale investigation of the lipoprotein composition of serum [141], made it possible to visualize hyperlipemias as hyperlipoproteinemias, and served as a basis for their differentiation into six different groups. Preparative ultracentrifugation allowed the isolation of lipoproteins and the subsequent examination of the protein part [198]. The new focus on apolipoproteins opened up the way for a more accurate classification system of serum lipoproteins according to differing apolipoprotein compositions of different lipoprotein particles [4]. This new understanding of lipid transport in the blood led to the detection and description of abnormal lipoproteins, to investigations regarding the interactions of cells with lipoproteins, and finally to the definition of some of the hyper- or hypolipoproteinemias on a molecular level and even on the level of the gene of an apolipoprotein, an enzyme, or a cellular receptor. The impact of molecular biology is not restricted to the investigation of the genes of the proteins that play a direct role in lipid metabolism, but also extends to mediatory intracellular regulatory proteins or DNA sequences. The first step in the diagnosis of a dyslipidemia remains the chemical determination of cholesterol, triglycerides, and high-density lipoprotein (HDL) cholesterol in the fasting state. The visual inspection of serum should not be neglected. For screening purposes, nonfasting cholesterol is acceptable. The majority of lipid disorders do not lead to hyperlipidemia. Instead, they consist of unfavorable combinations of concentrations of normal or slightly abnormal serum lipoproteins, a condition known as dyslipoproteinemia. The cause of the majority of dyslipoproteinemias is frequently not known. Most of them develop against an unfavorable genetic background comprising mutation either of a single gene or a combination of different genes favoring dyslipoproteinemia.

Since lipids are transported as lipoproteins, the investigatiion of a lipid disorder involves quantification and examination of the lipoproteins present in the plasma or serum.

Analytical Concepts

In order to be able to interpret correctly a clinical chemical test result, it is necessary to have a basic knowledge of some analytical concepts. The performance of any analytical method can be described by its performance characteristics, which include the reliability characteristics, such as analytical range, impression, inaccuracy, detection limit, interference, and specificity. Of these, the most important concepts, imprecision and inaccuracy, and related factors will be explained.

Imprecision

If an analyst took a single specimen of serum and undertook 20 tests for cholesterol, the results would not all be exactly the same because of random variation. Random variation is called imprecision. This variation arises from several sources, such as different amounts of specimens in the pipette, different volumes of reagents, different length of incubation, and different spectrophotometer settings. Imprecision is inherent in all analytical methods. It can be minimized, but cannot be eliminated. The distribution of the slightly different values follows a Gaussian distribution. Random errors have this type of distribution in contrast to biological variation, which does not necessarily have such symmetry.

The sum of all 20 cholesterol values divided by the number of all the results will give the mean cholesterol concentration.

An estimate of the dispersion of the distribution is the standard deviation (SD), which can be calculated by subtracting the mean value from each of the 20 values, squaring each difference and adding up the squares. This sum is then divided by (n-1) and finally the square root is taken to give the standard deviation. If all the results were the same, then they would equal the mean, the differences would be zero, and SD would also be zero. If the test results were widely scattered around the mean, then SD would be large. SD reflects the variability in the data. The standard deviation has the property that if the mean value ± 1 SD is taken, the central 67% of the distribution is selected. The mean value ± 2 SD and mean value ± 3 SD encompass 95% and 99.7%, respectively.

The standard deviation can be expressed as a percentage of the mean value, and this is termed the coefficient of variation (CV). If plasma glucose and cholesterol analyses both had an imprecision (SD) of 6 mg/dl, then if this is determined at a glucose level of 70 mg/dl and a cholesterol level of 220 mg/dl, the CV of glucose assay is $6{:}70 \times 100 = 8.6\%$, but the CV of cholesterol assays is $6{:}220 \times 100 = 2.7\%$. Thus the CV is useful when considering SD at different absolute values.

Inaccuracy

If the measured value of the given specimen analyzed 20 times were to yield exactly the true value, then the method would have no inaccuracy. If it were different from the true value, however, the method would have inaccuracy or bias. The reference method for cholesterol is the Abell-Kendall method [3, 40]. This method has been confirmed by isotope dilution/mass spectrometry [38]. Inaccuracy is due to systemic variation. This variation arises from sources such as using a pipette not delivering the correct volume of specimen or reagents, incubation at a wrong temperature, measuring at wrong wavelengths, or using a standard which does not actually have the value assigned. Inaccuracy may be constant (always inaccurate by the same amount at all levels) or proportional (inaccurate by the same relative amount at different levels). Inaccuracy of both types may occur at the same time and both types can be positive or negative.

Clinical Relevance of Standard Deviation

At a standard deviation of 6 mg/dl, a reported cholesterol concentration of 200 mg/dl has a 7% chance of lying between 194 and 206 mg/dl, a 95% chance of lying between 188 and 212 mg/dl, and a 97% chance of lying between 182 and 218 mg/dl. All single values have this possible range of values, and this is particularly important when comparing results with cutoff values necessitating therapeutic interventions.

Imprecision data can also provide an assessment of whether an analytically significant change has occurred in two results from specimens obtained sequentially from an individual, as is usually the case during treatment of hyperlipoproteinemias. If two results differ by more than 2.8 SD, there is a 95% chance that the difference is analytically significant. At a SD of 6 mg/dl, a serum cholesterol concentration is only significantly lower than 240 mg/dl if it is lower than 227 mg/dl.

The serum cholesterol concentration of an individual is subject to considerable variations. Precision and accuracy of the cholesterol determination depend critically on the pipetting step, the reaction mechanism of the method, composition of the reagents, interfering substances (drugs or biological substances), control material, standardization, and last but not least the person who does the work. The importance of most of these imponderabilities has considerably declined with the advent of modern clinical chemical analyzers using standardized methods. Using this technology, it is possible to achieve a CV no higher than 3% at 200 mg/dl.

However, it is vital to recognize that, in addition to analytical variation, biological variation has to be taken into account in the interpretation of single numerical results and in the assessment of the significance of changes in serial results from an individual.

Biological Variation

Biological variation includes diurnal, monthly, and annual rhythms, hormonal influences, and influences such as nutrition and disease. The normal day to day variations for cholesterol amount to about 15%, for triglycrides 20%, for HDL cholesterol 10%, and for the "Friedewald LDL" 8% [69].

Obtaining a blood sample from patients while they are consuming their habitual diet is particularly important. Decreasing intake of calories, cholesterol, or alcohol may allow lipid and lipoprotein levels to be normal or closer to normal than usual. Weight loss acutely lowers triglyceride concentrations and may transiently elevate cholesterol and low-density lipoprotein (LDL) levels. Any acute febrile illness, trauma, or recent surgical procedure may affect plasma lipid concentrations, often by elevating triglyceride levels and depressing cholesterol and LDL cholesterol concentrations. Chronic or debilitating illness may severely decrease LDL and intermediate-density lipoprotein concentrations. Finally, patients may be taking drugs that either lower lipid levels or substantially affect lipid metabolism. Young women often do not consider oral contraceptives as drugs.

Even if it is possible to minimize analytical and biological variation, another source of error has to be considered, i.e., the preanalytical phase.

Preanalytical Sources of Variation

Of the three sources of variation - analytical, biological, and those due to the preanalytical phase - the analytical and preanalytical sources can be influenced, and the biological source can be taken into account by standardizing some aspects of the method of obtaining blood and proper patient preparation. Influences on the preanalytical phase are at least of the same magnitude as methodological influences. They apply to the determination of both lipids and lipoproteins and apolipoproteins and are therefore considered here together. The concentration of triglycerids is subject to considerable biological variations; nevertheless, since it is often used to calculate LDL cholesterol, all the precautions also apply to the determination of triglycerides. Utmost precision and accuracy in the methods used to determine lipids and lipoproteins will have been in vain if they give nonrepresentative results. The preanalytical phase therefore has to be standardized.

Patient Factors

Intraindividual variations in cholesterol concentrations over a period of 1 year can reach 11%. In order to obtain a cholesterol value as accurate as possible, it is recommended that two samples be obtained within 2 months at least 1 week apart and that the mean value be taken before a medical decision is made about further action. If the difference between the two values exeeds 30 mg/dl, another sample should be collected 1 month later in order to obtain a new mean value. The daily variation of the concentration of triglycerides is approximately 35%. The CV of intraindividual variation within 1 month is 25%. For a reliable estimation of the triglyceride status, several samples drawn at monthly intervals are necessary.

In order to standardize biological variation, the corresponding factors have to be kept as constant as possible. These factors include diet, exercise, obesity, cigarette smoking, alcohol, and drugs.

After a meal, the concentration of triglycerides rises within 2 h and reaches a peak after 4 h. To measure cholesterol only, either fasting or nonfasting samples can be used; for triglyceride and lipoprotein measurements, a 12-h fasting sample is required. Even if the total cholesterol is largely unaffected by the presence of chylomicrons (CM); a pronounced hypertriglyceridema may cause erroneously high results in the colorimetric determination of cholesterol.

During the fasting period, consumption of water is allowed, but not of coffee. Lipids and liproteins should be measured only when the subject's metabolic state is steady. Individuals should consume their usual diet, and their weight should be stable for at least 2 weeks before lipids or lipoproteins are measured. In obese persons, weight loss causes variations in blood lipids.

Abstinence from alcohol is indicated for at least 2 days before blood sampling. The results can be better interpreted when it is known whether the patient is an habitual smoker. Smoking affects LDL and HDL unfavorably in opposite directions. Drug consumption should be recorded, since drugs can affect the test results by altering lipid metabolism or by interfering with the measurement.

Patients should not engage in vigorous physical activity within the 24 h before measurement. Exercise can increase total cholesterol by up to 6%.

An important aspect of the standardization of the preanalytical phase is the standardization of method of obtaining blood. Most important is the position of the body before and during the drawing of blood. The position of the body (upright or lying), together with venous congestion, can lead to deviations from the "true" cholesterol in both directions of up to 5%–10%. If the patient lies down from an upright position, hemodilution can cause a reduction in cholesterol of 10%–15% within 15 min. Even assuming a sitting position can reduce the cholesterol concentration by up to 6% within the same time frame. For optimal standardization, the patient should be in a relaxed sitting position for 15 min. Also important are the site from which the sample is obtained and the extent and duration of venous congestion before venipuncture. The cholesterol concentration in the serum of capillary blood is about 5% higher than in venous serum [19]. The tourniquet leads to a hemoconcentration. It should not be applied for more than 1 min before sample collection and should be released immediately after blood enters the collecting tube.

Technical Factors

The ideal sample for the determination of lipids and lipoproteins stems from a properly prepared patient and has been obtained taking the necessary precautions. The question arises whether serum or plasma should be used and how long it can be stored prior to examination.

Cholesterol, triglyceride, and HDL cholesterol levels can be measured in either serum or plasma. The anticoagulants fluoride, citrate, and oxalate lead to a considerable shift of water out of the erythrocytes into plasma. Ethylenediaminetetraacetic acid (EDTA) leads to an hemodilution of about 3%, whereas that caused by heaprin is negligible. Despite the slight hemodilution caused by EDTA, this is the anticoagulant of choice, since it chelates heavy metals such as Cu^{2+}. This helps to delay the auto-oxidation of triglycerides and prolongs the integrity of all lipoproteins. For reasons of standardization, however, serum is the recommended material.

Coagulated blood should be centrifuged after being kept for 2 h at room temperature. When complete lipoprotein fractionation or certain apolipoprotein measurements are to be performed, it may be necessary to use plasma, in which case the preferred anticoagulant is dry EDTA. In this case, the results should be multiplied by 1.03.

The plasma should be immediately cooled to 2–4°C to prevent changes in composition due to the transfer of cholesterol between the membranes of red cells and the plasma. The anticoagulated blood should be centrifuged as soon as possible. CM begin fo float on the surface of the liquid within 30 min. Therefore, the specimen has to agitated beford determination of triglycerides.

If the sample cannot be processed immediately, the specimen can be stored at 4°C for 4 days. Samples for cholesterol analysis only may be stored at -20°C; otherwise, samples should be stored frozen at -70°C or lower, provided the tube is properly sealed to avoid evaporation of water. When the sample is thawed, an inhomogenous specimen may result, which requires adequate mixing.

Practical Considerations

The detailed guidelines for clinicians established by the National Cholesterol Education Program (NCEP) [65] for measuring, treating, and monitoring cholesterol values were developed on the premise that serum cholesterol measurement by clinical laboratories is both precise and accurate. Measurements of lipids and lipoproteins are among the more difficult and exacting clinical laboratory tests. Although analytical precision continues to improve, proficiency surveys and research studies indicate that inaccuracy remains a problem. The determination of HDL cholesterol in particular, is sensitive to differences in methodology [161, 184].

In practice, however, inaccuracy may be a less important problem. In individuals undergoing either dietary or drug therapy, long-term precision of laboratory methods in monitoring plasma lipid and lipoprotein concentrations is clearly indispensable. The fact that there are so many possible sources of variation (analytical, biological, and preanalytical) raises serious questions about the reliability of any cholesterol or lipoprotein value. Only if the cholesterol concentration does not exceed 185 mg/

dl can one be sure that the true cholesterol does not exceed 200 mg/dl. A measured value of 255 mg/dl definitely reflects a true cholesterol level of over 240 mg/dl. LD: cholesterol measured as being below 116 mg/dl is certainly below 130 mg/dl, and LDL cholesterol measured as being over 174 mg/dl is definitely over 160 mg/dl. If a cholesterol value lies close to a cutoff point, the mesurement should be repeated. For example, to be able to decide whether a change of at least 10% has occurred, at least six determinations measurements would theoretically be necessary at either time [238]. Of the three most common errors leading to incorrect diagnosis and classification of disturbances in lipoproteins metabolism, two have been adressed, i.e., unreliable labarotory determination and improper sampling. The third is failure to repeat sampling. Errors in diagnosis and therapy for lipoprotein abnormalities may be the result of a single nonrepresentative sample. If an abnormal lipid or lipoprotein concentration is detected, it is extremely important that the finding be confirmed on at least two occasions, preferably 2–4 weeks apart.

In view of the difficulties regarding accuracy and precision of cholesterol determination and the marked influences of biological variation, one may ask whether a single cholesterol measurement is of any value at all. From prospective studies, we know that single cholesterol determinations are better than expected [104]. The coefficient of correlation between initial values and control values after 2 years is 0.66 in men [218]. In the Lipid Research Prevalence Study, two thirds of the subjects remained in the upper quintile [112].

Lipids

Most chemical substances produced by living organisms are soluble in water. Lipids are the exception, since they are only soluble in organic solvents such as ethanol, methanol, acetone, chloroform, hexane, or diethylether. Lipids include a variety of compounds that have different physiological and metabolic functions; they are commonly referred to as fats.

The importance of lipids in medicine was recognized long before the individual classes of lipids were quantitatively determined. By extracting all the lipids with organic solvents from definite serum sample, evaporating the organic solvent, and determining the weight of the extractable material, the total lipid concentration of serum have been determined. This value reflects the concentrations of all four major serum lipids, i.e., cholesterol, cholesteryl esters (CE), triglycerides, and phosphlipids, and of the free fatty acids of the serum. These various classes of lipids can now be determined separately.

Structure

The common structural element of lipids is a linear chain of carbon atoms (fatty acid). This chain can also form ring structures (e.g., cholesterol).

Upon hydrolysis, lipids yield either only fatty acids or complex alcohols, which can form esters with fatty acids. The lipids can be divided into simple and complex lipids. Simple lipids are electrically neutral and are therefore called neutral lipids. Neutral lipids include cholesterol, esters of cholesterol with fatty acids (CE), and triglycerides. Glycerophospholipids and sphingolipids are complex lipids exhibiting a negative charge due to a phosphoric acid residue and a positive charge caused by a quarternary nitrogen base. Complex lipids also contain sialic acid, sulfate or amino groups. Lipids can be divided into five major classes: sterols, fatty acids, glycerol esters, sphingolipids, and terpenes (Table 1).

Table 1. Classes of lipids

Sterols	Fatty acids	Glycerol esters	Sphingo-lipids	Terpenes
Cholesterol and cholesteryl-ester	Short chain (2–4 C atoms)	Triglycerides	Sphingomyelin	Vitamin A
Steroidhormones	Medium chain (6–10 C atoms)	Phosphoglycerides	Glycosphingolipid	Vitamin E
Bile acids	Long chain (12–26 C atoms)	–	–	Vitamin K
Vitamin D	Prostaglandins	–	–	–

Fatty Acids

A very small fraction of plasma lipids are unesterified fatty acids. They are predominantely associated with albumin and lipoproteins. If they are present in high concentrations, they influence the surface charge of lipoproteins, especially of HDL.

Fatty acids consist of a carboxyl group and an aliphatic chain of two to 23 carbon atoms. Almost all natrually occuring fatty acids contain an even number of carbon atoms. Those with 16 (palmitic acid) and 18 (stearic acid) carbon atoms are the most abundant. Humans can only synthesize fatty acids with an even number of carbon atoms.

According to the degree of saturation of the aliphatic carbon chain, fatty acids are divided into saturated and unsaturated fatty acids. Saturated fatty acids contain no double bond and are the principal type of fatty acid in human tissues. The general formula for a saturated fatty acid is:

$$CH_3\text{-}(CH_2)_n\text{-}COOH$$

The saturated fatty acids containing 12–24 carbon atoms and are solid at room temperature.

Unsaturated fatty acids contain one or more double bonds. They are liquid at room temperature. Monounsaturated fatty acids contain only a single double bond and are described according to the following general formula:

$$CH_3\text{-}(CH_2)_n\text{-}CH{=}(CH_2)_n\text{-}COOH$$

The physiologically most important monounsturated fatty acids are palmitoleic acid and oleic acid. The primary physiological function of long-chain fatty acids is to provide energy to cells by an oxidative process referred to as β-oxidation.

The polyunsaturated fatty acids contain several double bonds. These double bonds are never next to each other, but always separated by a single bond:

$$\text{-}CH{=}CH\text{-}CH_2\text{-}CH{=}CH\text{-}$$

Linoleic acid (two double bonds) and linolenic acid (three double bonds) are two essential polyunsaturated fatty acids of plant origin. In the brain, they serve as precursors for even longer and more unsaturated fatty acids. Linoleic acid is also the precursor of arachidonic acid, which is the precursor of prostaglandins and leukotrienes. Prostaglandins function as metabolic mediators and play a vital role in regulating a wide variety of physiological functions. The presence of a double bond has a significant influence on the spatial configuration of an aliphatic chain. In long-chain saturated fatty acids, the carbon atoms show a linear arrangement and can rotate freeely. Double bonds restrict the rotation at the site of the bond and can cause a kink in the line of atoms. Double bonds can exist either as a *cis* or a *trans* isomer. In the *cis* configuration, each of the remaining hydrogen atoms of the carbon atoms connected by the double bond are on the same side of the bond. *cis* causes a kink in the carbon chain and *trans* only a small deviation. In humans, all unsaturated fatty acids exist as *cis* isomers.

Fats can be solidified by hydrogenation of the double bonds of some of the unsaturated fatty acids. During this process, *trans* fatty acids can be formed.

Plants, fish, and bacteria are excellent sources of polyunsaturated fatty acids.

The plasma concentration of free fatty acids is only rarely determined in a routine laboratory. The concentration normally lies between 0.3 and 1.1 mmol/l. The levels can be markedly increased by injection of heparin (unleashes lipoprotein lipase from the capillary wall) or in circumstances when increased lipolysis leads to a rapid release of free fatty acids from the adipose tissue e.g., release or administration of adrenocorticotrophic hormone (ACTH), epinephrine, norepinephrine.

Triglycerides

Triglycerides consist of three long-chain fatty acids esterified to glycerol. Within a triglyceride, the three fatty acids may be identical, but more often they are different. Figure 1 illustrates the formation of tristearol, the major constituent of beef fat. Triglycerides with a high content of saturated fatty acids are solid at room temperature and are referred to as fats. With increasing content of unsaturated fatty acids, fats become more and more liquid, and in a liquid state they are called oils. Fats are usually of animal origin, whereas oils are of plant origin. Fats

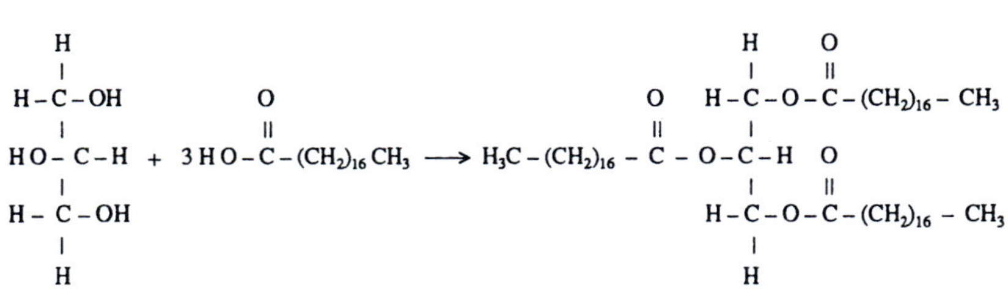

Fig. 1. Formation of tristearol

are stored within the adipocytes in the form of droplets occupying almost the entire volume of the cell. In contrast to glycogen, fats can be stored in the body in unlimited amounts. Triglycerides are the major component of glycerides in circulating blood and tissues. Small quantities of both mono- and diglycerides are also present and contain one or two fatty acids, respectively. Mono- and diglycerides are intermediate products of both biosynthesis and degradation of triglycerides.

Phospholipids

Phospholipids (phosphoglycerides) are structurally related to the triglycerides. Both contain glycerol and long-chain fatty acids. However, phospholipids contain a phosphate group attached to the α-hydroxyl group. A series of small nitrogen-containing alcohols or carbohydrates containing nitrogen are esterified to the phosphate group of these phosphatidic acis, forming a family of phosphoglycerolipids. The hydroxyl group of the alcohol can be provided by choline (lecithin) or ethanolamine, serine, and inositol (cephalins). Figure 2 illustrates the principal structure of phospholipids.

Phosphoglycerides are amphipathic molecules, i.e., molecules with both hydrophobic and hydrophilic properties. Because of their phosphoric acid-containing polar head group, they are water soluble. However, they can mix with other lipids because of their hydrophobic tails consisting of two fatty acids. Phospholipids therefore provide an ideal interface between neutral lipids and water, behaving like soaps. The ability to form a charged outer surface covering a hydrophobic core is the basis of lipoprotein structure. The same property is partly responsible for the fact that cholesterol remains solubilized in the lumen of the gut and in the bile.

An even more important function of phospholipids is their structural role in cell membranes. Phospholipids are present in considerable amounts in the cells of the nervous tissue. The phospholipids of the plasma are almost exclusively glycerophosophopholipids. Like triglycerides, they all originate from glycerol. Lecithin (phosphatidylcholine) is the major phospholipid in the plasma and the extracellular fluid. It is found in high concentrations in cellular membranes.

In the plasma, the fatty acid bound to the middle carbon atom of glycerol can be transferred to the free 3-hydroxyl group of cholesterol. This is the major in vivo reaction for the formation of CE. It is catalyzed by the lecithin: cholesterol acyltransferase (LCAT). The reaction products are CE and monoacyl glycerophospholipids (or lysophospholipids), termed lysolecithin. The lysophospholipids derive their name from their detergent properties, leading to the lysis of cell membranes.

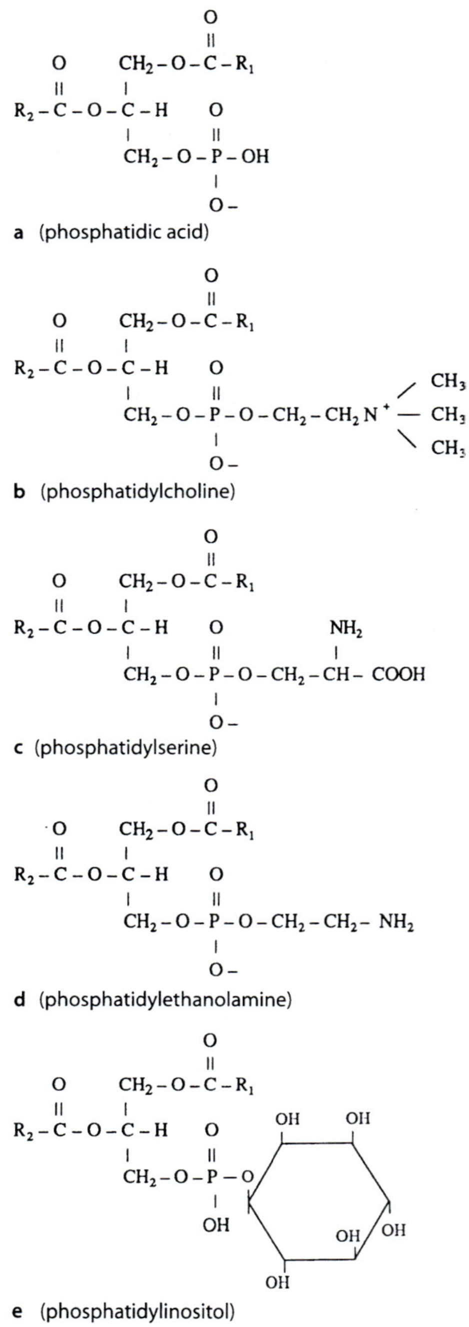

Fig. 2 a–e. Principal phospholipids

In addition to lecithin, other phospholipids are also found in cell membranes. Some of these are derived from the alcohol sphingosine instead of glycerol (sphingophospholipids). The major representatives of this group are the sphingomyelins.

Cholesterol

Sterols are compounds characterized by steroid core carrying an hydroxyl group. The molecule consists of 27 carbon atoms, which are arranged and numbered as indicated in Fig. 3. The carbon atom 3 to which the hydroxyl group is attached is asymmetric. This cholest-5-ene-3β-ol is a member of a class of 3β-hydroxysterols which share this basic steroidal structure. Mixtures of 3β-hydroxysterols can be isolated from plants, fish, and other living organisms. Cholesterol is the principal sterol in all higher forms of life. In animals, cholesterol can be found in all tissues. If the sterol core is considered as planar, the hydroxyl group extends towards the viewer. It is said to be in β-configuration.

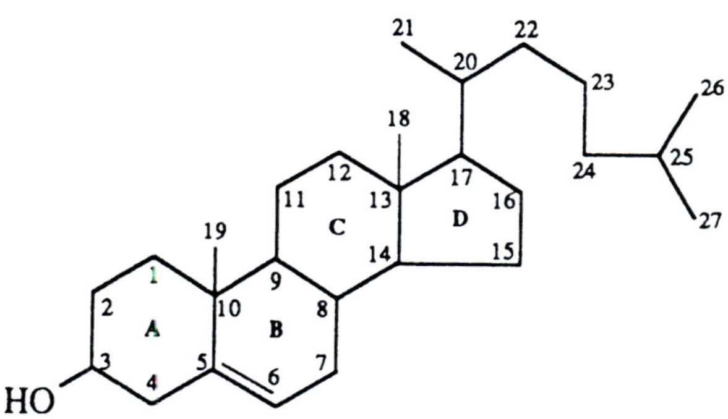

Fig. 3. Structure of cholesterol

Via this 3β-hydroxyl group, cholesterol can be esterified to a fatty acid. The correspondig fatty acids are oleic acid (predominantly) and stearic acid or palmitic acid. In plasma, esterified cholesterol makes up 75% – 85% of the total cholesterol. CE are the most hydrophobic lipids and serve as storage or transport forms of cholesterol.

The numbering of the sterol ring is also important for endocrinologists. Cholesterol is the starting point of many biosynthetic processes. These include the biosynthesis of vitamin D, steroid hormones, and bile acids. Enzymes working on the sterol ring are designated according the mode of action and the location of the catalyzed reaction (e.g., 21-hydroxylase plays an important role in the biosynthesis of cortisol). Approximately 0.5 cholesterol are converted into bile acids daily. In contrast to triglycerides and phospholipids, the sterol ring cannot be degraded by the human organism. Thus cholesterol cannot be used as an energy source for human cells.

Cholesterol is absent in plants. The most abundant plant sterol is sitosterol. The structural difference between cholesterol and sitosterol is the side chain attached at C17, which is longer by two carbon atoms in cholesterol. Plant sterols are absorbed by humans only in the very rare cases of sitosterolemia.

Metabolism of Triglycerides

In humans, triglycerides are the most important storage form of energy and are stored predominantly in the adipocytes of the adipose tissue. These specialized cells store triglycerides within a single large vacuole, which may constitute up to 90% of the adipocyte. Whenever energy is needed, triglycerides within the adipocyte are hydrolyzed and the fatty acids are released. During anabolism, adipocytes synthesize triglycerides from fatty acids delivered by CM from the intestine or very low density lipoproteins (VLDL) from liver.

Triglycerides from the diet cannot pass directly into the bloodstream. They are hydrolyzed in the intestine in two molecules of free fatty acids and one molecule of 2-acylglycerol, which are themselves powerful emulsifying agents. The hydrolysis is catalyzed by pancratic lipase and is favored by the presence of other emulsifying agents, the bile salts. Together with other minor components of the diet, such as cholesterol and fat-soluble vitamins, these compounds form micelles. These micelles diffuse to the brush border of the cells lining the intestinal lumen, where their contents are taken up. Fatty acids containing less than 12 carbon atoms are taken up directly, enter the portal vein, and travel tightly bound to albumin to the liver, where they are incorporated into newly formed triglycerides. Monoglycerides and long-chain fatty acids together with glucose are used for the resynthesis of triglycerides in the mucosal cells. Intestinal mucosa secretes into the lymph two types of lipid particles, CM and VLDL. They enter the circulation via the thoracic duct. In the circulation, the triglycerides of these particles are again hydrolyzed into monoglycerides and fatty acids. This time, hydrolysis is catalyzed by the lipoprotein lipase. This enzyme is attached to the endothelium lining the capillaries, particularly those of muscle and adipose tissue, by a heparin-like polysaccharide. The adipocytes take up the monoglycerides and the fatty acids fromt he circulation and store them in the form of newly synthesized triglycerides.

Triglyceride-Synthesis

The amount of glucose which can be stored in form of glycogen is limited. Surplus glucose is converted into triglycerides by the liver.

The components necessary for triglyceride synthesis are dihydroxyacetone phosphate and acetyl-coenzyme A (acetyl-CoA). The dihydroxy acetone phosphate is derived from glycolysis and serves as a precursor of the glycerol moiety of triglycerides; the fatty acids are assembled from acetyl-CoA stemming from the decarboxylation of pyruvate.

The synthesis of fatty acids is accomplished via the successive addition of 2-carbon fragments derived from acetyl-CoA. This is why fatty acids generally consist of an even number of carbon atoms. Synthesis is catalyzed by fatty acid synthetase, a complex consisting of seven enzymes.

Fatty acid synthesis take place in the cytoplasm. Acetyl-CoA originates from the mitochondria. Only in the presence of an excess of energy-rich compounds does the transport of acetyl-CoA out of the mitochondrium and its subsequent activation in the cytoplasm take place.

Glucose and glycolysis provide dihydroxyacetone phosphate for triglyceride synthesis to adipocytes owing to their lack of glycerol kinase and their inability to utilize glycerol as a substrate. Adipocytes contain insulin-sensitive glucose transporters. Glucose provides pyruvate for acetyl-CoA and malonyl-CoA for adipocyte fatty acid synthesis, which is quantitatively less important than in liver. Adipocytes derive most of their energy from fatty acid oxidation. During catabolism, adipocytes hydrolyze triglycerides and release fatty acids.

Breakdown of Triglycerides

Whenever there is an insufficient amount of glucose available to fulfil the energy needs of the organism, the triglycerides stored in the adipocytes are hydrolyzed. The reaction is catalyzed by the hormone-sensitive lipase. This enzyme is activated by cyclic adenosine monophosphate (cAMP) and consequently by the hormones using this compound as intracellular second messenger (epinephrine, ACTH, growth hormone, and glucagon). The glycerol reaches the liver and enters glycolysis, and the fatty acids are bound to albumin and are taken up rapidly by the most tissue except the brain, where they are oxidized.

Oxidation

As the principal route for catabolizing fatty acids, β-oxidation occurs in the mitochondria. It is called β-oxidation because in its course the β-carbon atom of a fatty acid is oxidized to a β-keto acid. The pathway of β-oxidation begins with acyl-CoA dehydrogenase oxidization of the fatty acid to create a *trans* double bond between carbons 2 and 3, the α- and β-carbon atoms. This monoenoic compound is named enoyl-CoA. A hydratase then hydrates this double bond, yielding 3-hydroxyacyl-CoA. A second dehydrogenase oxidizes this 3-hydroxy group to a 3-keto group, creating 3-ketoacyl-CoA. Finally, a thiolase uses the SH binding of CoA-SH to cleave the bond between carbons 2 and 3, liberating acetyl-CoA. The remaining fatty acyl-CoA, with two less carbon atoms than the original, can then reenter β-oxidation.

The complete oxidation of palmitic acid to CO_2 and water yields 129 molecules of ATP. Fat is an important energy source. In contrast to glucose, fatty acids cannot be oxidized anaerobically. Fats can be synthesized from glucose, but the reverse is not true. There is no significant pathway by which acetyl-CoA could be reconverted into pyruvate.

Ketogenesis

The liver produces ketone bodies when the rate of acetyl-CoA formation exceeds that of acetyl-CoA utilization by the citric acid cycle. Acetoacetic acid, β-hydroxybutyric acid, and acetone are classified as ketone bodies. The term ketone bodies is inaccurate, since β-hydroxybutyrate lacks a keto group.

Acetoacetic acid is the principal ketone body synthesized by the liver mitochondria. Acetate from acetyl-CoA is dimerized to yield acetoacetyl-CoA. This CoA cannot be readily removed to produce acetoacetic acid. Instead, another acetyl-CoA must first be added to the acetoacetyl-CoA to yield the six-carbon intermediate β-hydroxy-βmethylglutaryl-CoA (HMG-CoA). Acetyl-CoA is then removed from HMG-CoA in the liver to liberate acetoacetic acid; β-hydroxybutyrate dehydrogenase reduces much of this acetoacetic acid to β-hydroxybutyric acid. In addition, a decarboxylase converts some of the acetoacetate to acetone. Acetone is metabolized very slowly. Because of its volatility, it can evaporate through the lungs.

Extrahepatic tissues, such as skeletal muscle and heart muscle, utilize the other two ketone bodies as fuel. After a period of adaption, the cells of the nervous tissue can also utilize ketone bodies.

Cholesterol Metabolism

Approximately 40% of the cholesterol in the body is derived from the diet. In the intestine, the esterified cholesterol is hydrolyzed by the pancreatic cholesterol esterase. The cholesterol is then emulsified by its own degradation products, the bile salts. In the mucosal cells, the cholesterol is packed togehter with newly formed triglycerides and phospholipids into CM and VLDL and released in the intestinal lymphatics. The organism absorbs between 30% and 60% of the dietary cholesterol. The cholesterol of the CM is not only of dietary origin, but also may be derived from bile or can be synthesized or gained from lipoproteins incorporated by the mucosal cells.

Fat absorption always promotes the secretion of cholesterol by the intestine in the form of lipoproteins (CM and VLDL).

Most of the cholesterol in the body has been synthesized within the organism. Synthesis takes place in the smooth endoplasmic reticulum predominantly of liver cells, cells of the intestine, and the adrenal cortex. All atoms of cholesterol were once part of an acetyl-CoA molecule. Hepatic cholesterol synthesis is regulated by influx of lipoproteins such as LDL and remnants of CM or VLDL.

The final stage of the metabolism of cholesterol transported by lipoproteins takes place in the liver, since this is the only organ capable of excreting the sterol core of cholesterol. When cholesterol has not yet been excreted, it can be used for regeneration of plasma membranes or for synthesis of steroid hormones and bile acids. Cholesterol can be intracellularly stored in the form of droplets of CE. The esterification of intracellular cholesterol is catalyzed by the enzyme acyl-CoA: cholesterol acyltransferase (ACAT). The stored esters can be hydrolyzed by a neutral CE hydrolase. The CE within lysosomes (first station after cellular uptake of LDL) are hydrolyzed by an acid lipase.

Cholesterol cannot be oxidized to CO_2. It is eliminated from the body by excretion into the bile in equal parts either unchanged or converted into bile acids. If cholesterol is not reabsorbed during fat absorption, it is reduced by intestinal bacteria to coprosterol, which is eliminated in the feces. More than 95% of the bile acids are reabsorbed in the terminal ileum and can be reused after they have been transported back to the liver via the portal vein (enterohepatic circulation).

CM contain at least 2% cholesterol by weight. Since a normal person absorbs up to 150 g fat per day, almost 3 g cholesterol undergo a similar enterohepatic circulation. Under normal circumstances, equilibrium exists between ingestion, absorption, synthesis, and excretion of cholesterol.

Factors Affecting Total Cholesterol Concentration

All factors increasing the concentration of LDL also increase total cholesterol. However, not every increase in total cholesterol is brought about by an increase in LDL choleserol. Increases in total cholesterol may be due to a rise in HDL cholesterol, to the presence of LP-X, to a moderate increase in the concentration of VLDL, or to a marked increase in Lp(a). In addition, extreme hypertriglyceridemias due to chylomicronemia or type V hyperlipoproteinemia can also caus marked hypercholesterolemia. In these cases, the serum is extremely turbid. The highest concentrations of cholesterol in a clear serum are found in some cases of obstructive jaundice (especially biliary atresia) and in some homozygote forms of familial hypercholesterolemia.

If an increase in LDL cholesterol is accompanied by a marked decrease in HDL cholesterol, this highly atherogenic constellation may go unnoticed if HDL cholesterol has not been determined.

Lipoproteins

Lipoproteins are macromolecular complexes consisting of lipids and proteins. Serum lipoproteins differ mainly in their lipid composition and protein to lipid ratio. With the exception of free fatty acids, all lipids of the plasma (cholesterol, CE, phospholipids, and triglycerides) are exclusively constituents of plasma lipoproteins. Each lipoprotein contains all the lipids, the amount of which, however, varies considerably. The larger the protein part of a lipoprotein is, the higher its hydrated density. Correspondingly, HDL contain the largest proportion of protein (50%), while CM contain only of 1% protein. With increasing density, the particle size decreases. The largest lipoproteins are CM (diameter, 1 µm) followed by VLDL. Both contain a high proportion of triglycerides. The smalles lipoproteins are HDL (diameter, 30 nm). The major constituents of LDL are cholesterol and CE. Correspondingly, the LDL level markedly influences the total cholesterol concentration of the serum.

Lipoproteins consist of nonpolar core (triglycerides and CE) surrounded by a polar shell. The oldest classification of the lipoproteins present in plasma or serum is based on differences in the hydrated density of these particles, which can be exploited by analytical [138] or preparative [102] ultracentrifugation.

The major lipoprotein density classes are VLDL, LDL, and HDL. The hydrated density of CM is less than the density of water. During ultracentrifugation, LDL and HDL sediment at the density of the plasma water, but not VLDL and CM. Due to their low density, the latter float even without any centrifugation. Increasing the density of the plasma to that of a saturated solution of NaCl leads to sedimentation during ultracentrifugation of only the HDL. LDL, VLDL, and, of course, CM float to the surface of the centrifugation tube. HDL can be brought to floatation at a density of 1.22 g/ml, the approximate density of the Dead Sea.

All the different density classes of lipoproteins can be isolated from serum or plasma by ultracentrifugation after sequentially increasing the density of the plasma water to suitable densities [102]. Using density gradient ultracentrifugation, it is possible to achieve a continuous separation.

Lipoproteins can further be separated by electrophoretical methods. Serum lipoproteins have different electrophoretical mobilites. CM do not migrate, and the remaining lipoproteins are distributed within three different bands, i.e., α_1 (HDL), α_2 (VLDL), or pre-β and β (LDL). Only albumin and the γ-globulins are almost lipid free.

Since the most relevant serum lipids, cholesterol and triglycerides, occur only in the form of lipoproteins, the serum concentrations of these lipids reflect the concentrations of corresponding serum lipoproteins. An exception is lipoprotein (a) (Lp(a)), which is only rarely present in concentrations sufficient to cause hyperlipemia.

Metabolic Function and Apolipoproteins

Although the major function of lipoproteins is to facilitate the transport of lipids in the plasma, the lipids themselves are far from being passive passengers. They undergo vivid interlipoprotein exchange processes and diffuse from lipoproteins to cell membranes and vice versa. The lipoproteins are therefore integral parts of lipid metabolism. Rather than being simple transport vehicles, the apolipoproteins have active roles in metabolic pathways. They mediate synthesis and secretion of lipoproteins, regulate enzymatic activities, and attach to lipoprotein receptors at the surface of specific cells. So far, 15 different apolipoproteins have been identified and characterized (Table 2).

Table 2. Apolipoproteins of human plasma

Apoprotein	Lipoproteins in which present	Molecular weight	Serum concentration (mg/dl)	Function
A-I	HDL	28 016	80–160	Activator of LCAT
A-II	HDL	17 414	20–55	Possible activator of hepatic lipase?
A-IV	CM	46 000	<5	Participates in triglyceride metabolism
B_{100}	VLDL, IDL, LDL, and Lp(a)	550 000	60–160	Structural protein, ligand for receptor
B_{48}	CM	264 000	0–2	Necessary for synthesis and secretion of CM
C-I	CM, VLDL, IDL, HDL	6 600	3–11	Unknown
C-II	CM, VLDL, IDL, HDL	8 850	1–7	Activates LPL
$C\text{-}III_{0-2}$	CM, VLDL, IDL, HDL	8 800	3–23	Inhibits hepatic take-up
D	HDL	22 000	8–10	
E_{2-4}	CM, VLDL, IDL, HDL	34 100	2–6	Hepatic clearance of remnants
F	HDL	30 000	<5	–
G	VLDL	72 000	<5	–
H	CM	45 000	–	–
Apo(a)	Lp(a)	500 000	<30	–

HDL, high-density lipoproteins; CM, chylomicrons; VLDL, very low density lipoproteins; IDL, intermediate-density lipoproteins; LDL, low-density lipoproteins; LCAT, lecithin: cholesterol acyltransferase

Apo A consists of the two peptides A-I and A-II. A-I and A-II are almost exclusively found in the HDL density class. A-III is a misnomer for apo D, and A-IV is predominantely present in the *d* 1.21 g/ml infranatant. It plays a role in the reverse cholesterol transport process. Apo B is the major structural protein of VLDL, CM, and Lp(a) and almost the sole apolipoprotein of LDL. Apo B is necessary for the assembly of triglyceride-rich lipoproteins. It exists in two isoforms, a apo B_{100} and apo B $_{48}$. Apo B_{100} is synthesised by the liver and is part of VLDL, LDL, and Lp(a); apo B_{48} stems from the small intestine and is exclusively part of CM and their remnants. Both isoforms are derived from the same gene. Apo B_{48} constitutes the amino-terminal 48 % of apo B_{100}. The different expression in different tissues is achieved by alternative splicing of the mRNA.

Apo C consists of three different peptides (C-I, C-II, C-III). The physiological role of two of them is not entirely clear. C-II is an activator of the enzyme lipoprotein lipase, which hydrolyzes the core of triglyceride-rich lipoproteins, C-III apparently inhibits the premature uptake of triglyceride-rich lipoproteins in the liver, and C-I activates LCAT.

Apo E is one of the biologically most important apolipoproteins. Although it is present in the HDL density class, its major function is together with apo-B-containing lipoproteins. It can attach the carrier lipoproteins to two different receptors, LDL receptor and LDL receptor-related protein (LRP). One of the functions of the latter is the chaneling of CM remnants to the liver. Apo E exists in three different isoforms (E_2, E_3, and E_4), exhibiting different affinities to the receptors.

In addition to the apolipoproteins, two enzymes present in the plasma deserve mention. The lipoprotein lipase (LPL) catalyzes hydrolysis of triglycerides into monoglycerides and free fatty acids. LCAT catalyzes esterification of free cholesterol.

Chylomicrons

The major function of CM is the transport of triglycerides of dietary origin (exogenous triglycerides). CM are assembled within mucosal cells and released into the intestinal lymph. They enter the bloodstream together with other constituents of the thoracic duct. Within the mucosal cell, the dietary fatty acids are reesterified to triglycerides, and these triglycerides, together with a few molecules of CE and phospholipids and one molecule of apoB_{48}, assemble into a CM particle. This particle is secreted by the mucosal cell in the surrounding lymph, where it picks up apo C and apo E, both members of the HDL density class. Because of their size, CM scatter light and render the serum or plasma turbid. Clearing of the plasma is due to the action of LPL. This enzyme punches a small hole in the outer phospholipid layer of CM and hydrolyzes the triglycerides in the core of the particle into monoglycerides and free fatty acids. LPL is attached to the capillaries (muscle and adipose tissue) and is normally not present in the bloodstream. The capillaries of the liver do not contain LPL, but a different lipase (hepatic triglyceride hydrolase, HTGL). Both lipases can be freed by intravenous injection of heparin.

The CM is caught by the lipase and, when immobilized on the capillary wall, loses most of its core lipids. The CM is attached to the capillary wall partly by binding to LPL via the activator protein C-II (part of apo C) and partly by apo E, which also has a general affinity to heparin sulfate present on the surface of endothelial cells. The majority of the liberated fatty acids are taken up by the corresponding cells (muscle and adipose tissue), where they are either oxidized or reesterified to triglycerides. Some fatty acids escape cellular uptake and are transported in the plasma bound to albumin. Fatty acids inhibit the activity of LPL. This ensures that hydrolysis only proceeds as fast as the reaction products can be disposed of.

During hydrolysis of the core lipids, CM shrink, lose C-II from the surface, and may detach from the capillary wall. After several consecutive attachments and detachments, the CM has lost most of its triglycerides. The CM remnant has only half the volume of the original CM and consists mainly of CE, apo B_{48}, and apo E. During its journey in the bloodstream, it gains additional CE and is finally taken up by the liver via LRP recognizing apoE. The CE (core lipids) are split in fatty acids and cholesterol. The latter can be reutilized for lipoprotein synthesis or degraded to bile acids. A side effect of the temporary increase of the cholesterol content of the liver cell is the downregulation of the LDL receptor (B_{100}: E receptor). This leads to an increased residence time of LDL in the blood and also to an increased conversion of VLDL remnants (IDL) into LDL.

During shrinkage, the particle loses surface constituents, precursors of HDL. Thirty minutes following their assembly, half of the CM have already disappeared.

Very low Density Lipoproteins

Although it remains unclear whether the liver is also able to secrete LDL, VLDL are at present presumed to be the only apo B-containing lipoproteins secreted by the liver. LDL particles are derived from VLDL particles via the intravasal delipidation cascade. VLDL do not sediment in the ultracentifuge at the density of serum water (*d*=1.006 g/ml). Since they are relatively large, they scatter light and cause turbidity in the serum sample.

Nascent VLDL contain one molecule of a apo B_{100} per particle, some apo C, and some apo E. The core of the VLDL particles consist mostly of triglycerides (50% of the particle) and a few CE. The shell is made up of phospholipids, fee cholesterol, and the apolipoproteins. Upon release into the circulation, the particle is enriched with apo C and apo E. VLDL are synthesized in the liver predominantly from preformed fatty acids derived either from adipose tissue or from CM remnants and to a minor proportion also from fatty acids synthesized de nove from glucose.

Metabolism

The VLDL particles circulating in the plasma interact with the enzyme lipoprotein lipase, located on the surface of capillary endothelial cells, and their triglycerides are progressively removed in the process. Lipoprotein lipase is activated by apo C-II. After 6–12 h, half of the newly synthesized VLDL has been removed from the blood stream. During intravasal delipidation, fatty acids are delivered to adipocytes and muscle cells, and the surface constituents (apo C, phospholipids, and free cholesterol) are transferred to the HDL-density class. The remaining particles, the VLDL remnants, are called IDL.

Factors Determining the Concentration of Very Low Density Lipoproteins and Triglycerides

Three factors determine the steady state concentrations of the VLDL triglycerides: secretion, lipolysis, and remnant removal. Removal is due to uptake by the liver and conversion to LDL. Hepatic secretion of triglycerides can be enhanced by either increased production of VLDL particles or production of particles rich in triglycerides. The former appears to be the case in familial combined hyperlipidemia [37, 113, 125, 177], and the latter may be one of the causes of familial hypertriglyceridemia [29, 37].

Defective lipolysis is the cause of the most severe forms of familial chylomicronemia. Less marked deficiencies of LPL are typically manifested by moderately severe hypertriglyceridemia. Defective processing of VLDL remnants occurs in familial dysbetalipoproteinemia. Their prolonged circulation leads to cholesterol accumulation and to conversion into β-VLDL. Less severe increases in VLDL remnants occur in the absence of HTGL. This enzyme is likely necessary in the conversion of VLDL to LDL.

Dietary factors which influence serum triglycerides are dietary fat, dietary carbohydrate, alcohol, and obesity. ω-6-Polyunsaturated fatty acids have a pronounced triglyceride-lowering effect.

High-carbohydrate diets may promote synthesis of triglycerides in the liver and lead to the secretion of triglyceride-rich VLDL, but may also inhibit synthesis of lipoprotein lipase in the adipose tissue [111].

Alcohol is a high-calorie beverage and also leads to the secretion of triglyceride-rich VLDL. In patients with a preexisting hypertriglyceridemia, this may lead to excessively high serum triglycerides, a condition potentially associated with acute pancreatitis.

Obese people frequently have high triglyceride levels as a consequence of VLDL overproduction by the liver. However, this type of hypertriglyceridemia is fundamentally different from the hypertriglyceridemia induced by carbohydrates or alcohol.

Intermediate-Density Lipoproteins

IDL are VLDL remnants. They are found in the density range between 1.006 and 1.019 g/ml. IDL are smaller than VLDL and contain only half as many triglycerides. This increases the proportion of CE. They still contain some apo C, but apoE and apo B_{100} are predominant. The catabolism of IDL proceeds at a fast rate. IDL are taken up rapidly by liver cells (B_{100}: E receptor), where the lipids are recycled in VLDL genesis or the cholesterol is excreted in the bile unchanged or converted to bile acids. According to the prevailing theory, the majority of IDL particles are taken up by liver cells via the B_{100}: E receptor. The fraction of IDL whcih escapes hepatic uptake becomes devoid of apo E and ends up in the bloodstrem als LDL particles. The concentration of IDL in the plasma is normally very low. IDL have a half-life of 2–6 h.

Lipoproteins found in the density range of IDL are termed LDL_1. The "true" LDL are found in the range of 1.019 to 1.063 g/ml. The correct name would be LDL_2. IDL are considered to be atherogenic [131, 132].

Low-Density Lipoproteins

LDL (LDL_2) are derived from the catabolism of precursor lipoproteins (VLDL and IDL) and represent the end products of the delipidation cascade. The LDL consist mainly of CE and one single molecule of apo F_{100}. CE are densely packed in the core of the particle. Almost 50 % of the LDL mass is made up by CE and free cholesterol. They are too small to scatter light. Since they contain lipid-soluble vitamins, such as vitamin E and vitamin A, they appear yellow. Most of the LDL_2 density class (d=1.019 – 1.063 g/ml) consists of apo B in its lipid-binding form (LpB), i. e., particles exclusively containing apo B as apolipoprotein. Some particles also contain apo C and/or apo E. These particles are found predominantly in the LDL_1 density class (d=1.006 – 1.019 g/ml).

Metabolism

The intravasal mechanism of conversion of IDL in LDL is not fully understood. The elimination of LDL from the circulation proceeds via the B_{100}:E receptor, which under normal conditions is mainly expressed on hepatocytes, mucosal cells, gonadal cells, and cells of the adrenal cortex. The B_{100}:E receptor recognizes apo B_{100} and apo E. The receptor binds to the C-terminal half of apo B_{100}. Thus apo B_{48} goes undetected. The B_{100}:E receptor recognizes all lipoproteins containing apo B_{100} (VLDL, IDL, and LDL) except Lp(a), which binds to apo E with a much higher affinity than to apo B_{100}. Under normal conditions, binding of lipoproteins to the B_{100}:E receptor is rapidly followed by internalization of the bound lipoprotein via an endocytotic vesicle which fuses with a lysosome. The receptor escapes degradation within the lysosome, but the lipoprotein is completely degraded except for cholesterol, which may escape and leave the lysosome.

Endothelial cells can bind, but cannot internalize LDL in healthy states. However, follwing injury the endothelial cells regain this capability. The half-life of LDL is 2 – 3 days.

Factors Influencing Concentration

Humans have higher LDL cholesterol levels than most other primates. The total cholesterol of a normal 20-year-old man on a standard diet is approximately 140 mg/dl [121, 126], corresponding to an LDL cholesterol concentration of 75 – 90 mg/dl. There are populations which maintain such cholesterol levels in middle age. The major determinant of the concentration of LDL is the ratio of LDL production to LDL elimination. Since both processes are linked to hepatic expression of the B_{100}:E receptor (especially the latter), any condition influencing this variable will also influence the concentration of LDL. Consequently, apo B metabolism affects serum LDL levels in several ways. The liver secretes apo B-containing lipoproteins, and a certain fraction of these lipoproteins are converted to LDL. LDL and their precursors are taken up in the liver by the B_{100}:E receptor. The extent of these activities determines the concentration of lipoprotein particles present in the LDL density class.

The synthetic rate of the B_{100}:E receptor is backregulated by the intracellular excess of free cholesterol. Intracellular accumulation of cholesterol suppresses the transcription of the receptor gene. Since the liver is the predominant elimination site for LDL and the elimination takes place via the B_{100}:E receptor, any downregulation will delay LDL catabolism and increase the fraction of IDL converted to LDL with consecutive increases in LDL concentration.

A very important cause of receptor downregulation is the hepatic uptake of CM remnants via LRP. Any time fat is ingested and absorbed, the liver will be enriched with cholesterol and the LDL concentration increases. Consequently, the diet plays a major role in setting the LDL plasma concentration.

Dairy products and meat contain both saturated fatty acids and cholesterol. The impact of dietary cholesterol is limited. For example, 100 mg dietary cholesterol per 1000 calories per day will increase total plasma cholesterol by approximately 8 mg/dl. The major cause of high plasma cholesterol is acid. A reduction in dietary fatty acids of 50 % should lower plasma cholesterol levels by 20 mg/dl. Fatty acids are ingested mainly as triglycerides. These give rise to cholesterol-rich CM remnants, which are taken up rapidly by the liver, thereby reducing the hepatic expression of B_{100}:E receptors.

Obesity can adversely affect serum cholesterol levels in several ways. It can enhance hepatic secretion of VLDL and thereby increase VLDL levels and those of their conversion product LDL [48, 49, 119].

Being 10 kg overweight will raise total cholesterol by about 7 mg/dl. Since HDL cholesterol will be lowered by 3 mg/dl, VLDL and LDL cholesterol will increase by 10 mg/dl. The coronary risk is increased via lipoprotein disorders by approximately 16% (10% by increased VLDL and LDL and 6% by a decrease in HDL cholesterol).

The extent of dietary-induced changes in total plasma cholesterol depends on the hepatic expression of B_{100}:E receptors. Individuals also vary in their LDL cholesterol response to changes in body weight, probably due to their genetic make-up. In some people VLDL secretion may be stimulated more than in others; on the other hand, there is almost certainly genetic variability in inherent LDL receptor activity.

Cholesterol levels above 240 mg/dl are due to the above-mentioned factors working in concert with genetic factors, two of which are of major importance: a constitutive reduction in B_{100}:E receptor activity [84, 231] and a greater secretion of apo B-containing lipoproteins by the liver. Hypercholesterolemia is occasionally due to defective familial apo B_{100}. Sometimes an enhanced conversion of VLDL to LDL must be considered as the genetic cause of hypercholesterolemia.

Borderline high cholesterol (200–239 mg/dl) concentrations are mainly due to obesity, dietary habits, aging, estrogen deficiencies, and possibly a genetic predisposition. Dietary factors and obesity may each contribute up to 25 mg/dl (together 50 mg/dl total cholesterol). Aging per se brings about another increment of 20–30 mg/dl LDL cholesterol. Estrogen loss in women raises LDL cholesterol by another 20 mg/dl. Obesity alone does not influence hepatic expression of B_{100}:E receptor [61, 62, 82, 147, 166, 170, 204, 205].

Another factor affecting LDL cholesterol levels is the amount of cholesterol carried in each LDL particle [2]. Only one molecule of apo B is present in each LDL particle, but the quantity of cholesterol in each particle can vary. Normally the weight-to-weight ratio of cholesterol to apo B in an LDL particle is about 1.5. Even within the normal range of LDL cholesterol, this ratio can vary from 1.3 to 1.7 [28]. However, variations in LDL cholesterol levels are primarily due to variations in LDL apo B metabolism and not variations in protein lipid ratios.

Clinical Importance of Low-Density Lipoprotein Cholesterol

Among genetically determined hyperlipoproteinemias, the greatest risk of premature CHD occurs in those individuals in whom elevated LDL cholesterol is the only significant abnormality [84, 109, 180, 220, 230]. Moreover, in epidemiological studies, LDL cholesterol typically conveys the highest risk of CHD. In clinical trials in which LDL levels were lowered, a reduction in the risk of CHD was demonstrated [144, 145], and progression of atherosclerosis was retarded [22, 25, 30]. Thus LDL cholesterol is the major serum cholesterol fraction linked to CHD. LDL cholesterol is therefore the major target of diagnostics and lipid-lowering therapy. In order to standardize the clinical evaluation and treatment of patients with high LDL cholesterol in the United States, guidelines for detection and treatment in adults have been issued by an expert panel of the NCEP [65] (Table 3).

Table 3. National Cholesterol Education Program (NCEP) Adult Treatment Panel's decision cutoff points for low-density lipoprotein (LDL) cholesterol levels (mg/dl)

	Diet treatment	Drug treatment	Treatment goal
Risk factor absent	> 160	> 190	< 160
Risk factor present	> 130	> 160	< 130
CHD present	> 100	> 130	< 100

CHD, coronary heart disease.

Small, Dense Low-Density Lipoproteins

In hypertriglyceridemia, some CE in the core of the particle are replaced by triglycerides. This decreases the ratio of cholesterol to apo B in these particles. The subsequent hydrolysis of these triglycerides by HTGL increases the hydrated density and diminishes the size of these particles. Such "small, dense LDL" appear to be more atherogenic than normal LDL [14, 15, 17]. In addition, cholesterol-enriched LDL, as encountered in familial hypercholesterolemia and in cholesterol-fed primates, may produce more severe atherosclerosis compared to normal-sized LDL [186].

High-Density Lipoproteins

The HDL density class consists almost exclusively of all normal lipoproteins not containing apo B. All proteins capable of binding lipids have a lower density than the serum proteins, and most probably end up in their lipid-binding form in the HDL density class. Correspondingly, this class is the reservoir of most other minor apolipoproteins. Newly formed HDL stem either from secretion by the liver or the small intestine or are a byproduct of intravasal lipolysis of triglyceride-rich lipoproteins (surface remnants [60]). They always have a discoidal shape. Such HDL contain phospholipids, free cholesterol, and some apolipoproteins, but lack neutral lipids. Such discs are excellent substrates for LCAT, leading to the generation of CE and the conversion of discoidal structures into spherical particles.

Structure

Plasma HDL are small, dense lipid-protein complexes typically consisting of 45%–55% protein, 30% phospholipid (phosphatidylcholine), and 18% cholesterol, of which five sixths are esterified. Small amounts of glycerides are found in most preparations [68]. The two main structural apolipoproteins are A-I (28 kDa) and A-II (17 kDa). In addition, the HDL density class contains all other apolipoproteins with the exception of apo B. These include apo C (consisting of the constitutive peptides C-I, C-II, and C-III), apo E, and A-IV and trace quantities of the CE transfer protein (CETP), phospholipid transfer protein (PLTP), and LCAT. These minor components play an important role in the regulation of lipoprotein metabolism.

The density range of the HDL dnesity class is 3.3 times greater than that of LDL_2. Almost all the different HDL possess A-I. A lipoprotein containing only A-I as apolipoprotein (LpA-I) may be present, but most of the A-I is associated with other apolipoproteins [55, 70]. Some of these are devoid of A-II. Most particles contain more than one single apolipoprotein, especially apo C. Many particles contain in addition or instead apo E.

The HDL density class can be further fractionated by a variety of methods, including gel chromatography, isoelectric focusing, chromatofocusing, isatachophoresis, capillary electrophoresis, gradient gel electrophoresis polyanion precipititation, and gradient ultracentrifugation.

Subfractions

The earliest method of further fractionating the HDL density class was analytical ultracentrifugation. This technique gave clues about the presence of HDL_2 and HDL_3, but could not be used on a preparative scale. A preparative fractionation of HDL was accomplished by ultracentrifugation at a density of 1.125 g/dl, giving rise to the floating HDL_2 fraction and the sedimenting HDL_3 fraction. HDL_2 contain 40% protein, and HDL_3 55%. By gradient polyacrylamide gel electrophoresis, a much finer separation of the HDL density class can be achieved. However, none of these fractions is distinguished by a markedly different content of apolipoproteins.

The difference between HDL_2 and HDL_3 is that the latter are smaller and denser and have a higher content of A-II. HDL_2 contain all the apo E of the HDL fraction and A-I and A-II in a ratio of 3:1. The ratio of A-I to A-II in HDL_3 is 2:1.

Epidemiological studies suggest that it is the HDL_2 fraction which exhibits antiatherosclerotic effects [88, 142]. This is in contrast to the cholesterol-mobilizing property of HDL_3. The HDL_2 density class is increased in women and endurance athletes. The HDL_2 concentration bears a direct relationship to the ability of an individual to metabolize triglyceride-rich particles [97, 175].

As already mentioned, the HDL density class can also be divided based ont he content of apolipoprotein A, with lipoproteins containing either both major apolipoproteins A-I and A-II or only A-I [55, 70]. Only the latter fraction can originate in both the liver and the intestine. The former particles make up the majority of HDL_3. Plasma levels of HDL particles containing both A-I and A-II are generally higher and more constant than plasma levels of particles containing only A-I (these particles are different from LpA-I).

It is assumed that the protective effects of HDL reside in the particles possessing only A-I. However, HDL_2 contain relatively more HDL devoid of A-II. The lower HDL level in men than in women is reflected by the lower concentration of HDL devoid of A-II. Low HDL cholesterol concentrations are associated with lower levels of both lipoprotein species, but the decrease in HDL particles lacking A-I predominates.

HDL can also be classified according to different mobilities in agarose gel. It is possible to separate three distinct size populations of particles lacking A-II [55]. These exhibit different electrophoretic mobilities. Large subpopulations possess both pre-β and α-migrating components and the small fraction has only pre-β mobility (pre-β-1 HDL), accounting for up to 2%–5% of the plasma HDL. In addition to pre-β-1 HDL, there is also pre-β-2 HDL, which is larger and richer in phospholipids than pre-β HDL-1; it is disc shaped and contains no other apolipoproteins except three molecules of apo A-I per disc [115]. A significant proportion of A-I is therefore found in the pre-β region [33, 45]. This fraction can account for up to 10 % of the HDL density class and may be formed during incubation of the plasma. It is converted into α-lipoproteins by LCAT, whereas CETP activity converts α-HDL into pre-β HDL. Pre-β HDL may have particular importance in mediating cellular cholesterol efflux. Differentiation of the HDL particles based on apo A-I and A-II is achieved by a sandwich enzyme-linked immunosorbent assay (ELISA). If the particle is bound via A-II to the wall of the test tube and detected in this immobilized form by an antibody to A-I, the measured amount of A-T corresponds to the fraction of A-I associated with A-II.

Metabolism of High-Density Lipoproteins and Their Subfractions

Native HDL consist of free cholesterol, lecithin, A-I, and A-II. Regardless of origin, they always display a disc-like structure. The discs consist of a phosolipid bilayer circumscribed by a peripheral ring of apolipoproteins. Such discs are excellent substrates for LCAT. This enzyme catalyzes the transformation of lectithin into lysolecithin and the concomitant transformation of free cholesterol in CE. The LCAT enzyme is synthesized in the liver and is activated by A-I.

LCAT transfers fatty acids from the HDL phospholipids to the hydroxyl group of the free cholesterol, leading to the generation of CE and the conversion of discoidal structures into spherical particles. Thus newly secreted or newly formed HDL are rapidly converted into mature spherical HDL. LCAT is responsible for the scavenger functions of HDL.

Unesterified cholesterol is a very dynamic molecule that is constantly exchanged between different lipoproteins and between lipoproteins and cells. This migration comes to an end when the molecule becomes part of an HDL particle.

After esterification by LCAT, the molecule becomes hydrophobic and escapes into the core of the particle. Its original place on the surface of the disc can be occupied by an additional molecule of free cholesterol originating from cells or other lipoproteins. This molecule too, will proceed to the core of the particle after esterification. This process gives rise to an oil droplet that splits the bilayer and generates the mature HDL particle consisting of a neutral lipid core and surface monolayer of phospholipids containing the intercalated apolipoproteins between the splayed head groups.

A-I is synthesized in equal proportions by the liver and small intestine, whereas A-II stems exclusively from the liver. A major portion of HDL precursors is initially secreted on large VLDL or CM. During lipolysis of these particles by LPL, surface lipids (phospholipids and cholesterol) and proteins (A-I, A-II, and apo C) are released and end up in the HDL density class. From these precursors, either nascent discoidal HDL may be formed, which are typically subject to rapid LCAT action or can be incorporated into preexisting HDL particles. The latter process leads to an increase in size and a decrease in density, i. e., transformation of HDL_3 to HDL_2. HDL can likely be formed and secreted directly by enterocytes and hepatocytes. Such HDL are either spherical particles (containing neutral lipids) or dicoidal structures. Secretory cells contain only spherical particles, and the discs probably arise after the secretion of apolipoproteins.

Part of the HDL lipids stems from lipolysis (phospholipids) and from other lipoproteins and part from erythrocytes or endothelial cells (cholesterol). LCAT action removes both lipids and drives the influx of additional lipids into HDL. Lipid transfer proteins of the plasma transfer phospholipids is facilitated by a corresponding transfer protein (PLTP), replenishing HDL with unsaturated phospholipids necessary for the LCAT reaction.

Instead of hiding in the core of HDL particles, the newly formed CE can also be transferred to large, triglyceride-rich particles by the action of CETP. CETP delivers triglycerides in exchange of CE to the core of the HDL particle, resulting in CE depletion and triglyceride enrichment of HDL and representing the major pathway of LDL enrichment with CE. HDL devoid of A-II move in a circular pathway. A-I enters the cycle from the liver and small intestine and becomes incorporated into existing HDL particles. These smaller particles acquire core CE (LCAT). In this process, HDL_3 are expanded into HDL_{2a}. This species of HDL_2 contains mainly CE in its core. As HDL_{2a} circulate, some of the CE become replaced by triglycerides (CETP). This transforms HDL_{2a} into HDL_{2b}. Finally, HDL_{2b} are degraded back to HDL_3. HTGL plays an important role in this process. HTGL is an enzyme found primarily on the endothelial cells of the liver sinusoids and has both triglyceride hydrolase and phospholipase activity and results in a depletion of HDL triglycerides and phospholipids and a decrease in HDL size. As both the surface phospholipids and the core triglycerides of HDL_{2b} are hydrolyzed, HDL_3 are regenerated, allowing uptake of other cholesterol molecules from endothelial cells or macrophages.

During each cycle, some of the surface apo A-I is lost. Presumably the more rapid this cycle, the greater the amount of A-I lost. A rapid turnover causes a shrinkage of the HDL pool followed by a decrease in HDL cholesterol. LDL favor the deposition of cholesterol in cells, they are regarded as a major risk factor for atherosclerosis. As HDL can remove cholesterol from cells, they are regarded as being antiatherogenic. The first stop in the reverse cholesterol transport is the transfer of free cholesterol from endothelial cell membranes to HDLf [89, 173, 185, 194]. The cell-derived cholesterol is rapidly transferred to small, lipid-poor HDL containing no A-II and having pre-β-1 mobility. It is then rapidly transferred from pre-β-1 HDL to pre-β-2 HDL, pre-β-3 HDL, α-HDL, and finally LDL. LCAT directly esterifies a minor proportion of cell-derived cholesterol [66] during its passage via pre-β-3 HDL. Most of the cholesterol is esterified in the HDL after retransfer from LDL [106]. Thus the primary acceptors are pre-β-migrating discs; however, the substrate for LCAT may also be the spherical particles (HDL_3). The "blown-up" HDL_3 particles may acquire apo E and travel rather slowly to the liver [153]. Such particles belong partially to the LDL_2 density class, and their misnomers include HDLc and HDL_1. The intestinal mucosa may be a major source of HDL precursors but cannot synthesize A-II [107].

The mechanisms by which the discs and the regenerated HDL particles take up free cholesterol from the membranes of peripheral cells are poorly understood. It has been explained in terms of diffusion [66] along a concentration gradient [118], a process not mediated by a binding site at the cell surface, but rather dependent on the physical state of the acyl chains in phospholipids. Shorter and more unsaturated chains favor cellular efflux of free cholesterol [46]. The particles are not likely to interact with the presumptive HDL receptors (HDL-R). Since these receptors also bind apo E-free HDL, they are clearly different from the B_{100}:E receptor and the LRP. The expression of these receptors, whose function is not known, can be stimulated by preincubation with cholesterol [172].

The human LCAT gene is found on chromosome 16q22 [18] and encompasses six exons. LCAT mRNA is mainly expressed in the liver. The LCAT enzyme is responsible for almost all of the CE found in human serum.

CETP is a heavily glycosylated 476-amino acid protein. CETP mRNA is expressed in liver, intestine, spleen, adipose tissue, and a variety of other organs. CETP levels in the blood can be induced by a high cholesterol diet.

Clinical Importance

The mechanisms whereby low HDL levels enhance risk are not well understood. Since the physiological functions of HDL are largely unknown, it is difficult to speculate on their protective role in atherogenesis. Low HDL levels may impair reverse cholesterol transport from the arterial wall to the liver [89, 185, 229]. HDL may prevent oxidation and self-aggregation of LDL within the arterial wall and thereby reduce the atherogenicity of LDL [208]. Low HDL levels perhaps serve only an indicator of increased levels of atherogenic lipoproteins, such as IDL [182, 214] or small dense LDL [14, 15, 17].

HDL cholesterol plasma concentrations may therefore mainly rellect the ability to dispose of triglycoride-rich particles such as VLDL and CM remnants, which may be rendered more atherogenic by CETP due to their long residence time in the blood.

Factors Affecting Concentration

Differences in HDL cholesterol are mainly due to the different concentrations of HDL_2 cholesterol. About half the variation of HDL cholesterol levels is explained by genetic variability [103]. Nongenetic factors acting on an individual's genetic constitution appear to account for most of the low HDL levels in the population. Other CHD risk factors such as cigarette smoking, obesity, and lack of exercise are accompanied by low HDL, levels. These are the three major nongenetic factors leading to low HDL levels.

Low HDL levels result predominantly from an increased catabolism of A-I and not from a decreased synthesis. One mechanism for an enhanced catabolism of A-I could be an increased conversion rate of HDL_{2a} to HDL_{2b}. This can have several underlying causes, such as an increased exchange of triglycerides with CE in hypertriglyceridemia or an increased activity of hepatic triglyceride hydrolase [20]. There is a general inverse relationship between HDL cholesterol and serum triglycerides.

A significant proportion of the low HDL levels in industrialized civilizations is likely due to obesity. Obesity stimulates the synthesis of VLDL [57, 120] and independently the catabolism of A-I. In most obese patients, weight reduction restores HDL cholesterol to normal.

HDL can also be lowered by drugs such as beta blockers, gestagens, androgens, and low-fat diets. Endogenous androgens at puberty lead to a marked drop of HDL levels.

The highest HDL levels are found in populations that consume diets high in saturated fatty acids [126, 163]. These diets also produce the highest LDL cholesterol concentrations. The *cis* monounsaturated fatty acids (i.e., oleic acid) may yield slightly higher levels of HDL cholesterol than do saturated fatty acids. *Trans* mononusaturated fatty acids cause a significant reduction in HDL levels [162]. The ω-6-polyunsaturated fatty acids (linoleic acid) lower HDL cholesterol.

If dietary fat is replaced by carbohydrates, HDL levels decline [94, 95, 111].

Alcohol is one of the known substances to raise HDL cholesterol; however, the mechanism remains unclear.

High estrogen levels as induced by postmenopausal estrogen replacement can result in an increase of HDL cholesterol by about 10–20 mg/dl.

A rare genetic condition leads to markedly elevated levels of HDL cholesterol of up to 150–300 mg/dl. In these patients, LDL cholesterol and triglyceride levels are low. The reason for the high HDL levels in these individuals is a homozygous CETP deficiency. These individuals are clinically normal and have no signs of premature CHD. Heterozygotes show elevated HDL_2 cholesterol levels [108, 212].

Lipoprotein (a)

Lp(a) was first described in 1963, when immunological methods suggested polymorphism in LDL [21]. Lp(a) does not have a well-defined hydrated density and is found over a relatively wide density range [98, 176, 190]. The size of naturally occurring Lp(a) particles varies between 2000 and 10 000 kDa.

Structure

Lp(a) is a modified LDL particle. This modification consists in the association of the particle with another large protein, apo(a). The association is stabilized by a covalent bond via one disulfide bridge between apo(a) and apo B. This modification is sufficient to change almost all characteristic properties of LDL particles such as hydrated density, electrophoretic mobility, and interaction with receptors.

The structure of an apo(a) molecule can be derived from the corresponding cDNA. It is closely related to that of plasminogen [117, 139] and specifies a peculiarly monotonous protein. It consists of a variable number (up to 40) kringle-4 domains, one kringle-5 domain, and a protease domain of the plasminogen molecule. Kringles 1–3 of plasminogen are not found in Lp(a). Lp(a) was first considered to be a genetic variant of LDL [30]. Its hydrated density is typically slightly higher than that of LDL [58, 73, 192, 199, 241] and it electrophoretically migrates considerably faster than the β-migrating LDL (β-lipoproteins). It shares its pre-β mobility with VLDL, but in contrast to these particles it sediments during ultracentrifugation at serum density, leading to the designation "sinking pre-β-lipoprotein." As might be expected. Lp(a) dissociates under reducing conditions spontaneously in apo(a) and an LDL particle [59, 221].

Metabolism

The metabolism of Lp(a) in humans is largely unknown. Lp(a) is possibly synthesized by the liver [130]. In vitro it is possible to reconstitute Lp(a) from recombinant apo(a) and LDL. Lp(a) catabolism in vivo proceeds somewhat slower than that of LDL [133]. The different concentrations found in different individuals are presumably mainly due to different rates of synthesis [134]. The site in the organism where Lp(a) is catabolized is not known. The major route of catabolism is certainly not via the apo B_{100}:E receptor, since therapeutic increases of its expression do not lead to a decreasod Lp(a) level in the blood. Lp(a) has a much lower affinity to the apo B_{100}:E receptor than LDL [67, 134]. It seems possible that apo(a) partially masks the receptor-binding domain of apo B_{100} [10, 11].

L(a) is ubiquitously present. However, interindividually strikingly different levels are genetically determined [6, 101, 167, 193]. Caucasians exhibit a distribution which is strongly skewed toward the left [4]. It is assumed that the Lp(a) concentration is regulated by the apo(a) locus on chromosome 6 [52]. At least 20 allelic forms of apo(a) are now known, ranging between 320 and 838 kDa [75,

225–227]. The major difference between the isoforms is the number of copies homologous to the kringle-4 of plasminogen [129]. The apo(a) isoforms can be differentiated by polyacrylamide gel electrophoresis. They are associated with the serum concentrations of Lp(a) [225, 228]. The higher the molar mass of the isoform, the lower the concentration. The underlying mechanism of this correlation of isoform and serum concentration is largely unknown.

Clinical Importance

Lp(a) has been measured with a variety of immunological methods in a large number of clinical and epidemiological studies. These studies lend support to the opinion that elevated Lp(a) concentrations are associated with an increased risk of cardiovascular and cerebrovascalar disease. Lp(a) is believed to have a high affinity to subendothelial structures and to be oxidized rather easily. The association with vascular disease is probably much stronger than assumed, since the majority of studies were performed before reliable methods to determine Lp(a) had become available.

Lipoprotein-X

The lipids of the bile are predominantly free cholesterol and phospholipids. If bile comes in contact with blood, these insoluble lipids form a bilayer, which becomes eventually a vesicle [159]. This vesicle has a hydrated density of LDL and has been termed Lp-X [196]. The coat of the vesicles consists of free cholesterol and lipids, and the core is a droplet of plasma. The surface acquires some apolipoproteins, predominantly C-III. The electric charge of the particle is the lowest of all serum lipoproteins. Consequently, Lp-X can be separated and identified by electrophoretic techniques. The best method is agar electrophoresis (not agarose electrophoresis), whereby it is transported by electroendosmosis toward the cathode. Since it is the only lipoprotein with this property, it can be demonstrated in this position by nonspecific methods for the determination of lipoproteins, such as lipid staining or precipitation. Lp-X is a sensitive and very specific indicator of obstructive jaundice.

Determination of Lipids

Cholesterol

The clinical evaluation of the blood lipids can be approached by two different ways:

1. The concentration of total cholesterol and total triglycerides in the serum or plasma is determined. However, this approach involves destruction of all lipoproteins.
2. The individual proteins are measured based on the properties of apolipoproteins; the structural integrity of lipoproteins is preserved.

Methods

As recently as 20 years ago, serum cholesterol was routinely measured using methods that required caustic materials such as concentrated sulfuric acid, acetic anhydride, and acetic acid. Cholesterol and CE were ionized to form species that can be quantified by light absorption at wave lengths between 560 and 620 nm. These methods were mostly performed on "continuous flow" autoanalyzers. These methods have now been replaced by enzymatic methods, due to easy handling, ease of automation, and ability to use small sample volumes.

The most important enzymatic method employs cholesterol oxidase. In the first step, CE are hydrolyzed by the enzyme cholesterol esterase to yield free cholesterol. To avoid incomplete hydrolysis, two different esterases of different origins (animal and microbial) should be used. In the second step, the now completely free cholesterol reacts with oxygen in the presence of cholesterol oxidase. The products are cholestenone and H_2O_2. Cholestenone (cholest-4}en-3-one) is an oxidized form of cholesterol in which the hydroxyl group at C-3 has been converted to a keto group.

Assays for cholesterol quantitation with enzymes have used both consumption of oxygen and formation of hydrogen peroxide as indicators. The majority of commercial procedures measure peroxide formation by coupling the enzymic reaction to a second peroxide marker system. In the third step, the H_2O_2 formed in the previous reaction is then reduced to H_2O by an indicator substance in the presence of peroxidase. In the course of the peroxidase reaction, the usually colorless indicator is reduced to a colored substance, which can be quantitated spectrophotometrically. For example, in the "Trinder" reaction [219] peroxidase catalyzes the oxidative coupling of 4-aminoantipyrene and phenol by H_2O_2 to form a quinone imine dye and water. This quinone imine dye absorbs maximally at 500 nm and may be quantitated spectrophotometrically:

1. Cholesterolester + $H_2O \rightarrow$ cholesterol + fatty acid
2. Cholesterol + $O_2 \rightarrow \beta^4$-cholestenone + H_2O_2
3. 2 H_2O_2 + 4-aminophenazon + phenol $\rightarrow$ 4-(*p*-benzochinone-monoimino)-phenazone + H_2O

Enzymatic methods typically use serum or plasma directly. Hemolysis may therefore lead to interferences. Because of competition with the chromogen for hydrogen peroxide, bilirubin and ascorbate may also interfere with the measurements.

Accuracy and Precision

The causal relationship between the cholesterol concentration of the serum or the LDL cholesterol concentration and premature CHD appears to have been confirmed. A reduction in total or LDL cholesterol by 10% significantly reduces the risk of future myocardial infarction. In order to be able to evaluate correctly the coronary risk and the probability of future cardivascular events, accurate measurements of cholesterol are mandatory. In addition to adherence to properly established procedures of internal quality assurance, laboratories should also participate regularly in external surveys.

To improve the precision and accuracy of cholesterol testing in the United States. the NCEP has issued the following recommendations:

1. Clinical laboratories should adopt the uniform cholesterol decision criteria issued by the Adult Treatment Panel of the NCEP [65].
2. Laboratories should minimize method-specific biases and achieve precision of cholesterol measurements.
3. Cholesterol methods used in clinical laboratories should be calibrated to allow comparison with the reference method at the Center of Disease Control (CDC) in Atlanta, Georgia or with the detinitive method at National Institute of Standardization (NIST).
4. Laboratories must meet performance goals for all cholesterol testing: specifically, an overall precision consistent with a CV of 3% or less and a bias not exceeding 3% from the true value. The well-characterized reference material must exhibit the same properties as native serum. Since pure cholesterol can only be solubilized in organic solvents, the reference material has to be serum free of interfering substances. Since reconstituted lyophilized sera are not equivalent to native sera, their further use as reference material is not encouraged.

A Working Group on Lipoprotein Measurement of the NCEP made the recommendations summarized in Table 4. These recommendations distinguish between present and future goals for HDL cholesterol measurements.

Table 4. National Cholesterol Education Program (NCEP) performance criteria for triglyceride, high-density lipoprotein (HDL), and low-density lipoprotein (LDL) assays

Analyte	Bias (% of true value)	Imprecision (CV as %)[a]	Single-point total error (%)[b]
Triglyceride	±5	< 5.0%	< 14.8
HDL cholesterol	±10	(Interim) > 42 mg/dl; < 6.0% < 42 mg/dl; SD < 2.5 mg/dl	< 21.8
		(in 1998) < 42 mg/dl; SD < 1.7 mg/dl	< 12.8
LDL cholesterol	±4	< 4.0%	< 11.8

[a] Interlaboratory imprecision as % coefficient of variation (CV).
[b] Calculations for total error: linear model, two-tailed; total error = bias + (1.96 × interlaboratory CV), where 1.96 = *Z* for 95% of normally distributed population.

Reference Values

The serum cholesterol concentration varies according to age, gender, the season of the year, and the dietary habits of the individual. It slowly increases with age, starting at adolescence and reaching a plateau at the age of 60. During adult life, men exhibit a 10% higher cholesterol concentration than women. After the menopause, the difference between the sexes disappears. In both sexes, the serum cholesterol during winter is approximately 3% higher tban during summer.

Reference values are usually obtained from an apparently healthy population. This approach to the definition of normality is not valid for cholesterol concentrations if it is considered to be an indicator for risk of premature CHD. Values above 4.6 mmol/L (180 mg/dl) are associated with an increased coronary risk.

The concept of reference values has therefore be replaced by the concept of cuttoff points. Cholesterol concentrations beyond the cutoff point are associated with an inacceptable risk of CHD. The scientific community has agreed upon 5.2 mmol/l (200 mg/dl) as the cutoff point independent of age or sex. This cutoff point, however, should be modified according to the inevitable increase with age. Below the age of 30, it should be 4.6 mmol/l, and above 65 years 6.2 mmol/l is sufficient.

Triglycerides

Methods

The determination of triglycerides consists of two crucial enzymatically catalyzed steps. The first step is the complete hydrolysis of triglycerides, yielding three fatty acids and one molecule of glycerol, catalyzed by the lipases. The second step consists of the enzymatic quantitation of glycerol using either glycerol kinase or glycerol oxidase. Since all methods are based on the determination of glycerol, hydrolysis has to be complete. Since lipases exhibit different activities to fatty acids of different chain lengths, they should consist of a mixture of different microbial lipases. Since triglycerides in serum are components of lipoproteins, complete access of the lipases to their substrate can be facilitated by the incorporation of proteases in the assay. The microbial lipases themselves exhibit some proteolytic activity.

Glycerol kinase catalyzes the phosphorylation of glycerol to glycerol-3-phosphate. In this reaction, ATP is converted to ADP.

Glycerol can be determined either by measuring ADP or by determining glycerol-3-phosphate. To determine ADP, it is necessary to convert phosphophenol pyruvate and ADP into pyruvate and ATP. The pyruvate can then be used to consume NADH + H^+ during its reduction to lactate by the enzyme lactate dehydrogenase (LDH).

The enzymatic determination of glycerol-3-phosphate uses either glycerol-3-phosphate dehydrogenase or glycerol-3-phosphate oxidase. In the first case, the concentration of glycerol-3-phosphate is equal to the rate of appearance of NADH + H^+ as detected by ultraviolet spectroscopy. In the second case, H_2O_2 is generated, which can be quantified by the "Trinder" reaction:

1. Triglycerides + 3 H_2O $\rightarrow$ glycerol + three fatty acids
2. Glycerol + ATP $\rightarrow$ glycerol-3-phosphate + ADP
3. Glycerol-3-phosphate + O_2 $\rightarrow$ dihedroxyacetonphosphate + H_2O_2
4. ${}_2O_2$ + 4-aminophenazone + 4-chlorphenol $\rightarrow$ 4-(*p*-benzochinone-monoimino)-phenazone + 2 H_2O + HCl

The glycerol oxidase is not entirely specific for glycerol. Propylene glycol and other glycols can also react. Ethylene glycol is often used to stabilize control materials. A possible source of error is the presence of alkaline phosphatase in the sample. The enzyme reacts with glycerophosphate, dihydroxyacetone phosphate, phosphoenol pyravate, and even ATP. Samples with an increased activity of alkaline phosphatase therefore deserve special attention.

Another source of error is the presence of glycerol in the sample. The concentration of endogenous glycerol can be increased by stress, diabetes mellitus, liver diseases, and ingestion of glycerol-containing preparations. The problem can be solved by using a sample blank containing all reagents except the lipases. Since part of the glycerol is also derived from the spontaneous hydrolysis of triglycerides, the substraction of the blank value may lead to an underestimation of the triglyceride concentration. As in the case of cholesterol, the calibrator must be very similar to native serum.

Reference Values

Triglyceride concentration varies according to age and sex. Beginning in childhood it increases in both sexes with age. In males, the maximum is reached at the age of 50 and is followed by a considerable decrease. In women, the maximum is reached in the late 50s. During adult life, women exhibit lower triglyceride concentrations than men.

The etiologic role of the serum triglyceride concentration in the development of premature CHD remains uncertain, and definite cutoff points have not yet been established. Triglyceride concentrations below 260 mg/dl are considered desirable. The range between 250 and 500 mg/dl bears a potential risk, and values over 500 mg/dl are considered highly abnormal. It is reasonable to assume that the normal triglyceride concentration lies below 200 mg/dl.

Total Cholesterol and Total Triglycerides

Determination of total cholesterol or total triglycerides does not take into account the fact that these lipids are all part of different lipoproteins. At a first glance, this seems to be a disadvantage. However, the precise and accurate determination of these lipids together with a thorough visual inspection of the serum usually allows the assignment of a certain lipid constellation to an increase in specific lipoproteins. Hypertriglyceridemia without hypercholesterolemia can only be due to a moderate elevation of CM or VLDL. If the serum is kept for at least 12 h undisturbed in a refrigerator, CM can be detected as a cloudy surface layer. If this layer develops over a clear serum, the hypertriglyceridemia is due to the presence of considerable amounts of CM. If no layer develops and the serum remains turbid, the hypertriglyceridemia is due to an increase in the number of VLDL particles. Increased VLDL and the presence of CM can be detected by a creamy layer over turbid serum. This condition is only rarely associated with a normal cholesterol concentration. It normally leads to a strong increase in triglycerides accompanied by a moderate increase in cholesterol.

An increased cholesterol concentration at a normal triglyceride concentration is always accompanied by clear serum and is the result of an increased LDL concentration or the presence of Lp-X. If cholesterol and triglycerides are both moderately increased by roughly the same amount (in mg/dl), the serum is never highly turbid. This condition can be due either to the presence of abnormal lipoproteins rich in cholesterol and in triglycerides (familial dysbetalipoproteinemia) or to a concomitant increase in both VLDL and LDL. These two cases can only be differentiated by lipoprotein analysis.

Phospholipids

Serum or plasma phospholipids are occasionally measured in the clinical laboratory; in particular, phosphatidylcholine and sphingomyelin ratios are used to assess fetal lung maturity. Basic phospholipid measurements are performed to give a more complete analysis of individual lipoprotein structure.

Serum phospholipids are increased together with free cholesterol in the case of obstructive jaundice. This is due to the presence of the abnormal lipoprotein Lp-X.

Methods

Determination of total serum phospholid is performed by several modifications of two different approaches. Enzymic procedures involve hydrolysis of choline-containing phospholipids (which constitute 91%–97% of total phospholipids) by microbial phospholipase D. This enzyme splits phospholipids in choline and phosphatidic acids. Choline is oxidized to betaine. The resulting H_2O_2 is utilized in a color-generating "Trinder" reaction:

1. Phospholipids + $H_2O \rightarrow$ choline + phosphatidic acids
2. Choline + $2O_2$ + $H_2O \rightarrow$ betaine + $2H_2O_2$
3. $2H_2O_2$ + 4-aminophenazon + phenol $\rightarrow$ 4-(*p*-benzochinone-monoimino)-phenazone + H_2O

Older techniques for measuring serum total phospholipids required separation of organic from inorganic phosphorus, followed by digestion of organic material and subsequent phosphorus determination. These methods measure total phospholipid phosphorus, and not only the fraction containing choline. Phospholipids can be separated according to their polarity by thin-layer chromatography or high-pressure liquid chromatography (HPLC) and subsequently quantitated.

Free Fatty Acids

Determination of free fatty acids is performed either by titration of the total free acid or by measurement of the amount of copper reagent complexed by free fatty acids. Both of these procedures require the extraction of fatty acids from the serum either free or complexed with copper.

Two enzymatic approaches are now possible. Both methods require as a first step the formation of a CoA-fatty acid. One method then uses AMP (a byproduct of the first reaetion) which, together with Acyl-CoA and one additional ATP, gives two molecules of ADP. The reaction is catalyzed by myokinase. ADP is subsequently measured by its participation in the conversion of phosphoenol pyruvate in pyruvate, a reaction catalyzed by pyruvate kinase. This reaction reconstitutes ATP from ADP. During this reaction, NADH is oxidized by lactate dehydrogenase. The decrease in absorption at 340 nm is proportional to the amount of ADP present in the reaction mixture.

The second enzymatic approach to the determination of free fatty acids first requires the elimination of all the CoA not utilized in the first step. This can be achieved by complexion with *N*-ethylmaleimide. The fatty acid-CoA complex is then oxidized by acyl-CoA oxidase to form 2,3-trans-enol-CoA and H_2O_2. The latter can be determined by the "Trinder reaction".

Determination of Lipoproteins

If one excludes the time-consuming and complicated analytical ultracentrifugation, the methodological spectrum for the clinical investigation of the plasmalipoprotein system consists of ultracentrifugation, lipoprotein electrophoresis, precipitation techniques, and the determination of apolipoproteins. The fact that the concentration of LDL increases the risk of CHD and that the concentration of HDL cholesterol seems to be protective justifies the quantitative determination of these lipoproteins.

Techniques

Techniques for the separate determination of the concentrations of serum lipoproteins rely on the usual techniques for lipoprotein separation followed by quantitative determination of a lipid (preferably cholesterol) or an apolipoprotein. Separation is achieved by taking advantage of different physicochemical properties of lipoproteins, such as size, hydrated density, or surface charge. Sometimes separation techniques are applied sequentially.

An additional possibility for the separation of lipoproteins is affinity chromatography using immobilized antibodies to apolipoproteins (immunoabsorption). Using this method, lipoprotein particles can be isolated, containing a specific combination of apolipoproteins, lacking specific apolipoproteins, or containing only one single specilic apolipoprotein, such as apo B or AI.

More sophisticated methods for the preparative separation of lipoproteins such as preparative isoelectric foeusing, chromatofocusing, capillary electrophoresis, or isotachophoresis are not widely used in the routine clinical laboratory.

Ultracentrifugation

Lipoproteins were originally isolated by preparative ultracentrifugation [102]. This technique is now occasionally used for differential diagnosis of unusual or severe hyperlipoproteinemias often secondary to other diseases such as obstructive jaundicezor nephrotic syndrome. Analytical ultracentrifugation was the first method used to investigate the connection between lipid metabolism and atherosclerosis [78,79]. It is now used only for research purposes. The same is true of zonal centrifugation and density gradient centrifugation. The latter techniques yield lipoprotein fractions which can be further analyzed. In both methods, a density gradient is established either in a whole rotor (zonal centrifugation) or in a single centrifugation tube. Lipoproteins are separated according to their hydrated density along this gradient and are then recovered by slowly emptying the rotor or tube into an fraction collector; the optical absorbance of the solution can be monitored simultaneously.

Isolation of lipoproteins by preparative ultracentrifugation involves their sequential flotation after sequential adjustment of the density of the specimen by addition of salts [102]. In order to achieve densities beyond 1.063 g/ml, salts other than NaCl have to be employed, including NaBr, KCl, and KBr. VLDL are isolated at d=1.006 g/ml, IDL at d=1.019 g/ml, LDI, at d=1.063 g/ml, and HDL at d=1.21 g/ml. The centrifugal force depends on the type of rotor and the speed of centrifugation. In the common types of rotors and ultracentrifuges, it is approximately 100 000 times the g force. The centrifugation for the isolation of VLDL under the usual conditions (50 000 rpm at 10°C) takes approximately 18 – 24 h. The isolation of LDL takes 36 h and that of HDL 48 h. At the end of each run, the lipoproteins concentrated in the top fourth of the tube (supernatant) are harvested by a tube slice technique using a special horizontal guillotine or by aspiration with a syringe. The density of the infranatant is then adjusted to the desired higher value and transferred to another tube and subjected to ultracentrifugation again. The harvested lipoprotein fraction is then further analyzed for lipid and apolipoprotein content. Analysis of the lipoprotein system by preparative ultracentrifugation requires 500 ml serum or plasma. This amount has to be pipetted bubble free in a polycarbonate tube. The weight of the filled tube is determined and the sample is then carefully layered with 100 µl saline (d= 1.006 g/ml) in order to obtain a greater space between the separated VLDL and the rest of the serum. This makes the aspiration of the VLDL fraction easier and keeps contamination of LDL by VLDL and vice versa at a minimum. In order to obtain reproducible separations, time, temperature, and speed of the centrifugation have to be standardized. To separate VLDL from the rest of the serum, 18 h at 50 000 × g at 10°C is sufficient. During centrifugation, the VLDL float to the top of the tube and appear as a white layer beneath the surface. The LDL and HDL fraction can be seen as yellow layers underneath. The VLDL layer can be completely removed by aspiration using a syringe and transferred into a small test tube for further examination. Traces of VLDL contaminating the wall of the ultracentrifugation tube can be removed using a cotton stick. The remaining fraction contains LDL, HDL, and all the other proteins of the sample. After adjustment of the weight of the tube to its initial value and thorough mixing of its contents, an aliquot of the now VLDL-free serum is subjected to polyanion precipitation of the LDL using phosphotungstic acid as the polyanion and $MgCl_2$ as the divalent cation [146]. The concentration of the specific VLDL lipids is calculated as the difference between the total concentration of the corresponding lipid in the sample and in the corresponding VLDL-free serum. The isolated VLDL fraction can be used to determine the concentration ratios of the different VLDL lipids, the electrophoretic mobility of the VLDL, or the isoforms of apo E.

The concentration of LDL lipids is obtained as the difference between the concentrations in the VLDL-free sample and the LDL-free sample. In addition to the distribution of the lipids, the distribution of any other measurable compound over the serum fractions obtained by this kind of fractionation can also be determined.

Discontinuous density gradient ultracentrifugation provides a means of separating all the major lipoprotein density classes in a single run in a swinging bucket rotor and involves the creation of a stepwise gradient by manual addition of solutions of differing density. It can also be used to isolate LDL subfractions.

Since the time required for separation of density classes by ultracentrifugation is a function of the diameter of the tube as long as the tube lies horizontal during centrifugation, attempts have been made to increase the area through which the lipoproteins have to migrate horizontally by keeping the tube at a fixed angle to the axis of rotation during centrifugation. This has culminated in the development of vertical spin density gradient ultracentrifugation. In this technique, the density of the plasma is increased by addition of solid KBr using a formula based on the partial specific volume of that salt. The sample is then overlayered with a solution of less dense NaCl. This two-step gradient is then centrifuged in a vertical rotor. It takes about 2 h to isolate LDL. The initial and the final phases are particularly critical, since conversion of horizontal layers into vertical layers and vice versa takes place during these phases. A major part of Lp(a) can also be isolated in this way.

Precipitation

It has long been known that lipoproteins can be precipitated from the serum using polyanions and divalent cations. Burstein and Scholnick have undertook a systematic approach to this phenomenon and found several combinations of polyanions and divalent cations useful for the differential precipitation of plasma lipoproteins [31, 32]. The most widely used procedure has been the precipitation of LDL and VLDL by heparin and $MnCl_2$ in order to obtain a serum sample free of these lipoproteins for the determination of HDL cholesterol. Unfortunately, the enzymatic methods for cholesterol determination usually employ a phosphate buffer which develops turbidities with the manganese ions. The appropriate polyanions for the non-interfering magnesium ions are phosphotungstic acid or dextrane sulfate.

Dextrane sulfate (MW, 50 000) and $MgCl_2$ are only rarely used in Europe nowadays. The phosphotungstic acid/$MgCl_2$ [146] method is the most widely used method for the precipitation of VLDL and LDL from whole serum.

The separation of HDL_2 and HDL_3 can in theory only be achieved by ultracentrifugation at a density of 1.125 g/ml. Attempts have been made to achieve a similar separation using sequential precipitation methods. After precipitation of the apo B-containing lipoproteins with any precipitation method, the addition of low or high molecular weight dextrane sulphate precipitates HDL_2, selectively. Alternatively, all lipoproteins except HDL_3 can be precipitatcd using polyethylene glycol. The HDL_2 lipids can then be calculated by substraction of thc HDL_3 lipids from the HDL lipids. These methods have not found wide acceptance because the determination of the HDL_2 lipids is not sufficiently accurate. The appropriate conditions may vary considerably between different individuals, and the specificity of the precipitation methods also differs from that of ultracentrifugation. The HDL_2 and HDL_3 density classes do not differ dramatically in their apolipoprotein contents. Because HDL apolipoproteins are present in both density classes, it seems questionable whether such a differentiation will become clinically valuable.

Lipoprotein Electrophoresis

The major classes of lipoproteins migrate electrophoretically according to both their charge and their size, shape, and interaction with the supporting medium. Agarose gel and paper produce similar separations of the lipoproteins, with the agarose gel offering increased resolution and, occasionally, increased separation within classes. The separation in both supporting materials has been improved by adding albumin [140]. Cellulose acetate may be inadequate to detect CM that comigrate with VLDL and is therefore not recommended.

The electrophoretic separation of lipoproteins on a strip of filter paper and subsequent staining with Sudan black [114] was the basis of the typing system of hyperlipidemias according to Fredrickson and Lees [68]. Using this technique, it was possible to translate hyperlipidemias into different forms of hyperlipoproteinemias.

Lipoproteins separated by lipoprotein electrophoresis (LPE) are classified according to the serum protein band of corresponding mobility. On agarose gel and paper, HDL are conventionally associated with the α_1-globulin region, VLDL with the α_2-globulin region, and LDL with the β-globulin region; CM remain at the origin (Fig. 4).

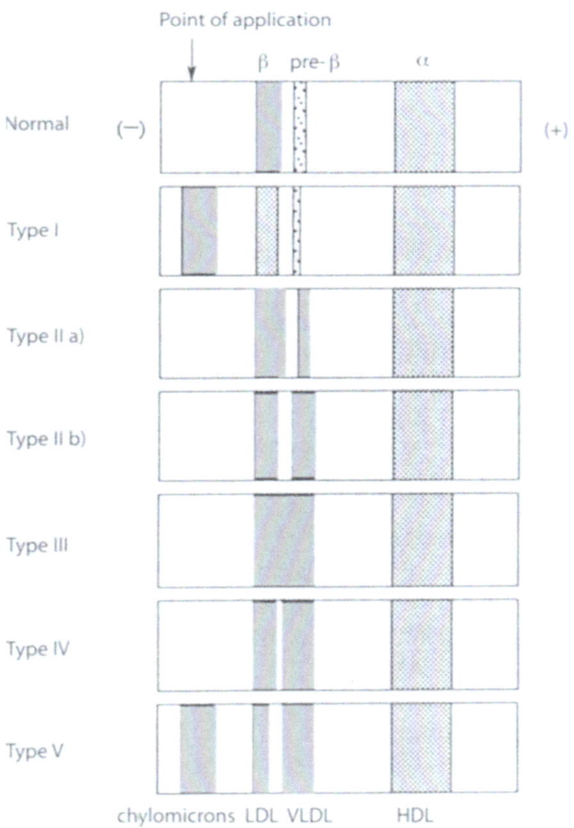

Fig. 4. Electrophoretic classification of hyperlipoproteinemias. *LDL*, low-density lipoprotein; *VLDL*, very low density lipoprotein; *HDL*, high-density lipoprotein

The change from paper to agarose gel [171] as supporting material led to a considerable shortening of the time required for the analysis.

However, in a number of studies quantitative densitometry has been found to be unreliable. The lipid stains Sudan Black or Oil Red O are two azodyes that preferentially stain triglycerides and CE, whereas free cholesterol and phospholipids are not stained well. The α-lipoproteins band is therefore faint and has not been considered in the typing system, which was originally predominantly a means to differentiate the lipoproteins of a turbid serum sample. Since protein bands stained for lipids do so inconsistently with changing intensity, this type of LPE could not serve as a basis for quantitative LPE.

The first successful quantitative LPE was based on polyanion precipitation after electrophoretic separation of the serum lipoproteins in agarose gel [197, 242]. It has now been superseded by enzymatic staining (cholestcrol dehydrogenase) of the cholesterol moiety of the separated lipoproteins using a formazane dye [13]. This is a very convenient method for lipoprotein quantification, requiring less than 5 μl of sample and available on a large scale. In addition, it allows separate quantification of Lp(a) cholesterol [169].

LPE of native serum can identify Lp-X; on most support media, Lp-X migrates with the β-lipoproteins, but in agar gels, in which electroendosmosis is strong, Lp-X moves in the opposite direction cathodically. Lp-X is found in sera of patients with obstructive jaundice. A typical electrophoretic pattern of obstructive jaundice is a single broad β-band. The α-band is missing, and pre-β-lipoproteins exhibit a slower mobility. Sometimes, a bilirubin-stained albumin band is clearly visible.

LPE of native serum is also helpful in evaluating postheparin lipolytic activity. Blood specimens are obtained before injection of heparin and 15 min later (100 U/kg body weight), and both sera are subjected to LPE. Evidence of heparin-releasable LPL consists in greater mobility and smearing of bands in the postheparin sample as compared with the preheparin sample.

The combination of preparative ultracentrifugation and quantitative LPE is a very powerful tool to detect and to quantify abnormal lipoproteins. Under certain conditions, Lp-X can be clearly separated from Lp-B. In VLDL-free serum, Lp(a) is clearly detectable as a pre-β-band.

The hallmark of type III hyperlipoproteinemia is a lipoprotein in the VLDL fraction exhibiting not pre-β, but β-mobility (β-VLDL). In comparison to normal VLDL, this particle is enriched with apo E (E_2 with poor ligand characteristics) and CE. It is derived from CM remnants and VLDL and leads to a broad β-band in serum.

Since CM do not migrate, even postprandial samples can be investigated. In addition to the enzymatic staining for cholesterol, the separated bands can also be enzymatically stained for other lipids, e.g., for instance free cholesterol, triglycerides, and choline-containing phospholipids. By this method, the lipid composition of lipoproteins can be determined in minute samples. In addition, this method allows reliable quantitation of the amount of triglycerides present in β-lipoproteins. LDL triglyceride concentration appears to be closely associated with the presence of angiographically proven coronary artery disease (CAD).

Since HDL are considered to be protective and LDL are indicative of future CAD, the ratio of LDL cholesterol to HDL cholesterol is more meaningful than either concentration alone. Since the determination of LDL cholesterol is less accurate and less precise than that of total cholesterol, the preferred ratio is that of total cholesterol to HDL cholesterol. However, it requires four pipetting steps (three for HDL cholesterol) and two cholesterol determinations. Since the total cholesterol to HDL cholesterol ratio is independent of hemoconcentration or hemodilution, the only problem is the comparatively poor precision of the HDL cholesterol method. Since HDL cholesterol is the denominator of the fraction, it has a considerable influence on the value of this ratio. This drawback is overcome by quantitative LPE, because the ratio of β-lipoproteins to α-lipoproteins requires only one enzymatic staining for cholesterol and one densitometric scan of the electrophoresis and no quantitative pipetting step at all.

The value of LPE as part of the routine profile has been debated for a number of years. Experts now discourage the use of LPE in the primary assessment of lipid or lipoprotein disorders. They recommend instead quantitative assays for triglycerides, total cholesterol, and HDL cholesterol, calculation of VLDL cholesterol and LDL cholesterol inspection of plasma, and follow-up of abnormal findings with ultracentrifugation to establish the phenotype. In its semiquantitative form, however, LPE continues to be important for assesing postheparin lipolytic activity. In addition, a small CM band at the origin in LPE signals a nonfasting state in a patient and LPE detects Lp-X, an abnormal lipoprotein that is a marker in obstructive jaundice.

Quantitative LPE is a very useful second step in lipoprotein diagnostics, since it bears all the advantages of the semiquantitative form and via the contribution to total cholesterol, also provides a precise and accurate quantitation of all normal and abnormal lipoproteins, provided they can be separated electrophoretically.

Measurement of Serum Lipoproteins

High-Density Lipoprotein

In addition to total cholesterol and triglycerides, the first step of lipid diagnostics should also include the determination of HDL cholesterol. In the fasting state, this serves as a basis for the calculation of LDL cholesterol by Friedewald's formula [69]; in the nonfasting state, at least the ratio of total cholesterol to HDL cholesterol can be determined. Some cases of borderline hypercholesterolemia may be due to increased HDL cholesterol at perfectly safe LDL cholesterol concentrations. HDL cholesterol itself has some prognostic value and influences the treatment goals. HDL cholesterol below 35 mg/dl is considered as a risk factor for CHD.

Methods

HDL cholesterol is determined most precisely and conveniently after removal of all apo B-containing lipoproteins (and posssibly Lp-X) from the serum or plasma by precipitation methods. These methods do not all exhibit the same specificity, and the remaining fraction does not correspond in every aspect to the HDL density class. The latter contains relatively large particles rich in apo E, which are precipitated and do not contribute to HDL cholesterol. The HDL density class can be further subdivided in HDL_1, HDL_2, and HDL_3.

The hydrated density of HDL_1 is between 1.055 and 1.085 g/ml. This range also contains apo B-containing lipoproteins and Lp(a) (1.051–1.082 g/ml). HDL_1 concentration can be increased by cholesterol feeding. It might play a role in reverse cholesterol transport. A measure of HDL_1 is the concentration of apo E in the HDL density class (not in the fraction obtained after precipitation of apo B-containing lipoproteins).

The HDL subfractions are usually quantified using analytical ultracentrifugation or zonal centrifugation. Because of the uncertain clinical implications of the corresponding values and the different principle of separation most likely giving different fractions than ultracentrifugation, the dual precipitation methods have not found widespread acceptance.

The major difficulty with the determination of HDL cholesterol is that there is insufficient laboratory quality control. The HDL cholesterol measurement must be performed on serum or plasma before freezing. This somewhat hampers standardization. In addition, HDL are a mixture of many different molecular species of different origins, composition, and physical properties. Different methods for their isolation may thus give different results, and the particular physical chemical properties of the particles on which the different isolation procedures prior to quantitation are based may be altered in disease states.

Most of the epidemiological studies establishing the inverse relationship between low HDL cholesterol and the rate of incidence of CHD have used heparin/manganese precipitation followed by a nonenzymatic cholesterol method or a variant of this procedure. If EDTA plasma is used, the manganese concentration has to be doubled; if manganese ions are present in a sample undergoing an enzymatic cholesterol determination, it will form precipitates with the phosphate buffer and cause an interfering turbidity. This can be avoided by either chelating the manganese ions or by centrifugation of tube before reading.

The most popular method for HDL cholesterol measurement, the precipitation of apo B-containing lipoproteins (and Lp-X) by sodium phosphotungstate/magnesium chloride, gives lower values than heparin/$MnCl_2$ (more complete precipitation of apo E containing lipoproteins). Since guidelines for the interpretation of lipid values are based on the heparin procedure, the results of the phosphotungstate procedure have to be interpreted with caution. In addition to the two mentioned, precipitation methods already dextran sulfate and $MgCl_2$ are also sometimes used. Apo B-containing lipoproteins can also be precipitated by suitable concentrations of polyethyleneglycol (PEG). With all these methods, slightly different HDL cholesterol measurements are obtained, even if the same cholesterol assay is used. Interlaboratory standardization is therefore difficult.

PEG can also be used to precipitate, in addition to apo B-containing lipoproteins, a fraction roughly corresponding to HDL_2. HDL_3-like lipoproteins remain in the supernatant and their lipids can be quantitated. Such a differential precipitation can also be achieved by different concentrations of dextrane sulfate. HDL_2 lipid concentrations can then be calculated as the difference between total HDL lipids and HDL_3 lipids. The quantifiable lipids are predominantly cholesterol and phospholipids. HDL triglycerides or HDL_3 triglycerides cannot be reliably quantitated without concomitant determination of the free glycerol concentration in the samples, since, in addition to the corresponding lipoproteins these fractions contain all other constituents of the serum under investigation.

The PEG method is suitable for clinical use. However, there is considerable variation in the reference ranges for HDL subfractions with the different methods and from various laboratories. This indicates that there is no universally valid definition of HDL_2 or HDL_3 subfractions.

Evaluation of Concentrations

For men aged 45–49 years, the average HDL cholesterol level is 45 mg/dl, with the bottom decile below 33 mg/dl and the top decile above 66 mg/dl. For women, the average is 56 mg/dl, and the corresponding deciles are below 39 mg/dl and above 78 mg/dl. Up to puberty, both sexes show the same avcrage level (58 mg/dl); after puberty, the level drops by about 10–15 mg/dl and stays in that region throughout adult llfe (testosterone effect). Physiological estrogen levels are apparently not a major factor contributing to differences in HDL cholesterol between the sexes, since women retain the same levels throughout their lives.

Levels of HDL cholesterol are inversely correlated with the risk of CHD [80, 85, 165]. This inverse relationship has been noted in many epidemiological studies and is particularly strong in high-risk populations, such as in the United States and Northern Europe. In these populations, low HDL cholesterol levels and high LDL cholesterol concentrations are equally important predictors of CHD. Prospective studies in the United States [87] showed taht, for every decrease of 1 mg/dl in HDL cholesterol concentrations, the risk of CHD increases by 2%–3%. Because of the growing evidence for a link between low HDL levels and CHD, the NCEP has acknowledged low HDL cholesterol as a major risk factor and has recently [65] put increased emphasis on HDL levels for identifying and treating high-risk patients. An increased risk of CHD is associated with an HDL cholesterol concentration below 35 mg/dl (for women, 45 mg/dl) [64].

Very low Density Lipoprotein Cholesterol

VLDL cholesterol concentration is the best measure of an endogenous hypertriglyceridemia. It is largely unaffected by the presence of CM and its direct determination is a prerequisite for the precise and accurate determination of LDL cholesterol using the LRC procedure. Measurement of VLDL cholesterol is best performed by ultracentrifugation and not by the common form of quantitative LPE, since Lp(a) also migrates in the pre-β-position. The calculation of VLDL cholesterol by dividing the total triglycerides by 5 is a rough estimate of the VDL cholesterol concentration. It is strongly dependent on the absence of CM and on the presence of sufficient LDL and HDL to account for at least 40 mg/dl triglycerides, otherwise the calculated value is too low, since the ratio of triglycerides to the enzymatically determined cholesterol in VLDL is approximately 4.2. The VLDL cholesterol concentration does not normally exceed 30 mg/dl.

Low-Density Lipoprotein Cholesterol

A positive relationship between total serum cholesterol levels and risk of CHD has been established [207]. Many studies on experimental animals, including primates, have shown that diet-induced hypercholesterolemia produces arterial lesions resembling human atherosclerosis [9, 151, 209, 210]. Several epidemiological studies, including those carried out between different populations [122, 124], within populations [8, 86], and in migrating populations [116], subsequently revealed a positive association between serum cholesterol and rates of CHD.

The causal relationship between the total cholesterol concentration in serum and premature CHD is mainly due to the concentrations of the atherogenic lipoproteins LDL, IDL. and Lp(a). The inclusion of the protective HDL cholesterol in the total cholesterol concentration weakens this relationship somewhat. However, since the HDL cholesterol concentration in comparison to total cholesterol remains fairly constant, the overall effect is limited. In some cases, however, it is highly desirable to know the concentrations of LDL cholesterol and HDL cholesterol. Since LDL are found in a density class between VLDL and HDL, they cannot be isolated in a single-step procedure by ultracentrifugation. The most laborious procedure for the determination of LDL cholesterol involves elimination of VLDL by floatation in the ultracentrifuge at the density of serum water (d=1.006 g/ml) followed by floation of the LDL density class at a density of 1.063 g/ml. This leads to the isolation of all lipoproteins present in the density range between 1.006 and 1.063 g/ml and allows an estimate of the contribution of the lipoproteins of the LDL density class to the total serum cholesterol concentration. However, to this end these lipoproteins have to be recovered completely, burt complete recovery is difficult to achieve with sequential ultracentrifugation. Thus precision and accuracy of this expensive procedure are rather poor. A generally accepted procedure consists in elimination of VLDL by ultracentrifugation, followed by determination of the relevant lipids and apolipoproteins in the infranatant [158]. The LDL are then eliminated from this fraction by polyanion precipitation [31, 32], and the same measurements are performed on the same serum specimen after removal of VLDL and LDL. The concentrations of the corresponding parameters of the LDL fraction are determined by subtraction. This method for the determination of LDL cholesterol has been recommended by the National Institutes of Health (NIH) in the United States and the World Health Organization (WHO) worldwide. In addition to the concentration of the LDL parameters, those of HDL (directly) and VLDL (by subtraction of the values obtained in VLDL-free serum from those of the corresponding whole serum) can also be determined. The isolated VLDL fraction is most suitable for determining concentration ratios of VLDL lipids and proteins. In addition, its examination by isoelectric focusing allows simple and inexpensive determination of the apo E phenotype. Using sodium dodecyl sulfate (SDS) gel electrophoresis for the detection of apo B_{48}, the VLDL fraction can be examined for the presence of CM or their remnants. However, similar to sequential ultracentrifugation, this procedure also does not yield Lp-B, the major lipoprotein of the LDL density class. This lipoprotein corresponds to apo B in its lipid-binding form and does not contain apo C, apo E, or any other apolipoproteins.

The fraction is contaminated with Lp(a) and other lipoproteins of the LDL density class, mainly IDL. A fraction free of Lp(a) can, however, be obtained electrophoretically, since Lp(a) does not exhibit β-mobility [168].

The determination of LDL cholesterol alone, but not of the other LDI lipids and apolipoproteins, can be further simplified by calculation instead of determination. To this end, the total cholesterol, total triglycerides, and HDL cholesterol concentrations are required. Assuming that the cholesterol present in the VLDL density class (formerly eliminated by ultracentrifugation) can be estimated by dividing the trigylceride concentration by 5, this calculated value together with the HDL cholesterol can be subtracted from total cholesterol to obtain the LDL cholesterol concentration (Friedewald formula [69]).

Examination of many thousands of isolated VLDL fractions has showed that the ratio of triglycerides to cholesterol is relatively constant, provided CM are absent. CM, if present, are usually ultracentrifugally coisolated together with VLDL. Since the majority of serum triglycerides are usually found within the VLDL fraction, division of triglycerides by a constant (e.g., 5.0) gives a good estimate of VLDL cholesterol. The ratio of triglycerides to cholesterol in the VLDL fraction is below 5, however, and not all triglycerides are exclusively present in this fraction. Nevertheless, the contribution of all other serum lipoproteins to the total triglyceride concentrationlies is fairly reproducible (range, 30–40 mg/dl). The division of the serum triglyceride concentration by 5 therefore establishes the VLDL cholesterol concentration fairly accurately, provided abnormal triglyceride-rich lipoproteins and CM are absent from the serum.

The ratio of triglycerides to cholesterol in CM lies over 20. Thus in postprandial states, LDL cholesterol concentrations calculated with the Friedewald formula will be underestimated. In addition, in patients with a serum triglyceride concentration above 400 mg/dl, the VLDL are enriched in triglycerides and the Friedewald formula is not applicable.

A further simple method for the determination of LDL cholesterol is based on the simple, semiselective precipitation of LDL from the serum. LDL cholesterol can then be calculated as the difference between the cholesterol concentrations of the serum before and after precipitation. Alternatively, it can be directly determined after dissolving the precipitate in a buffer with a volume corresponding to the volume of the precipitated serum. Determination of the triglyceride concentration in the precipitate, however, reveals that varying amounts of VLDL are coprecipitated. If one has to rely on a simple procedure, calculation of LDL cholesterol according to the Friedewald formula is far superior, since in this case the precipitation step separates LDL and VLDL from HDL and gives at least one pure, clinically significant lipoprotein fraction.

The LDL cholesterol concentration can easily be determined along with other lipoproteins, provided that the lipoproteins can be separated from each other by quantitative LPE.

LDL cholesterol should always be determined when total cholesterol exceeds 200 mg/dl.

Increases in the LDL cholesterol concentration are due to primary and secondary causes. The primary genetic causes include familial hypercholesterolemia, familial defective B_{100}, and combined familial hyperlipemia. Most causes of increased LDL cholesterol concentrations are polygenic [213], including homozygosity for E_4 [47, 63] and a genetic polymorphism at apo B locus [1].

Secondary causes include hypothyroidism (especially in postmenopausal women), nephrotic syndrome, and cholestatic liver diseases. In children, familial hypercholesterolemia can be mimicked by sitosterolemia.

Calibration and quality control of the methods for the determination of LDL cholesterol are not easy to carry out, since there is no standard exhibiting higher concentrations of native LDL. Such a standard would, however, be a prerequisite for quality control of the separation steps. Control sera which have been freeze-dried very gently, are available. These materials are suitable for quality control of quantitative LPE.

Standard materials for the determination of HDL cholesterol usually contain only trace amounts of LDL and cannot be used as a control in LDL measurements. The separation step and the cholesterol determination together show day to day variation in CV of more than 3%. Determining LDL cholesterol with an accuracy of ± 5 mg/dl is therefore hardly feasible.

Intermediate-Density Lipoproteins

IDL are found in the density range of 1.006–1.019 g/ml. During normal ultracentrifugation, they sediment together with LDL. The only way to determine IDL cholesterol is by sequential ultracentrifugation. In LPE they form the front of the β-band or trail behind the pre-β-band. The concentration of LDL triglycerides provides a rough estimate of the IDL concentration.

Low-Density Lipoprotein Triglycerides

LDL triglycerides have been found to be a sensitive discriminator between patients with angiographically proven CHD and matched controls without angiographically demonstrable CHD. Patients with atherogenic conditions such as non-insulin-dependent diabetes mellitus (NIDDM) and chronic hemodialysis typically have relatively high concentrations of LDL triglycorides (> 40 mg/dl). LDL triglycerides are determined by ultracentrifugation in exactly the same way as LDL cholesterol. In our laboratory, LDL cholesterol is always determined together with LDL triglycerides. An increase in the LDL triglyceride concentration can also be due to the presence of considerable amounts of small, dense LDL. Since both IDL and small, dense LDL can be considered atherogenic lipoproteins, the determination of LDL triglycerides is very meaningful, provided it can be done with sufficient precision. The upper limit of the reference range is 28 mg/dl.

Since the LDL triglyceride concentration is determined by subtraction of two concentrations before and after polyanion precipitation of the same sample, interfering substances such as free glycerol are present in both samples and will cancel each other out. The method is therefore sufficiently precise.

LDL triglycerides are not very stable and cannot be determined in frozen serum.

Interpretation of Lipid and Lipoprotein Concentrations

Even in normal populations, the concentrations of lipoproteins cover a wide range. The normal range is usually defined as cholesterol values less than a maximum or greater than a minimum of 2.5% (mean ± 2 SD) of all values determined in an apparently healthy population, respectively. Based on this definition, a serum cholesterol level of 260 mg/dl would still be considered normal in our society. In contrast, the majority of factory workers in Wuhan would "suffer" from abnormally low cholesterol values (the upper limit there is 150 mg/dl).

Since it is not the concentration of total cholesterol, but the concentration of LDL cholesterol which conveys the risk of CHD, a threshold value for LDL cholesterol of 155 mg/dl has been established by the guidelines of the European Atherosclerosis Society [64]. An increased risk of CHD is also attributed to an HDL cholesterol concentration below 35 mg/dl (for women, 45 mg/dl) [64].

This LDL cholesterol value is exceeded by about 40% of 40–60-years-old Germans (male and female). The combination of increased LDL and decreasod HDL less frequent, affecting an additional 7% of the population.

The most recent guidelines regarding the clinical management of lipid disorders have been published in the United States as part of the second report of the NCEP Expert Panel on Detection, Evaluation, and Treatment of High Blood Cholesterol in A [65]. The guidelines are based on the determination of total cholesterol triglycerides and HDL cholesterol. The subsequent determination of LDL cholesterol is recommended if HDL cholesterol is below 35 mg/dl or total cholesterol above 240 mg/dl ("high blood cholesterol"). The LDL cholesterol concentration should ideally be below 130 mg/dl, and "high-risk" LDL cholesterol starts at 160 mg/dl. Depending on accompanying risk factors (two or more), an LDL cholesterol concentration of between 130 and 160 mg/dl is also considered to require lipid-lowering therapy. For symptomatic patients, the optimal LDL cholesterol eoneentration is below 100 mg/dl. The triglyceride concentration is considered normal if it is below 200 mg/dl; 1000 mg/dl is considered very high, with 400 mg/dl representing the borderline value.

Atherogenic Lipoproteins

Since the concomitant elevation of both cholesterol and triglycerides is predictive of future atherosclerotic disease, atherogenic lipoproteins containing either cholesterol or triglycerides or both must be present in these patients. The paradigm of such lipoproteins are β-VLDL, one of the most atherogenic lipoprotein known today [26]. β-VLDL originates from CM and VLDL, and its concentration in blood is increased due to overproduction of VLDL in combination with a decreased clearance of remnants of VLDL and CM.

In additon to an elevation of single lipoprotein species such as β-VLDL and LDL cholesterol, the chemical nature of serum lipoproteins not present in high concentrations or the presence of combinations of particular lipoprotein patterns also appear to predispose individuals to premature CHD. An example of such an atherogenic dyslipoproteinemia is the combination of increased IDL, elevated small, dense LDL, and low HDL cholesterol.

A hallmark of this condition is an elevated concentration of LDL triglycerides, since both IDL and small dense LDL contain relatively more triglycerides compard to normal LDL. Consistent with this observation is the fact that the LDL triglyceride concentration shows a strong correlation with the presence of CHD and that individuals without CHD show low concentrations of LDL triglycerides. The major causes of secondary atherogenic dyslipoproteinemias such as chronic renal failure with hemodialysis, hemofiltration, or continuous ambulatory peritoneal dialysis and diabetes mellitus are associated with an increase in the LDL triglyceride concentration.

The normal range of LDL triglycerides is below 28 mg/dl. When LDL triglycerides are increased in hypertriglyceridemia, this condition has to be regarded as atherogenic. LDL triglycerides are typically increased when the concentrations of LDL_2 and/or IDL and/or small, dense LDL are increased. The presence of β-VLDL, which is in also part found in the LDL_1 range, leads to a marked increase in LDL triglycerides. Small, dense LDL particles are relatively enriched in triglycerides and are associated with an increased risk of CHD. However, their atherogenic role has still to be confirmed by prospective cohort studies. These particles also appear to be an integral feature of the atherogenic insulin resistance syndrome. The concentration of IDL and of small, dense LDL can best be measured by density gradient ultracentrifugation.

LDL triglycerides can be determined by the LCR procedure and by quantitative LPE (β-triglycerides).

A number of prospective and case-control studies suggest that serum triglyceride levels are positively correlated with CHD. In multivariate analyses, total cholesterol and HDL cholesterol are dominant because of their closer links with CHD. Triglycerides retain their independent risk factor status only in a limited number of studies [16].

Fasting triglyceride levels mainly reflect the concentration of VLDL particles. Some of these particles may be more atherogenic than others. Large triglyceride-rich VLDL appear less atherogenic than small, relatively cholesterol-rich VLDL. The latter are increased in familial combined hyperlipidemia [132] and in NIDDM [28].

Hypertriglyceridemia may also indirectly induce atherogenic conditions [96]. Elevated VLDL may cause a delay in the hydrolysis of CM triglycerides or compete for apo E, thereby promoting a longer residence time of CM remnants, which, when enriched with CE, may become atherogenic. Hypertriglyceridemia also promotes the formation of the atherogenic small, dense LDL [29–31] and is associated with low levels of HDL cholesterol.

LDL particles are considered the major culprit for the development of myocardial infarction as exemplified by the premature death of patients with familial hypercholesterolemia. In addition to their concentration, composition also appears relevant in atherogenesis. The content of antioxidants, triglycerides, and hydrophobic substances not yet identified should be considered. A reduction in the LDL concentration induced by either changes in lifestyle or by drugs has been shown to reduce the frequency of coronary events in symptomatic patients. LDL are best quantified by the LRC procedure or by quantitative LPE. The Friedewald formula is best suited for an initial estimate of the LDL cholesterol concentration. Subsequent therapeutic efforts should be monitored by more direct methods that also allow the composition of LDL to be investigated.

Lp(a) considerably increases coronary risk, particularly in familial hypercholesterolemia patients [195], indicating that, at low levels of LDL cholesterol, Lp(a) may be less atherogenic.

Lp(a) promotes CHD by a number of possible mechanisms. It binds to plasminogen-binding sites on blood clots and cell surfaces, thereby inhibiting the activation of plasminogen and possibly preventing clot lysis to some extent. Inhibition of plasminogen prevents activation of the proteinase plasmin. Plasmin can activate transforming growth factor-β (TGF-β), a multipotential cytokine that, in its activated form, inhibits cell proliferation [90, 127]. By this mechanism, Lp(a) contributes to cell proliferation in the vessel wall and to migration of cells in the atherosclerotic plaque. Lp(a) can also contribute to lipid uptake by macrophages.

Determination of Apolipoproteins

Some authors believe that measurement of apolipoproteins may be as reliable as measurement of lipoproteins in assessment of the risk of CHD. Supporting evidence has been provided by studies suggesting that patients with atherosclerosis may be better distinguished by increased plasma apo B levels rather than by decreased HDL cholesterol and increased LDL cholesterol levels.

Besides the possible value of measurement of the four major apolipoproteins A-I, A-II, apo B, and apo E, the measurement of a number of minor apolipoproteins may have clinical uses. For example, studies on patients with chronic renal failure and consequently an increased risk of CHD seem to suggest that apo A-IV and B_{48}, as well as an abnormal distribution of apo C and E, have a role in the atherogenic process.

The apolipoproteins of clinical interest are apo B, A-I, apo E, and apo(a). Apo B and apo A-I are present in the serum in quite high concentrations (approximately 100 mg/dl). Apo B is the major structural apolipoprotein of VLDL and LDL. Except in type V hyperlipoproteinemia, up to 90% of the total apo B in the plasma is present in the the LDL density class. Approximately 70% of apo B occurs as Lp-B, the major apo B-containing lipoprotein.

The concentration of apo E bears a close relationship with familial dysbetalipoproteinemia. In this condition, the concentration of apo B-containing serum lipoproteins enrichcd in apo E prevails over that of those poor in apo E. Consequently, the ratio of apo E to apo B in the serum is increased.

Apo(a) is the part of Lp(a) which differentiates these particles from Lp-B. Consequently, the immunological determination of Lp(a) is based on the immunoassay of apo(a).

Although it is also a component of CM, apo A-I is almost exclusively confined to the HDL density class.

Apo B and apo A-I can easily be determined by turbidimetric assays performed by routine clinical chemical analyzers.

Production of specific antibodies and calibration of the assays is, however, not a trivial matter [39]. All the relevant apolipoproteins show polymorphisms, and an antiserum may not react identically with all the isoforms. In addition, it is questionable whether all apolipoproteins of a given lipoprotein are accessible for the antibody. This 90%–95% of the apo A-I in HDL may be masked by lipids.

Apolipoproteins in solution (if they are completely solubilized at all) tend to self-aggregate. This makes them difficult calibrators and tracers, and secondary calibrators are necessary.

In our opinion, the concentration of apolipoproteins is not a better predictor of the risk of CHD than the concentration of lipoprotein lipids. Due to the lack of reference values and the lack of prospective studies, the determination of apolipoproteins has not yet found widespread use in routine laboratories.

Methods

Apolipoprotein assays can be performed by a number of established immunochemical techniques. These include radial immunodiffusion (RID), electroimmunoassay ("rocket" electrophoresis), enzyme-linked immunosorbentassay (ELISA), fluorescence immunoassay (FIA), radioimmunoassay (RIA), immunonephelometry (INA), and turbidometric immunoasay (TIA).

Radial Immunodiffusion

RID is a slow, unprecise, and rather insensitive procedure. It needs comparatively large sample volumes, and pretreatment of samples is often advisable. The diffusion process takes 2–3 days. Since the gel has no true properties of a molecular sieve, in the case of determination of apo B, the outer rim of the not yet fully developed diffusion ring by no means consists of a precipitate of only LDL apo B and the antibody. Using this technique, a condition called hyperapobetalipoproteinemia (LDL with an unusual high content of apo B) has been postulated and introduced in the literature. However, in our opinion the true occurrence of this condition appears questionable.

Electroimmunoassay

EIA is a much more rapid and slightly more sensitive immunoprecipitation technique than RID. It is, however, more complicated, since rocket formation depends on the duration of electrophoresis, properties of the agarose gel (electroendosmosis), the buffer, and the concentration of polyethyleneglycol. The need to pretreat samples depends on the properties of the antibody. The precision for A-I and apo B in the reference range is not satisfactory (CV of 10%). For apo E and other apolipoproteins found in lower concentrations, the CV is between 10% and 15%.

Enzyme-linked Immunosorbentassay

ELISA procedures have been developed for all relevant apolipoproteins and Lp(a). The competitive assays require a labeled apolipoprotein with the concomitant problems of self-aggregation and instability. Sandwich procedures, in which the second antibody is labeled, avoid these problems. In contrast to most other immunoassays, monoclonal antibodies can be used. The assay does not require much time, sample volume, or antiserum. The precision is acceptable (CV usually less than 10%). Because the ELISA depends on several dilution steps, temperature, and other imponderabilities, it is not the method of choice in routine evaluations. With the sandwich ELISA, it is possible to measure the concentration of lipoprotein particles characterized by the presence of two different apolipoproteins. For instance, in order to determine the amount of particles containing both apo B and apo E (present mostly in the VLDL class, but also in the LDL class), the particles can be isolated from the specimen by immobilization to a surface by the first antibody (e.g., anti-apo-E). Quantitation is then accomplished by the second antibody (e.g., anti-apo B). Using this technique, Lp(a) particles can be quantified irrespective of the number of kringles. The further quantitative subdivision of HDL in particles containing or lacking A-II has also become possible using this technique [5].

Immunonephelometry and Turbidimetric Assays

Antigen-antibody complexes (AAC) scatter or absorb light. The intensity of the two optical phenomena depends on the number of insoluble AAC complexes, which at fixed antibody concentrations reflects the amount of apoliprotein present in the sample. This technique can be performed in two different modes, at equilibrium or by a kinetic mode. In the equilibrium mode, antigen must be in excess, while the kinetic mode requires an excess of antibody. The most commonly used assay for apo A and apo B is the turbidimetric method, since it can easily be automated.

Lipoprotein (a)

The determination of Lp(a) presents some peculiar difficulties. Size and structural heterogeneity of apo(a) have confounding effects on the measurement of Lp(a). In spite of the proliferation of attempts to determine Lp(a), the standardization of methods is still in its infancy. Proper and reliable standardization, however, is a prerequisite to determine the relationship between Lp(a) levels and the risk of CHD in different populations and to establish population-based reference values.

Initially, Lp(a) was determined qualitatively using immuno double diffusion [42, 44, 234], countercurrent immunoelectrophoresis, and electrophoretically as "sinking pre-β lipoprotein" [24, 43, 183] or as pre-β lipoprotein [41, 42, 44, 110, 178]. The antisera were obtained by immunization with Lp(a)-positive human sera with subsequent absorption of all undesired antibodies using Lp(a)-negative sera. At this time, an indidividual was either Lp(a) positive or Lp(a) negative. Later, quantitative immunological methods were employed, such as RID [5, 6, 42], electroimmunoassay [34, 58, 73, 74, 99, 128, 174] and enzyme immunoassay [56, 74, 136, 233].

The immunological quantitation of Lp(a) only measures the apo(a) part. Since the size of this component of the particle can vary considerably, it is not feasible to base any conclusions concerning the amount of Lp(a) particles in any material on the apo(a) value [75, 225]. In addition, all limitations regarding the determination of apolipoproteins have to be taken in account. Since there is a strong cross-reactivity of older antisera against Lp(a) with plasminogen, older reports in the literature concerning the quantitation of Lp(a) have to be interpreted with caution.

At present, Lp(a) is mostly determined by EIA (rocket electrophoresis), ELISA, and RIA. All methods are commercially available. Recently, turbidimetric assays have been developed, which can be performed on any modern clinical chemical analyzer. The cutoff point considered to be associated with increased risk of atherosclerosis is 30 mg Lp(a)/dl. As outlined above, it is difficult to assign to this value a certain number of Lp(a) particles, mainly for two reasons: (1) the amount of apo(a) per particle is variable and (2) no analytical method has thus far been sufficiently standardized.

The antibodies used in the assay must be characterized carefully, including the documentation of apo(a) domain specificity. In order to estimate the number of Lp(a) particles, the apo B content of Lp(a) has to be determined or antibodies have to be used detecting only the nonvariable epitopes of Lp(a). Assays that principally identify the repeat kringles of apo(a) should be expressed in terms of apo(a) mass. Suitable reference materials and reference methods need to be developed to harmonize Lp(a) values in terms of either Lp(a) particle number or apo(a) mass.

Using quantitative LPE, Lp(a) cholesterol can be easily quantitated. It remains to be seen whether Lp(a) cholesterol has the same clinical significance as the particle number. Since Lp(a) transports per particle as much cholesterol as Lp-B, the Lp(a) cholesterol concentration may be an adequate measure for the number of Lp(a) particles. All Lp(a) isoforms migrate with pre-β-mobility.

Hyperlipoproteinemias

Some hyperlipoproteinemias are due to abnormalities in the metabolism of lipoproteins. the so-called primary hyperlipoproteinemias. Other hyperlipoproteinemias are only one of many manifestations of a metabolic disorder. so-called secondary hyperlipoproteinemias.

Primary disorders are either genetic (familial) or nongenetic (sporadic). The genetic hyperlipoproteinemias are either monogenic or polygenic.

For practical purposes, several consecutive classification systems of hyperlipoproteinemias have been advanced in recent years. The most recent was published in March 1994 [65].

The first step in diagnosis of hyper- and hypolipoproteinemias is to define a phenotype or plasma lipoprotein pattern by chemical analysis of plasma for lipids and lipoproteins. The information obtained by this analytic step will not define a homogeneous disease entity and additional testing will be necessary to establish a more precise diagnosis and the individual risk of atherosclerotic disease.

Classification of Dyslipoproteinemias

The classification of lipoprotein disorders began with the system of Fredrickson and Lees [68]. Since then, it has been declared obsolete several times, but in our experience Fredrickson's types continue to be important tools because (a) they allow sharp focus on a diverse groups of metabolic abnormalities related to the hyperlipoproteinemias, (b) they identify hyperlipoproteinemias not as specific disease states, but as disorders that affect concentrations of particular lipoproteins in a similar way, (c) they associate a majority of lipoprotein types with certain distinct clinical features, and (d) they provide a basis for successful approaches to diet and drug therapy for a majority of lipoprotein disorders regardless of the etiology.

The major limitation of Fredrickson's system is its tendency to group etiologically heterogeneous disease states together. For example, hyperchylomicronemia (Fredrickson's type I) can be due to either LPL deficiency or C-II deficiency.

In addition, the system neither assigns roles for HDL or individual apolipoproteins nor does it take into account significant changes in plasma phenotypes that occur with alterations in diet, use of drugs or alcohol, or state of general health. The major reason for the recommendation of its discontinuation were the somewhat pretentious Roman numerals, which imply a well-defined separate genetic origin of each type, as is the case, for example, in glycogen storage diseases.

Despite these shortcomings, the underlying rationale of Fredrickson's system, with its emphasis on plasma lipoprotein concentrations, remains an important element of classification.

The hallmark of a hyperlipidemia is a turbid serum sample. Turbidity is caused by triglyceride-rich lipoproteins, and the major triglyceride-rich lipoproteins exhibit different electrophoretic mobilities (Fig. 4). Five of the six different pheno types of hyperlipidemia are characterized by a turbid serum.

The phenotypes (I–V) identified by lipid measurements and a visual evaluation of an electrophoretic pattern are by no means all genetic entities; type I (CM present because of a hereditary lack of the LPL or the activating C-II) and type III (broad β-band caused by a delayed catabolism of remnants of CM and VLDL and hence their accumulation in the serum due to homozygosity of E_2 and an unknown additional condition) come close to it. What remains are type II, type IV, and type V. In type II, the most slowly migrating lipoproteins accumulate (β-lipoproteins, LDL), all associated with hypercholesterolemia. In addition to hypercholesterolemia, accumulation of VLDL also lead to hypertriglyceridemia (type IIb in contrast to the normotriglyceridemic type IIa). Type IV is due to an accumulation of VLDL (pre-β-lipoproteins migrating one step further than β-lipoproteins), and type V represents a combination of type IV and type I.

It soon became clear that the different phenotypes do not represent genotypes and that hyperlipoproteinemias can also be secondary to other diseases. Since a classification of dyslipoproteinemias should lead to clear therapeutical concepts and therapy often must start at lipid concentrations not yet characteristic of a distinct hyperlipoprotenemia, other classification systems have evolved.

A contemporary classification of dyslipoproteinemias is shown in Table 5. It is an extension of Fredrickson's or the National Heart, Lung, and Blood Institute (NHLB) classification, which describes particular patterns of lipid and lipoprotein levels that have strong associations with clinical disease.

Table 5. Classification and characterization of primary hyperlipoproteins

Type	Genetic classification	Affected lipoprotein	Appearance of serum	Triglycerides (mg/dl)	Cholesterol (mg/dl)	CHD risk
I	Familial defect of LDL or of CII	Chylomicrons	Lactescent; clear with creamy layer[a]	> 1000	< 500	No
IIa	Familial hypercholesterolemia Familial combined hyperlipemia	LDL	Clear	Normal	230–600 (heterozygote) 600–1200 (homozygote)	Yes
IIb	Familial combined hyperlipemia	LDL and VLDL	Clear or slightly turbid	200–500	300–600	Yes
III	Familial dysbetalipoproteinemia	IDL	Turbid	300–900	295–500	Yes
IV	Familial hypertriglyceridemia Familial combined hyperlipemia	VLDL	Turbid	250–1000	Normal or slightly elevated	Yes together with other risk factors
V	-	VLDL and chylomicrons	Turbid; turbid with a creamy layer[a]	> 1000	> 250	-

LDL, low-density lipoproteins; VLDL, very low density lipoproteins; IDL, intermediate-density lipoproteins; CHD, coronary heart disease.
[a] First appearance when fresh; second appearance when left overnight in a refrigerator.

Primary Hyperlipoproteinemias

The different genetic backgrounds of primary hyperlipoproteinemias lead to different ages of patients at manifestation of the disorder. Monogenic conditions such as defects of the enzyme LPL, a deficiency of the activator of this enzyme (apo C-II), and a defect in the proper binding and internalization of LDL by hepatocytes and other cells are rare causes of a hyperlipemia and already become manifest in infancy. The same is true for deficiencies of other enzymes such as LCAT or HTGL. Deficiencies of apolipoproteins (except apo E,) usually lead to hypolipidemias. The vast majority of dyslipidemias develop in middle-aged patients. The earlier they are detected, the more likely is a genetic background. Diseases such as familial combined hyperlipidemia, familial hypertriglyceridemia, and familial dysbetalipoproteinemia (type III hyperlipoproteinemia) are hyperlipemias with a strong genetic component. They still comprise only a minority of dyslipidemias. In many common diseases of middle life such as diabetes mellitus, hypertension, and CHD, genetic factors are operative. The same probably holds true for dyslipidemias. It is assumed that many unspecified genes acting together with environmental factors are operative in the etiology of these disorders. The biologic action of the involved genes remains largely unknown. In addition to these polygenic hyperlipidemias, sporadic forms also occur. The most common monogenic forms are familial deficiency of LPL, familial C-II deficiency, familial type III hyperlipoproteinemia, familial hypercholesterolemia, familial defective apo B_{100}, familial hypertriglyceridemia, and familial combined hyperlipoproteinemia.

Monogenic Primary Hyperlipoproteinemias

Familial Deficiency of Lipoprotein Lipase. Autosomal recessive deficiency of LPL leads to a defect in the catabolism of triglyceride-rich lipoproteins and to an excessive hypertriglyceridemia (types I und V) [188]. The fasting serum contains CM, VLDL, are slightly elevated, and HDL markedly decreased. Heterozygotes have decreased activity of LPL, but mostly normal serum lipids. The diagnosis is established by determining the postheparin lipolytic activity (injection of heparin and subsequent exmination of the ability of the serum to hydrolyze an artificial substrate). The concentration of C-II is normal. The disease is clearly not associated with an increased risk for atherosclerotic disease. The major symptoms are abdominal cramps.

A deficiency of C-II, one of the three peptides of apo C, can also lead to the persistence of CM [23, 187]. The concentration of VLDL is also increased. The disease is inherited as an autosomal recessive trait. Heterozygotes have normal lipids, but decreased C-II. Treatment consists in the infusion of normal serum (containing sufficient quantities of C-II). Best known mutations cause a decrease or a complete lack of C-II. Only one missense mutation at the C-II locus is known so far (Thr-50), associated with chylomicronemia.

The clinical symptoms are indistinguishable from LPL deficiency. Many carriers of the LPL deficiency trait show no abnormality in the serum lipids. A thorough investigation of several large families with different mutations in the LPL gene indicate that some of the more common hyperlipidemias may indeed be due to heterozygosity for LPL deficiency [50, 164, 189/. A significant association exists between the carrier state and familial hypertriglyceridemia [72], familial combined hyperlipidemia [243], and postprandial lipemia [51].

Heterozygosity for LPL deficieney is as common as and in some areas even more prevalent [71] than the heterozygous state for familial hypercholesterolemia. The relatively high frequency of the carrier state of LPL deficiency may account – through mutations in LPL alone or additional interactions with either environmental or genetic factors – for a significant proportion of hyperlipidemias. It is unclear whether the carrier states predispose to premature CHD. Reduced activity in macrophages of the atherosclerotic lesion may reduce foam cell formation, since incorporated lipoproteins are degraded more slowly. The presence of LPL may promote the binding of atherogenic lipproteins to the subendothelial matrix. On the other hand, LPL-mediated lipoprotein uptake in the liver may enhance the catabolism of atherogenic lipoproteins.

Familial Dysbetalipoproteinemia (Type III Hyperlipoproteinemia) Familial dysbetalipoproteinemia is an autosomal recessive disorder characterized by the presence of an abnormal lipoprotein population. This population consists of remnants of CM and VLDL not normally present in the plasma [35, 36, 181]. Consequently, the serum concentration of apo E is increased.

The genetic defect lies in the homozygosity for apo E_2. Apo E is a ligand for the B_{100}:E receptor and for LRP. E_2 contains two cysteines at positions 112 and 158 and is therefore a poor ligand for these receptors. The triglyceride-rich particles accumulate in the circulation and are further enriched with CE. This apparently renders them atherogenic. β-VLDL are best detected by LPE. Their presence is confirmed by the demonstration of homozygosity for E_2.

The relatively long residence time of these abnormal triglyceride-rich particles in the blood leads to their marked enrichment with CE by CETP. Consequently, both triglycerides and cholesterol are elevated to values of up to 600 mg/dl. Since the abnormal particles are smaller than CM or VLDL, the turbidity of the serum is less pronounced. If the serum is kept in a glass tube which is held close to a newspaper, the text can usually still be read.

In LPE these lipoproteins lead to the formation of a large confluent zone in the β-region comprising the abnormal particles as well as LDL, IDL, and VLDL (broad β- disease). During ultracentrifugation at plasma density, the remnants partially float like VLDL, but still retain their slower electrophoretic mobility ("floating beta").

The disorder becomes apparent in early adulthood and is considered highly atherogenic [154, 155]. More than 90% of patients are homozygous for apo E_2. Although the prevalence of E_2 homozygotes in the population is about 1%, only 5% of these subjects develop type III hyperlipoproteinemia. The overall prevalence is therefore 0.05%. Thus it appears that, in addition to E_2 homozygosity, there must be other metabolic conditions predisposing patients to the full-blown disease [47, 91, 92, 155, 221, 223, 224]. Such conditions may either be other genetic defects of lipoprotein metabolism (e.g., familial combined hyperlipemia; see below) or secondary causes such as obesity, diabetes mellitus, hypothyroidism, or oral contraceptives.

The diagnosis can be made most easily by LPE and can be confirmed by determination of the VLDL lipids. The ratio of cholesterol to triglycerides is characteristically higher than 0.45.

A major feature of the disease is the rapid disappearance of the remnants after drug therapy with clofibrate or its derivatives. This, together with the homozygosity for apo E_2, is sufficient proof. Sometimes even a clear-cut type III hyperlipoproteinemia is not associated with this genetic trait. In all these cases, apo E of the particles has been found to be either nonexistent or a poor ligand for the receptors. It appears that in these patients apo E is abnormal and has a decreased affinity to the receptors 77, 149, 150, 156, 157, 160, 179, 211, 235–237, 239]. In addition to these rare mutants, two families have been found exhibiting a complete absence of apo E [76, 148, 191].

In these cases, the diagnosis is very likely made by isolation of the VLDL fraction and demonstration of enrichment in cholesterol (ratio of cholesterol to triglycerides in the VLDL fraction, > 0.45; normal, 0.25).

Type III hyperlipoproteinemia can also be due to a deficiency in hepatic lipase.

Familial Hypercholesterolemia. Familial hypercholesterolemia is one of the most common inherited metabolic disorders (frequency of heterozygotes, 1/500) [27]. It is inherited as an autosomal dominant trait. The defect lies in a malfunction of the LDL receptor [81]. About 5% of all patients with myocardial infarction before the age of 60 years are heterozygous for familial hypercholesterolemia. This corresponds to a 25-fold increased risk of premature CHD. However, 85% of heterozygotes have already had one myocardial infarction before the age of 60. The LDL cholesterol concentration of homozygotes is over 600 mg/dl (in heterozygotes, 230 – 450 mg/dl). The concentration of triglycerides is normal (Fredrickson's type IIa). The defect leads to impaired catabolism of LDL and to an increased production rate.

About 100 [105] different mutations of the receptor gene are now known [105]. Besides structural mutations of the receptor protein impairing the binding of lipoproteins, every stage of the metabolism of the receptor can be defective (synthesis, migration to the cell surface, anchoring in the cell membrane, and internalization) [83]. Because of this large number of possible defects, most "homozygotes" are actually "compound" heterozygotes [83].

In homozygous patients, the severity of the disease is mostly a consequence of the nature of the mutation at the LDL receptor locus [206, 217]. In heterozygous patients, many exogenous factors (age, gender, diet) and genetic polymorphisms of the two ligands of the receptor, apo E [63, 100, 224] and apo B [2, 100], exert additional effects.

Familial hypercholesterolemia is likely if the serum cholesterol concentration ranges between 350 and 450 mg/dl, xanthomas of the tendons are present, and half of the first-degree relatives suffer from hypercholesterolemia. The diagnosis can be definitively established by studying the interaction of LDL with cultivated skin fibroblasts of the patient. The heterogeneity of the disease and the complex structure of the gene make the DNA diagnosis difficult. Recently, a method has been developed for screening all 18 polymerase chain reaction (PCR)-amplified exons for mutations using denaturing gradient gel electrophoresis. Heterozygotes have to exhibit at least one mutation in one of the 18 exons.

Familial Defective Apo B_{100}. A mutation at position 3500 of apo B 100 leads to an autosomal dominant condition with a markedly lower (80%) affinity of apo B to the LDL receptor (familial defective apo B_{100} FDB) [109, 152, 220]. The low affinity is due to a substitution of glutamine for arginine at this position. FDB is one of the most common point mutations with metabolic consequences (prevalence, 2/1000). Heterozygotes have only moderate hypercholesterolemia (250 – 350 mg/dl). The serum cholesterol of the few homozygotes described so far is not much higher. Apparently, as long as the particles contain apo E they are recognized by the LDL receptor and the LDL precursors are eliminated sufficiently rapidly to avoid increased LDL production. This is in contrast to the form of familial hypercholesterolemia which is due to a receptor dysfunction.

The condition can be identified by partially defective binding of patients' LDL to normal fibroblasts or by allele-specific PCR.

Familial Hypertriglyceridemia. Familial hypertriglyceridemia is inherited as an autosomal dominant trait. It appears most frequently in the form of Fredrickson's type IV and rarely as type V hyperlipoproteinemia. Its frequency is about the same as that of familial hypercholesterolemia (1/500). The VLDL of the patients are enriched with triglycerides. This is probably due to an overproduction of triglycerides not accompanied by concomitant overproduction of apo B. This condition is frequently associated with impaired glucose tolerance, hyperuricemia, and arterial hypertension. The pathomechanism and genetic defect have not yet been determined. The diagnosis of familial hypertriglyceridemia is established only after exclusion of a secondary hypertriglyceridemia together with a corresponding family history. Since in these families hyperlipoproteinemias of Fredrickson's types IIa and IIb are absent, it is considered to be a separate entity and not a form of combined familial hyperlipemia.

Familial Combined Hyperlipemia. Familial combined hyperlipidemia (FCH) is one of the most common monogenetic disorders in humans, with a gene frequency assuming a single defect as high as 3 – 5/1000 [52, 54, 56, 212]. The clinical features of FCH are usually expressed after the third decade. A characteristic feature is the presence of multiple lipoprotein profiles in the patient and his or her affected relatives. This leads to Fredrickson's types IV, IIa, and IIb. According to the opinion of some authors, the characteristic features of the condition are elevated levels of apo B (> 130 mg/dl) and the presence of "dense" LDL particles relatively enriched in cholesterol (cholesterol to apo B ratio higher than 1.3). If hypertriglyceridemia prevails, HDL cholesterol is low.

The most important clinical sequela of FCH is the development of premature CHD, which is similar in severity and clinical course to the cardiovascular disease present in familial hypercholesterolemia heterozygotes. FCH is found in about 10 % of all survivors of myocardial infarction. Obesity, impaired glucose tolerance, and hyperuricemia are common. The disease is inherited as an autosomal dominant trait; however, the underlying cause is not known. An increased secretion of VLDL might play an important role. The diagnosis is established by family examination. Xanthomas almost never occcur.

No homozygotes for FCH have been identified. Many affected subjects may be patients with genetic compounds, containing two defective genes, one for FCH and another underlying genetic dyslipoproteinemia.

Polygenic ("Common") Hyperlipoproteinemia. In most cases of hypercholesterolemia (80 %), it is impossible to establish a molecular cause for the disease. Although it is called polygenic hypercholesterolemia, the underlying cause may still be an unknown monogenic one with a low expressivity. Probable candidate genes are those of all proteins involved with synthesis, secretion, and catabolism of lipoproteins. The relative contributions of these genes to hypercholesterolemia may vary from individual to individual. There is no sharp distinction between normocholesterolemia and polygenic hypercholesterolemia. The risk of premature CHD starts to increase markedly in both instances at serum cholesterol levels of 200 mg/dl [207].

Hyperapobetalipoproteinemia: "Small, Dense" Low-Density Lipoproteins. According to reports in the literature, patients with CHD often exhibit LDL particles with an unusually high content of apo B in comparison to their cholesterol content. This condition is called hyperapobetalipoproteinemia [93, 135, 137, 200, 201, 203]. According to our current knowledge, these particles have to be either lipid poor or the cholesterol must have been replaced by another lipid, most probably triglycerides. This leads to the formation of small, dense LDL. These particles rarely predominate sufficiently to markedly incrase the ratio of apo B to cholesterol in the LDL fraction. This condition can be induced by hypertriglyceridcmia [201, 215, 216], by continuos ambulatory pertoneal hemodialysis (CAPD) [202, 216], or by diabetes mellitus [93].

Based on the current recommendations, it is evident that Fredrickson's types are in the regions of high-risk LDL cholesterol and high triglycerides and that the recent guidelines also extent to lower-level lipid disorders not included in the typing system.

Roughly one third of all men between 40 and 60 years of age suffer from some type of hyperlipoproteinemia; the prevalence of hyperlipoproteinemias in women is about 20 %. In men, type IV hyperlipoproteinemia (pre-β-lipoprotein cholesterol above 30 mg/dl) accounts for 50 % of all cases of hyperlipoproteinemia; in women, it accounts only for 15 % of all cases. The type most frequently found in women is Fredrickson's type IIa (70 %). Type IIb is found in 10 % of men and 15 % of women. In men, 40 % of the hyperlipoproteinemias are of type IIa.

The prevalence of hyperlipoproteinemias in the general population is the sum of primary and secondary disturbances of lipid metabolism.

Secondary Hyperlipoprotinemias

There are several forms of secondary hyperlipoproleinemias. They originate from different pathologic conditions, from intake of certain drugs, or from certain habits, including overalimentation leading to obesity and alcohol abuse. They lead predominantly to type IV hyperlipoproteinemia. In severe alcoholics, HDL cholesterol is increased and drops within 2 weeks of cessation. It is a sensitive indicator of relapse. Fredrickson's type IV is commonly also found in diabetics and in patients suffering from chronic renal insufficiency or from the nephrotic syndrome. It is also a common consequence of chronic hemodialysis or continuous ambulatory peritoneal dialysis. It is sometimes due to oral contraceptives.

Secondary type IIa disease is often due to hypothyroidism or the nephrotic syndrome. In obstructive jaundice, a hypercholesterolemia can be found. The presence of Lp-X leads to an increase in free cholesterol and phospholipids.

The differentiation in secondary and primary hyperlipoproteinemias is sometimes not clear-cut. An acquired hyperlipoproteinemia may reveal some predisposing genetic factors. For instance, overnutrition manifests itself as hyperlipoproteinemia only in genetically susceptible subjects. Roughly 40% of all hyperlipoproteinemias are secondary forms.

Hypolipoproteinemias

Like hyperlipoproteinemias, hypolipoproteinemias can also be divided into primary and secondary forms. Whereas hyperlipoproteinemias are seldom due to an increase in HDL, hypolipoproteinemias are more often due to a decrease in HDL concentration.

A complete lack of HDL is a common feature of obstructive jaundice. It is sometimes also found in hepatic failure. Malaria can cause extremely low HDL levels.

Primary causes of lacking HDL are Tangier disease, LCAT deficiency, and defects in the gene for apo A-I.

A-I deficiency is a very rare disease. It is associated with premature CHD, planar xanthomas, and corneal opacifications. Levels in heterozygotes are significantly lower than normal [12]. To date, more than 50 different mutations have been found in the A-I gene on chromosome 11. Approximately 50 interfere with the synthesis of normal A-I. Mutations in the A-I gene occur at a frequency of 1:1000.

The genetically determined lack of LCAT activity in the blood leads to two different clinical conditions: LCAT deficiency and fish-eye disease. In these cases, dramatic corneal opacifications develop. LCAT deficiency also affects red blood cells and kidney cells, leading to hypochromic anemia with target cells and to renal failure. Both conditions are characterized by very low levels of HDL cholesterol and A-I. Interestingly, in fish-eye disease the diminished LCAT activity does not lead to a very low ratio of CE to free cholesterol, since the enzyme esterifies abnormally free cholesterol in VLDL and LDL.

The most nebulous cause of a deficiency of HDL is that underlying Tangier disease. To date, up to 50 patients with this disease are known. The major clinical signs are hyperplastic orange tonsils, neuropathy, and hepatosplenomegaly. Other clinical signs include corneal opacifications and abnormal erythrocytes (stomatocytes). HDL and A-I are deficient or almost deficient, total cholesterol is low, and triglycerides are slightly increased. This is accompanicd by CE accumulation in histiocytes.

Low levels of apo B containig lipoproteins are usually the consequence of severe illnesses. Critically ill patients or patients receiving parenteral nutrition show markedly decreased levels of LDL cholesterol.

Although the liver eliminates most of the LDL, in severe liver diseases the synthesis and secretion of apo B containing lipoproteins is apparently even more impaired. A common cause of a secondary decrease in LDL cholesterol is hyperthyroidism.

Deficieny of apo B-containing lipoproteins is either due to impaired synthesis of apo B or defective secretion of apo B-containing lipoproteins by intestine or liver. The former is the case in homozygous hypobetalipoproteinemia, and the latter in abetalipoproteinemia. Both conditions are very rare, but their study has provided valuable insights into the normal metabolism of apo B-containing lipoproteins.

Abetalipoprotcinemia (Bassen-Kornzweig syndrome) is characterized by acanthozytes (spiculated red blood cells) in the peripheral blood smear. The intestine is incapable of synthezing and secreting CM. This results in fat malabsorption and a deficiency of fat-soluble vitamins. The relative deficiency of vitamin E causcs neurological, muscular, and ocular symptoms and abnormalities (cerebellar ataxia). Patients are unable to walk by their mid-20s. Abetalipoproteinemia is caused by a deficiency of the microsomal triglyceride transfer protein, which usually transfers triglycerides into the lumen of the endoplasmic reticulum of cells of liver and intestinal mucosa [240]. Within the endoplasmic reticulum, the apo B of CM and VLDL is supplied with lipids in order to form lipoproteins.

Abetalipoproteinemia is characterized by extremely low concentrations of plasma lipids together with fat malabsorption or fat intolerance. Apo B is absent from the serum. The parents of children with abetalipoproteinemia have normal values for serum lipids and apo B.

In the other condition characterized by absence of apo B, the parents are heterozygous and show familial hypobetalipoproteinemia. The clinical presentation of the homozygotes is in most cases milder than that of abetalipoproteinemia. Hypobetalipoproteinemia results from mutations in the apo B gene which prevent the synthesis of a protein containing all the 4536 amino acids. The shorter the polypeptides, the poorer the capacity to bind lipids is. The lipid and lipoprotein concentrations are dependent on the length of the truncated molecules. The severe cases are similar to abetalipoproteinemia.

Another rare form of low concentrations of lipoproteins is the selective failure of enterocytes to form lipoproteins. In these patients, low concentrations of HDL and LDL are detected (Andersen's disease).

Recommendations

In all individuals over 30 years of age, at least total cholesterol, triglycerides, HDL cholesterol, and Lp(a) should be determined. If HDL cholesterol is below 35 mg/dl or if total cholesterol is above 240 mg/dl, further lipoprotein diagnostics are indicated. The LDL cholesterol has to be evaluated according to the most recent NCEP guidelines [65]. Elevated Lp(a) has likely to be considered as an additional risk factor. Marked hypercholesterolemias or hypertriglyceridemias should be characterized at the molecular level whenever possible. Therapy should be monitored at intervals of 3–6 months in order to evaluate the therapeutic response.

References

1. Aalto Setälä K, Gylling H, Helve E, Kovanen P, Miettinen TA, Turtola H, Kontula K (1989) Gentic ppolymorphism of the apolipoprotein B gene locus influences serum LDL cholesterol level in familial hypercholesterolemia. Hum Genet 82: 305–307
2. Abate N, Vega GL, Grundy SM (1993) Variability in cholesterol content and physical properties of lipoproteins B-100. Atherosclerosis 104: 159–171
3. Abell LL, Levey BB, Brodie BB, Kendall (1952) A simplified method for the estimation of total cholesterol in serum and demonstration of its specificity. J Biol Chem 195: 357–366
4. Alaupovic P, Lee DM, McConathy WJ (1972) Studies on the composition and structure of plasma lipoproteins. Distribution of lipoprotein families in major density classes of normal human plasma lipoproteins. Biochim Biophys Acta 260: 689–707
5. Albers JJ, Hazzard WR (1974) Immunochemical quantification of human plasma Lp(a) lipoprotein. Lipids 9: 15–26
6. Albers JJ, Wahl P, Hazzard WR (1974) Quantitative genetic studies of the human plasma Lp(a) lipoprotein. Biochem Genet 11: 4754–4786
7. Albers JJ, Adolphson JL, Hazzard WR (1977) Radioimmunoassay of human plasma Lp(a) lipoprotein. J Lipid Res 18: 331–338
8. Anderson KM, Castelli WP, Levy DL (1987) Cholesterol and mortality: 30 years of follow-up from the Framingham Study. JAMA 257: 2176–2180
9. Anitschkow N, Chalatow S (1913) Über experimentelle Cholesterinsteatose und ihre Bedeutung für die Entstehung einiger pathologischer Prozesse. Zbl Allg Pathol Pathol Anat 24: 1–9
10. Armstrong VW, Walli AK, Seidel D (1985) Isolation, characterization, and uptake in human fibroblasts of an apo(a)-free lipoprotein obtained on reduction of lipoprotein(a). J Lipid Res 26: 1314–1323
11. Armstrong VW, Harrach B, Robenek H, Helmhold M, Walli AK, Seidel D (1990) Heterogeneity of human lipoprotein Lp(a): cytochemical and biochemical studies on the interaction of two Lp(a) species with the LDL receptor. J Lipid Res 31: 429–441
12. Assmann G, von Eckardstein A, Funke H (1992) The role of apolipoprotein mutants in HDL metabolism. In: Rosseneu MY (ed) Structure and function of apolipoproteins. CRC, Boca Raton, pp 85–121
13. Aufenanger J, Haux P, Weber U, Kattermann R (1988) A specific method for the direct determination of lipoproteincholesterol in electrophoretic patterns. Clin Chim Acta 177: 197–208
14. Austin MA, Breslow JL, Hennekens CH, Buring JE, Willett WC, Krauss RM (1988) Low-density lipoprotein subclass patterns and risk of myocardial infarction. JAMA 260: 1917–1921
15. Austin MA, King MC, Vranizan KM, Newman B, Krauss RM (1988) Inheritance of low-density lipoprotein subclass patterns: results of complex segregation analysis. Am J Hum Genet 43: 838–846
16. Austin MA (1989) Plasma triglyceride as a risk factor for coronary heart disease. The epidemiologic evidence and beyond. Am J Epidemiol 29: 249–259
17. Austin MA, King MC, Vranizan KM, Krauss RM (1990) Atherogenic lipoprotein phenotype: a proposed genetic marker for coronary heart disease risk. Circulation 82: 495–506
18. Azoulay M, Henry I, Tata F, Weil D, Grzeschik KH, Chaves ME, McIntyre N, Williamson R, Humphries SE, Junien C (1987) The structural gene for lecithin: cholesterol acyl transferase (LCAT) maps to 16q22. Ann Hum Genet 51(2): 129–136
19. Bachorik PS, Cloey TA, Finney CA, Lowry DR, Becker DM (1991) Lipoprotein-cholesterol analysis during screening: accuracy and reliability. Ann Intern Med 114: 741–747
20. Blades B, Vega GL, Grundy SM (1993) Activities of lipoprotein lipase and hepatic triglyceride lipasein postheparin plasma of patients with low concentrations of HDL cholesterol. Arterioscler Thromb 13: 1227–1235
21. Berg K (1963) New serum type system: Lp system. Acta Pathol Miocrobiol Scand 59: 369–382
22. Blankenhorn DM, Nessim SA, Johnson RL, Sanmarco ME, Azen SP, Cashin-Hemphill L (1987) Bebeficial effects of combined colestipol-niacin therapy on coronary atherosclerosis and coronary venous bypass grafts. JAMA 257: 3233–3240
23. Breckenridge WC, Little JA, Steiner G, Chow A, Poapst M (1978) Hypertriglyceridemia associated with deficiency of apolipoprotein C-II. N Engl J Med 298: 1265–1273
24. Breckenridge WC, Maquire GF (1981) Quantification of sinking pre beta lipoprotein in human plasma. Clin Biochem 14: 82–86
25. Brown G, Albers JJ, Fisher LD, Schaefer SM, Lin JT, Kaplan C, Zhao XQ, Bisson BD, Fitzpatrick VF, Dodge HT (1990) Regression of coronary artery disease as a result of intensive lipid-lowering therapy in men with high levels of apolipoprotein B. N Engl J Med 323: 1289–1298

26. Brown MS, Goldstein JL, Fredrickson DS. Familial type 3 hyperlipoproteinemia (dysbeta lipoproteinemia). In: Stanbury JB, Wyngaarden JB, Fredrickson DS, Goldstein JL, Brown MS (eds) The metabolic base of inherited disease, 5th edn. McGraw-Hill, New York, pp 665-671
27. Brown MS, Goldstein JL (1986) A receptor-mediated pathway for cholesterol homeostasis. Science 232: 34-47
28. Brunzell JD, Schrott HG, Motulsky AG, Bierman EL (1976) Myocardial infarction in familial forms of hypertriglyceridemia. Metabolism 25: 313-320
29. Brunzell JD, Albers JJ, Chait A, Grundy SM, Groszek E, McDonald GB (1983) Plasma lipoproteins in familial combined hyperlipidemia and monogenic familial hypertriglyceridemia. J Lipid Res 24: 147-155
30. Buchwald H, Varco RL, Matts JP et al (1990) Effect of partial ileal bypass surgery on mortality and morbidity from coronary heart disease in patient with hypercholesterolemia. Report of the Program on the Surgical Control of Hyperlipidemias (POSCH). N Engl J Med 323: 946-955
31. Burstein M, Samaille J (1960) Sur un dosage rapide du cholesterol lié aux α-et aux β-lipoprotéines du sérum. Clin Chim Acta 5: 609-615
32. Burstein M, Scholnick HR, Morfin R (1970) Rapid method for the isolation of lipoproteins from human serum by precipitation with polyanions. J Lipid Res 11: 583-595
33. Castro GR, Fielding CJ (1988) Early incorporation of cell-derived cholesterol into pre-β-migrationg high density lipoprotein. Biochemistry 27: 25-29
34. Cazzolato G, Prakasch G, Green S, Kostner GM (1983) The determination of lipoprotein Lp(a) by rate and endpoint nephelometry. Clin Chim Acta 135: 203-208
35. Chait A, Brunzell JD, Albers JJ, Hazzard WR (1977) Type-III hyperlipoproteinaemia ("remnant removal disease"). Lancet II: 1176-1178
36. Chait A, Hazzard WR, Albers JJ, Kushwaha RP, Brunzell JD (1978) Impaired very low density lipoprotein and trigylceride removal in broad beta disease. Comparison with endogenous hypertriglyceridaemia. Metabolism 27: 1055-1066
37. Chait A, Albers JJ, Brunzell JD (1980) Very low density lipoprotein overproduction in genetic forms of hypertriglyceridemia. Eur J Clin Invest 10: 17-22
38. Cohen A, Hertz HS, Mandel J et al (1991) Total serum cholesterol by isotope dilution/mass spectrometry: a candidate definitive method. Clin Chem 26: 854-861
39. Cooper GR, Henderson LM, Smith SJ, Hannon WH (1991) Clinical application and standardization of apolipoprotein measurements in the diagnostic workup of lipid disorders. Clin Chem 37: 319-320
40. Cooper GR, Smith SJ, Duncan JW et al (1986) Interlaboratory testing of transferability of a candidate reference method for total cholesterol in serum. Clin Chem 32: 921-929
41. Dahlén G, Ericson C, Furberg C. Lindkvist L, Svardsudd K (1972) Studies on an extra pre-beta lipoprotein fraction. Acta Med Scand [Suppl] 531: 1-29
42. Dahlén G (1974) The pre-beta lipoprotein phenomenon in relation to serum cholesterol and triglyceride levels, the Lp(a) lipoprotein and coronary disease. Acta Med Scand [Suppl] 570: 1-45
43. Dahlén G, Berg K, Gillnas T, Ericson C (1975) Lp(a) lipoprotein/pre-beta-lipoprotein in Swedish middle-aged males and in patients with coronary heart disease. Clin Genet 7: 334-341
44. Dahlén G, Frick MH, Berg K, Valle M, Woljasalo M (1975) Further studies of Lp(a) lipoprotein/pre-betal-lipoprotein in patients with coronary heart disease. Clin Genet 8: 183-189
45. Davidson WS, Sparks DL, Lund-Katz, Phillips MC (1994) The molecular basis for the difference in charge between pre-β and a-migrating high density lipoproteins. J Biol Chem 269: 8959-8965
46. Davidson WS, Gillotte KL, Lund-Katz S, Johnson WJ, Rothblat CH, Phillips MC (1995) The effect of high density lipoprotein phospholipid acyl chain composition on the efflux of cellular free cholesterol. J Biol Chem 270: 5882-5890
47. Davignon J, Gregg RE, Sing CF (1988) Apolipoprotein E polymorphism and atherosclerosis. Arteriosclerosis 8: 1-21
48. Denke MA, Sempos CT, Grundy SM (1993) Excess body weight: an underrecognized contributor to high blood cholesterol in Caucasian American men. Arch Intern Med 153: 1093-1103
49. Denke MA, Sempos CT, Grundy SM (1994) Excess body weight: an underrecognized contributor to dyslipoproteinemia in white American women. Arch Intern Med 154: 401-410
50. Devlin RH, Deeb S, Brunzell J, Hayden MR (1990) Partial gene duplication involving exon-Alu interchange results in lipoprotein lipase deficiency. Am J Hum Gene 46: 112-119
51. Dionne C, Gagne C, Julien P, Murthy MR et al (1992) Genetic epidemiology of lipoprotein lipase deficiency in Saguenay-Lac-St-Jean. Ann Genet 35: 89-92
52. Drayna DT, Hegele RA, Hass PE, Emi M, Wu LL, Eaton DL, Lawn RM, Williams RR, White RL, Lalouel JM (1988) Genetic linkage between lipoprotein(a) phenotype and a DNA polymorphism in the plasminogen gene. Genomics 3: 230-236
53. Dunning AM, Houlston R, Frostegard J, Revill J, Nilsson J, Hamsten A, Talmud P, Humphries S (1991) Genetic evidence that the putative receptor binding domain of apolipoprotein B (residues 3130 to 3630) is not the only region of the protein involved in interaction with the low density lipoprotein receptor. Biochim Biophys Acta 1096: 231-237
54. Durrington PN, Ishola M, Hunt L, Arrol S, Bhatnagar D (1988) Apolipoproteins (a), AI, and B and parental history in men with early onset ischaemic heart disease. Lancet 1: 1070-3107
55. Duverger N, Rader D, Duchateau P, Fruchart J-C, Castro G, Brewer HB Jr (1993) Biochemical characterization of the three major subclasses of lipoprotein A-I preparatively isolated from human plasma. Biochemistry 32: 12372-12379
56. Duvic CR, Smith G, Sledge WE, Lee LT, Murray MD, Roheim PS, Gallaher WR, Thompson JJ (1985) Identification of a mouse monoclonal antibody, LHLP-1, specific for human Lp(a). J Lipid Res 26: 540-548
57. Egusa G, Beltz WF, Grundy SM, Howard BV (1985) Influence of obesity on the metabolism of apolipoprotein B in man. J Clin Invest 76: 596-603

58. Ehnholm C, Garoff H, Simons K, Aro H (1971) Purification and quantitation of the human plasma lipoprotein carrying the Lp(a) antigen. Biochim Biophys Acta 236: 431-439
59. Ehnholm C, Garoff H, Renkonen O, Simons K (1972) Protein and carbohydrate composition of Lp(a)lipoprotein from human plasma. Biochemistry 11: 3229-3232
60. Eisenberg S (1991) High density lipoprotein metabolism. J Lipid Res 25: 1017-1058
61. Ericsson S, Ericsson M, Vitol S, Einarsson K, Berglund L, Angelin B (1991) Influence of age on the metabolism of plasma low density lipoprotein metabolism in healthy males. J Clin Invest 87: 591-596
62. Eriksson M, Berglund L, Rudling M, Henriksson P, Angelin B (1989) Effects of estrogen on low density lipoprotein metabolism in males: short-term and long-term studies during hormonal treatment of prostatic carcinoma. J Clin Invest 84: 802-810
63. Eto M, Watanabe K, Chonan N, Ishii K (1988) Familial hypercholesterolemia and apolipoprotein E4. Atherosclerosis 72: 123-128
64. European Atherosclerosis Society (1988) Carmena R, Crepaldi G, De Backer G, de Gennes JL, Eisenberg S, Galton D, Gotto AM, Goodwin JF, Greten H, Hanefeld M, Huttunen JK, Jacotot B, Katan MB, Mann JL, Miettinen TA, Norum KR, Oganov RG, Olsson AG, Paoletti R, Pometta D, Pyorala K, Schettler G, Shepherd J, Schwandt P, Tikkanen MJ (1988) The recognition and management of hyperlipidaemia in adults: a policy statement of the European Atherosclerosis Society. Eur Heart J 9: 571-600
65. Expert Panel on Detection, Evaluation, and Treatment of High Blood Cholesterol in Adults (1994) National Cholesterol Education Program: second report of the Expert Panel on Detection, Evaluation, and Treatment of High Blood Cholesterol in Adults (Adult Treatment Panel II). Circulation 89: 1329-1445
66. Fielding CJ, Fielding PE (1995) Molecular physiology of reverse cholesterol transport. J Lipid Res 36: 211-228
67. Floren CH, Albers JJ, Bierman EL (1981) Uptake of Lp (a) lipoprotein by cultured fibroblasts. Biochem Biophys Res Commun 102: 636-639
68. Fredrickson DS, Levy RI, Lees RS (1967) Fat transport in lipoproteins - an integrated approach to mechanisms and disorders. N Engl J Med 276: 34-42
69. Friedewald WT, Levy RJ, Fredrickson DS (1972) Estimation of the concentration of low density lipoprotein cholesterol in plasma, without use of preparative ultracentrifuge. Clin Chem 18: 499-509
70. Fruchart JC, Ailhaud G (1992) Apoliprotein A-containing particles: physiological role, quantification and clinical significance. Clin Chem 38: 793-797
71. Gagne C, Brum LDF, Julien P, Moorjani S, Lupien PJ (1989) Primary lipoprotein lipase activity deficiency: clinical investigation of a French Canadian population. Can Med Assoc J 140: 405-411
72. Gagne C, Brun D (1993) Primary lipoprotein lipase deficiency. Presse Med 22: 212-217
73. Gaubatz JW, Heideman C, Gotto AM Jr, Morrisett JD, Dahlén GH (1983) Human plasma lipoprotein (a). Structural properties. J Biol Chem 258: 4582-4589
74. Gaubatz JW, Cushing GL, Morrisett JD (1986) Quantitation, isolation, and characterization of human lipoprotein (a). Methods Enzymol 129: 167-186
75. Gaubatz JW, Ghanem KI, Guevara J Jr, Nava ML, Patsch W, Morrisett JD (1990) Polymorphic forms of human apolipoprotein(a): inheritance and relationship of their molecular weights to plasma levels of lipoprotein(a). J Lipid Res 31: 603-613
76. Ghiselli G, Schaefer EJ, Gascon P, Brewer HB Jr (1981) Type-III hyperlipoproteinemia associated with apolipoprotein E deficiency. Science 214: 1239-1241
77. Ghiselli G, Gregg RE, Brewer HB Jr (1984) Apolipoprotein E Bethesda. Isolation and partial characterization of a variant of human apolipoprotein E isolated from very low density lipoproteins. Biochem Biohpys Acta 794: 333-339
78. Gofman JW, Lindgren FT, Elliott H (1949) Ultracentrifugal studies of lipoproteins of human serum. J Biol Chem 179: 973-979
79. Gofman J, Lindgren FT, Elliott H, Mantz W, Hewitt J, Strisower B, Hering V (1950) The role of lipids and lipoproteins in atherosclerosis. Science 111: 166-171
80. Goldbourt U, Holtzman E, Neufeld HN (1985) Total and high density lipoprotein cholesterol in the serum and risk of mortality: evidence of a threshold effect. Br Med J 290: 1239-1243
81. Goldstein JL, Brown MS (1973) Familial hypercholesterolaemia: identification of a defect in the regulation of 3-hydroxy-3-methylglutaryl coenzyme. A reductase activity associated with overproduction of cholesterol. Proc Natl Acad Sci USA 70: 2804-2808
82. Goldstein JL, Brown MS (1977) The low density lipoprotein receptor and its relation to atherosclerosis. Annu Rev Biochem 46: 879-930
83. Goldstein JL, Brown MS (1984) Progress in understanding the LDL receptor and HMG-CoA reductase, two membrane proteins that regulate the plasma cholesterol. J Lipid Res 25: 1450-1461
84. Goldstein JL, Brown MS. Familial hypercholesterolemia. In: Scriver CR, Beaudet AL, Sly WS, Valle D (eds) The metabolic basis of inherited diseases. McGraw-Hill, New York, pp 1215-1250
85. Gordon T, Castelli WP, Hjortland MC, Kannel WB, Dawber TR (1977) High density lipoprotein as a protective factor against coronary disease. The Framingham study. Am J Med 62: 707-714
86. Gordon T, Kannel WB, Castelli WP, Dawber TR (1981) Lipoproteins cardiovascular disease and death: the Framingham Study. Arch Intern Med 141: 1128-1131
87. Gordon DJ, Probstfield JL, Garrison RJ, Neaton JD, Castelli WP, Knoke JD, Jacobs DR Jr, Bangdiwala S, Tyroler HA (1989) High-density lipoprotein cholesterol and cardiovascular disease. Four prospective American studies. Circulation 79: 8-15
88. Gotto Am Jr (1983) High-density lipoproteins: biochemical and metabolic factors. Am J Cardiol 52: 2B-4B
89. Glomset JA (1968) The plasma lecithin: cholesterol, acyltransferase reaction. J Lipid Res 9: 155-167
90. Grainger DJ, Kirschenlohr HL, Metcalfe JC, Weissberg PL, Wade DP, Lawn RN (1993) The proliferation of human smooth muscle cells is promoted by lipoprotein(a). Science 260: 1655-1658
91. Gregg RE, Zech LA, Schaefer EJ, Brewer HB (1981) Type-III hyperlipoproteinemia defective metabolism of an abnormal apolipoprotein E. Science 211: 584-586
92. Gregg RE, Brewer HB Jr (1988) The role of apolipoprotein E and lipoprotein receptors in modualating the in

vivo metabolism of apolipoprotein B-containing lipoproteins in humans. Clin Chem 34: B28 - 32
93. Grundy SM, Vega GL, Kesianiemi YA (1985) Abnormalities in metabolism of low density lipoproteins associated with coronary heart disease. Acta Med Scand [Suppl] 701: 23 - 37
94. Grundy SM (1986) Comparison of monounsaturated fatty acids and carbohydrates for lowering plasma cholesterol. N Engl J Med 314: 745 - 748
95. Grundy SM, Florentin L, Nix D, Whelan MF (1988) Comparison of monounsaturated fatty acids and carbohydrates for reducing raised levels of plasma cholesterol in man. Am J Clin Nutr 47: 965 - 969
96. Grundy SM, Vega GL (1992) Two different views of the relationship of hypertriglyceridema to coronary heart disease: implications for treatment. Arch Intern Med 94: 119 - 127
97. Gunby P (1983) High HDL2 levels lower postprandial lipids (news). JAMA 249: 1250
98. Guo HC, Chapman MJ, Bruckert E, Farriaux JP, De Gennes JL (1991) Lipoprotein Lp(a) in homozygous familial hypercholesterolemia: density profile, particle heterogeneity and apolipoprotein(a) phenotype. Atherosclerosis 86: 69 - 83
99. Guyton JR, Dahlén GH, Patsch W, Kautz JA, Gotto AM Jr (1985) Relationship of plasma lipoprotein Lp(a) levels to race and to apolipoprotein B. Arteriosclerosis 5: 265 - 272
100. Gylling H, Aalto-Setälä K, Kontula K, Miettinen TA (1991) Serum low density lipoprotein cholesterol level and cholesterol absorption efficiency are influenced by apolipoprotein B and E polymorphism and by the FH-Helsinki mutation of the low density lipoprotein receptor gene in familial hypercholesterolemia. Arterioscler Thromb 11: 1386 - 1375
101. Harvie NR, Schultz JS (1973) Studies on the heterogeneity of human serum Lp lipoproteins and on the occurrence of double Lp lipoprotein variants. Biochem Genet 9: 235 - 245
102. Havel RJ, Eder HA, Bragdon JH (1955) Distribution and chemical composition of ultracentrifugally separated lipoproteins in human serum. J Clin Invest 43: 1345 - 1353
103. Heller DA, de Faire U, Petersen NL, Dahlen G, McClern GE (1993) Genetic and environmental influences on serum levels in twins. N Engl J Med 328: 1150 - 1164
104. Hetland ML, Haarbo J, Christiansen C (1992) One measurement of serum total cholesterol is enough to predict future levels in healthy postmenopausal women. Am J Med 92: 25 - 28
105. Hobbs HH, Brown MS, Goldstein JL (1992) Molecular genetics of the LDL receptor gene in familial hypercholesterolemia. Hum Mutat 1: 445 - 466
106. Huang Y, von Eckardstein A, Assmann G (1993) Cell derived cholesterol cycles between different HDLs and LDL for its effective esterification in plasma. Arterioscler Thromb 13: 445 - 458
107. Hussain MM; Zannis VI (1990) Intracellular modification of human apolipoprotein AII (apoAII) and sites of apoAII mRNA synthesis: comparison of apoAII with apoCII and apoCIII isoproteins. Biochemistry 2: 209 - 217
108. Inazu A, Brown ML, Hesler CB, Agellon LB, Koizumi J, Takata K, Marahuma Y, Mabuchi H, Tall AR (1990) Increased high density lipoprotein levels caused by a common cholesteryl ester transfer protein gene mutation. N Engl J Med 323: 1234 - 1238
109. Innerarity TL, Mahley RW, Weisgraber KH, Bersot TP, Krauss RM, Vega GL, Grundy SM, Friedl W, Davignon J, McCarthy BJ (1990) Familial defective apolipoprotein B-100: a mutation of apolipoprotein B that causes hypercholesterolemia. J Lipid Res 31: 1337 - 1349
110. Iselius L, Dahlén G, de Faire U, Lundman T (1981) Complex segregation analysis of the Lp(a)/pre-beta 1-lipoprotein trait. Clin Genet 20: 147 - 151
111. Jackson RL, Yates MT, McNerney CA, Kashyap ML (1987) Diet and HDL metabolism: high carbohydrate vs. high fat diets. Adv Exp Med Biol 210: 165 - 172
112. Jacobs DR Jr, Barrett-Connor E (1982) Retest reliability of plasma cholesterol and triglyceride. The Lipid Research Clinics Prevalence Study. Am J Epidemiol 116: 878 - 885
113. Janus ED, Nicoll AM, Turner PR, Magill P, Lewis B (1980) Kinetic bases of the primary hyperlipidaemias: studies of apolipoprotein B turnover in genetically defined subjects. Eur J Clin Invest 10: 161 - 172
114. Jencks WP, Hyatt MR, Jetton MR, Mattingly TW, Durrum FL (1956) Studies of serum lipoproteins in normal and atherosclerotic patients by paper electrophoretic techniques. J Clin Invest 35: 980 - 990
115. Jonas A, Wald JH, Zoohill KL, Krul ES, Kedzy KE (1990) Apolipoprotein A-I structure and lipid properties in homogeneous reconstituted spherical and discoidal high density lipoproteins. J Biol Chem 256: 22123 - 22129
116. Kagan A, McGee DL, Yano K, Rhoads GG, Nomura A (1981) Serum cholesterol and mortality in a Japanese-American population: the Honolulu Heart program. Am J Epidemiol 114: 11 - 20
117. Karàdi I, Kostner GM, Gries A, Nimpf J, Romics L, Malle E (1988) Lipoprotein (a) and plasminogen are immunochemically related. Biochim Biophys Acta 960: 91 - 97
118. Karlin JB, Johnson WJ, Benedict CR, Chacko GK, Phillips MC, Rothblat GH (1987) Cholesterol flux between cells and high density lipoprotein. Lack of relationship to specific binding of the lipoprotein to the cell surface. J Biol Chem 262: 12557 - 12564
119. Kesaniemi YA, Grundy SM (1983) Increased low density lipoprotein production associated with obesity. Arteriosclerosis 3: 170 - 177
120. Kesaniemi YA, Beltz WF, Grundy SM (1985) Comparisons of metabolism of apolipoprotein B in normal subjects, obese patients, and patients with coronary heart disease. J Clin Invest 76: 586 - 595
121. Kesteloot H, Huang DX, Yang XS (1985) Serum lipids in the People's Republic of China: comparison of western and eastern populations. Arteriosclerosis 5: 427 - 433
122. Keys A (1980) Seven countries: a multivariate analysis on death and coronarty heart disease. Harvard University Press, Cambridge, p 132
123. Keys A, Menotti A, Aravanis C, Blackburn H, Djordevic BS, Buzina R, Dontas AS, Fidanza F, Karvonen MJ, Kimura N et al (1984) The seven countries study: 2,289 deaths in 15 years. Prev Med 13: 141 - 154
124. Keys A, Toshima H, Koga Y, Blackburn H (1994) Lessons for science from the seven countries study: a 35-

year collaborative experience in cardiovascular disease epidemiology. Springer, Berlin Heidelberg New York
125. Kissebah AH, Alfarsi S, Evans DJ (1984) Low density lipoprotein metabolism in familial combined hyperlipidemia. Mechanism of the multiple lipoprotein phenotypic expression. Arteriosclerosis 4: 614-62
126. Knuiman JT, West CE, Katan MB, Hautvast JGA (1987) Total cholesterol and high density lipoprotein levels in populations differing in fat and carbohydrate intake. Arteriosclerosis 612-619
127. Kojima S, Harpel PC, Rifkin DB (1991) Lipoprotein(a) inhibits the generation of transforming growth factor beta: an endogenous inhibitor of smooth muscle cell migration. J Cell Biol 113: 1439-1445
128. Kostner GM, Avogaro P, Cazzolato G, Marth E, Bittolo-Bon G, Qunici GB (1981) Lipoprotein Lp(a) and the risk for myocardial infarction. Atherosclerosis 38: 51-61
129. Koschinsky ML, Beisiegel U, Henne-Bruns D, Eaton RM (1990) Apolipoprotein(a) size heterogeneity is related to variable number of repeat sequences in its mRNA. Biochemistry 29: 640-644
130. Kraft HG, Menzel HJ, Hoppichler F, Vogel W, Utermann G (1989) Changes of genetic apolipoprotein phenotypes caused by liver transplantation. Implications for apolipoprotein synthesis. J Clin Invest 83: 137-142
131. Krauss RM (1987) Relationship of intermediate and low-density lipoprotein subspecies to risk of coronary artery disease. Am Heart J 113: 578-582
132. Krauss RM, Lindgren FT, Williams PT, Kelsey SF, Brensike J, Vranizan K, Detre KM, Levy RI (1987) Intermediate-density lipoprotein and progression of coronary artery disease in hypercholesterolaemic men. Lancet 2: 62-66
133. Krempler F, Kostner GM, Bolzano K, Sandhofer F (1980) Turnover of lipoprotein (a) in man. J Clin Invest 65: 1483-1490
134. Krempler F, Kostner GM, Roscher A, Haslauer F, Bolzano K, Sandhofer F (1983) Studies on the role of specific cell surface receptors in the removal of lipoprotein (a) in man. J Clin Invest 71: 1431-1441
135. Kwiterovich PO Jr (1988) HyperapoB: a pleiotropic phenotype characterized by dense low-density lipoproteins and associated with coronary artery disease. Clin Chem 34: B71-77
136. Labeur C, Michiels G, Bury J, Usher DC, Rosseneu M (1989) Lipoprotein(a) quantified by an enzyme-linked immunosorbent assay with monoclonal antibodies. Clin Chem 35: 1380-1384
137. Ladias JA, Kwiterovich PO Jr, Smith HH, Miller M, Bachorik PS, Forte T, Lusis AJ, Antonarakis SE (1980) Apolipoprotein B-100 Hopkins (arginine 4019-tryptophan). A new apolipoprotein B-100 variant in a family with premature atherosclerosis and hyperapobetalipoproteinemia. JAMA 262: 1980-1988
138. de Lalla OF, Gofman JW (1954) Ultracentrifugal analysis of serum lipoproteins. In: Glick D (ed) Methods of biochemical analysis. Interscience, New York p 469
139. Lawn R (1987) cDNA sequence of human apolipoprotein(a) is homologous to plasminogen. Nature 330: 132-137
140. Lees RS, Hatch FT (1963) Sharper separation of lipoprotein species by paper electrophoresis in albumin-containing buffer. J Lab Clin Med 61: 518-528
141. Lees RS, Fredrickson DS (1965) The differentiation of exogenous and endogenous hyperilipemia by paper electrophoresis. J Clin Invest 44: 1968-1977
142. Lewis B (1983) Relation of high-density lipoproteins to coronary artery disease. Am J Cardiol 52: 5B-8B
143. Lindgren FT, Nichols AV (1960) Structure and function of human serum lipoproteins. In: Putnam FW (ed) The Plasma proteins, vol 2. Academic, New York, p 1
144. Lipid Research Clinics Program (1984) The Lipid Research Clinics Coronary Primary Prevention Trial results. I. Reduction in the incidence of coronary heart disease. JAMA 251: 351-364
145. Lipid Research Program (1984) The Lipid Research Clinics Coronary Primary Prevention Trial results. II. The relationship of reduction in incidence of coronary heart disease to cholesterol lowering. JAMA 251: 365-374
146. Lopes-Virella MF, Stone P, Ellis S, Colwell JA (1977) Cholesterol determination in high-density lipoproteins separated by three different methods. Clin Chem 23: 882-884
147. Ma PT, Yamamoto T, Goldstein JL, Brown MS (1986) Increased mRNA for low density lipoprotein receptor in livers of rabbits treated with 17 a-ethinyl estradiol. Proc Natl Acad Sci USA 83: 792-796
148. Mabuchi H, Itoh H, Takeda M, Kajinami K, Wakasugi T, Koizumi J, Takeda R, Asagami C (1989) A young type-III hyperlipoproteinemic patient associated with apolipoprotein E deficiency. Metabolism 38: 115-119
149. Maeda H, Nakamura H, Kobori S, Okada M, Niki H, Ogura T, Hiraga S (1989) Molecular cloning of a human apolipoprotein E variant: E5 (Glu3-Lys3). J Biochem (Tokyo) 105: 491-493
150. Maeda H, Nakamura H, Kobori S, Okada M, Mori H, Niki H, Ogura T, Hiraga S (1989) Identification of human apolipoprotein E variant gene: apolipoprotein E7 (Glu244,245-Lys244,245). J Biochem (Tokyo) 105: 51-54
151. McGill HC Jr, McMahan CA, Kruski AW, Mott GE (1981) Relationship of lipoprotein cholesterol concentrations to experimental atherosclerosis in baboons. Arteriosclerosis 1: 3-12
152. März W, Ruzicka C, Pohl T, Usadel KH, Gross W (1992) Familial defective apolipoprotein B-100: mild hypercholesterolaemia without atherosclerosis in a homozygous patient (letter). Lancet 340: 1362
153. Mahley RW, Hui DY, Innerarity TL, Weisgraber KH (1981) Two independent lipoprotein receptors on hepatic membranes of dog, swine, and man. Apo-B,E and apo-E receptors. J Clin Invest 68: 1197-1206
154. Mahley RW (1988) Apolipoprotein E: cholesterol transport protein with expanding role in cell biology. Science 240: 622-630
155. Mahley RW, Hui DY, Innerarity TL, Beisiegel U (1989) Chylomicron remnant metabolism. Role of hepatic lipoprotein receptors in mediating uptake. Arteriosclerosis [1, Suppl I): 14-18
156. Mailly F, Xu CF, Xhignesse M, Lussier-Cacan S, Talmud PJ, Davignon J, Humphries SE, Nestruck AC (1991) Characterization of a new apolipoprotein E5 variant

detected in two French-Canadian subjects. J Lipid Res 32: 613 - 620
157. Mann WA, Gregg RE, Sprecher DL, Brewer HB Jr (1989) Apolipoprotein E-1 Harrisburg: a new variant of apolipoprotein E dominantly associated with type-III hyperlipoproteinemia. Biochim Biophys Acta 1005: 239 - 244
158. Manual of laboratory operations (1974) Lipid research clinics program, vol I: lipid and lipoprotein analysis. DHEW Publ (NIH) 75 - 628
159. Manzato E, Fellin R, Baggio G, Walch S, Neubeck W, Seidel D (1976) Formation of lipoprotein-X. J Clin Invest 57: 1248 - 1260
160. McLean JW, Elshourbagy NA, Chang DJ, Mahley RW, Taylor JM (1984) Human apolipoprotein E mRNA. cDNA cloning and nucleotide sequencing of a new variant. J Biol Chem 259: 6498 - 6504
161. McQueen MJ, Henderson AR, Patten RL, Krishnan S, Wood DE, Webb S (1991) Results of a province-wide quality assurance program assessing the accuracy of cholesterol, triglycerides, and high-density lipoprotein cholesterol measurements and calculated low-density lipoprotein cholesterol in Ontario, using fresh human serum. Arch Pathol Lab Med 115: 1217 - 1222
162. Mensink RP, Katan MB (1990) Effect of dietary trans fatty acids on high-density and low-density lipoprotein cholesterol levels in healthy subjects. N Engl J Med 323: 439 - 445
163. Mensink RP, Katan MB (1992) Effects of dietary fatty acids on serum lipids and lipoproteins: a meta analysis of 27 trials. Arteriosclerosis 12: 91 - 919
164. Miesenboeck G, Hoelzl B, Foeger B, Brandstätter E, Paulweber B, Sandhofer F (1993) Heterozygous lipoprotein lipase deficiency due to a missense mutation as the cause of impaired triglyceride tolerance with multiple lipoprotein abnormalities. J Clin Invest 91: 448 - 455
165. Miller GJ, Miller NE (1975) Plasma high density lipoprotein cholesterol concentration and development of ischemic heart disease. Lancet i: 16 - 19
166. Miller NE (1984) Why does plasma low density lipoprotein concentration in adults increase with age? Lancet 1: 263 - 266
167. Morton NE, Gulbrandsen CL, Rhoads GG, Kagan A (1978) The Lp(a) lipoprotein in Japanese. Clin Genet 14: 207 - 212
168. Nauck M, Winkler K, Wittmann C, Mayer H, Luley C, März W, Wieland H (1995) Direct determination of Lipoprotein(a) cholesterol. A combination of ultracentrifugation and agarose gel electrophoresis with enzymatic cholesterol staining. Clin Chem 41: 731 - 738
169. Nauck M, Winkler K, März W, Wieland H (1995) Quantitative determination of high-, low-, and very-low-density lipoproteins and lipoprotein(a) by agarose gel electrophoresis and enzymatic cholesterol staining. Clin Chem 41: 1761 - 1767
170. Nicolosi RJ, Stucchi AF, Kowala MC, Hennessy LK, Hegsted DM, Schaefer EJ (1990) Effect of dietary fat saturation and cholesterol on LDL composition and metabolism. Arterisclerosis 10: 119 - 128
171. Noble RD (1968) Electrophoretic separation of plasma lipoproteins in agarose gel. J Lipid Res 9: 693 - 700
172. Oram JF, Brinton EA, Bierman EL (1983) Regulation of high density lipoprotein receptor activity in cultured human skin fibroblasts and human arterial smooth muscle cells. J Clin Invest 72: 1611 - 1621
173. Oram JF, Johnson CJ, Brown TA (1987) Interaction of high density lipoprotein with its receptor on cultured fibroblasts and macrophages: evidence for reversible binding at the cell surface without internalization. J Biol Chem 262: 2405 - 2410
174. Pagnan A, Kostner G, Braggion M, Ziron L, Bittolo-Bon G, Avogaro P (1983) Familial study on "sinking pre-beta", the Lp(a) lipoprotein, and its relationship with serum lipids, apolipoprotein A-I and B and clinical atherosclerosis. J Clin Chem Clin Biochem 21: 267 - 272
175. Patsch JR, Prasad S, Gotto AM Jr, Bengtsson-Olivecrona G (1984) Postprandial lipemia: a key for the conversion of HDL2 into HDL3 by hepatic lipase. J Clin Invest 74: 2017 - 2023
176. Pfaffinger D, Schuelke J, Kim C, Fless GM, Scanu AM (1991) Relationship between apo(a) isoforms and Lp(a) density in subjects with different apo(a) phenotype: a study before and after a fatty meal. J Lipid Res 32: 679 - 683
177. Pooling Project Research Group (1978) Relationship of blood pressure, serum cholesterol, smoking habit, relative weight and ECG abnormalities to incidence of major coronary events: Final report of the Pooling Project. J Chron Dis 31: 201 - 306
178. Postle AD, Darmady JM, Siggers DC (1978) Double pre-beta lipoprotein in ischaemic heart disease. Clin Genet 13: 233 - 236
179. Rall SC Jr, Newhouse YM, Clarke HR, Weisgraber KH, McCarthy BJ, Mahley RW, Bersot TP (1989) Type-III hyperlipoproteinemia associated with apolipoprotein E phenotype E3/3. Structure and genetics of an apolipoprotein E3 variant. J Clin Invest 83: 1095 - 1101
180. Rauh GH, Keller C, Kormann B, Spengel F, Schster H, Wolfram G, Zöllner N (1992) Familial defective apolipoprotein B_{100}: clinical characteristics of 54 cases. Atherosclerosis 92: 233 - 241
181. Reardon MF, Poapst ME, Steiner G (1982) The independent synthesis of intermediate density lipoproteins in type-III hyperlipoproteinaemia. Metabolism 31: 421 - 427
182. Reardon MF, Nestel PJ, Craig IH, Harper RW (1985) Lipoprotein predictors of the severity of coronary artery disease in men and women. Circulation 71: 881 - 888
183. Rhoads GG, Morton NE, Gulbrandsen CL, Kagan A (1978) Sinking pre-beta lipoprotein and coronary heart disease in Japanese-American men in Hawaii. Am J Epidemiol 108: 350 - 356
184. Rivin AU (1989) Total and high-density lipoprotein cholesterol measurements. Hazards in clinical interpretation. West J Med 151: 289 - 291
185. Rothblat GH, Bamberger M, Phillips MC (1986) Reverse cholesterol transport. In: Albers JJ, Segrest JP (eds) Method in enzymology, vol 129. Academic, London pp 628 - 644
186. Rudel LL, Pitts LL II, Nelson CA (1977) Characterization of plasma low density lipoproteins of nonhuman primates fed dietary cholesterol. J Lipid Res 18: 211 - 222
187. Santamarina-Fojo S, de Gennes JL, Beisiegel U (1991) Molecular genetics of apoC-II and lipoprotein lipase deficiency. Adv Exp Med Biol 285: 329 - 333

188. Santamarina-Fojo S, Brewer HB (1992) Hypertriglyceridaemia due to genetic defects in lipoprotein lipase and apolipoprotein C-II. J Intern Med 231: 669-677
189. Santamarina-Fojo S, Dugi K (1994) Structure, function and role of lipoprotein lipase in lipoprotein metabolism. Curr Opin Lipidol 5: 117-125
190. Scanu AM (1990) Lipoprotein(a): a genetically determined cardiovascular pathogen in search of a function. J Lab Clin Med 116: 142-146
191. Schaefer EJ, Gregg RE, Ghiselli G, Forte TM, Ordovas JM, Zech LA, Brewer HB Jr (1986) Familial apolipoprotein E deficiency. J Cli Invest 78: 1206-1219
192. Schultz JS, Shreffler DC, Harvie NR (1968) Genetic and antigenic studies and partial purification of a human serum lipoprotein carrying the Lp antigenic determinant. Proc Natl Acad Sci USA 61: 963-970
193. Schultz JS, Schreffler DC, Sing CF, Harvie NR (1974) The genetics of the Lp antigen. I. Its quantification and distribution in a sample population. Ann Hum Genet 38: 39-46
194. Schmitz G, Robenek H, Lohmann U, Assmann G (1985) Interaction of high density lipoproteins with cholesterylester laden macrophages: biochemical and morphological characterization of cell surface binding, endocytosis and resecretion of high density lipoproteins by macrophages. EMBO J 4: 613-622
195. Seed M, Hoppichler F, Reaveley D, McCarthy S, Thompson GR, Boerwinkle E, Utermann G (1990) Relation of serum lipoprotein(a) concentration and apolipoprotein(a) phenotype to coronary heart disease in patients with familial hypercholesterolemia. N Engl J Med 322: 1494-1499
196. Seidel D, Alaupovic P, Furman RH (1969) A lipoprotein characterizing obstructive jaundice. I. Method for quantitative separation and identification of lipoprotein in jaundiced subjects. J Clin Invest 48: 1211-1223
197. Seidel D, Wieland H, Ruppert C (1973) Improved techniques for assessment of plasmalipoprotein patterns. I. Precipitation in gels after electrophoresis with polyanionic compounds. Clin Chem 19: 737-739
198. Shore V, Shore B (1962) Protein subunit of human serum lipoproteins of density 1.125-1.200 gram/ml. Biochem Biophys Res Commun 9: 455-460
199. Simons K, Ehnholm C, Renkonen O, Bloth B (1970) Characterization of the Lp(a) lipoprotein in human plasma. Acta Pathol Microbiol Scand [B] Microbiol Immunol 78: 459-466
200. Sniderman A, Shapiro S, Marpole D, Skinner B, Teng B, Kwiterovich PO Jr (1980) Association of coronary atherosclerosis with hyperapobetalipoproteinemia (increased protein but normal cholesterol levels inhuman plasma low density (beta) lipoproteins). Proc Natl Acad Sci USA 77: 604-608
201. Sniderman AD, Wolfson C, Teng B, Franklin FA, Bachorik PS, Kwiterovich PO Jr (1982) Association of hyperapobetalipoproteinemia with endogenous hypertriglyceridemia and atherosclerosis. Ann Intern Med 97: 833-839
202. Sniderman A, Cianflone K, Kwiterovich PO Jr, Hutchinson T, Barre P, Prichard S (1987) Hyperapobetalipoproteinemia: the major dyslipoproteinemia in patients with chronic renal failure treated with chronic ambulatory peritoneal dialysis. Atherosclerosis 65: 257-264
203. Solakivi T, Salo MK, Puska P, Nikkari T (1988) Plasma apolipoprotein B in middle-aged Finnish men. Evidence for a regional gradient of apo B and lack of negative correlation between apo B and dietary linoleate in hyperapobetalipoproteinemia. Atherosclerosis 72: 55-61
204. Sorci TM, Wilson MD, Johnson FL, Williams DL, Rudel LL (1989) Studies on the expression of genes encoding apolipoprotein B 100 and B48 and the low density lipoprotein receptor in nonhuman primates. Comparison of dietary fat and cholesterol. J Biol Chem 264: 9039-9045
205. Spady DK, Dietschy JM (1985) Dietary saturated triglycerides suppress hepatic low density lipoprotein receptors in hamster. Proc Natl Acad Sci USA 82: 4526-4530
206. Sprecher DL, Hoeg JM, Schaefer EJ, Zech LA, Gregg RE, Lakatos E, Brewer HB Jr (1985) The association of LDL receptor activity, LDL cholesterol level, and clinical course in homozygous familial hypercholesterolemia. Metabolism 34: 294-299
207. Stamler J, Wentworth D, Neaton JD (1o86) Is the relationship between serum cholesterol and risk of premature death from coronary heart disease contionuous and graded? Finding sin 356222 primary screenes of the Multiple Risk Factor Intervention Trial (MRFIT). JAMA 256: 2823-2828
208. Steinberg D, Parthasarathy S, Carew TE, Khoo JC, Witztum JL (1989) Beyond cholesterol: modifications of low-density lipoprotein that increase its atherogenicity. N Engl J Med 320: 915-923
209. Strong JP, McGill HC (1967) Diet and eperimntal atheroscleosis in baboons. Am J Pathol 50: 669-690
210. Strong JP (1976) Atherosclerosis in primates. Introduction and overview. Primates Med 9: 1-15
211. Tajima S, Yamamura T, Yamamoto A (1988) Analysis of apolipoprotein E5 gene from a patient with hyperlipoproteinemia. J Biochem (Tokyo) 104: 48-52
212. Tall AR (1990) Plasma high density lipoproteins. Metabolism and relationship to atherosclerosis. J Clin Invest 86: 379-384
213. Talmud PJ, Barni N, Kessling AM, Carlsson P, Darnfors C, Bjursell G, Galton D, Wynnn V, Kirk H, Hayden MR et al (1987) Apolipoprotein B gene variants are involved in the determination of serum cholesterol levels: a study in normo- and hyperlipidaemic individuals. Atherosclerosis 67: 81-89
214. Tatami R, Mabuchi H, Ueda K, Ueda R, Haba T, Kametani T, Ito S, Koizumi J, Ohta M, Miyamoto S, Nakayama A, Kanaya H, Oiwake H, Genda A, Takeda R (1981) Intermediate-density lipoprotein and cholesterol-rich very low density lipoprotein in angiographically determined coronary artery disease. Circulation 64: 1174-1118
215. Teng B, Thompson GR, Sniderman AD, Forte TM, Krauss RM, Kwiterovich PO Jr (1983) Composition and distribution of low density lipoprotein fractions in hyperapobetalipoproteinemia, normolipidemia, and familial hypercholesterolemia. Proc Natl Acad Sci USA 80: 6662-666
216. Teng B, Sniderman AD, Soutar AK, Thompson GR (1986) Metabolic basis of hyperapobetalipoproteinemia. Turnover of apolipoprotein B in low density lipoprotein and its precursors and subfractions compared

with normal and familial hypercholesterolemia. J Clin Invest 77: 663-672
217. Thompson GR, Seed M, Niththyananthan S, McCarthy S, Thorogood M (1989) Genotypic and phenotypic variation in familial hypercholesterolemia. Arteriosclerosis [1 Suppl I]: 75-80
218. Tornberg SA, Jakobsson KF, Eklund GA (1988) Stability and validity of a single serum cholesterol measurement in a prospective cohort study. Int J Epidemiol 17: 797-803
219. Trinder P (1969) Determination of glucose in blood using glucose oxidase with an alternative oxygen acceptor. Ann Clin Biochem 6: 24-27
220. Tybjaerg-Hansen A, Humphries SE (1992) Familial defective apolipoprotein B-100: a single mutation that causes hypercholesterolemia and premature coronary artery disease. Atherosclerosis 96: 91-107
221. Utermann G, Lipp K, Wiegandt H (1972) Studies on the Lp(a)-lipoprotein of human serum. IV. The disaggregation of the Lp(a)-lipoprotein. Humangenetik 14: 142-150
222. Utermann G, Hees M, Steinmetz A (1977) Polymorphism of apolipoprotein E and occurrence of dysbetalipoproteinaemia in man. Nature 269: 604-607
223. Utermann G, Canzler H, Hees M, Jaeschke M, Mühlfellner G, Schoenborn W, Vogelberg KH (1977) Studies on the metabolic defect in Broad-beta disease (hyperlipoproteinaemia type-III). Clin Genet 12: 139-154
224. Utermann G (1987) Apolipoprotein E polymorphism in health and disease. Am Heart J 113: 433-440
225. Utermann G, Menzel HJ, Kraft HG, Duba HC, Kemmler HG, Seitz C (1987) Lp(a) glycoprotein phenotypes. Inheritance and relation to Lp(a)-lipoprotein concentration in plasma. J Clin Invest 80: 458-465
226. Utermann G, Kraft HG, Menzel HJ, Hopferwieser T, Seitz C (1988) Genetics of the quantitative Lp(a) lipoprotein trait. I. Relation of Lp(a) glycoprotein phenotypes to Lp(a) lipoprotein concentrations in plasma. Hum Genet 78: 41-46
227. Utermann G, Duba C, Menzel HJ (1988) Genetics of the quantitative Lp(a) lipoprotein trait. II. Inheritance of Lp(a) glycoprotein phenotypes. Hum Genet 78: 47-50
228. Utermann G (1989) The mysteries of lipoprotein(a). Science 246: 904-910
229. Van Tol A (1989) Reverse cholesterol transport. In: Steinmetz A, Kaffarnik H, Schneider J (eds) Cholesterol transport systems and their relation to atherosclerosis. Springer, Berlin Heidelberg New York, pp 85-91
230. Vega GL, Grundy SM (1986) In vivo evidence for reduced binding of low density lipoproteins to receptors as a cause of primary moderate hypercholesterolemia. J Clin Invest 78: 1410-1415
231. Vega GL, Denke MA, Grundy SM (1991) Metabolic basis of primary hypercholesterolemia. Circulation 84: 118-128
232. Vu-Dac N, Chekkor A, Parra H, Duthilleul P, Fruchart JC (1985) Latex immunoassay of human serum Lp(a+) lipoprotein. J Lipid Res 26: 267-269
233. Vu-Dac N, Mezdour H, Parra HJ, Luc G, Luyeye I, Fruchart JC (1989) A selective bi-site immunoenzymatic procedure for human Lp(a) lipoprotein quantification using monoclonal antibodies against apo(a) and apoB. J Lipid Res 30: 1437-1443
234. Walton KW, Hitchens J, Magnani HN, Khan M (1974) A study of methods of identification and estimation of Lp(a) lipoprotein and of its sigificance in health, hyperlipidaemia and atherosclerosis. Atherosclerosis 20: 323-346
235. Wardell MR, Brennan SO, Janus ED, Fraser R, Carrell RW (1987) Apolipoprotein E2-Christchurch (136 Arg-Sr). New variant of human apolipoprotein E in a patient with type-III hyperlipoproteinemia. J Clin Invest 80: 483-490
236. Wardell MR, Weisgraber KH, Havekes LM, Rall SC Jr (1989) Apolipoprotein E3-Leiden contains a seven-amino acid insertion that is a tandem repeat of residues 121-127. J Biol Chem 264: 21205-21210
237. Wardell MR, Rall SC Jr, Schaefer EJ, Kane JP, Weisgraber KH (1991) Two apolipoprotein E5 variants illustrate the importance of the position of additional positive charge on receptor-binding activity. J Lipid Res 32: 521-528
238. Wasenius A, Stugaard M, Otterstad JE, Froyshov D (1990) Diurnal and monthly intra-individual variability of the concentration of lipids, lipoproteins and apolipoprotein. Scand J Clin Lab Invest 50: 635-642
239. Weisgraber KH, Rall SC Jr, Innerarity TL, Mahley RW, Kuusi T, Ehnholm C (1984) A novel electrophoretic variant of human apolipoprotein E. Identification and characterization of apolipoprotein E1. J Clin Invest 73: 1024-1033
240. Wetterau JR, Aggerbeck LP, Bouma M-E, Eisenberg C, Munck A, Hermier B, Schmitz J, Gay DJ, Rader DJ, Gregg RE (1992) Absence of microsomal triglyceride-transfer protein in individuals with abetalipoproteinemial. Science 258: 999-1001
241. Wiegandt H, Lipp K, Wendt GG (1968) Identifizierung eines Lipoproteins mit Antigenwirksamkeit im Lp-System. Hoppe Seylers Z Physiol Chem 349: 489-494
242. Wieland H, Seidel D (1987) Quantitative lipoprotein electrophoresis. In: Lewis LA (ed) Handbook of electrophoresis, vol II. CRC, Boca Raton
243. Wilson DE, Emi M, Iverius P-H, Hata A, Wu LL, Hillas E (1990) Phenotypic expression of heterozygous lipoprotein lipase deficiency in the extended pedigree of a proband homozygous for a missense mutation. J Clin Invest 86: 735-750
244. Yamamura T, Yamamoto A, Sumiyoshi T, Hiramori K, Nishioeda Y, Nambu S (1984) New mutants of apolipoprotein E associated with atherosclerotic diseases but not to type-III hyperlipoproteinemia. J Clin Invest 74: 1229-12237

Assessment of Homocysteine

P.M. Ueland, H. Refsum, H.J. Blom, and M.R. Malinow

Introduction

Patients with the inborn error homocystinuria have extremely high levels of total plasma homocysteine (tHcy). Deficiency of the enzyme cystathionine β-synthase (CS) is the most common cause, but other enzymic defects have been described in a minority of these patients. Notably, all forms of homocystinuria, irrespective of enzymic defect, are associated with a high incidence of cardiovascular disease, which often occurs in early adolescence and even in childhood [57]. The high incidence of vascular disease in these patients led to the Hcy theory of atherosclerosis, which states that moderate elevation of tHcy is a risk factor for early cardiovascular disease in the general population [53, 54]. During the last 20 years, more than 25 retrospective and two prospective studies totaling more than 4000 patients have provided ample evidence that tHcy is a risk factor for atherosclerotic occlusive disease in the coronary, cerebrovascular, and peripheral vascular beds, as well as the extracranial carotid vessels [16]. A relation between elevated tHcy and venous thrombosis has been demonstraded in some [10, 25, 26] but not all studies [20].

Conservative estimates of the odds ratios for coronary artery disease and cerebrovascular disease associated with a 5 μmol/l tHcy increment are about 1.6 and 1.8, respectively. For cornary artery disease, this increment elevates risk as much as does a 0.5 mmol increase in cholesterol [16]. Elevated plasma tHcy is at least as strong a risk factor for vascular disease as hypercholesterolemia, smoking, or hypertension; it is a graded, independent risk factor, but shows a particularly strong interactive effect with smoking and hypertension [32].

Biochemistry

Homocysteine is a sulfur amino acid formed from methionine as a product of *S*-adenosylmethonine-dependent transmethylation. Intracellular Hcy is salvaged to methionine by remethylation. The reaction is in most tissues catalyzed by the enzyme methionine synthese (EC 2.1.1.13), which requires methylcobalamin as cofactor and 5-methyltetrahydrofolate as methyl donor. Hcy is also remethylated by the enzyme betaine-homocysteine transmethylase (EC 2.1.1.5), which is confined to the liver and, possibly, kidney. An alternative route of Hcy disposal is conversion to cystein, and the first step of this pathway is catalyzed by the vitamin B_6-dependent enzyme cystathionine β-synthase (EC 4.2.1.22), which completes the trans-sulfuration pathway [30].

Methionine synthase has a low K_m for Hcy and its activity increases at low dietary methionine intake. These features suggest that the enzyme conserves methionine [30].

One of the substrates of the methionine synthase reaction, 5-methyltetrahydrofolate, is produced by the enzyme methylenetrhydrofolate reductase (EC 1.1.1.69, MTFR). This enzyme represents another regulatory locus of Hcy remethylation [30].

Cystathionine β-synthase has a high K_m for Hcy; its activity increases in response to a high intake of methionine, and the enzyme probably controls the catabolism of excess Hcy [30].

Cellular export of Hcy represents an additional mechanism regulating intracellular Hcy content. This process becomes important under conditions of imbalance between Hcy production and metabolism [74]. Increased Hcy production (induced by methionine loading) or inhibition of Hcy metabolism (during folate or cobalamin deficiencies, or a defect of cystathionine β-synthase) causes export of Hcy into the extracellular fluid. This is the biochemical basis for plasma Hcy as a marker of folate or cobalamin deficiency or inborn errors of Hcy metabolism [76].

Homocysteine Species and Concentrations in Plasma or Serum

Hcy is probably released into the extracellular fluid and plasma in its reduced form, but only trace amounts of reduced Hcy can be detected in plasma under physiological conditions [73]. In plasma, Hcy undergoes oxidation and disulfide exchange reactions. In freshly prepared plasma, about 70% of Hcy exists as albumin-Hcy mixed disulfide, and this fraction is referred to as protein-bound Hcy [38]. When whole plasma or serum is deproteinized with acid, the soluble, free Hcy is obtained, and most Hcy in this fraction has been identified as Hcy-cysteine mixed disulfide. The sum of all Hcy species in plasma/serum is designated tHcy [76].

The tHcy concentrations show a skewed distribution towards higher values in healthy subjects. The arithmetic means were 11.3 µmol/l in 5918 healthy men and 9.6 µmol in 6348 women aged 40-years [58].

Plasma tHcy levels are also dependent on age, gender, and in women, possibly menopausal status. Normal mean values are about 1 µmol lower in premenopausal women than in postmenopausal women, and there seems to be a significant increase (about 1-2 µmol/l) in the mean values as a function of age (from 20 to 70 years) in both sexes [5, 58].

Good correlation between tHcy measurements performed in different laboratories and with different methodes has been obtained, and values between 5 and 15 µmol/l are usually considered as normal [59, 76].

Causes of Hyperhomocysteinemia

"Hyperhomocysteinemia" means "elevated tHcy in blood" [49]. Hyperhomocysteinemia has been classified as moderate, intermediate, and severe. Moderate hyperhomocysteinemia is defined by a fasting tHcy concentration in plasma/serum of 15-30 µmol/l, intermediate by concentrations between 31 and 100 µmol/l, and severe by concentrations higher than 100 µmol/l [44].

Hyperhomocysteinemia is either interited or acquired (Table 1). Genetic variants include the homozygous form of cystathionine β-synthase deficiency, which is the most common cause of homocystinuria [57]. Rare forms are severe genetic defects of methylenetetrahydrofolate reductase, and inborn errors of cobalamin metabolism, classified as cblC, cblD, cblF, cblG, and cblE mutations [65].

Table 1. Causes of acquired and genetic hyperhomocyst(e)inemia

	Hyperhomocysteinemia	Prevalence as cause of hyperhomocyst(e)inemia
Acquired:		
Cobalamin deficiency	M, I, S	Common
Folate deficiency	M, I	Common
Vitamin B_6 deficiency	(M)	Probably common
Renal failure	M, I	Common
Malignancy	M	Not common
Psoriasis	M	Fairly common
Hypothyroidism	M	Fairly common
Drugs	M	Fairly common
Methotrexate		
Nitrous oxide		
Antiepileptic agents		
Colestipol plus niacin		
Vitamin B_6 antagonists (azaribin, isoniazide)		
Genetic:		
Homozygous for CS deficiency	I, S	Rare
Homozygous for MTFR deficiency	I, S	Rare
Cobalamin mutations (C, D, E, F, G)	I	Rare
Homozygous for the C677T MTFR mutation[a]	M	Common (5%-10%)
Heterozygous for CS deficiency	M	Probably rare
Heterozygous MTFR deficiency	M	Rare
Compound heterozygosity (MTFR deficiency and thermolabile MTFR)	I	-

M, moderate hyperhomocyst(e)inemia, 15-30 µmol/l; I, intermediate hyperhomocysteinemia, 30-100 µmol/l; S, severe hyperhomocyst(e)inemia, > 100 µmol/l; CS, cystathionine β-synthese; MTFR, methylenetetrahydrofolate reductase.
[a] This mutation causes the thermolabile enzyme variant.

Heterozygosity for cystathionine β-synthase deficiency is present in 0.3%-1%, or 2% at most, of the general population [57]. Although heterozygosity for cystathionine β-synthase was postulated earlier as the main cause of moderate hyperhomocysteinemia [12, 23], this has recently been called into question by enzymic and molecular genetic studies that demonstrated no heterozygotes for cystathionine β-synthase among vascular patients with moderate hyperhomocysteinemia [27, 47, 48].

A (C677T) mutation of methylenetetrahydrofolate reductase, characterized by thermolability and a 50% reduction in activity of the enzyme, occurs in 5%-10% of the general population, and these subjects have a tendency towards moderate hyperhomocysteinemia [20, 41-43]. This C677T mutation may cause a redistribution of the folates [77], and the homozygous subjects probably need more folate to keep their tHcy levels within acceptable ranges.

Subjects with compound heterozygosity of methylenetetrahydrofolate reductase deficiency and the thermolabile enzyme have also been described.

These have intermediate hyperhomocysteinemia [42]. Thus, heterozygosity for various forms of homocystinuria may explain the observation that tHcy is a genetic trait [60].

Among the acquired conditions causing elevated tHcy, folate [40] or cobalamin deficiency [1, 18] are most often encountered. Folate deficiency is associated with moderate and intermediate hyperhomocysteinemia. In cobalamin-deficient patients, severe hyperhomocysteinemia is occasionally observed [1]. Elevation of tHcy is also observed in disease states such as renal failure [15, 79], acute leukaemia, psoriasis, and hypothyroidism [75], and is induced by some drugs, e.g. methotrexate, nitrous oxide, antiepileptic agents, colestipol plus niacin [11], and some agents acting as vitamin B_6 antagonists [61].

Analytical Methods

There is a continuous redistribution of Hcy species in plasma/serum, so that after storage for days (at room temperature) or months (frozen), most Hcy becomes associated with plasma proteins. Reliable measurement of free Hcy therefore requires immediate deproteinization of plasma/serum, which is impractical in the clinical routine. It has therefore been largely abandoned and tHcy is measured instead [76].

Measurement of tHcy, which includes all Hcy species, is now widely recommended since the values remain stable during storage of plasma/serum. tHcy is measured by procedures including treatment of whole plasma/serum with a reductant. The Hcy disulfides are then quantitatively converted into reduced Hcy [76].

The methods used for separation and quantitation of reduced Hcy vary. The Hcy assays can be categorised into five types according to the nature of the method: (1) enzymic assays, (2) gas chromatography-mass spectrometry (GC-MS), (3) assays based on precolumn derivatization, high-performance liquid chromatography (HPLC), and fluorescence detection, (4) HPLC and electrochemical detection, and (5) assays based on liquid chromatography and postcolumn derivatization, including the amino acid analyzer.

The Enzymic Assays

These methods are based on the conversion of Hcy to *S*-adenosylhomocysteine, catalyzed by the enzyme *S*-adenosylhomocysteine hydrolase. *S*-adenosylhomocysteine is quantitated by HPLC [62], paper chromatography [21], or thin-layer chromatography [22].

Low instrumental cost of the modification based on thin-layer chromatography is the main advantage of this assay. However, these assays are laborious and the linearity may be limited by consumption of the cosubstrate (adenosine) used for the enzymic derivatization of Hcy.

A fluorescence polarization immunoassay for tHcy, run on an Abbott IMx analyzer, uses monoclonal antibodies against *S*-adenosylhomocysteine [66]. This is a homogenous assay characterized by high sample throughput, and may be particularly useful in laboratories with no chromatographic expertise. However, data on performance and experience with this assay are limited.

Gas Chromatography

In the GC-MS assay developed by Stabler and coworkers, deuterated Hcy is used as internal standard, the sample is subjected to solid-phase extraction, and Hcy is derivatized with *N*-methyl-*N*(*t*-butyldimethylsilyl)trifluoroacetamide. The *t*-butyldimethylsilyl derivatives are seperated and quantitated by capillary GC and selected ion monitoring [68, 69]. Attractive features of this method are codetermination of other metabolites such as methylmalonic acid. This technique has been simplified from the initial version [69], but it is still a cumbersome procedure. Furthermore, expensive equipment and technical skill are required.

tHcy and other sulfur amino acids in plasma have also been measured by GC with flame photometric [45, 46]. The assay is fast and simple, but again, experience with the assay is limited.

Precolumn Derivatization, HPLC, and Fluorescence Detection

Hcy can be derivatized with the thiol-specific fluorogenic reagents monobromobimane (mBrB) [31, 36, 37, 51, 64] or ammonium-7-fluoro-2, 1, 3-benzoxadiazole-4-sulfonate (SBD-F) [8; 70; 78] or 7-fluorobenzo-2-oxa-1.3-diazole-4-sulfonamide (ABD-F) [24], followed by separation of the adducts with HPLC. These tags also label cycsteine and cysteinylglycine, which are codetermined in these assays.

mBrB is a reactive agent and the derivatization is completed within minutes. Assays based on this reagent can be fully automated [64]. The automatization results in high precision. The composition and pH of the mobile phase are critical for the separation of the Hcy adduct from hydrolysis products and other interfering material [31].

Among the halogenosulfonylbenzofurazans, SDB-F has low reactivity (derivatization is carried out at 60°C for 30–60 min) whereas ABD-F reacts more rapidly (50°C for 5–10 min). Slow derivatization prevents automatization. the separation of the thiol adducts is simple and fast since the reagents themselves are not fluorogenic and there is no interfering material [8, 24, 70, 78].

Methods have been published which are based on precolumn derivatization with thiol-reactive maleimide derivatives [3, 80] or with *o*-phthaldialdehyde [29, 34], but these assays have not yet gained widespread use.

HPLC and Electrochemical Detection

In this assay, plasma/serum samples are subjected to HPLC immediately after treatment with reductant, and Hcy is detected with an electrochemical detector equipped with a gold-mercury electrode, which affords great specificity towards thiols. Simple sample processing, short run time, and high sample output are attractive features of this technique [49, 67]. However, particular attention must be paid to maintenance of flow cell and the gold-mercury electrode, since deterioration of the these parts of the detector system may cause baseline fluctuations and variable electrochemical response. Pulsed integrated amperometry may offer a solution to these problems since the electrode is self-cleaning and degradation of the electrode surface is minimized [28].

Amino Acid Analyzer and Postcolumn Derivatization

Hcy can be analyzed using an amino acid analyzer, either following reduction [2] or after the sulfhydryl group has been carboxymethylated using iodoacetic acid [39]. The free sulfhydryl is quantitated on an ion-exchange column eluted with the standard program [35] or with a mobile phase optimized for Hcy determiniation [2]. Even the optimized program results in long retention time (about 25 min), which is followed by column regeneration [2]. This seriously restricts sample output, which is low compared to the HPLC methods. Other disadvantages are relatively high imprecision, and formation of interfering ninhydrin-positive material upon storage of samples at −20°C [76].

A method for tHcy determination based on HPLC and postcolumn derivatization with thiol-specific chromophor 4,4'-dithiodipyidine has been published [7]. Critical measures to reduce baseline noise have been worked out, and the method may turn out to be useful.

Procedures for Sample Collection and Processing

Plasma tHcy increases slowly to a maximum increase of 15%–20% 6–8h after a protein-rich meal. The increased tHcy level persists for several hours [76]. This effect from food intake is small relative to the Hcy levels caused by some acquired or genetic diseases (see, Table 1), and does not interfere with interpretation of data. However, in a recent prospective study a 41% increase in risk of myocardial infarction has been found for each 4μ*M* increase in Hcy concentration [9]. Thus, when plasma/serum Hcy is used as a parameter to evaluate cardiovascular risk, measurement of fasting levels is preferable.

tHcy is increased in plasma/serum when whole blood is left at room temperature. This is caused by a temperature- and time-dependent release of Hcy from the blood cells secondary to its synthesis mainly in the erythrocytes [6, 50]. After 1 h at 22°C, there is a significant (10%) increase in plasma tHcy [4, 31, 71, 78]. A release of Hcy from the blood cells before aspiration explains the observation that tHcy is slightly higher in serum than in plasma [78].

The artificial elevation is markedly reduced when the samples of whole blood are placed on ice. Under these conditions (0–2°C), plasma tHcy is stable tHcy is stable for at least 4h [31]. The release of Hcy from blood is also inhibited by fluoride [72]. To stabilize plasma tHcy, it is recommended that whole blood is kept on ice and the blood cells removed from the plasma fraction within 1 h. Serum must be aspirated immedialy after clot retraction.

Collection of blood into standard tubes with fluoride and with heparin as an anticoagulant is a practical procedure to reduce artifical elevation of tHcy [56], but inference from fluoride with the assay procedure must be ruled out.

tHcy in serum/plasma is stable for at least 4 days at room temperature, and for several weeks when stored at 0–2°C. In frozen samples kept at −20 C, it is stable for years [76].

Methionine Loading Test

The methionine loading test involes oral intake of a standard dose of methionine (0.1 g/kg or 3.8 g/m^2), and tHcy is measured after a fixed time interval, usually 4 or 6 h [3, 17, 19, 63, 75].

An abbreviated version of the oral methionine loading test, measuring tHcy 2 h post-load, seems to identify the same individuals as those who had an abnormal 4 h post-load value. The 2-h loading test is advantageous in terms of practicality and logistics [14].

The methionine loading test has been used to find possible defects in methionine metabolism in patients with cardiovascular disease. An abnormal response has been defined as a postload tHcy concentration or postload increase in tHcy exceeding the 95th or 90th percentile, the mean plus 2 standard deviations for controls, or the highest control value [13, 75].

Subjects with impaired ability to remethylate Hcy due to cobalamin deficiency or defective methylenetetrahydrofolate reductase have hyperhomocysteinemia during fasting, but a normal increase in tHcy after methionine loading. In contrast, obligate heterozygotes for cystathionine β-synthase deficiency have normal tHcy but are methionine-intolerant [19]. This is in accordance with studies in rats showing that folate deficiency causes fasting hyperhomocysteinemia whereas B_6 deficiency results in postload hyperhomocysteinemia [55]. However, there are indications that the discriminative power of fasting versus postload tHcy is an oversimplification, since erythrocyte folate has been found to be related to both parameters [32].

There is a significant positive correlation between fasting and postload tHcy; the two parameters have similar ability to discriminate between vascular patients and controls, but do not provide completely overlapping results [52]. A recent report indicates that fasting tHcy alone fails to identify more than 40 % of subjects with an abnormal tHcy response to a methionine loading test [13]. Thus, determination of tHcy after methionine loading is a laborious but valuable adjunct to fasting tHcy in cardiovascular risk assessment.

Conclusion

There is ample evidence that hyperhomocysteinemia is a strong risk factor for cardiovascular disease. A moderately elevated tHcy concentration of 4–5 μmoL/l, which represents a less than 50 % increase above normal values, conveys a significantly increased risk. Thus, precautions must be taken during blood sampling and processing to avoid any artificial increase in tHcy when this parameter is used for cardiovascular risk assessment. This is in contrast to the more flexible procedures sufficient to detect the massive elevation of tHcy caused by severe vitamin deficiencies or inborn errors of Hcy metabolism.

Numerous techniques for analysis of tHcy in serum or plasma have been described, but HPLC methods based on precolumn derivatization using SBD-F or mBrB, electrochemical assay, and GC-MS have been most extensively used. Comparison of methods have showed good interassay agreement, and the choise of method should be based on the personnel and instrumental resources available and the training of the staff.

References

1. Allen RH, Stabler SP, Savage DG, Lindenbaum J (1994) Metabolic abnormalities in cobalamin (vitamin-B12) and folate deficiency. FASEB J 7: 1344–1353
2. Andersson A, Brattström L, Isaksson A, Israelsson B, Hultberg B (1989) Determination of homocysteine in plasma by ion-exchange chromatography. Scand J Clin Lab Invest 49: 445–450
3. Andersson A, Brattström L, Israelsson B, Isaksson A, Hultberg B (1990) The effect of excess daily methionine intake on plasma homocysteine after a methionine loading test in humans. Clin Chim Acta 192: 69–76
4. Andersson A, Isaksson A, Brattström L, Israelsson B, Hultberg B (1991) Influence of hydrolysis on plasma homocysteine determination in healthy subjects and patients with myocardial infarotion. Atherosclerosis 88: 143–151
5. Andersson A, Brattström L, Israelsson B, Isaksson A, Hamfelt A, Hultberg B (1992) Plasma homocysteine before and after methionine loading with regard to age, gender, and menopausal status. Eur J Clin Invest 22: 79–87
6. Andersson A, Isaksson A, Hultberg B (1992) Homocysteine export from erythrocytes and its implication for plasma sampling. Clin Chem 38: 1311–1315
7. Andersson A, Isaksson A, Brattström L, Hultberg B (1993) Homocysteine and other thiols determined in plasma by HPLC and thiol-specific postcolumn derivatization. Clin Chem 39: 1590–1597
8. Araki A, Sako Y (1987) Determination of free and total homocysteine in human plasma by high-performance liquid chromatography with fluorescence detection. J Chromatogr 422: 43–52
9. Arnesen E, Refsum II, Bønaa KH, Ueland PM, Førde OH, Nordrehaug JE (1995) Serum total homocysteine and coronary heart disease. Int J Epidemiol 24: 704–709

10. Bienvenu T, Ankri A, Chadefaux B, Montalescot G, Kamoun P (1993) Elevated total plasma homocysteine, a risk factor for thrombosis. Relation to coagulation and fibrinolytic parameters. Thromb Res 70: 123-129
11. Blankenhorn DR, Malinow MR, Mack WJ (1991) Colestipol plus niacin therapy elevates plasma homocyst(e)ine levels. Coron Art Dis 2: 357-360
12. Boers GHJ, Smals AGH, Trijbels FJM, Fowler B, Bakkeren JAJM, Schoonderwaldt HC, Kleijer WJ, Kloppenborg PWC (1985) Heterozygosity for homocystinuria in premature peripheral and cerebral occlusive arterial disease. N Engl J Med 313: 709-715
13. Bostom AG, Jacques PF, Nadeau MR, Williams RR, Ellison RC, Selhub J (1995) Post-methionine load hyperhomocysteinemia in persons with normal fasting total plasma homocysteine: initial results from the NHLBI family heart study. Atherosclerosis 116: 147-151
14. Bostom AG, Roubenoff R, Dellaripa P, Nadeau MR, Sutherland P, Wilson PWF, Jacques PF, Selhub J, Rosenberg 111 (1995) Validation of abbreviated oral methionine-loading test. Clin Chem 41: 948-949
15. Bostom AG, Shemin D, Lapane KL, Miller JW, Sutherland P, Nadeau M, Seyoum E, Hartman W, Prior R, Wilson PWF, Selhub J (1995) Hyperhomocysteinemia and traditional cardiovascular disease risk factors in end-stage renal disease patients on dialysis: a case-control study. #therosclerosis 114: 93-103
16. Boushey CJ, Beresford SAA, Omenn GS, Motulsky AG (1995) A quantitative assessment of plasma homocysteine as a risk factor for vascular disease: probable benefits of inoreasing folic acid intakes. JAMA 274: 1049-1057
17. Brattström L, Israelsson B, Hultberg B (1988) Impalred homocysteine metabolism - a possible risk factor for arteriosclerotic vascular disease. In: Smith U, Eriksson S, Lindgärde F (eds) Genetic susceptibility to environmental factors a challenge for public intervention. Almqvist and Wiksell, Stockholm, pp 25-34
18. Brattström L, Israelsson B, Lindgärde F, Hultberg B (1988) Higher total plasma homooysteine in vitamin B 12 deficiency than in heterozygosity for homocystinuria due to cystathionine β-synthase deficiency. Metabolism 37: 175-178
19. Brattström L, Israelsson B, Norrving B, Bergqvist D, Thörne J, Hultberg B, Hamfelt A (1990) Impaired homocysteine metabolism in early-onset cerebral and peripheral occlusive arterial disease-effects of pyridoxine and folic acid treatment. Atherosolerosis 81: 51-60
20. Brattström L, Tengborn L, Israelsson B, Hultberg B (1991) Plasma homocysteine in venous thromboembolism. Haemostasis 21: 51-57
21. Chadefaux B, Coude M, Hamet M, Aupetit J, Kamoun P (1989) Rapid determination of total homocysteine in plasma. Clin Chem 35: 2002
22. Chu RC, Hall CA (1988) The total serum homocysteine as an indicator of vitamin B12 and folate status. Am J Clin Pathol 90: 446-449
23. Clarke R, Daly L, Robinson K, Naughten E, Cahalane S, Fowler B, Graham I(1991) Hyperhomocysteinemia: an independent risk factor for vascular disease. N Engl J Med 324: 1149-1155
24. Comwell PE, Morgan SL, Vaughn WH (1993) Modification of a high-performance liquid chromatographic method for assay of homocysteine in human plasma. J Chromatogr 617: 136-139
25. Den Heijer M, Blom HJ, Gerrits WBJ, Rosendaal FR, Haak HL, Wijermans PW, Bos GMJ (1995) Is hyperhomocysteinaemia a risk factor for recurrent venous thrombosis? Lancet 345: 882-885
26. Den Heijer M, Koster T, Blom HJ, Bos GMJ, Briet E, Reitsma PHR, Vandenbroucke W, Rosendaal FR (1996) Hyperhomocysteinemia: a risk factor for deep-vein thrombosis. Leiden thrombophilia study. N Engl J Med 334: 759-762
27. Engbersen AMT, Franken DG, Boers GHJ, Stevens ENIB, Trijbels FJM, Blom HJ (1995) Thermolabile 5,10-methylenetetrahydrofolate reductase as a cause of mild hyperhomocysteinemia. Am J Hum Genet 56: 142-150
28. Evrovski J, Callaghan M, Cole DEC (1995) Determination of homocysteine by HPLC with pulse integrated amperometry. Clin Chem 41: 757-758
29. Fermo I, Arcelloni C, Devecchi E, Vigano S, Paroni R (1992) High-performance liquid chromatographic method with fluorescence detection for the determination of total homocyst(e)ine in plasma. J Chromatogr 593: 171-176
30. Finkelstein JD (1990) Methionine metabolism in mammals. J Nutr Biochem 1: 228-237
31. Fiskerstrand T, Refsum H, Kvalheim G, Ueland PM (1993) Homocysteine and other thiols in plasma and urine: automated determination and sample stability. Clin Chem 39: 263-271
32. Graham I, Daly LE, Refsum HM, Robinson K, Brattström L, Leland PM, Palma-Reis RJ, Boers GHJ, Sheahan RG, Israelsson B et al (1996) Plasma total homocysteine: a risk factor for vascular disease with interactions with smoking, hypertension and hypercholesterolemia. The European concerted action project. (in press)
33. Haj-Yehia AI, Benet LZ (1995) 2-(4-N-maleimidophenyl)-6-methoxybenzofuran: a superior derivatizing agent for fluorimetric determination of aliphatic thiols by high-performance liquid chromatography. J Chromatogr 666: 45-53
34. Hyland K, Bottiglieri T (1992) Measurement of total plasma and cerebrospinal fluid homocysteine by fluorescence following high-performance liquid chromatography and precolumn derivatization with orthophthaldialdehyde. J Chromatogr 579: 55-62
35. Israelsson B, Brattström LE, Hultberg BJ (1988) Homocysteine and myocardial infarotion. Atherosclerosis 71: 227-234
36. Jacobsen DW, Gatautis VJ, Green R (1989) Determination of plasma homocysteine by high-performance liquid chromatography with fluorescence detection. Anal Biochem 178: 208-214
37. Jacobsen DW, Gatautis VJ, Green R, Robinson K, Ji J, Savon SR, Otto JM, Taylor LM (1994) Rapid HPLC determination of total homocysteine and other thiols in serum and plasma: sex differences and correlation with cobalamin and folate levels in normal subjects. Clin Chem 40: 873-881
38. Kang S-S, Wong PWK, Becker N (1979) Protein-bound homocyst(e)ine in normal subjects and in patients with homocystinuria. Pediatr Res 13: 1141-1143
39. Kang S-S, Wong PWK, Curley K (1982) The effect of D-penicillamine on protein-bound homocyst(e)ine in homocystinurics. Pediatr Res 16: 370-372
40. Kang S-S, Wong PWK, Norusis M (1987) Homocysteinemia due to folate deficiency. Metabolism 36: 458-462

41. Kang S-S, Wong PWK, Zhou J, Sora J, Lessick M, Ruggie N, Grcevich G (1988) Thermolabile methylenetetrahydrofolate reductase in patients with coronary artery disease. Metabolism 37: 611-613
42. Kang S-S, Wong PWK, Bock H-GO, Horwitz A, Grix A (1991) Intermediate hyperhomocysteinemia resulting from compound heterozygosity of methylenetetrahydrofolate reductase mutations. Am J Rum Genet 48: 546-551
43. Kang S-S, Wong PWK, Susmano A, Sora J, Norusis M, Ruggie N (1991) Thermolabile methylenetetrahydrofolate reductase: an inherited risk factor for coronary artery disease. Am J Hum Genet 48: 536-545
44. Kang S-S, Wong PWK, Malinow MR (1992) Hyperhomocyst(e)inemia as a risk factor for occlusive vascular disease. Annu Rev Nutr 12: 279-298
45. Kataoka H, Tanaka H, Fujimoto A, Noguchi I, Makita M (1994) Determination of sulphur amino acids by gas chromatography with flame photometric detection. Biomed Chromatogr 8: 119-124
46. Kataoka H, Takagi K, Makita M (1995) Determination of total plasma homocysteine and related aminothiols by gas chromatography with flame photometric detection. J Chromatogr 664: 421-425
47. Kluijtmans LAJ, VandenHeuvel LPWJ, Boers GHJ, Frosst P, VanOost BA, den Heijer M, Stevens EMB, Trijbels JMF, Rozen R, Blom RJ (1996) Molecular genetic analysis in mild hyperhomocysteinemia: a common mutation in the methylenetetrahydrofolate reductase gene is a genetic risk factor for cardiovascular disease. Am J Rum Genet 58: 35-44
48. Kozich V, Kraus E, DeFranchis R, Fowler B, Boers GRJ, Graham I, Kraus JP (1995) Hyperhomocysteinemia in premature arterial disease: examination of cystathionine beta-synthase alleles at the molecular level. Rum Mol Genet 4: 623-629
49. Malinow MR, Kang SS, Taylor LM, Wong PWK, Inahara T, Mukerjee D, Sexton G, Upson B (1989) Prevalence of hyperhomocyst(e)inemia in patients with peripheral arterial occlusive disease. Circ Res 79:1180-1188
50. Malinow MR, Axthelm MK, Meredith MJ, MacDonald NA, Upson BM (1994) Synthesis and transsulfuration of homocysteine in blood. J Lab Clin Med 123: 421-429
51. Mansoor MA, Svardal AM, Ueland PM (1992) Determination of the in vivo redox status of cysteine, cysteinylglycine, homocysteine and glutathione in human plasma. Anal Biochem 200: 218-229
52. Mansoor AM, Bergmark C, Svardal AM, Lønning PE, Ueland PM (1995) Redox status and protein-binding of plasma homocysteine and other aminothiols in patients with early-onset peripheral vascular disease. Arteriosclerosi Thromb Vasc Biol 15: 232-240
53. McCully K5 (1992) Homocystinuria, arteriosclerosis, methylmalonic aciduria, and methyltransferase deficiency - a key case revisited. Nutr Rev 50: 7-12
54. McCully KS, Wilson RB (1975) Homocysteine theory of arteriosclerosis. Atherosclerosis 22: 215-227
55. Miller JW, Nadeau MR, Smith D, Selhub J (1994) Vitamin B-6 deficiency vs folate deficiency - comparison of responses to methionine loading in rats. Am J Clin Nutr 59: 1033-1039
56. Møller J, Rasmussen K (1994) Homocysteine in plasma: stabilization of blood samples with fluoride. Clin Chem 41: 758-759
57. Mudd SH, Levy HL, Skovby F (1995) Disorder of transsulfuration. In: Scriver CR, Beaudet AL, Sly WS, Valle D (eds) The metabolic basis of inherited disease. McGraw-Hill, New York, pp 1279-1327
58. Nygård O, Vollset SE, Refsum H, Stensvol I Tverdal A, Nordrehaug JE, Ueland PM, Kvå(1995) Total plasma homocysteine and cardiovascular risk profile. The Hordaland homocysteine study. JAMA 274:1526-1533
59. Poelepothoff MTWBT, Vandenberg M, Franken DG, Boers GHJ, Jakobs C, Dekroon IFI, Eskes TKAB, Trijbels JMF, Blom HJ (1995) Three different methods for the determination of total homocysteine in plasma. Ann Clin Biochem 32: 218-220
60. Reed T, Malinow MR, Christian JC, Upson B (1991) Estimates of heritability for plasma homocyst(e)ine levels in aging adult male twins. Clin Genet 39: 425-428
61. Refsum H, Leland PM (1990) Clinical significance of pharmacological modulation of homocysteine metabolism. Trends Pharmacol Sci 11: 411-416
62. Refsum H, Helland S, Ueland PM (1985) Radioenzymic determination of homocysteine in plasma and urine. Clin Chem 31: 624-628
63. Refsum H, Helland S, Ueland PM (1989) Fasting plasma homocysteine as a sensitive parameter to antifolate effect. A study on psoriasis patients receiving low-dose methotrexate treatment. Clin Pharmacol Ther 46: 510-520
64. Refsum H, Ueland PM, Svardal AM (1989) Fully automated fluorescence assay for determining total homocysteine in plasma. Clin Chem 35: 1921-1927
65. Rosenblatt DS, Cooper BA (1990) Inherited disorders of vitamin-B 12 utilization. Bioessays 12: 331-334
66. Schipchandler MT, Moore EG (1995) Rapid, fully automated measurement of plasma homocyst(e)ine with the Abbott IMx analyzer. Clin Chem 41: 991-994
67. Smolin LA, Benevenga NJ (1982) Accumulation of homocyst(e)ine in vitamin B-6 deficiency: a model for the study of cystathionine β-synthase deficiency. J Nutr 112:1264-1272
68. Stabler SP, Marcell PD, Podell ER, Allen RH (1987) Quantitation of total homocysteine, total cysteine, and methionine in normal serum and urine using capillary gas chromatography-mass spectrometry. Anal Biochem 162:185-196
69. Stabler SP, Lindenbaum J, Savage DG, Allen RH (1993) Elevation of serum cystathionine levels in patients with cobalamin and folate deficiency. Blood 81: 3404-3413
70. Ubbink JB, Vermaak WJH, Bissbort S (1991) Rapid high-performance liquid chromatographic assay for total homocysteine levels in human serum. J Chromatogr 565: 441-446
71. Ubbink JB, Vermaak WJH, Vandermerwe A, Becker PJ (1992) The effect of blood sample aging and food consumption on plasma total homocysteine levels. Clin Chim Acta 207: 119-128
72. Ubbink JB, Vermaak WJH, van der Merwe A, Becker PJ (1993) Vitamin B-12, vitamin B-6, and folate nutritional status in men with hyperhomocysteinemia. Am J Clin Nutr 57: 47-53
73. Ueland PM (1995) Homocysteine species as components of plasma redox thiol status. Clin Chem 41: 340-342
74. Ueland PM, Refsum H (1989) Plasma homocysteine, a risk factor for vascular disease: plasma levels in health, disease, and drug therapy. J Lab Clin Med 114: 473-501

75. Ueland PM, Refsum H, Brattström L (1992) Plasma homocysteine and cardiovascular disease. In: Francis RB Jr (eds) Atherosclerotic cardiovascular disease, hemostasis, and endothelial function. Dekker, New York, pp 183-236
76. Ueland PM, Refsum H, Stabler SP, Malinow MR, Andersson A, Allen RH (1993) Total homocysteine in plasma or serum. Methods and clinical applications. Clin Chem 39: 1764-1779
77. VanderPut NMJ, Steegers-Theunissen RPM, Frosst P, Trijbels FJM, Eskes TKAB, van den Heuvel LP, Mariman ECM, den Heijer M, Rozen R, Blom HJ (1995) Mutated methylenetetrahydrofolate reductase as a risk factor for spina bifida. Lancet 346: 1070-1071
78. Vester B, Rasmussen K (1991) High performance liquid chromatography method for rapid and accurate determination of homocysteine in plasma and serum. Eur J Clin Chem Clin Biochem 29: 549-554
79. Wilcken DEL, Gupta VJ, Betts AK (1981) Homocysteine in the plasma ofrenal transplant recipients: effects of cofactors for methionine metabolism. Clin Sci 61: 743-749
80. Winters RA, Zukowski J, Ercal N, Matthews RH, Spitz DR (1995) Analysis of glutathione, glutathione disulfide, cysteine, homocysteine, and other biological thiols by high-performance liquid chromatography following derivatization by n- (1 -pyrenyl)maleimide. Anal Biochem 227: 14-21

Immunological Assessments

J. Kekow and W.L. Gross

Introduction

With the availability of autoantibody assays, immunologic laboratory evaluations have become an important component of the diagnostic work-up of patients with systemic vascular disorders. Relevant autoantibodies are immunoglobulins of different isoforms directed against autologous intracellular, cell surface, and extracellular antigens. The intracellular antigens include nuclear components (antinuclear antibodies, or ANA) and cytoplasmic components (anti-neutrophilic cytoplasmic, or ANCA). In some vascular disorders the detection of autoantibodies is specific and its significance may be compared with that of histomorphological findings.

Autoantibodies are detected by a variety of techniques including indirect immunofluorescence, passive hemagglutination, particle agglutination, immunodiffusion, counter immunoelectrophoresis, radioimmunoassay, and enzyme-linked immunosorbent assay. At present there is no standardization of either the assay method or the units in which the results are reported. Therefore, comparison of data between laboratories is difficult. In addition, low autoantibody titers are present in a small proportion of the normal population. Thus, a diagnosis of systemic vasculitis cannot be based solely on serology.

In this chapter we will focus on diagnostic laboratory methods available to assess autoantibodies relevant to vascular diseases and briefly describe the pathophysiological role of these antibodies in the development of the latter.

Nomenclature and Overview

General Definition and Nomenclature of Vasculitides

Systemic vasculitides form a heterogeneous group of disorders whose common pathological feature is an inflammatory reaction of blood vessels of varying size and at varying sites. Vasculitis is a feature of many different diseases and is referred to as secondary vasculitis in disease with a know etiology (e.g. virus infection) or when vasculitis develops in a preexisting disease (e.g., systemic lupus erythematosus, SLE). Idiopathic vasculitides are called primary vasculitides. Since little is know of the precise pathogenesis of these conditions, the morphological features are still one of the most important aspects in classifying vasculitides (type of blood vessels involved and granuloma formation; see Tables 7 and 8). When the possible mechanisms of blood vessel injury and the occurrence of vasculitis secondary to other diseases are included, vasculitides can be further distinguished in to at least five groups (Table 1).

Table 1. Nomenclature of vasculitides based on presumed pathogenesis

Immune vasculitis
Pauci-immune vasculitis
Autoantibody-associated:Wegener's granulomatosis, microscopic polyangiitis, Kawasaki's disease
Immune complex-mediated vasculitis
Autoantigen/autoantibody associated: systemic lupus erythematosus
In infectious diseases: HBV infection in polyarteritis nodosa
In cryoglobulinemia: HCV infection, myeloma
Granulomatous form of vasculitis with rich T-helper cell infiltrates
Giant cell arteritis (arteritis temporalis)
Others
Vasculitis in infectious diseases
Viral: cytomegalovirus
Bacterial: tyhpus, Lyme disease
Vasculitis in neoplasms
Infiltration of vessels by tumor cells: lymphomatoid granulomatosis, hairy cell leukemia

HBV, HCV, Hepatitic B, C viruses.

Autoantibodies: Pathophysiological Implications for Vasculitis

Antinuclear Antibodies

Immune complex deposits are thought to be the pivotal aspect of vasculitis in SLE, representing the type III immune reaction of the Gell and Coombs classification. Circulating immune complexes per se do not cause vasculitis until immune complex deposition in the vessel wall activates the complement cascade. Important factors leading to immune complex deposition include (1) moderate antibody production with antigen excess, resulting in intermediate-sized immune complexes which are not efficiently cleared, (2) formation of small immune complexes that are slowly eliminated, (3) production of IgM-containing immune complexes, (4) blockade of the reticuloendothelial system by large amounts of immune complexes, (5) alterations in vascular permeability, and (6) regional differences in hydrostatic pressure, e.g., in the glomeruli [17]. Once immune complexes attached to the vessel wall activate the complement cascade, complement fragments promote chemotaxis of polymorphonuclear cells (PMN) and expression of complement receptor 3 adhesion molecules. This enables adherence to the endothelium and entry into the vessel wall. Tissue necrosis is the consequence of enzymes and oxygen radicals released by the PMN.

Antineutrophilic Cytoplasmic Antibodies

In contrast to the immune complex-mediated mechanisms found in collagen diseases such as SLE, the pathophysiology of ANCA-associated vasculitides is less well understood. It is know at any rate that different mechanisms than in ANA-mediated responses contribute to endothelial damage, because immune complexes are absent in primary vasculitides such as Wegener's granulomatosis, microscopic polyangiitis, and Churg-Strauss syndrome. The current theories favor a loss of self-tolerance to granule proteins, the ANCA targets, but the cause of this presumed altered self-tolerance remains unknown. Both humoral and cellular autoimmune mechanisms may be involved. Based on defferent observations in vivo and in vitro, a model for the development of cANCA (proteinase 3-positive) vasculitis has been introduced, according to which ANCA, normally present in granules of PMN and not accessible to the autoantibodies, are expressed on the cell surface in response to inflammatory cytokines. The binding of ANCA to proteinase 3 (PR3) further activates the PMN, resulting in endothelial cell damage due to enzyme release and the generation of oxygen radicals [12, 13]. This model is supported by various animal studies in which ANCA and the corresponding antigens were able to induce vasculitis [4, 8]. Other data indicate that ANCA can bind directly to the vessel wall since the corresponding antigen either sticks to endothelial cells or can be expressed on their surface.

Diagnosis of Vasculitis

Clinical Signs

The clinical picture in vasculitis varies depending on which particular type of vasculitis is involved (size of affected vessels, underlying disease). In primary vasculitis, first symptoms are directly related to vessel demage with subsequent organ failure or, in granuloma-forming vasculitis, are due to tumor-like lesions (e.g., protrusio bulbi in orbital granuloma). Important clinical features of primary vasculitides are given in Table 2 (Chapel Hill classification) [16]. In collagen diseases such as SLE, clinical signs of vasculitis are quite similar. Important clinical manifestations of SLE include leukocytoclastic angiitis, livedo vasculitis, subcutaneous nodules, livedo reticularis, coronary arteritis, mononeuritis multiplex, cerebral infarcts, mesenteric arteritis, and retinopathy. Table 3 lists important symptoms which are suggestive of vasculitis.

Laboratory Findings

Spectrum of ANA and ANA Assays

The term "anti-nuclear-antibody" is used to describe all (auto-)antibodies that react with nuclear cell components. The classical method for their detection (indirect immunofluorescence technique, IFT) has remained widely unchanged. Briefly, cells (human cell lines, e.g., Hep2 cells; tissue sections, e.g., from liver, either human or rat; sections from mouse kidney) are fixed to a slide and treated with patient serum. Then, the distribution of bound antibody is visualized with the help of a second, fluorescent anti-human immunoglobulin antibody. The fluorescent antibody staining is visualized by ultraviolet light microscopy (Fig. 1). The ANA finding is reported as positive at a defined screening dilution or endpoint dilution. A WHO reference for ANA is available.

The IFT readings are not uniform, differing in intensity (due to the amount of autoantibodies present) and in the appearance of the nuclear stain. This can be explained by the presence of antibody subsets of varying antigen specificity. In early stu-

Table 2. Names and definitions adopted by the Chapel Hill Consensus Conference on the Nomenclature of Systemic Vasculitides [16]

Large vessel vasculitis[a]	
Giant cell (temporal) arteritis	Granulomatous arteritis of the aorta and ist major branches, with a predilection for the extracranial branches of the carotid artery. *Often involves the temporal artery. Usually occurs in patients older than 50 and ist often associated with polymyalgia rheumatica.*
Takayasu arteritis	Granulomatous inflammation of the aorta and ist major branches. *Usually occurs in patients younger than 50.*
Medium-sized vessel vasculitis	
Polyarteritis nodosa[b]	Necrotizing inflammation of medium-sized or small (classic polyarteritis nodosa) arteries without glomerulonephritis or vasculitis in arterioles, capillaries, or venules.
Kawasaki's disease	Arteritis involving large, medium-sized, and small arteries, and associated with mucocutaneous lymph node syndrome. *Coronary arteries are often involved. Aorta and veins may bei involved. Usually occurs in children.*
Small vessel vasculitis	
Wegeners's granulomatosis	Granulomatous inflammation involving the respiratory tract (Wegener's granulomatosis), and necrotizing vasculitis affecting small to medium-sized vessels (i.e., capillaries, venules, arterioles, and arteries). *Necrotitzing glomerulonephritis is common.*
Churg-Strauss syndrome	Eosinophil-rich and granulomatous inflammation involving the respiratory tract, and necrotizing vasculitis affecting small to medium-sized vessels, and associated with asthma and eosinophilia.
Microscopic polyangiitis*	Necrotizing vasculitis, with few or no immune deposits affecting small vessels [i.e., capillaries, venules, or (microscopic polyarteritis)[b] arterioles]. *Necrotizing arteritis involving small and medium-sized arteries may be present. Necrotizing glomerulonephritis is very common. Pulmonary capillaritis often occurs.*
Henoch-Schönlein purpura	Vasculitis, with IgA-dominant immune deposits, affecting small vessels (i.e., capillaries, venules, or arterioles). *Typically involves skin, gut, and glomeruli, and is associated with arthralgias or arhritis.*
Essential cryoglobulinemic vasculitis	Vasculitis, with cryoglobulin immune deposits, affecting small vessels (i.e., capillaries, venules, or arterioles), and associated with cryoglobulins in serum. *Skin and glomeruli are often involved.*
Cutaneous leukocytoclastic angiitis	Isolated cutaneous leukocytoclastic angiitis without systemic vasculitis or glomerulonephritis

[a] "Large vessel" refers to the aorta and the largest branches directed toward major body regions (e.g., to the extremities and the head and neck); "medium-sized vessels" refers to the main visceral arteries (e.g., renal, hepatic, coronary, and mesenteric arteries); "small vessel" refers to venules, capillaries, arterioles, and the intraparenchymal distal arterial radicals that connect with arterioles. Some small and large vessel vasculitides may involve medium-sized arteries, but large and medium-sized vessel vasculitides do not involve vessels smaller than arteries. Essential components are represented by normal type; italicized type represents common, but not essential components.

[b] Preferred term. Strongly associated with antineutrophil cytoplasmic autoantibodies.

Table 3. Clinical symptoms and signs suggestive of vasculitis

General signs:
- Constituional symptoms, fatigue
- Rheumatic complaints such as polymyalgia, polymyositis, arthraglia, arthritis

Complications indicating small vessel involvement:
- Episcleritis, otitis media, vertigo, hemoptysis, microhematuria, peripheral, polyneutropathy, palpable purpura, perimyocarditis

Complications indicating medium-sized vessel involvement:
- Infarction: heart, central nervous system, kidney, gasbrointestinal tract, extremities, aneurysm bleeding

Complications indicating large vessel involvement:
- Claudication, thrombosis

Laboratory findings:
- Acute-phase reactants (erytrhocyte sedimentation rate, C-reactive protein)
- Increased white blood cell and platelet counts

dies, partial purification of the potential antigens was gained by protein extraction of nuclei from the thymus. The antigens isolated were called "extractable nuclear antigens" (ENAs). They represent different ribonucleoproteins (RNP) or nonhistone proteins (see Table 4 for details).

In SLE, certain ANA subset are highly specific for SLE, including anti-Sm (Smith) and anti-double-stranded DNA (dsDNA) antibodies. However, anti-Sm and anti-dsDNA antibodies are not sufficiently sensitive and measurements are subject to variability depending on the laboratory and the technique employed. The Farr assay is highly specific and sensitive for the detection of dsDNA. This is a soluble-phase radioligand binding assay, in which radiolabeled dsDNA is precipitated together with the patient's autoantibodies. Unfortunately it is technically demanding and imprecise. The IFT for dsDNA with *Crithidia luciliae* is a unique solid-phase technique similar to the ANA IFT. The dsDNA-containing kinetoplast of the protozoan is used as substrate. However, this assay has a low sensitivity, while the dsDNA enzyme-linked immunosorbent assay (ELISA) lacks specificity [28].

In active SLE ANA are present in at least 95% of patients, and a negative test argues against the diagnosis. However, as shown in Table 4, many other rheumatic disorders are also associated with a positive ANA test. Some antibody subsets are closely associated with distinct clinical entities. In addition, patients taking certain medications (procainamide, hydralazine, phenytoin) may test positive for ANA. Using IFT, serial dilutions are necessary to identify the spectrum of the staining pattern, since various antigens may contribute to the immunofluores-

Table 4. Association between antinuclear antibodies and collagen diseases.[a] (Adapted from [22, 26]

	SLE	MCTD	PSS	CREST	Srögen's Syndrome	Rheumatoid arthritis	Normal subjects
ANA	95%	95%	50%–90%	60%–90%	70%	15%–50%	<5%
Pattern of ANA staining[b]	PDSN	SD	SDN	S	DS	D	
Anti-dsDNA	20%–60%	Neg.	Neg.	Neg.	Neg.	Neg.	Neg.
Anti-Sm[c]	30%	Neg.	Neg.	Neg.	Neg.	Neg.	Neg.
Anti-RNP[c]	30%–50%	95%	30%	Neg.	15%	Rare	<5%
Anti-centromere	Rare	Rare	10%–15%	60%–90%	Neg.	Neg.	Neg.
Anti-Ro (SSA)[c]	30%	Rare	Rare	Neg.	50%–70%	Rare	<5%
Anti-La (SSB)[c]	15%	Rare	Rare	Neg.	25%–60%	Rare	Rare
Anti-nuclear	Common	Neg.	Neg.	Rare	Rare	Neg.	Neg.
Anti-Scl.70[d]	Neg.	Neg.	10%–20%	Neg.	Neg.	Neg.	Neg.
Anti-histone	60%	Neg.	Neg.	Neg.	Neg.	20%	Neg.

[a] Percentages represent the proportion of cases where staining is positive.
[b] Staining: P, peripheral; D, diffuse; S, speckled; N, nucleolar.
[c] Ribonucleoproteins
[d] Nonhistone proteins.
SLE, Systemic lupus erythematosus; MCTD, mixed connective tissue disease; PSS, progressive systemic sclerosis; CREST, calcinosis – Raynaud's phenomenon – esophageal dysfunction – sclerodactyly – telangiectasia

cence pattern. The intensity of IFT, defined as the highest dilution with positive readings, is an particularly important diagnostic tool because the disease activity often correlates with IFT titer.

Although detection of ANA and anti-dsDNA antibodies represents the laboratory hallmark of SLE diagnosis, other tests such as the erythrocyte sedimentation rate (ESR) and C-reactive protein (CRP) concentration are also useful. CRP levels are often within the normal range despite a high ESR. This is in contrast to findings in other inflammatory diseases, including ANCA-associated vasculitides. The determination of complement components such as C3 and C4, which may be reduced by immune complex formation, is also clinically useful. In addition, C3 and C4 levels are typically low in all active collagen diseases, whereas they remain unchanged in most ANCA-associated vasculitides. Total complement hemolytic

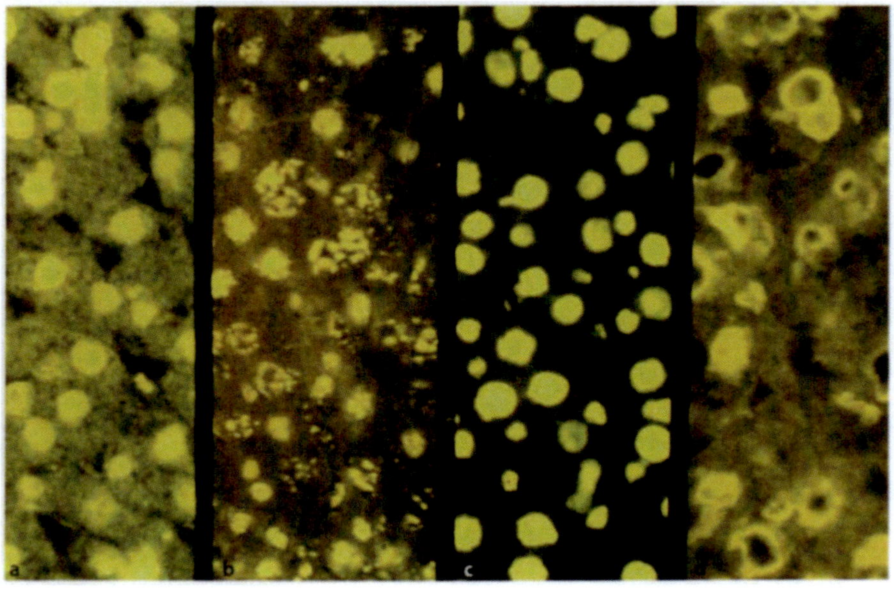

Fig. 1a–d. Typical immunofluorescence staining patterns of anti-nuclear antibodies (ANA). **a** Peripheral, **b** diffuse, **c** speckled, **d** nucleolar

activity (CH50) is an appropriate screening test for the presence of C1–9, assessing the integrity of the classical pathway of complement activation.

ANA-Associated Vasculitis

The classification criteria of SLE according to the 1982 revised American Rheumatism Association criteria are given in Table 5 [27]. ANA and anti-dsDNA are among the criteria listed. Note that, along with ANA autoantibodies, hematologic changes such as leukocytopenia and thrombocytopenia also caused by antibodies have been included. Vasculitis may occur independently of these antibodies. The incidences of vasculitic lesions in SLE reported in autopsy studies are as follows: skin 20%–30%, lung 18%–25%, gastrointestinal tract 10%–30%, central nervous system 7%–12%, and heart 3%–4%. Typically in SLE only small vessels are affected; involvement of large vessels is uncommon. However, the reported occurrence of vascular lesions varies depending on the organs investigated and on the study design (clinical diagnosis or autopsy) [17]. Other collagen diseases such as Sjögren's syndrome or scleroderma can also cause vasculitis. Secondary vasculitis is often misdiagnosed because of the symptoms of the underlying disease. For instance, motor neuropathy may not be suspected in patients with arthritis (SLE, rheumatoid arthritis) or with myalgia (viral infection). Amongst the inflammatory rheumatic diseases, rheumatoid arthritis may also be complicated by vasculitis: in rheumatoid arthritis autopsy series, vasculitis has been found in about 50% of cases [1].

Table 5. American Rheumatism Association criteria for classification of SLE[a] [25]

Criterion	Comments
1. Malar rash	
2. Discoid rash	
3. Photosensitivity	
4. Oral ulcers	
5. Arthritis	Nonerosive arthritis of ≥2 peripheral joints
5. Serositis	Pleuritis, pericarditis
7. Renal disorder	Proteinuria >0.5g/day, cellular casts
8. Neurologic disorders	Seizures, psychosis
9. Hematologic findings	Hemolytic anemia, WBC <4000/mm^3, Lymphopenia <15000/mm^3, Thrombocytopenia <100 000/mm^3
10. Immunologic findings	Positive LE cell preparation, anti-DNA, anti-Sm, false positive test for syphilis
11. ANA	ANA by IFT of an equivalent assay

[a] Interpretation: SLE ist defined by the resence of four or more criteria.

Spectrum of cANCA and pANCA Assays

While determination of ANA and of ANA subspecies have been well established as vascular diagnostic tools since 1957 [10], ANCAs represent a relatively new antibody group first described in necrotizing glomerulonephritis [7]. A Dutch-Danish collaboration [29] discovered a distinct granular cytoplasmic fluorescence pattern, first called anti-cytoplasmic antibodies (ACPA), and later termed "anti-neutrophil cytoplasmic antibodies" (ANCA). The IFT technique of ANCA determination is comparable with that used for ANA; only the antigen preparation is different. In spite of Hep2 cells, PMN are fixed to the slides. Two major patterns of fluorescence can be distinguished which have been assigned the acronyms cANCA (Cytoplasmic) and pANCA (Perinuclear) (Fig. 2). cANCA represents a special subset with a granular cytoplasmic pattern with accentuation of fluorescence intensity in the area within the nuclear lobes as a seromarker for Wegener's granulomatosis. Falk and Jenette [9] detected ANCA in the idiopathic form of pauci-immune necrotizing crescentic glomerulonephritis, now considered to be a renal limited form of microscopic polyarteritis (now renamed microscopic polyangiitis MPA). They showed that MPA was associated with a perinuclear fluorescence pattern (pANCA).

Today, the IFT is still the standard screening method for ANCA detection. Antibodies with different antigenic specificities are distinguished first by their patterns of immunoreactivity (Fig. 3) when analyzed by fluorescence microscopy on alco-

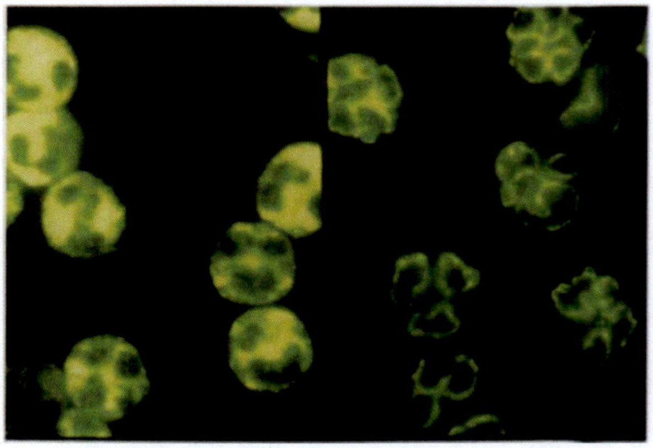

Fig. 2 a, b. Typical immunofluorescence staining patterns of anti-neutrophilic cytoplasmic antibodies (ANCA).
a cANCA with granular cytoplasmic pattern, **b** pANCA with perinuclear pattern.

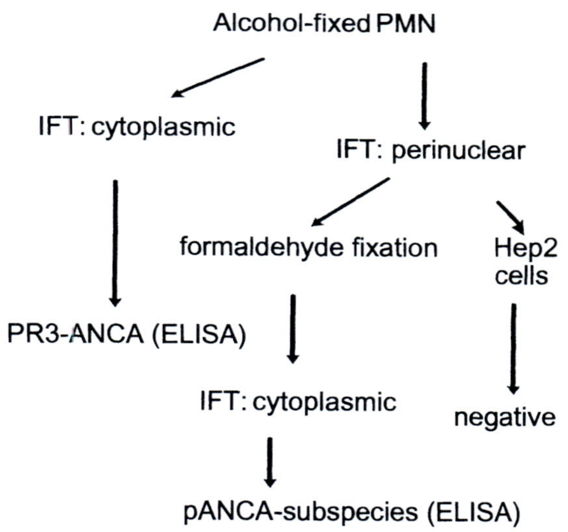

Fig. 3. Detection of cANCA and pANCA by indirect immunofluorescence and confirmation by ELISA.

hol-fixed cytospins of normal human PMN. The perinuclear pattern cannot always be distinguished from the nuclear staining pattern induced by ANA. The autoantibodies staining the nuclei or the perinuclear zone of PMN can be directed toward both nuclear antigens and cationic cytoplasmic proteins of PMN (e.g., myeloperoxidase, elastase), which migrate to the anionic components of the nucleus upon removal of lipids from granule membranes (permeabilization) by ethanol fixation. Cross-linking fixatives (e.g., formaldehyde) trap the proteins in their original locations, thereby preventing the perinuclear staining pattern. Further analysis is needed in order to distinguish between pANCA and antibodies specific to nuclei (ANA) and granulocyte nuclei ("true" granulocyte-specific ANA, GS-ANA). The GS-ANA is found in Felty's syndrome and in some cases of rheumatoid arthritis. Thus, in order to prevent false positive ANCA results, sera should be studied on both Hep2-cells (ANA) and formaldehyde/acetone-fixed PMN (pANCA). When PMN are fixed with the cross-linking fixative myeloperoxidase ANCA-positive sera produce a cytoplasmic staining pattern, whereas ANA-positive sera still display nuclear staining.

In addition to IFT, methods such as enzyme-linked immunosorbent assay (ELISA) and radioimmunoassay are also employed and can help to define ANCA subspecies. Although some concordance between the results of ELISA and IFT has been reported [20], most ELISAs – as reported in a European multicenter study – require strict standardization [14]. In practice, ELISAs (and/or additional Western blotting or immunoprecipitation procedures) are not suitable as screening procedures, but they can be used to identify the target antigen.

ANCA-Associated Vasculitis

ANCA have been reported in many diseases with and without vasculitis. However, ANCA gained special clinical importance in the group of primary vasculitides as defined by the Chapel Hill conferences (Table 2) [16]. Table 6 shows the association of cANCA and pANCA with these entities.

cANCA

In Wegener's granulomatosis, the cANCA pattern is usually (approximately 90% of cases) induced by PR3 antibodies (PR3-ANCA). cANCA, however, can also be found infrequently in vasculitides closely related to Wegener's granulomatosis, e.g., micro-

Table 6. ANCA association with primary systemic vasculitis

Disease	Vessels involved	ANCA association
Giant cell arteritis	Large	Rare
Takayasu arteritis	Large	Rare
Polyarteritis nodosa	Medium	Rare
Kawasaki's disease	Medium	Rare
Wegener's granulomatosis	Small	cANCA
Churg-Strauss syndrome	Small	cANCA
Microscopic polyarteritis	Small	pANCA >cANCA
Henoch-Schönlein purpura	Small	Rare
Essential cryoglobulinemic vasculitis	Small	Rare
Cutaneous leukocytoclastic angiitis	Small	Rare

Table 7. Forms of primary vasculitis shown according to vessel size, presence or absence of granuloma, and percentage of cases with a cANCA staining pattern

Vessel size	Granuloma present	Granuloma absent	cANCA pattern
Large	Giant cell arteritis		0% (0/155)
	Takayasu's arteritis		0% (0/40)
Medium	Churg-Strauss		15% (7/47)
		Polyarteritis nodosa	9% (12/130)
Small	Wegener's granulomatosis		81% (406/502)
		Microscopic polyangiitis	15% (32/179)

scopic polyangiitis, Churg-Strauss syndrome, (classic) polyarteritis nodosa [15], and rarely, in the giant cell arteritides – giant cell (temporal) arteritis and Takayasu's arteritis [2], in Henoch-Schönlein purpura [24], cutaneous leukocytoclastic angiitis [11], and cryoglobulinemic vasculitis [13] (Table 7). In many of these cANCA-positive sera the target antigen is still unknown.

As shown in Table 2, at least some of the primary vasculitides present with similar symptoms, which emphasizes the value of ANCA determination. Even more importantly, the ANCA assay is the only noninvasive diagnostic procedure with sufficient specificity and sensitivity, as demonstraded in Wegener's granulomatosis. The sensitivity of a positive ANCA assay for this disease ranges between 78% and 96%, and specificity is 86%–100%. Titer changes are found to correlate with disease activity in Wegener's granulomatosis and have predictive value. Although cANCA findings are rare in infectious disorders, one should always be aware of the possibility of a concomitant (secondary) vasculitis [25]. A homogeneous cANCA has been observed in symptomatic HIV-positive patients [18] and, more recently, in patients with amebic liver abscess [23].

pANCA

pANCA with myeloperoxidase (MPO) specificity are mainly found in MPA, formerly called microscopic polyarteritis (for review see [13]). Unlike MPA, polyarteritis nodosa has no or only weak association with ANCA (Table 8). pANCA also occur with variable but usually low frequency in Wegener's granulomatosis, polyarteritis nodosa, and Churg-Strauss syndrome, and are characteristically absent in Kawasaki's disease, Takayasu's arteritis, giant cell (temporal) arteritis, and Henoch-Schönlein purpura. It has be emphasized that pANCA are not specific for any single disease entity, and are found in several diseases other than vasculitides, most notably in inflammatory bowel disease, rheumatoid arthritis, dollagen vascular diseases, and infections [21]. For example, it was noticed that 50%–70% of patients with ulcerative colitis exhibited pANCA reactions (sometimes referred to as "atypical perinuclear with snow drift pattern"). Among these, particularly patients with primary sclerosing cholangitis exhibited the highest titers. With regard to the antigen specificity of the "atypical" ANCA in ulcerative colitis and primary biliary cirrhosis, there is agreement that they do not react to any significant extent with PB3 and MPO [13].

Table 8. Forms of primary vasculitis shown according to vessel size, presence or absence of granuloma, and percentage of cases with a pANCA staining pattern

Vessel size	Granuloma present	Granuloma absent	pANCA pattern
Large	Giant cell arteritis		3% (5/155)
	Takayasu's arteritis		0% (0/40)
Medium	Churg-Strauss		13% (6/47)
		Polyarteritis nodosa	15% (20/130)
Small	Wegener's granulomatosis		4% (20/502)
		Microscopic polyangiitis	42% (75/179)

Recently, pANCA reactions have also been reported in patients with HIV infection and cystic fibrosis and a relationship was suggested to associated vasculitic lesions (for review see [12]). In these circumstances ANCA induce an atypical homogeneous cytoplasmic pattern different from both cANCA and pANCA. Figure 4 summarizes antigens so far identified as being responsible for a positive pANCA stain. It has to be stressed that only MPO-ANCA is of clinical significance, because of its close association with MPA.

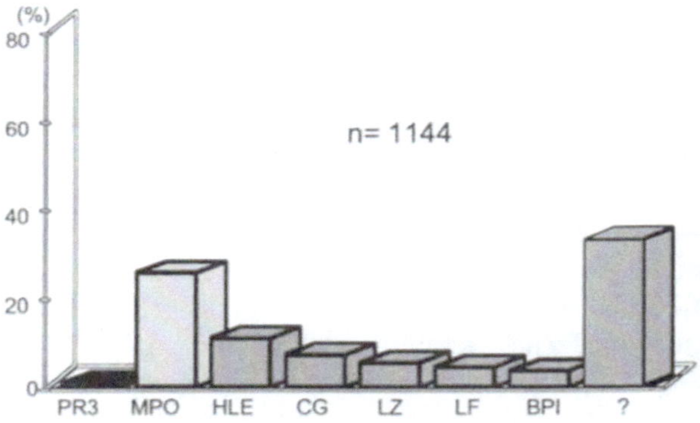

Fig. 4 Target antigens in pANCA-positive patients. *PR3*, proteinase 3; *MPO*, myeloperoxidase; *HLE*, human leukocyte elastase; *CG*, cathepsin G; *LZ*, lysozyme; *LF*, lactoferrin; *BPI*, bactericidal/permeability-increasing protein; *?* unknown antigens

MPO-ANCA have also been detected in Goodpasture's syndrome (30%–40%) and in hydralazine-induced glomerulonephritis, both conditions well known to be associated with small-vessel vasculitis. Interestingly, MPO-ANCA have also been detected in hydralazine-induced lupus [19]. However, in SLE and rheumatoid arthritis only low-level MPO-ANCA have been seen in ELISA [3].

pANCA induced by "non-MPO-ANCA," e.g., antibodies against cathepsin G, elastase, lysozyme etc. can be associated with MPA and diseases not complicated by vasculitis, e.g., collagen vascular diseases, rheumatoid arthritis, and chronic inflammatory bowel disease [13]. About 10% of pANCA-positive sera were shown to react with more than one target antigen, for example with lactoferrin, MPO, or elastase. It is unknown whether patients with several ANCA specificities differ clinically from patients with monospecific ANCA.

Recommendations

Autoantibody screening is recommended when the etiology of a vascular disorder is unclear and vasculitis is suspected (Table 4). Since many other diseases show vascular complications, further diagnostic procedures have to be employed to exclude the underlying conditions such as infectious diseases (viruses, bacteria, protozoans, fungi), neoplasms, other inflammatory diseases (inflammatory lung and bowel diseases), and drug intake. A complete diagnostic work-up of patients with systemic vasculitis often therefore requires a multidisciplinary approach. For practical purposes a laboratory program such as that indicated in Table 9 is suggested to establish the diagnosis.

Table 9. Recommended immunological evaluations in cases with suspected vasculitis

1. Basic laboratory tests: erythrocyte sedimentation rate; C-reactive protein
2. Complement analysis: C3, C4, CH50
   ANA, if positive: identification of ANA specificity (see Table 4)
4. ANCA: if cANCA-positive, confirmation by PR3 ELISA; if pANCA-positive, test for pANCA specificity (only MPO commercially available as yet)
5. Other: cryoglobulins, anti-endothelial cell antibodies, anti-glomerula membrane antibodies

Summary

Determination of autoantibodies is essential in patients in whom clinical and basic laboratory findings suggest an underlying inflammmatory process. The significance of a positive ANA result depends on the ANA titer, the underlying antigen specificity, and the assay system employed. Some ANA antibodies show a high disease specificity (e.g., anti-dsDNA antibodies) while other (e.g., RNP antibodies) do not. Quite similarly, ANCA comprise a heterogeneous group of autoantibodies targeting antigens in PMN, monocytes, and even endothelial cells. Comparable with ANA, ANCA are routinely detected by indirect immunofluorescence technique. At least two different patterns of fluorescence can be distinguished which have been assigned the acronyms cANCA and pANCA. cANCA is mostly induced by PR3 antibodies, and pANCA by MPO. While cANCA is highly specific for Wegener's granulomatosis, MPO-pANCA has a close association with microscopic polyangiitis. pANCA are frequently also seen in other vasculitides, in inflammatory diseases such as ulcerative colitis, and in viral and bacterial infections.

References

1. Bacon PA (1991 Vasculitic syndromes associated with other rheumatic conditions and unclassified systemic vasculitis. Curr Opin Rheumatol 3: 56–61
2. Baranger TAR, Audrain MAP, Castagne A, Barrier JH, Esnault VLM (1994) Absence of antineutrophil cytoplasmic antibodies in giant cell arteritis. J Rheumatol 21: 871–873
3. Braun MG, Csernok E, Schmitt WH, Flesch BK, Gross WL (1993) Incidence and specificity of P-ANCA in rheumatic diseases. Adv Exp Med Biol 336: 371–373
4. Brouwer E, Weening JJ, Klok PA, Huitema MG, Tervaert JWC, Kallenberg CGM (1992) Induction of an humoral and cellular (auto) immune response to human and rat myeloperoxidase (MPO) in Brown Norway (BN), Lewis and Wistar Kyoto (WKY) rat strains. In: Gross WL (ed) ANCA associated vasculitides: immunodiagnostic and pathogenetic value of antineutrophil cytoplasmic antibodies. Plenum, London
5. Cambridge G, Wallace H, Bernstein RM, Leaker B. (1994) Autoantibodies to myeloperoxidase in idiopathic and drug-induced systemic lupus erythematosus and vasculitis. Br J Rheumatol 33: 109–114
6. Cohen Tervaert JW, Limburg PC, Elema JD, Huitema MG, Horst G, The TH, Kallenberg CGM (1991) Detection of autoantibodies against myeloid lysosomal enzymes: a useful adjunct to classification of patients with biopsy-proven necrotizing arteritis. Am J Med 91: 59–66
7. Davies DJ, Moran JE, Niall JF, Ryan GB (1982) Segmental necrotizing glomerulonephritis with antineutrophil antibody: possible arbovirus aetiology. Br med J 285: 606
8. Ewert BH, Jennette JC, Falk RJ (1991) The pathogenic role of antineutrophil cytoplasmic autoantibodies. Am J Kidney Dis. 18: 188–195
9. Falk RJ, Jennette JC (1988) Antineutrophil cytoplasmic autoantibodies with specificity for myeloperoxidase in patients with systemic vasculitis and idiopathic and crescentic glomerulonephritis. N Engl J Med 318: 1651–1657
10. Friou G (1957) Clinical application of lupus-nucleoprotein reactions using fluorescent antibody technique. J Clin Invest 36: 890

11. Gross WL, Hauschild S, Mistry N (1993) The clinical relevance of ANCA in vasculitis. Clin Exp Immunol 93: 7-11
12. Gross WL, Schmitt WH, Csernok E. (1993) ANCA and associated diseases: immunodiagnostic and pathogenic aspects. Clin Exp Immunol 91: 1-12
13. Gross WL, Csernok E, Helmchen U (1995) Antineutrophil cytopplasmic autoantibodies, autoantigens, and systemic vasculitis. APMIS 103: 81-97
14. Hagen EC, Andrassy K, Csernok E, Daha MR, Gaskin G, Gross WL, Lesavre P, Lüdemann J, Pusey CD, Rasmussen N et al (1993). The value of indirect immunofluorescence and solid phase techniques for ANCA detection. A report on the first phase of an international cooperative study on the standardization of ANCA assays. J Immunol Meth ods 159: 1-16
15. Hauschild S, Csernok E, Schmitt WH, Gross WL (1994). Antineutrophil cytoplasmic antibodies in systemic polyarteritis nodosa with and without hepatitis B virus infection and Churg Strauss syndrome. J Rheumatol 21: 1173
16. Jennette JC, Falk R, Andrassy K, Bacon PA, Churg J, Gross WL, Hagen EC, Hoffman GS, Hunder GG, Kallenberg CGM et al (1994) Nomenclature of systemic vasculitides. Proposal of an international consensus conference. Arthritis Rheuma 37: 187-192
17. Kerr GS, Hofmann GS (1992). Systemic lupus erythematosus and the cardiovascular system: vasculitis. In: Lahita RG (ed). Systemic lupus erythematosus, 2nd edn. Churchill Livingstone New York; pp 719-729
18. Klaassen RJL, Goldschmeding R, Dolman K, Vlekke AWJ, Weigel HM, Eeftinck Schattenkerk JKM, Mulder JW, Westedt ML, von dem Borne AEGK (1992). Antineutrophil cytoplasmic autoantibodies in patients with symptomatic HIV infection. Clin Exp Immunol 87: 24-30
19. Leavitt RY, Fauci AS, Block DA (1990). Criteria for the classification of Wegener's granulomatosis. Arthritis Rheum 33: 1101-1106
20. Nölle B, Specks U, Lüdemann J, Rohrbach MS, De Remee RA, Gross WL (1989). Anticytoplasmic autoantibodies: their immunodiagnostic value in Wegener's granulomatosis. Ann Intern Med 111: 28-40
21. Peter HH, Metzger D, Rump A, Röther E (1993). ANCA in disease other than systemic vasculitis. Clin Exp Immunol 93: 12-14
22. Peter JB (1995). Use and interpretation of tests in clinical immunology, 8th edn. Specialty Laboratories, Santa Monica
23. Pudifin D, Duursma J, Gathiram V, Jackson T (1994). Invasive amoebiasis is associated with the development of anti-neutrophil cytopplasmic antibody. Clin Exp Immunol 97: 48-51
24. Ronda N, Esnault VLM, Layward L, Sepe V, Allen A, Feehelly J, Lockwood CM (1994). Antineutrophil cytoplasma antibodies (ANCA) of IgA isotype in adult Henoch-Schönlein purpura. Clin Exp Immunol 95: 49-55
25. Schmitt WH, Csernok E, Gross WL (1991). ANCA and infection. Lancet 337: 1416-1417
26. Shmerling RH, Liang MH (1993). Laboratory evaluation of rheumatic diseases. In: Schumacher HR (ed) Primer on the rheumatic disease, 10th edn, Arthritis Foundation Atlanta pp 64-66
27. Tan EMM, Cohen AS, Fries JF et al (1982). The 1982 revised criteria for the classification of systemic lupus erythematosus. Arthritis Rheum. 25: 1271
28. Teodorescu M, Froelich CJ (1992). Laboratory evaluation of systemic lupus erythematosus. In: Lahita RG (ed) Systemic lupus erythematosus, 2 nd edn. Churchill Livingstone New York, pp 345-368
29. Van der Woude FJ (1985). Anticytoplasmic antibodies in Wegener's granulomatosis. Lancet 7: 48

Part II: Diagnostics of Vascular Diseases: Work-in-Progress

Section I: Imaging Methods

Physics of High-Resolution Ultrasonography

K. Lindström and P.A. Olofsson

Introduction

Diagnostic medical ultrasound is on the point a major clinical breakthrough [8, 11]. The turnover of ultrasound equipment worldwide now amounts to more than 50% of that of the X-ray technology market. Further, diagnostic ultrasound is the only imaging modality which currently shows a significant growth rate, and it is exected to equal the X-ray market before the year 2000. While the 1970s focused on computed tomography (CT) and the 1980s on magnetic resonance imaging (MRI), the 1990s will most likely continue to focus on ultrasound. There are a number of reasons for this. Ultrasound is a real-time, versatile, low-cost, and safe procedure for patients. A unique feature with diagnostic ultrasound is that the sensor goes to the patient, whereas in all other imaging modalities it is the other way round. The first clinical application of diagnostic ultrasound, echocardiography, was introduced by Edler and Herz in 1953 [1] – 43 years ago! In spite of this, the technology of ultrasound is still immature. However, rapid improvements in transducer technology and digital signal processing will soon results in improved ultrasound scanners with a spatial resolution better than 100 μm.

Image quality is a measure of the diagnostic value of an ultrasound image for a physician. Generally, the physician uses ultrasound to examine the internal organs of a patient noninvasively. Hence, the scanned ultrasound image must accurately represent structures in the body [9]. Unfortunately, the human body is far from ideal as an ultrasonic medium in terms of its ability to propagate an undistorted ultrasound wave. Different layers of body tissue individually attenuate, scatter, and refract the ultrasound wave to different degrees. Objective measurements to judge the quality of the ultrasound image include different forms of resolution, such as detail resolution, contrast resolution, and temporal resolution, uniformity throughout the field of view, and depth of penetration.

In vascular imaging either the blood flow hemodynamics and/or vascular wall morphology and function are visualized. With increasing emphasis on vascular prevention, more subtle and detailed information regarding the definition of early atherosclerotic lesion and detection of impaired vasomotion are placing high demands on both spatial and temporal resolution.

Resolution

Detail Resolution

The spatial resolution of the ultrasound image is a measure of its ability to separate closely spaced individual structures with clarity. The spatial resolution for an ultrasound scanner can be divided into three distinct areas: (1) the resolution in the scanning plane perpendicular to the direction of pulse propagation, or *lateral resolution*, (2) the resolution in the scanning plane in the direction of pulse pro-

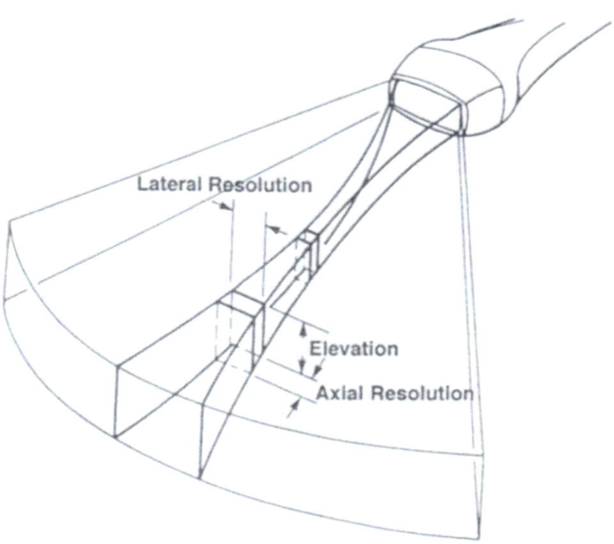

Fig. 1. Definition of an ultrasound scanner's spatial resolution. The ultrasound beam's lateral, elevation, and axial resolutions are functions of many different factors (see text)

pagation, or *axial resolution*, and (3) the resolution in the direction perpendicular to the plane of the scan, or *elevation resolution* (Fig.1). Improvements in detail resolution are relatively easy to recognize, for example using a standard tissue-equivalent phantom. A pattern of thin nylon reflecting threads is often embedded in the phantom gel to generate dots whose size provides a measure of detail resolution.

Beamplots provide the most accurate measure of detail and contrast resolution of an imaging system. Such plots are normally made in a water tank by moving a very small acoustic target, such as a small glass pellet, in an arc of constant radius in front of the transducer under investigation. The relative echo signal strength is monitored as a function of the angle. The 20-dB beam width has proven to be a useful practice measure of lateral resolution (Fig. 2).

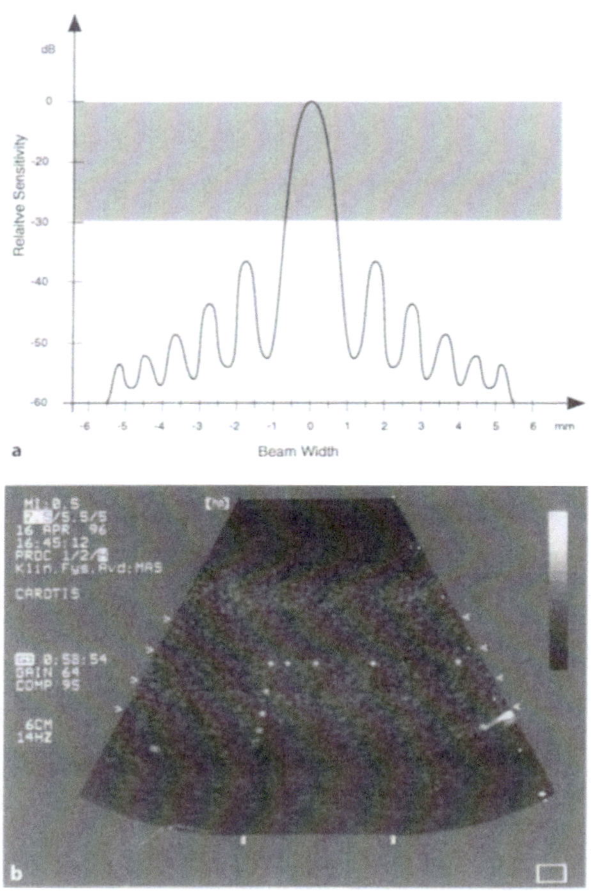

Fig. 2 a. The main lobe width in the *shaded area* 0 to −30 dB should be as small as possible to provide good lateral resolution. Detail resolution can easily be demonstrated by using a tissue-equivalent phantom with embedded nylon threads (diameter, 0.3 mm). **b** The ultrasound image demonstrates axial and lateral detail resolution

In pulse echo imaging, the echoes of two targets separated by *d*/2 have a path length difference of *d*. If the acoustic pulse length is *d*, then echoes of the two targets are just distinguishable. The axial resolution in a pulsed echo system is determined by system bandwidth and center frequency. Ultrasound transducers typically have a constant percentage bandwidth; thus the higher the center freuquency of the transducer, the wider the bandwidth (shorter acoustic pulse) and the better the range resolution. The bandwidth of the electronic receiver also affects resolution, as the time response of the receiver filter might broaden the returning echo pulses. Sometimes, especially in cardiology, electronic circuits are used to estimate the derivative of the received echo envelope complex for tissue edge enhancement.

Elevation resolution is normally worse than lateral or axial resolution. This is because the aperture of the acoustic transducer is rectangular, with one (smaller) dimension falling along the elevation direction and the other along the lateral dimension. Elevation resolution determines the thickness of the scanned image plane. All echoes within this plane are mapped together into the two-dimensional image. A thick image plane results in obscuring of some small details. Normally, a plastic lens is used to create an elevation focal point. Because there is no overall best choice of elevation focal point, several transducers with different elevation focal points are available. Thus users can select the transducer frequency and focal point most appropriate for their particular imaging application.

Contrast Resolution

Contrast resolution enables us to differentiate between tisue types and to see subtle structures in the presence of very bright reflectors. Contrast resolution is often overlooked when judging ultrasound image quality, but this tissue-differentiating ability supplies critical diagnostic information.

Information about contrast resolution requires scrutinous examination of the ultrasound transducer beamplot. The subtle, weaker echoes that determine the tissue texture are normally 40 – 60 dB below the brightest (0 dB) echoes (Fig. 3). Consequently, the 50-dB beam width provides a reasonable and objective measure of contrast resolution, i.e., of the ability of the system to resolve the echoes that indicate tissue character and permit visual tissue differentiation. The occurrence of transducer

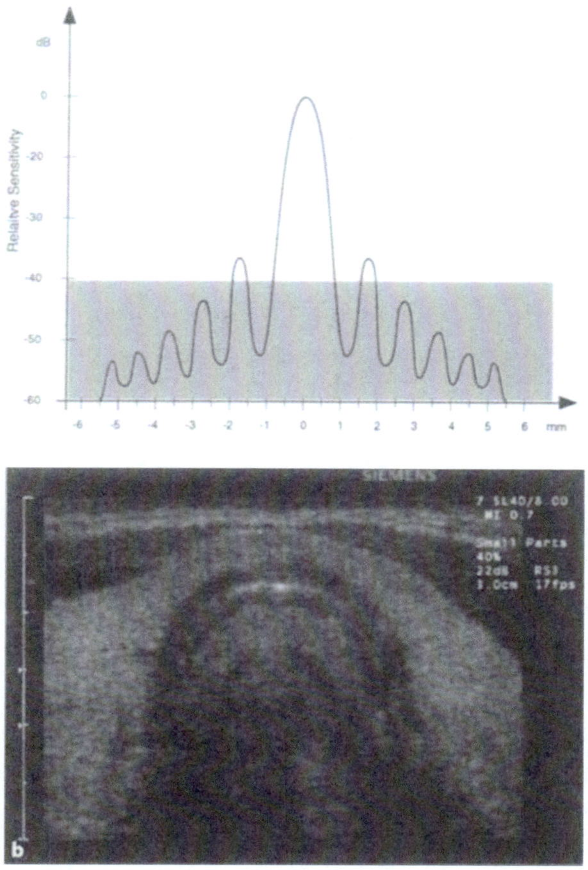

Fig. 3 a, b. Contrast resolution is the system's ability to differentiate between low-level echos and to permit visual tissue differentiation. A low sidelobe (grating lobe) level is of great importance to achieve high-quality tissue differentiation. **a** Low levels in the shaded range (–40 to –60 dB) of the beam plot indicate good contrast resolution. **b** Ultrasound image of normal thyroid glands, neck muscle, and trachea with low-level echo signals

sidelobes often decreases the contrast resolution that can be achieved.

The dynamic range of the system can also be reduced in the subsequent electronic signal processing. Modern ultrasound scanners utilize digital signal processing, where the analog signals from the ultrasound transducer head after suitable preamplification are analog to digital (A/D) converted. This conversion must be rapid (more than three to four times the highest ultrasound frequency used, typically 40 MHz) and must use as many bits as economically justificable (currently 10 bits). These data still imply undesired limitations to the ultrasound system.

Temporal Resolution

Temporal resolution is a measure of the ultrasound scanner's ability to follow tissue movement with time. The frame rate for normal two-dimensional real time images should be at least 20 per s in order to avoid image flicker. For certain cardiovascular applications, particularly for detecting abnormalities in the movement of the vessel walls or heart valves, much faster sampling is required.

The relation between the (one-way) distance d of an object that caused an echo from the transducer to the (round-trip) time delay t and the speed of sound in the medium c is given by

$$t = 2\, d/c$$

The speed of sound in soft body tissues lies in a fairly narrow range, i.e., 1450–1580 m/s. An average of 1500 m/s is often used for rough estimates of time of flight. For a longest-range measurement of 15 cm, this leads to a delay time of about 200 µs. To allow echoes and reverberations to die out, one might have to wait even longer before launching the next interrogating pulse. This leads to possible pulse repetition frequencies (PRF) in the order of a few kilohertz. The resulting frame rate will depend on the actual measurement range as well as on the image width (line density and number of lines in each frame). For a measurement range of 15 cm and 100 lines/frame, an image frame rate of 30 frames/s is quite feasible. For shallower measurements, i.e., blood vessels, this frame rate can be uprated correspondingly, whereas use of dynamic focusing, simultaneous Doppler measurements, or high-resolution M-mode recording might decrease the frame rate that can be achieved.

Methods To Improve System Performance

Lateral Resolution

Transmit Focus

The generated ultrasound beam can be focuced in order to reduce lateral width at certain parts of the beam. This is traditionally performed by suitable shaping of the transducer material or by the use of a properly designed ultrasound lens. Both these methods are actually only measures to change the specific transmission time for a sound pulse from a certain spatial position to different parts of the transducer array in order to sum up all ultrasound signals in phase. Such time delays can be imple-

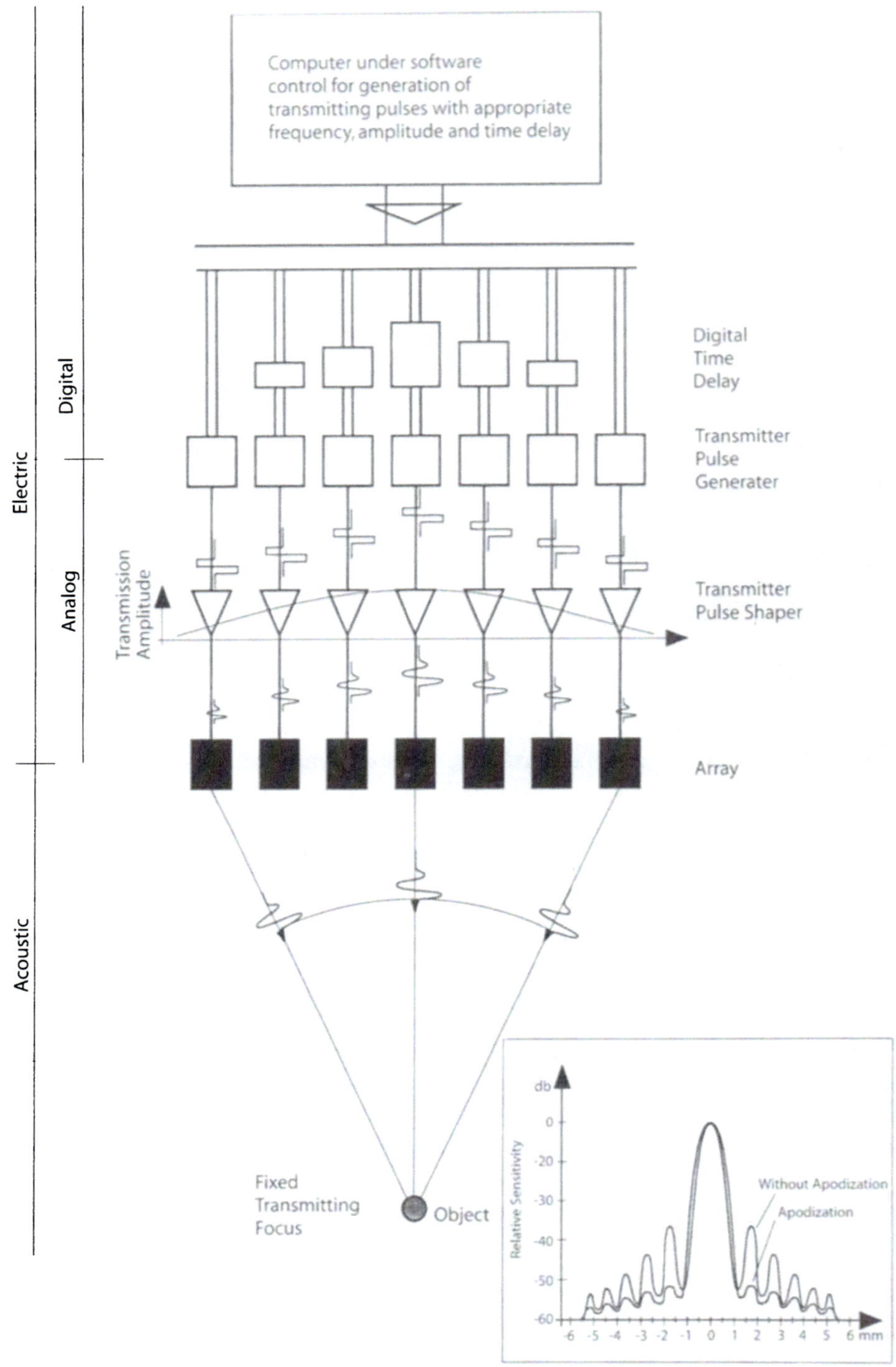

Fig. 4. The transmitted beam can be focused only at one focal point for each transmission. If two or more transmission focal points are required, new sets of pulses for every focal point with appropriate time delays have to be transmitted. Multifocal transmission reduces frame rate and increases spatial resolution. *Inset* apodization is done by individually controlling high voltage applied to all transmitter stages

mented electronically inside the ultrasound scanner. In fact, this technique is very well suited for use in a modern array transducer digital scanner.

A block diagram of a scanner, where the transmission ultrasound pulse is electronically focused, is shown in Fig. 4. In order to achieve focusing during transmission, digital time delay elements are introduced to each element before the signal enters the transmitter pulse generator. The delays are arranged so that there is a greater delay to the center

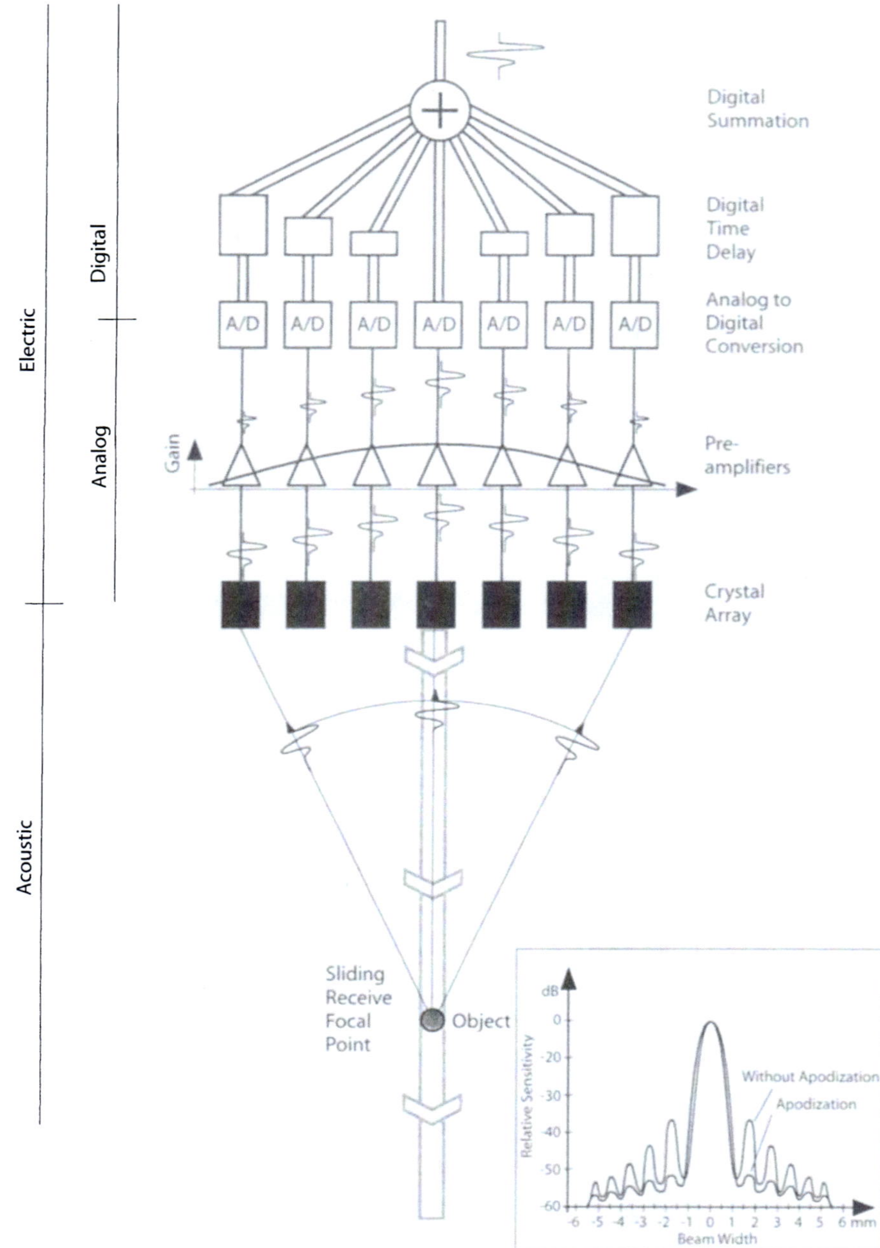

Fig. 5. In reception mode, focusing is dynamic, starting from the near zone and moving along the axis with the speed of ultrasound *Inset,* spatial filter function is applied for apodization to exclude grating and sidelobes. Analog to digital (A/D) conversion in modern ultrasound equipment is done after preamplification. The high sampling speed and high number of bits in A/D conversion is a challenge to implement without sacrificing image quality. Former analog delay lines are substituted by fast digital electronics to give time delays with high precision and resolution without signal distortion during summation

elements than to the outer elements. At any given instant, the part of the wavefront generated from the outer elements will then have traveled a greater distance than the part from the center elements, thereby producing a concave-shaped wavefront which will converge into a focus. The position of the focus can be changed by altering the delays (changing the curvature of the emitted wavefront). The closer the focus is to the transducer, the greater the difference in delay between center and outer elements.

When the ultrasound pulse leaves the transducer, it is focused at a specific spatial position. However, the total focusing effect can be improved if subsequent pulse are focused at different positions along the same line direction. All these beam shapes can be used together in a mode called multiple zone focusing, where the shaded area shows the equivalent beam shape (Fig. 4). It should be noted that the frame rate of the multiply focused beams is reduced by a factor $1/n$, where n is the number of focal zones.

Receive Focus
The receive focus can be implemented in a similar way (Fig. 5). The received signal from each transducer element is delayed before adding. Again, there is a focus at the point where the transit time of the echo pulse from the point plus ist electronic delay is the same for each transducer elements.

It is interesting to note that the focus can be altered during the scan in reception mode. The receiver delays are first adjusted to give a focus close to the transducer. When the origin of the received echoes moves from the first focal zone to the second focal zone, the delays are adjusted in accordance to focal zone 2. This continues for the following focal zones. In this case, there is no loss in pulse repetion frequency for this "dynamic focusing." The eqivalent beam shape is similar to that for multiple zone focusing.

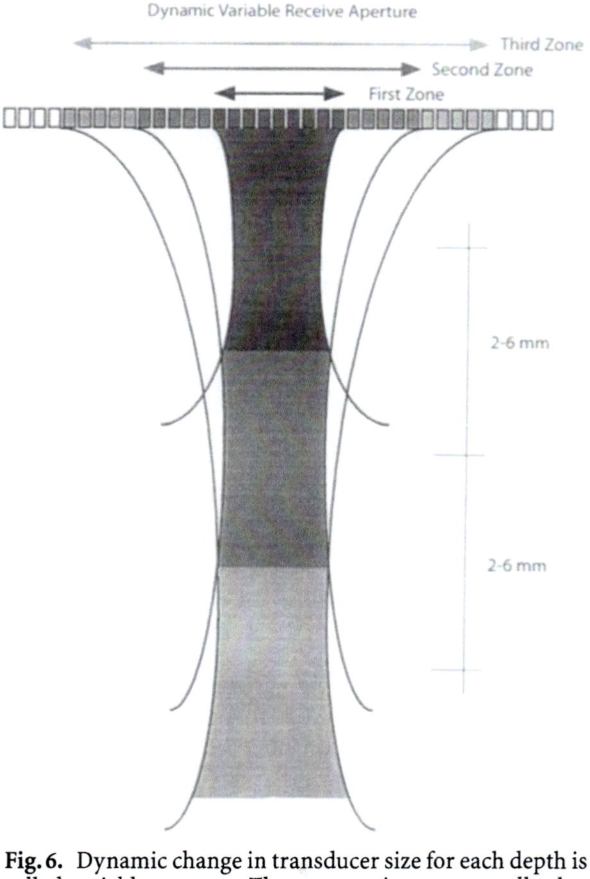

Fig. 6. Dynamic change in transducer size for each depth is called variable aperture. The aperture is set to a small value by using only few elements when echo arrives from the near zone. With increasing depth, more elements are connected, giving a wider aperture and as a result a longer focal zone

Variable Aperture
The beam shape can be further improved by dynamic aperture control (Fig. 6). By using only the inner elements of the transducer for ultrasound echoes close to the transducer surface, the resulting focal zone will be narrower over a longer distance. At greater depth, when the focal length is longer, the outer elements are included to improve the focusing ability of the transducer. This aperture change is normally performed in a number of steps, typically five to 30.

Axial Resolution

Frequency
A fundamental problem in ultrasound imaging is attenuation in soft tissue. For low ultrasound frequencies, attenuation increases roughly linearly with frequency. Human soft tissue attenuates ultrasound by about 0,5 dB/MHz cm; thus a 2-MHz pulse propagating down to a depth of 15 cm and back will be attenuated by 30 dB, whereas an 5-MHz pulse is attenuated by 75 dB. This is why deep imaging usually is done with lower ultrasound frequencies, and shallow imaging is done with higher ultrasound frequencies to take advantage of the superior image quality. The higher frequency actually does more to the image than just giving it better range resolution, as it also gives an improved tissue contrast detectability (due to the frequency dependence of the scatter intensity). Manufacture of high-frequency ultrasound transducer arrays is extremely laborious. A piezoelectric ceramic slab has to be cut in say, 256 pieces, each 100–200 μm wide. Typical ultrasound frequencies for vessel scanning are 7–10 Mhz. A 13-MHz ultrasound array has recently been launched on the market. Frequency-dependent attenuation has a peculiar effect on the frequency spectrum of the transmitted pulse. As higher frequencies are attenuated more than low frequencies, the center frequency of the transmitted spectrum is shifted down as the pulse propagates.

Pulse Length
A broad bandwidth of the ultrasound transducers corresponds to a possibility of generating short acoustic pulses and thus improved axial resolution. A narrow bandwidth improves both lateral and ele-

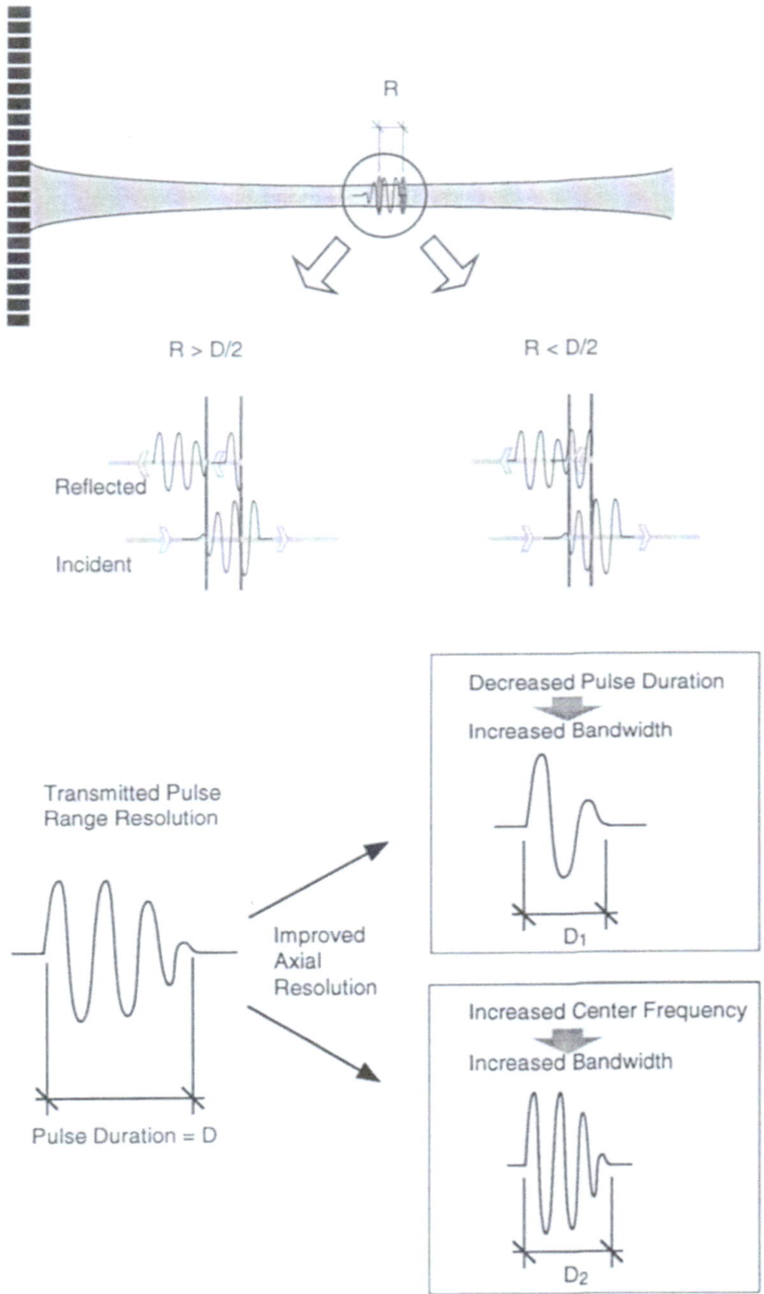

Fig. 7. Axial resolution is the system's ability to distinguish between two closely spaced targets in the axial direction. With decreased transmitted pulse length, which can be achieved either by increasing the transmitted frequency or by reducing the number of wavelengths, the resolving capacity of close reflectors is increased. Axial range resolution (R) equals half the pulse duration D ($R = D/z$). D^1 and D^2 are less than D

vation resolution and focusing at the expense of axial resolution (Fig. 7).

Tracking

Extreme axial resolution, i.e., to record the wall motion of the fetal aorta *in situ,* can be obtained using the phased-locked echo-tracking principle, first devised by Hokansson et al [5]. This principle involves locking on the zero-crossing of a selected echo complex, which makes the system independent of the echo amplitude, but also has the disadvantage of a limited maximum tracking velocity. Using a new digital measurement principle, Gennser et al. [3] managed to double the maximum tracking velocity. Using a 3.5-MHz ultrasound transducer, diameter changes of 7.8 μm can be detected. A further improvement was made by the introduction of a dual echo tracker, which allows recordings to be made at two levels of the vessel simultaneously, thereby including direct measurements of the pulse propagation velocity [7].

Temporal Resolution

For conventional ultrasound image formation, the ultrasound scanner system selects an image line, transmits an ultrasound pulse, and thereafter receives echoes from the corresponding direction inside the patient and presents the echo information along the corresponding image line on the display. Depending on the selected measurement depth, this puts an upper limit on the number of measurements which can be performed per time unit. This in turn limits the obtainable image frame rate, which is dependent on the number of individual lines in each image frame. In many clinical situations, such as in cardiovascular medicine, these limitations can be troublesome. A somewhat better situation can be obtained by reducing the scanned image width (number of image lines).

In sonar, in which propagation times for each ultrasound pulse might be in the order of seconds, this kind of problem is well known. Generating a 100-line ultrasound image usually takes 1–2 min, not exactly "real-time" scanning. However, recent progress in information technology has opened up new possibilities. In a modern ultrasound array scanner, the direction of the receiving ultrasound beam is set up in a special digital "beam-former" which add signals from the different transducer elements, after careful adjustment of time delays, into the receiving of the ultrasound scanner. However, depending on the width of the transmitted ultrasound beam, a number of such beam-formers can be connected in parallel to produce a corresponding number of simultaneously generated receiving lines (from different directions). This kind of technique has been implemented to generate more than 1000 receiving lines from different directions of the sea bottom for each transmission pulse.

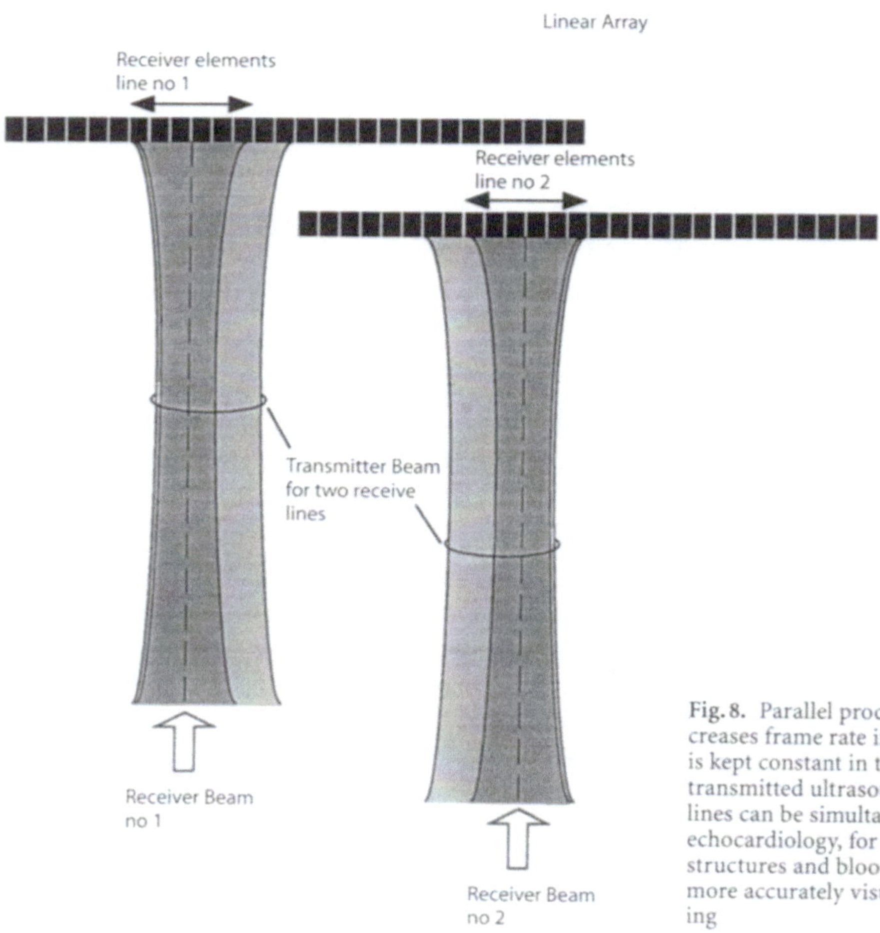

Fig. 8. Parallel processing in reception mode increases frame rate if the number of received lines is kept constant in the scanning field. For every transmitted ultrasound line, up to four parallel lines can be simultaneously received. In fetal echocardiology, for example very rapidly moving structures and blood flow velocity changes are more accurately visualized with parallel processing

In modern ultrasound scanners, an functional strategy often chosen is to receive two or four imaging lines for every transmission pulse (Fig. 8). In the case of four receiving lines, this can be used for a four fold increase in the resulting frame rate of the ultrasound scanner, for example (up to 200 frames/ for an echocardiograph or 50 frames/for a color Doppler), or for a two fold increase in both the frame rate and the line density. Such a method provides more diagnostic information and greater accuracy due to the higher number of sampling points.

Contrast Resolution

Apodization

If an ultrasound transducer array with excessively high sidelobe levels is used for scanning, the main lobe signal from a weak signal may be obscured by the sidelobe signal from a strong signal. Thus the dynamic range of the ultrasound image is reduced, which is often seen as noise signals in areas such as cysts, which should normally appear completely black. The best solution to this situation is to use an ultrasound transducer in which the signals to (transmission mode) or from (reception mode) the individual transducer elements are spatially weighted as a finite-length filter in a process called apodization.

A transducer with a rectangular apodization function can generate a narrow main lobe, but the maximum sidelobe level will only be decreased by about 20 dB. Other apodization weighting functions, such as the Blackman or Hanning functions, generate a much wider main lobe, but the sidelobes are decreased by almost 60 dB. The aim is to design a finite-length weighted filter with the lowest possible sidelobe level and the narrowest possible main lobe. Such a filter normally has a fairly close approximation to a Gaussian weighting [6].

Analog to Digital Converter

Dynamic range is a key issue in good contrast resolution. The practical amplitude range of echoes from the ultrasound transducer is between 1 μV and 1 V, i.e., a factor of $1-10^6$, corresponding to 20 digital bits, which is the optimal choice for the A/D converter. Due to the large number of transducer channels (256) and the required A/D conversion speed (> 40 Mhz), no realistic A/D converter is presently available on the market. For example, the approximate price of 40-MHz A/D converters is currently as follows: 8 bits, \$3; 10 bits, \$30; 12 bits, \$1500; 16 bits \$6000. Using present technology, the price of a 16-bit A/D converter is about \$1.5 million per scanner. The current solution is to use a 10-bit A/D converter in combination with a suitable time-gain compensation circuit (TGC) producing ultrasound images with a dynamic range of 60–90 dB. Practically working and economically justifiable A/D converters will probably be on the market within 5–10 years.

Beam Elevation

Linear Arrays

Linear sequential arrays have as many as 600 elements in current commercial scanners. A subaperture of up to 128 is selected to operate at a given time. The scanning lines are directed perpendicular to the face of the transducer; the acoustic beam is focused, but not steered. Linear array transducers have a large footprint to obtain an adequate field of view. Curvilinear or convex arrays have a different shape to sequential linear arrays, but they operate in the same manner. In both cases, the scan lines are directed perpendicular to the transducer surface. A curvilinear array, however, scans a wider field of view because of its convex shape [4].

The more advanced linear phased arrays have up to 256 elements. All the elements are used to transmit and receive each line of data. The scanners steer the ultrasound beam through a sector-shaped region in the lateral plane. Phase arrays scan a region which is significantly wider than the footprint of the transducer, making them suitable for scanning through restricted acoustic windows, e.g., in cardiac imaging.

1.5D Arrays

The so-called 1.5D array is similar to a 2D array in construction, but a 1D array in operation. It contains elements along both the lateral and the elevation dimension (Fig. 9, 10). Features such as dynamic focusing and apodization can be implemented in both dimensions to improve image quality. Since the 1.5D array contains a limited number of elements in the elevation dimension (e.g., three to five elements), steering is not possible in this direction. Due to symmetry, array elements in rows 1 and 5 and rows 2 and 4 can be connected in parallel to reduce the number of electronic channels.

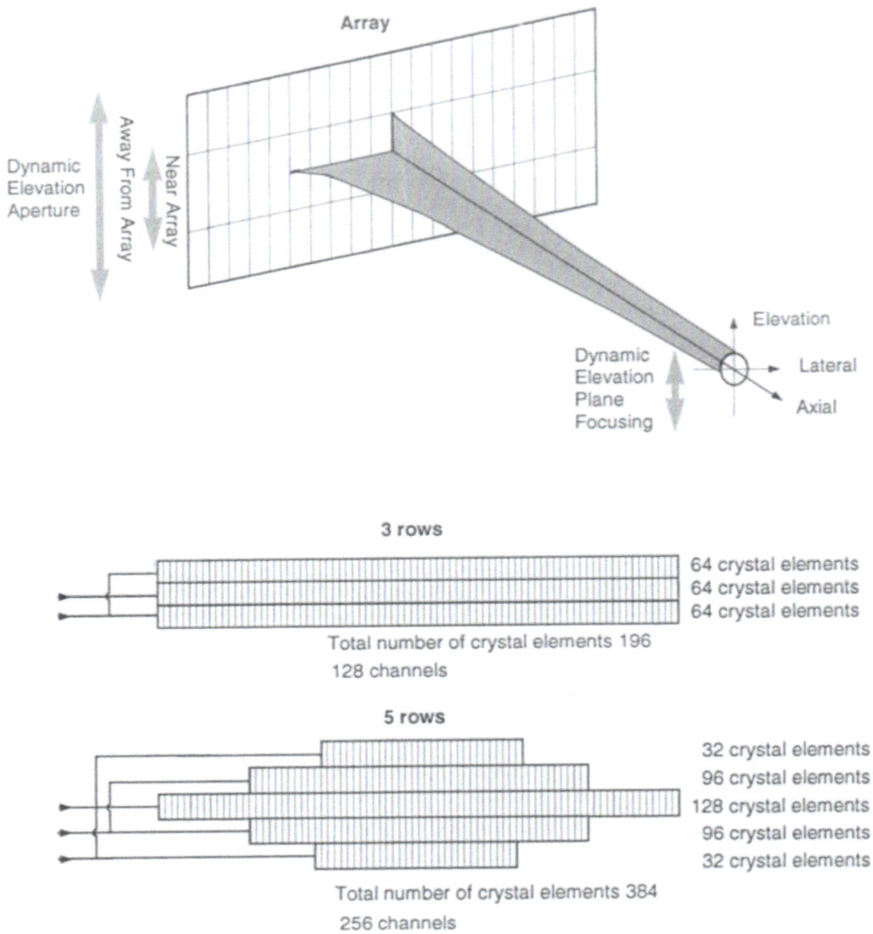

Fig. 9. In contrast to conventional single-line linear array with fixed focus in the elevation plane, 1.5 dimensional array maintains sharp focus at all depths. These arrays are cut into everal lines (three, five, or seven) and, by introducing time delays between center and outer elements, dynamic electronic focusing of layer thickness is accomplished. Compare lateral focusing described in text. Elevation focusing can also be applied to phased-array transducers

2D Phased Arrays

These have, a large number of transducer elements in both the lateral and the elevation dimension. Therefore, 2D arrays can electronically focus and steer the acoustic beam in both dimensions and scan over a pyramidal-shaped region in real time. Such instrumentation has the theoretical ability of providing improved volumetric determinations, more rapid appreciation of organ and structural contours, and better assessment of the 3D relationship of structures. Parallel processing in reception mode is often used to increase the data acquisition rate by a factor of 16 or more so that pyramidal volumes can be scanned in 1/20 of a second. Experimental in vitro validation demonstrates ±5% correlation with known volumes (below 200 ml) [10].

A prototype of a 2D array 20 x 20 mm^2 in size developed in the Siemens research center consists of 64 x 64 = 4096 elements. Since the individual elements, which are only 220 x 220 μm^2 in size, are supposed to transmit and receive independently of one another they must be contacted individually and connected with an independent electronic transmission and reception circuit. Extending the possibilities of the 1.5D array, the acoustic beam can be focused with the 2D array in both directions with consistently high quality. Such a system has the unique ability to depict anatomic structures from different directions simultaneously. Projectional, multiple cross-sectional, and stereoscopic pairs can be produced simultaneously from a single aperture. This electronic circuit is designed in a highly integrated form for integration in the transducer.

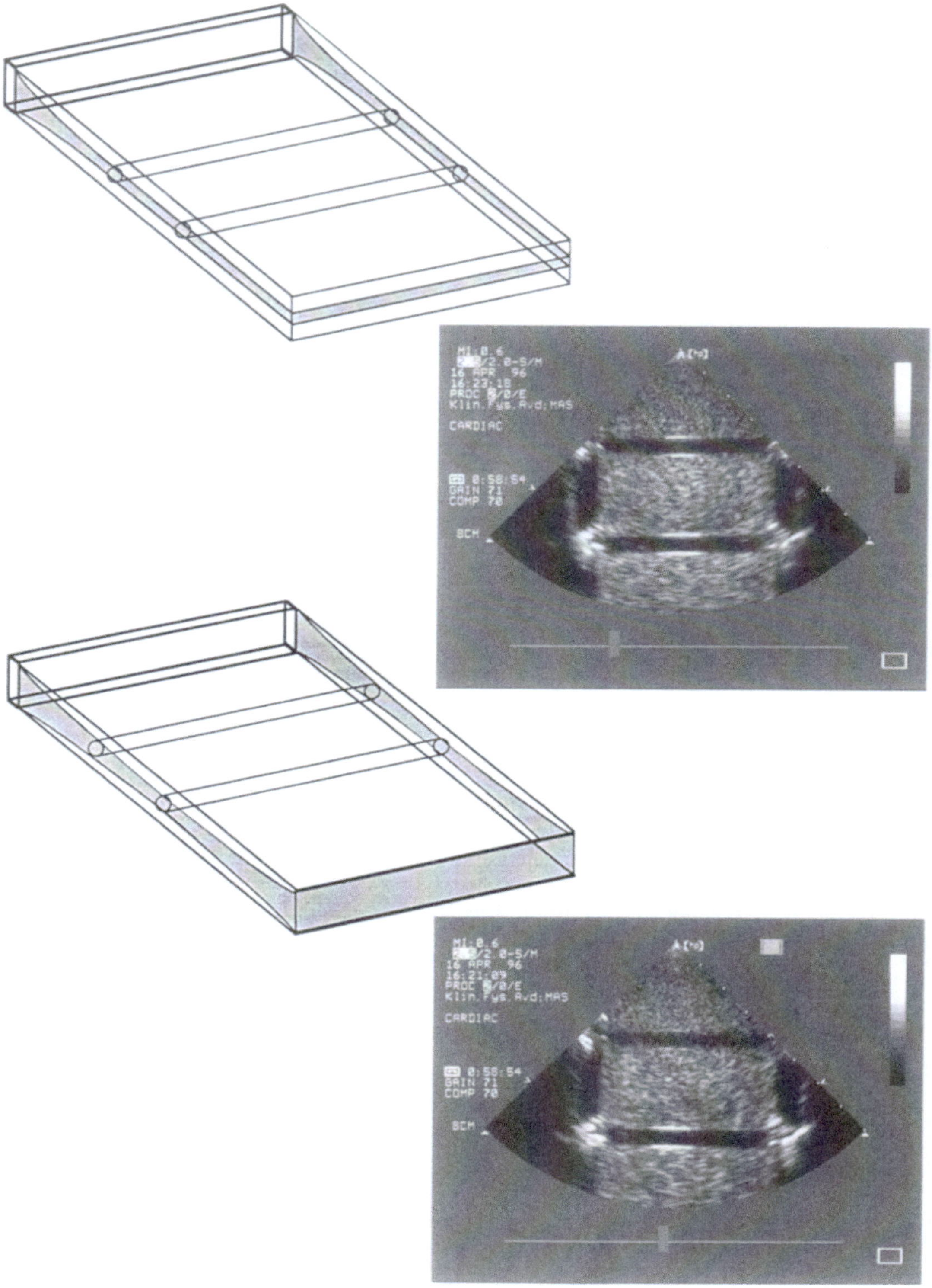

Fig. 10. Ultrasound images of a tissue-equivalent phantom with echo-free circular tubes at different depth, scanned longitudinally (simulated vessels). The *lower image* shows fixed focus in the elevation plane, and the *upper image* dynamic beam elevation. Improvements in image quality are notable in the near and far field. Variable apertures in the near field enhance image quality even further

Summary

The remarkable development of array transducer technology in recent years has formed the basis for high-resolution ultrasound imaging. Several hundred transducer elements, all of a thickness comparable to the human hair, can be cut out from a piezoelectric ceramic slab using a 20-μm-thick sawblade. The resulting array transducer, efficient and well damped, can transmit hundreds of time-controlled ultrasound pulses as well as receive hundreds of echo signals for further processing. All this effort is needed to be able to steer the direction and shape of the ultrasound beam as well as control the amplitude and phase of the received echo signals. This immense task can now be performed in realtime using modern information technology with massive parallel computerized signal and image processing.

The first generation of super high-resolution ultrasound scanners have now been launched to the market, and present ultrasound images with a real-time spatial resolution down to 0.1 mm. The near future will give us further improved spatial and temporal resolution in combination with 3D scanning and presentation of images. The information on morphology and function given in these images can be supplemented by the use of different forms of ultrasound Doppler technology such as color Doppler, power Doppler and harmonic Doppler (using special contrast agents), thereby showing not only blood flow in vessels but also perfusion flow in tissue. As a result, these new ultrasound techniques will bring us unprecedented diagnostic information, including new forms for noninvasive tissue quantification.

References

1. Edler I, Hertz CH (1953): The use of ultrasonic reflectoscope for the continuous recording of the movements of the heart. Kungl Fysiogr Sällskap Lund Förhandl 24(5): 1–19
2. Fish P (1990): Physics and instrumentation of diagnostic medical ultrasound. Wiley, Chichester
3. Gennser G, Lindström K, Dahl P, Benthin M (1981): A dual high-resolution 2-dimensional ultrasound system for measuring target movements. In: Kurjak A, Kratochwil A (eds.) Recent advances in ultrasound diagnosis. Excerpta Medica Amsterdam, pp 71–75
4. Goldberg RL Smith SW (1995) Transducers. In: Bronzino ID (ed) The biomedical engineering handbook. CRC and IEEE Press, Boca Raton, pp 1077–1092
5. Hokansson DE, Mozersky DJ, Sumner DS, Strandness DE Jr (1972) A phase-locked echo tracking system for recording arterial diameter changes in vivo. J Appl Physiol 32: 726–733
6. Kino GS (1987) Acoustic waves. Prentice Hall, Eaglewood Cliffs
7. Lindström K, Gennser G, Sindberg-Erikssen P, Benthin M, Dahl P (1987) An improved echo-tracker for studies of pulse waves in the fetal aorta. In: Rolfe P (e.d.) Fetal physiological neasurement. Butterworth London, pp 217–226
8. Maslak SH (1985) Computed sonography. In: Sanders RC, HiU MC (eds) Ultrasound annual, Raven, New York
9. Snyder RA, Conrad RJ (1983) Ultrasound image quality. Hewlett Packard 34(10): 34–40
10. von Ramm OT, Smith SW, Carroll BA (1994) Real-time volumetric US imaging. Radiological Society of North America, 100 years of progress. p 308 Radiology (Suppl) 193
11. Weill F (1994) The future of ultrasound. Eur Ultrasound 1: 105–109

Ultrasound Assessment of Endothelial Vasomotor Function

J.A. Vita and J.F. Keaney

Introduction

The normal vascular endothelium regulates vasomotor tone, fibrinolysis, thrombosis, platelet adhesion, intimal growth, and leukocyte recruitment to the vascular wall. Disturbances of these endothelial functions have been suggested to be important mechanisms in both the pathogenesis and the clinical expression of coronary atherosclerosis. Among the many regulatory functions of the endothelium, release of nitric oxide, a potent vasodilator and platelet-inhibitor, has been the focus of a large number of studies. Over the past decade, nitric oxide-dependent vasodilation has emerged as a readily measurable and clinically relevant marker of more generalized endothelial function in patients. Studies of nitric oxide action have been performed in the coronary and peripheral circulations and have examined both conduit arteries and the microcirculation using a variety of invasive techniques. However, the requirement for intra-arterial infusion of nitric oxide-dependent agonists in such studies has placed limits on the number of subjects that can be studied and the number of studies that can be performed in each individual. Recently, several groups developed noninvasive methods for examination of nitric oxide-dependent vasodilation in peripheral conduit arteries that use vascular ultrasound. The emergence of these methods has opened the door for studies of endothelial vasomotor function in large numbers of subjects, in patients early in the course of the disease process when invasive studies are difficult to justify, and for repeated examination of endothelial vasomotor function during a variety of interventions.

In this chapter, we will review the technical aspects of noninvasive examination of endothelial function using vascular ultrasound. We will describe the technique in detail as performed in our laboratory and compare and contrast the methods of several investigators. We will review the reproducibility of these methods, the dependence of the observed responses on nitric oxide release, and the evidence that such studies in the peripheral circulation are relevant to coronary artery disease. Finally, we will briefly touch on recent investigations using this technique that confirm its utility for examination of the effects of interventions on endothelial function and suggest future applications.

Overview of Endothelial Vasomotor Function

The vascular endothelium regulates vasomotor tone by releasing a number of substances that act locally in the vascular wall and adjacent vessel lumen. In 1980, Furchgott and Zawadzki [1] first described release of endothelial-derived relaxing factor (EDRF) from isolated rabbit aorta in response to acetylcholine. Subsequent studies have identified EDRF as nitric oxide [2] or a closely related compound [3]. Nitric oxide is synthesized from l-arginine in endothelial cells by a constitutive nitric oxide synthase [4]. Nitric oxide relaxes vascular smooth muscle and, thus, produces vasodilation by activating soluble guanylyl cyclase and increasing intracellular cyclic 3',5'-guanosine monophosphate (cGMP) concentration [5]. In addition to acetylcholine, a variety of other agents also stimulate release of nitric oxide from endothelial cells, including serotonin, thrombin, α2-adrenergic agonists, substance P, and bradykinin, all of which act through specific receptors on endothelial cells [6]. Importantly, nitric oxide release is also induced by changes in shear stress at the endothelial cell surface resulting from increased blood flow, a process that depends on activation of a shear-sensitive calcium-dependent potassium channel [7–9]. Flow-mediated nitric oxide release serves as the basis for the noninvasive methods described in this chapter since changes in arterial blood flow can be induced noninvasively. The vascular endothelium further controls vasomotor tone by producing a number of other vasoactive substances including the cyclooxygenase-derived vasodilator prostacyclin [10], which is also released in the setting of increased shear stress [11].

In patients with coronary risk factors or atherosclerosis, effective endothelial release of nitric oxide is impaired. This impairment has been demonstrated in the coronary arteries of patients with atherosclerosis [12], and in the coronary and peripheral circulations of subjects with hypercholesterolemia [13, 14], diabetes mellitus [15, 16], hypertension [17, 18], and cigarette smoking [19]. In these invasive studies of nitric oxide release, changes in epicardial coronary diameter were determined using quantitative coronary angiography, and changes in forearm microvascular tone were assessed using venous occlusion plethysmography. Using similar methods, impaired release of nitric oxide has been shown to precede the development of angiographic evidence of atherosclerosis, supporting the hypothesis that endothelial dysfunction may play a pathogenic role in the atherogenic process [13]. Furthermore, there is convincing evidence that impaired endothelial vasomotor function contributes to the pathophysiology of clinical ischemia in patients with stable [29] and unstable [21, 22] coronary syndromes. Recently, several studies have shown that endothelial vasomotor dysfunction could be improved with lipid lowering [23, 24] and possibly with the combination of lipid-lowering and antioxidant therapy [25]. On the basis of such studies, we and others have proposed that restoration of normal endothelial vasomotor and other functions may be an important mechanism for the reduction in cardiovascular events associated with such interventions [26, 27]. The growing appreciation of the clinical relevance of endothelial function and the desire to examine nitric oxide release in a greater number of subjects and repeatedly during interventions served as the stimulus for development of the noninvasive methods described below.

Noninvasive Methods for Examination of Endothelial Function

In noninvasive studies, nitric oxide release and consequent arterial dilation are stimulated by increasing blood flow in the conduit artery of interest (brachial or femoral artery). Flow is increased by inflating a standard blood pressure cuff on the limb for 2–10 min and then releasing the cuff. Using one of several ultrasound techniques, careful measurements of arterial diameter are made at baseline and again during the "reactive hyperemia" that occurs after cuff release (Fig. 1). In these studies, Doppler ultrasound is used to measure blood flow velocity in the vessel of interest, and brachial or femoral arterial flow is calculated from blood flow velocity determined by Doppler ultrasound and vessel cross-sectional area assuming a circular lumen. The specific details of the protocol vary somewhat according to investigator, but in recent years, relatively similar protocols have evolved at the major centers performing this work.

The first studies using cuff occlusion to stimulate reactive hyperemia and subsequent flow-mediated dilation were reported by Laurent and colleagues [28, 29]. These investigators determined brachial artery diameter using an 8-MHz pulsed Doppler velocimeter with an adjustable multiple range-gated system and double-transducer probe (Echovar Doppler pulse, Alvar Electronic) [30]. Briefly, with this technique, the vessel diameter is determined from the time delay of the earliest and latest Doppler signal detected in the vessel that correspond to the near and far wall of the vessel with correction made for the ultrasonic angle of incidence with the vessel axis. Using this method, these investigators examined flow-mediated dilation of the brachial artery at the antecubital crease in healthy 15 subjects [29]. Hyperemic flow was induced by a 2-min arterial occlusion with a wrist cuff, and vessel diameter was measured before and 30 s after cuff occlusion. They reported that flow velocity increased 8.2-fold following release of the cuff, was maximal immediately (within 5 s) after cuff release, and returned to baseline by 60–90 s. In response to this stimulus, the brachial artery dilated by a mean of 3.8% (4.45 $\pm$ 0.62 to 4.62 $\pm$ 0.65 mm, mean $\pm$ SD) with a wide range of responses (–8% to 30%). Increasing the period of cuff occlusion from 2 to 4 min significantly increased the hyperemic response, and there was a significant correlation between change in blood flow velocity and change in brachial artery diameter. Preventing the hyperemic response by only partially deflating the cuff eliminated the vasodilator response, further suggesting that dilation was a response to the flow increase, rather than a response to the discomfort of occlusion or some other unrelated mechanism. Shortly after this group's initial report [28], Anderson and Mark [31] reported that cuff release after a 10-min forearm occlusion in 23 healthy subjects induced a 2.9-fold increase in blood flow and 18% dilation of the brachial artery (4.74 $\pm$ 0.17 to 5.6 $\pm$ 0.16 mm) using the same range-gated Doppler methodology.

Although Laurent and colleagues established the precedent for study of endothelial function noninvasively, two additional groups, Deanfield and col-

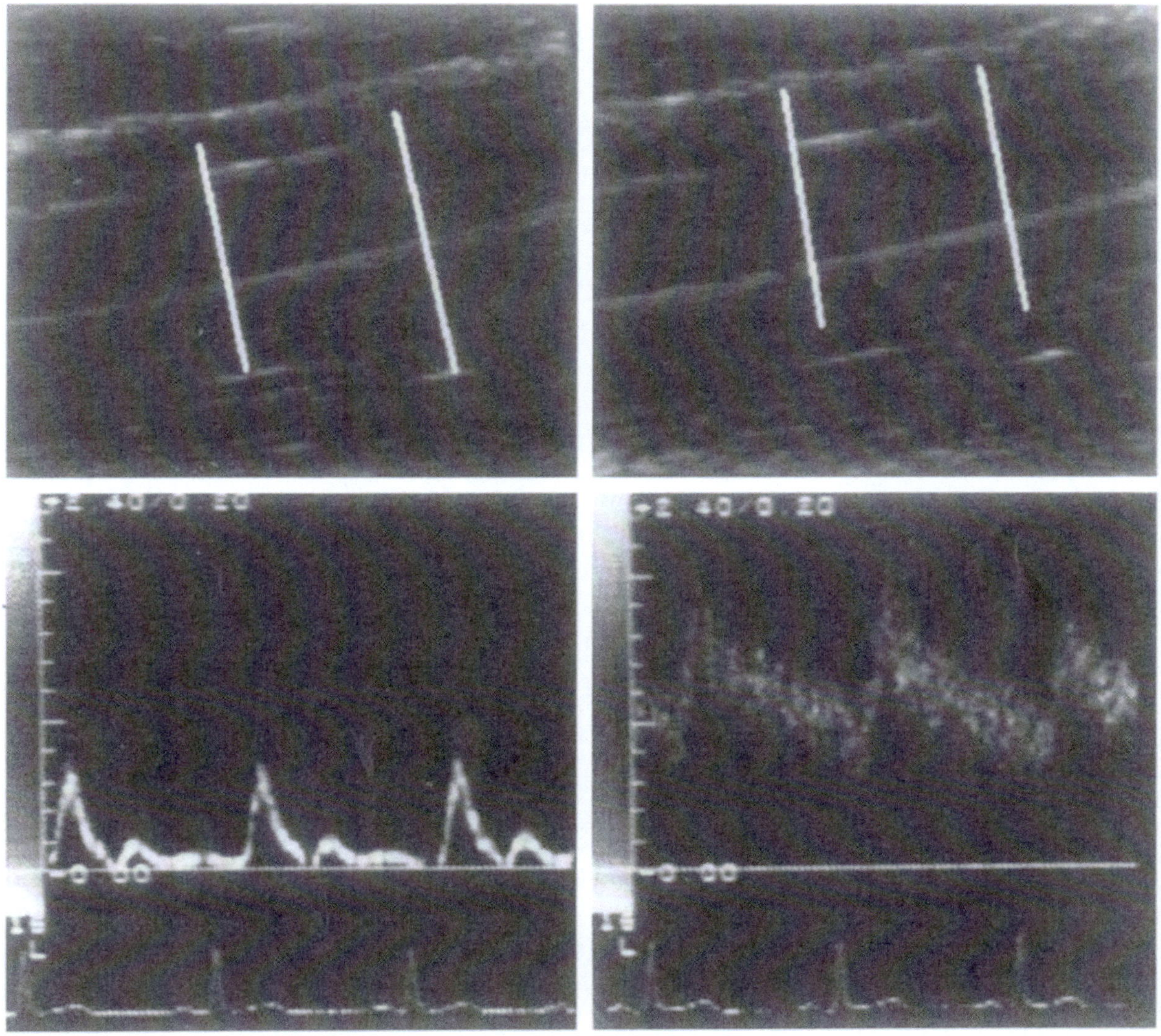

Fig. 1. Flow-mediated brachial artery dilation in a healthy individual. 2D *(upper panels)* and Doppler ultrasound images *(lower panels)* from a healthy individual were obtained using a Toshiba 140A ultrasound system with a 7.5-MHz linear array probe. Images at baseline are displayed in the left panels. The Doppler signal immediately after cuff release is displayed in the *lower right panel* and the 2D image obtained 1 min after cuff release is displayed in the *upper right panel*. Using customized image analysis software [48] to determine vessel diameter at baseline and after cuff release, flow-mediated dilation was found to be 8%

leagues [32–39] and Creager and colleagues [40–46], have more recently developed and utilized these methods to a much greater extent. In particular, the former group has the greatest published experience with the noninvasive assessment of endothelial function. Several other groups have also utilized and refined the methodology, and the different approaches to determination of vessel diameter and stimulating and measuring changes in blood flow will now be considered.

Assessment of Vessel Diameter

In contrast to the range-gated Doppler method developed by Safar and colleagues, we and several other groups determine vessel diameter from two-dimensional ultrasound images acquired with a 7.0 to 7.5-MHz linear array transducer and a standard ultrasound system, e.g., Acuson 128XP/10 (Acuson, Mountain View, CA) [32], Toshiba 140A or SSA-270 (Toshiba America Medical Systems, Tustin, CA) [45], HP Sonos 1500 (Hewlett-Packard, Andover,

MA) [47], or ATL Ultramark 9 (Advanced Technology Limited, Bothell, WA) [48]. Brachial artery diameter is measured from 2 to 20 cm above the antecubital crease; the optimal location must be identified in each subject. In our experience, imaging higher and more laterally provides a better image than imaging close to the antecubital crease. In this location, the vessel is also straighter and more parallel to the skin surface. It is most difficult to obtain optimal images in thinner individuals with small arteries. If repeated scans are required, it is useful to mark the identified skin location. In children, Deanfield's group [32, 34] also examined the superficial femoral artery just distal to the bifurcation of the common femoral. In all studies, the vessel is imaged longitudinally and anatomical landmarks such as branchpoints or adjacent tendons and tissue planes are used to consistently identify the arterial segment to be measured. It is important to examine vessel diameter at a specific point in the cardiac cycle because brachial artery diameter may vary as much as 6.6% between systole and diastole [49]. Typically, gating is accomplished by timing the image selection to a simultaneously recorded ECG signal. Deanfield's group [45, 48, 50] uses the R-wave to identify end-diastole, while we and other groups use the T-wave, which in the brachial artery corresponds to maximal distention. If an ECG signal is not available, it is possible to reproducibly select the point of maximal distention by advancing frame-by-frame through several cardiac cycles [48].

In our laboratory, the ultrasound system is a Toshiba 140A with a 7.5-MHz probe (Toshiba America Medical Systems, Tustin, CA). The focal zone was set at the depth of the near wall, which is more difficult to clearly delineate, and depth and gain setting are optimized to provide the clearest borders between lumen and vessel wall. For the Toshiba 140A the following settings are preset for these brachial artery studies: dynamic range 60 dB, persistence 4, edge enhancement 3, postprocessing curve 3, predepth gain compensator "on", and echo filter "resolution" (7.5 to 9.5 MHz). The television line width is 0.078 mm and the limit of resolution for the system is 0.2 mm. Once set for an individual patient, the settings remain constant throughout the study and are duplicated during follow-up studies.

Images are recorded on super-VHS video tape and analyzed off-line. Deanfields group [32, 37] used digital calipers to measure vessel diameter at a single point along the vessel wall and average the results from four images. The measurements are made from the "m-line", which is the interface between the media and adventitia, a point which is identified by the operator in a blinded fashion. Vogel's group [47] recorded images of a 5-cm segment of artery and measure the vessel diameter at five evenly spaced locations along the segment length using the digital calipers provided with the ultrasound system. We digitize images from the super-VHS tape for analysis using a video cassette recorder (Panasonic AG-7344) and a computer (Macintosh Quadra 840AV) containing a digitizing board (Scion LG-3). In some cases images are digitized on-line. A 10 to 20-mm segment is identified and diameter measurements are made in a blinded fashion using customized software that was developed by Joseph Polak, M.D. [40–42, 48]. In this system, the operator traces along the m-line for the near and far wall, and the computer then makes and averages 10–20 measurements along the traced segment [45].

Two other groups have examined endothelium-dependent dilation in the radial rather than the brachial artery [51, 52]. In these studies, the radial artery walls are detected using a 10-MHz ultrasound probe (NIUS 02, Asulab) and an A-mode echo-tracking device. In this system, the echoes from the anterior and posterior walls are visualized on a computer screen, tagged by electronic trackers, and continuously displayed. The probe is fixed in position using a sterotaxic arm and the vessel position is identified and optimized using the Doppler flow signal rather than two-dimensional ultrasound [51]. This system offers the advantage of a continuous and immediately available measurement of vessel diameter, but it provides only a single diameter measurement. In addition, it is not possible to use landmarks to precisely identify the segment during repeated examinations as is possible with systems based on the two-dimensional image. Although the details of image acquisition and analysis differ for each investigator, the reported reproducibility of these methods is quite comparable (Table 1).

Assessment of Change in Arterial Flow

In the noninvasive study of endothelial vasomotor function, we and other groups use Doppler ultrasound to measure brachial arterial flow [32, 47, 48]. Volume flow at baseline and during reactive hyperemia is calculated from vessel cross-sectional area and mean blood flowvelocity. Traditionally, venous occlusion plethysmography has been used to non-

Table 1. Reproducibility of arterial diameter determination using ultrasound

Group	Method (see text)	Mean difference between repeated measures (mm)	Coefficient of variation (%)
Laurent et al. [28]	Gated pulsed Doppler	–	3.0
Celermajer et al. [32]	2D/single caliper measurement	0.11 ± 0.10	2.6
Uehara et al. [40]	2D/computer-based software	0.00±0.07	2.9
Lieberman et al. [45]			
Coretti et al. [50]	2D/multiple caliper measurements	0.12± 0.10	2.6
Levine et al. [48]	2D/computer-based software	0.08 ± 0.01	1.7
Joannides et al. [51]	A-mode echo tracking	0.04 ± 0.01	–

invasively determine blood flow in the upper extremity, but this method requires an elaborate system of cuffs and timed inflation equipment, as well as calibrated strain gauges and physiological recording apparatus. It is appropriate to use venous occlusion plethysmography for studies of microvascular vasoreactivity since blood flow is the primary parameter of study and relatively small differences in flow must be detected. For example, in a study examining the effect of hypercholesterolemia on microvascular responses in the forearm, Creager and colleagues [14] observed group differences of 25%–50% in the flow response to methacholine infusion using this technique. However, for study of vasodilation of the brachial artery during reactive hyperemia, the increase in blood flow is typically 600%–1000% [32, 47, 48], and less precision is required to detect such large changes in flow. Further, Doppler methodology is only reliable for calculating the relative change in flow rather than absolute flow, since any introduced errors are present both at baseline and during hyperemia and thus cancel out. The extent of reactive hyperemia tends not to be affected by the presence of hypercholesterolemia and other risk factors [14], and flow determination is primarily performed as a control to ensure that the stimulus for conduit artery dilation remains constant.

Laurent and colleagues [29] used the electronically integrated Doppler velocity for the entire arterial lumen and calculated vessel cross-sectional area from diameter measurements. They report an average resting brachial artery flow of 47.7± 24.2 ml/min (mean ± SD) in a group of 15 healthy individuals, and coefficient of variation of 18±3% for their method of flow determination. Using the same method, Anderson and Mark [31] reported a resting brachial artery flow of 123 ± 96 ml/min. Celermajer and colleagues [32] calculated brachial artery flow using Doppler flow velocity measured at the center of the artery and the vessel cross-sectional area, and reported a resting value of 91 ± 44 ml/min. Other investigators report resting brachial artery blood flow in the range of 84 ± 26 [47] to 140 ± 102 ml/min [48] using lumen area and the integral of the Doppler flow velocity obtained with the range gate at the center of the artery to calculate flow. Corretti and colleagues [47] reported a coefficient of variation for measurement of baseline arterial flow of 9.9%.

Doppler ultrasound also provides a reliable and reproducible method for assessment of peak blood flow during reactive hyperemia. Following cuff occlusion for 2–10 min, flow peaks within 5–20 s of cuff release and then rapidly returns to baseline over 30–120 s depending on the duration of occlusion [29, 31, 32, 47, 48, 50, 53]. Since maximal flow velocity changes on a beat-to-beat basis, precise determination of peak flow following cuff release may be difficult. Deanfield's group and our group continuously record the Doppler signal during cuff occlusion and during the first 15–20 s following cuff release and calculate the peak flow from the flow velocity integral of the single beat with the maximal flow velocity [32, 48]. Vogels group [47] uses the velocity integral of five consecutive beats recorded immediately following cuff release. For a 4.5- to 5-min period of occlusion, peak flow determined by this method ranges from 628 ± 192% to 812 ± 548% in healthy individuals [32, 50]

Creager and colleagues [14, 45] have used venous occlusion plethysmography to examine blood flow to the forearm (excluding the hand) at rest and during reactive hyperemia. In healthy subjects, they report resting flow to be 2.9 ± 1.0 ml/100 mg tissue/min [14], and assuming a forearm volume of 1000 ml, brachial artery blood flow would be approximately 29 ml/min under these conditions. With this methodology, maximal flow during reactive hyperemia following 5-min cuff occlusion ranges from 717% to 900% [14, 45]. These studies with plethysmography examined forearm flow, while studies using Doppler examine brachial artery flow with circulation to the hand intact. Despite

Table 2: Techniques for noninvasive assessment of endothelium-dependent flow-mediated vascular dilation

Investigators	Normal subjects (*n*)	Artery	Cuff location	Occlusion duration (min)	Hyperemic flow (%)	Flow-mediated dilation (mean, ±SD, %)
Laurent et al. [28]	15	Brachial	Distal	2	783	3.8
Celermajer et al. [32]	50	Brachial	Distal	4.5	628	11 ± 8.7
Uehara et al. [40]	13	Brachial	Proximal	5	900	7.6 ±6.3
Lieberman et al.						
Corretti et al. [50] [45]	27	Brachial	Proximal	5	812	9.1 ± 6.0
Joannides et al. [51]	16	Radial	Distal	3	204	4.2
Levine et al. [48]	46a	Brachial	Proximal	5	680	5.4±4.7

[a] Subjects with angiographically documented coronary artery disease.

these methodological differences, the relative increases in blood flow during reactive hyperemia are comparable. Two small studies have used both Doppler ultrasound and venous occlusion plethysmography in the same individual to examine flow in the leg [54] and the arm [55]. These studies suggest that the two techniques are comparable for assessment of resting blood flow. Although the available studies suggest that comparable information is obtained, no careful study has compared venous occlusion plethysmography to Doppler ultrasound for assessment of changes in whole-arm blood flow during reactive hyperemia as is typically used for noninvasive study of endothelial vasomotor function.

Assessment of Flow-Mediated Dilation

In addition to the different methods used to measure arterial diameter and blood flow, the specific technique for inducing and measuring endothelium-dependent flow-mediated dilation of the brachial artery differs somewhat according to group. Protocol differences include duration of cuff inflation, location of the inflation cuff, and study of the brachial, radial, or femoral artery. Despite these differences, relatively similar protocols have been developed and similar findings have been reported (Table 2).

Regarding the duration of inflation, investigators have used 2–10 min occlusion to stimulate hyperemic flow, and in general, more prolonged occlusion produces a higher peak flow and a more sustained flow increase, with a maximal response produced at 10 min [53]. However, more prolonged cuff inflation is uncomfortable for the patient, and 4.5 [32] and 5 min [45, 47, 48] cuff inflation has been shown to reproducibly stimulate flow-mediated dilation of the brachial artery. In a study of seven normal subjects, Corretti and colleagues [47] examined brachial dilation after 1, 3, and 5 min cuff inflation and observed a significant change from baseline only after 5 min. On the basis of such studies, we use a 5-min cuff occlusion and find that it is well tolerated and produces reproducible flow-mediated dilation. In studies of the radial artery, Joannides and colleagues [51] obeserved significant, but more modest dilation following 3 min cuff occlusion (Table 2).

Deanfield's group [32] position the inflation cuff on the forearm, distal to the site of brachial artery imaging, while other investigators position the cuff on the upper arm, proximal to the site of imaging [45, 48, 47]. Deanfield's group argue that positioning the cuff proximal to the studied segment exposes the vessel to a period of ischemia that could alter vascular reactivity and induce vasodilation that is not related to endothelial release of nitric oxide. In addition, the degree of vessel collapse during distal cuff inflation is less, and it is easier to continuously image the vessel while the cuff is up. While these are realistic considerations, the available data do not support the view that cuff position is an important determination of brachial artery responses. For example, Corretti and colleagues [47] examined the effect of both a proximal and a distal cuff location in a group of seven normal subjects, and observed no significant effect on reactive hyperemia and flow-mediated dilation. Two groups, one using a proximal cuff (Fig. 2) [44] and the other using a distal cuff [51], have confirmed that flow-mediated dilation in these studies depends on nitric oxide synthesis by demonstrating that infusion on $N^{[G]}$-monomethyl-*L*-arginine (L-NMMA), a specific inhibitor of nitric oxide synthase, largely eliminates the vasodilator response during hyperemia. On the basis of these studies, we use the more proximal cuff location because it tends to be more comfortable for the patient.

The reproducibility of vessel measurement is well validated. Celermajer and colleagues [32] report a mean interobeserver difference for repeated measurement of flow-mediated dilation of 1.7 ± 1.4% with a coefficient of variation of 2.3%. The consistancy of responses within a particular patient (repeatability) of the method is also well validated. When 21 subjects underwent two studies of flow-mediated dilation on different days, the average difference between measurement of flow-mediated dilation was 2.8 ± 2.3% with a coefficient of variation of 2.3%. Sorensen and colleagues [37] further examined repeated measurement of flow-mediated dilation in a group of 40 healthy subjects with technically excellent studies. On the basis of the observed variance, they calculated that for an intervention study with a cross-over design, an improvement in flow-mediated dilation of 2.5% (i.e. from 7.0% to 9.5% dilation) could be detected with 80% power and 95% confidence in a study involving 10 subjects. For a parallel trial in which separate groups of subjects received treatment or placebo, an improvement of 3% could be detected with the same power and confidence with a sample size of approximately 25 subjects per group [37].

An important factor that influences the extent of flow-mediated dilation in this type of study is the baseline size of the vessel [32, 36, 38, 39, 46]. Studies have consistently demonstrated an inverse relationship between baseline vessel diameter and extent of flow-mediated dilation and extent of dilation in response to exogenous vasodilators such as nitroglycerin. In fact, the findings of an initial report that suggested better endothelium-dependent dilation in women in comparison to men [40] are probably explained by the smaller brachial artery diameter in women. Using multivariate analysis, Celemajer and colleagues carefully controlled for vessel size when examining the relationship between brachial dilation and age [36] and coronary risk factors [38]. In intervention studies, it is important to randomize treatment to ensure that there is no systematic group difference in brachial artery diameter.

Another potential methodological problem to consider is the issue of endothelial vasodilator function of the microvasculature, particularly in the setting of coronary risk factors. On the basis of studies with intra-arterial infusion of L-NMMA, several investigators have suggested that reactive hyperemia is, in part, dependent on endothelial release of nitric oxide in resistance vessels in the vascular bed rendered ischemic [53, 56]. Since the stimulus for brachial artery dilation is increased blood flow, a reduction in the extent of reactive hyperemia because of impaired nitric oxide release in the microvasculature might explain a reduced vasodilator response in the conduit artery. Alternatively, an impaired brachial dilator response could reflect the combined effects of impairment at both the conduit and resistance vessel levels, complicating attempts to correlate conduit vessel vasodilator responses with risk factors or the effects of an intervention. In practice, however, the extent of reactive hyperemia is not affected by the presence of coronary risk factors or atherosclerosis [14, 29, 32, 34, 39, 50]. Furthermore, inhibition of nitric oxide synthesis does not reduce peak hyperemic response [51, 53], but instead affects the total duration of elevated flow in the later stages of reactive hyperemia. The available studies suggest that the extent of brachial artery dilation 1 min after cuff release is largely determined by the peak flow.

In summary, Doppler ultrasound can be used to measure the change in blood flow that occurs during reactive hyperemia, and ultrasound methods

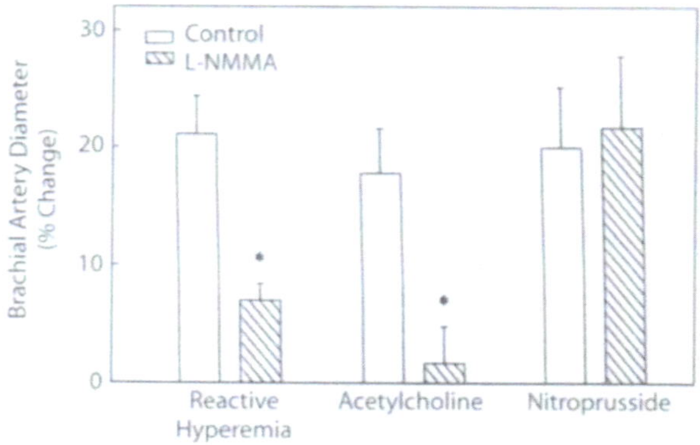

Fig. 2. Noninvasive assessment of endothelium-dependent vasodilation in the brachial artery. Using high-resolution brachial ultrasound as described in the text, brachial artery diameter was determined at baseline and during reactive hyperemia, intra-arterial infusion of the endothelium-dependent vasodilator acetylcholine, and during infusion of the endothelium-independent vasodilator sodium nitroprusside in 12 healthy subjects. Percent change in brachial artery diameter was calculated during control conditions *(open bars)*. After infusion of the nitric oxide synthase antagonist N^G-monomethyl-*L*-arginine l-NMMA; *(hatched bars)*, the vasodilation to hyperemia and acetylcholine is reduced, confirming the importance of nitric oxide synthesis in these responses [44]. *L*-NMMA did not affect endothelium-independent vasodilation caused by nitroprusside. (Data were kindly provided by Mark Creager, M.D.)

Table 3: Recommended protocol for ultrasound study of brachial artery endothelial vasomotor function

Stop all vasoactive medications for 18 – 24 h
Determine blood pressure and collect any blood samples from the contralateral arm (nonstudy arm)
Have patient in supine position resting quietly in a temperature-controlled environment for 15 min after blood sample collection
Position narrow blood pressure cuff on most proximal portion of the arm
Optimize 2D images of the brachial artery 2 – 20 cm proximal to antecubital crease, record images from three cardiac cycles, gated to ECG to systole or end-diastole. Record all images on super-VHS tape
Acquire Doppler flow signal from artery
Inflate the blood pressure cuff to suprasystolic pressure (220 mmHg) for 5 min while carefully maintaining transducer position
Release cuff and record first 15 – 20 s Doppler flow signal
At 1 min after cuff release record 2D images of vessel
Allow 10 – 15 min to re-establish resting conditions
Record 2D images before and 3 min after sublingual nitroglycerin 0.4 mg
Make diameter and flow measurements off-line in a blinded fashion

are available to reliably and reproducibly assess flow-mediated dilation, a response that is known to be endothelial-dependent. Previous work in animal models [7–9] and recent human studies [44, 51] confirm that these responses depend largely on synthesis of nitric oxide. On the basis of published studies and our own experience in study of over 150 subjects, a recommended protocol for ultrasound study of brachial artery endothelial vasomotor function is presented in Table 3.

Clinical Relevance of Brachial Artery Studies

Although the brachial artery is readily accessible for study, it is important to address the question of the relevance of vasomotor function in a peripheral artery to coronary artery disease. As noted above, there is convincing evidence that impairment of the vasomotor, antithrombotic, and other regulatory properties of the endothelium is relevant to the development and clinical expression of atherosclerosis, and we and others have recently reviewed this topic in detail [26, 27, 57]. Several lines of evidence suggest that it is reasonable to hypothesize that endothelial vasomotor function in the conduit brachial artery relates to endothelial function in epicardial coronary arteries. The brachial artery is similar in size to the proximal coronary artery (3–6 mm) [58] and although the brachial artery does not develop occlusive atherosclerosis, it does develop intimal atherosclerotic plaques. Systemic risk factors associated with coronary endothelial dysfunction are also associated with impaired brachial flow-mediated dilation measured noninvasively, including hypercholesterolemia [32, 34], cigarette smoking [32, 35], passive exposure to cigarette smoke [39], diabetes mellitus [42], older age [38], elevated α-lipoprotein level [34], and hyperhomocysteinemia [33].

To more directly address the issue of whether endothelial function in the brachial artery relates to endothelial function in the coronary circulation, Anderson and colleagues [46] recently examined brachial artery flow-mediated dilation and the coronary artery vasodilator response to intracoronary acetylcholine infusion in a group of 50 patients undergoing cardiac catheterization. They observed a close relationship between these different measures of endothelial vasomotor dysfunction in the two circulations. In fact, by multivariate analysis, coronary endothelial dysfunction was an independent predictor of brachial artery endothelial dysfunction. The positive predictive value of abnormal brachial dilation for coronary endothelial dysfunction was 95% [46]. This important study provides strong support for the contention that endothelial vasodilator function in the brachial artery is relevant to the coronary circulation.

Further evidence for the relevance of these noninvasive studies is provided by the observation that interventions associated with improved coronary endothelial function and reduced cardiovascular risk are also associated with improved brachial responses. For example, cholesterol-lowering therapy [59], estrogen replacement therapy [45], and exercise [52], therapies known to reduce cardiovascular risk [27], are all associated with improved flow-mediated dilation assessed noninvasively in the arm. We recently observed improved responses following an oral dose of ascorbic acid [48], providing the first evidence that increased oxidative stress may play a mechanistic role for impaired endothelial vasomotor function in patients with coronary artery disease. This methodology will likely provide further opportunities to define the pathophysiologic mechanisms of endothelial dysfunction and better understand the benefits of interventions for coronary artery disease.

Finally, the availability of a noninvasive method to assess endothelial function provides an opportunity to investigate the relationship between endothelial dysfunction and patient outcome. Using invasive methodology, it is not feasible to complete studies in the large number of subjects required to prospectively examine coronary events such as myocardial infarction and cardiac death. Studies using noninvasive ultrasound methodology to address the prognostic significance of endothelial dysfunction are currently in the planning stage.

Conclusion

Noninvasive evaluation of endothelial function using vascular ultrasound has great promise as a clinical and investigative tool. Over the past decade, it has become clear that simple examination of the anatomic severity of coronary artery stenoses fails to adequately describe pathophysiologic mechanisms of coronary artery disease. Instead, impaired regulation of vasomotion, thrombosis, and other functional abnormalities in atherosclerotic arterial wall appear to be more relevant to the development of ischemic events and more appropriate targets for new therapies. Study of endothelium-dependent vasomotion has emerged as an important surrogate for the more generalized abnormalities of vascular function that relate directly to cardiovascular risk. As described in this chapter, highly reproducible noninvasive studies can be performed repetitively and in large numbers of subjects using readily available equipment. These methods are well suited for intervention studies that may provide information about pathophysiologic mechanisms in human subjects and suggest possible therapies for vascular dysfunction. The methodology also lends itself well to larger studies of newly recognized coronary risk factors, interactions between risk factors, and patient prognosis. We anticipate that investigators will continue to use and refine this methodology and develop new applications that will further enhance care of patients with cardiovascular disease.

References

1. Furchgott RF, Zawadzki JV (1980). The obligatory role of endothelial cells in the relaxation of arterial smooth muscle by acetylcholine. Nature 288: 373-376
2. Ignarro LJ, Buga GM, Wood KS, Byrns RE, Chaudhuri G (1987) Endothelium-derived relaxing factor produced and released from artery and vein is nitric oxide. Proc Natl Acad Sci USA 84:9265-9269
3. Stamler JS, Singel DJ, Loscalzo J (1992) Biochemistry of nitric oxide and its redox-activated forms. Science 258: 1898-1902
4. Palmer RM, Ashton DS, Moncada S (1988) Vascular endothelial cells synthesize nitric oxide from l-arginine. Nature 333:664-666
5. Ignarro LJ, Burke TM, Wood KS, Wolin MS, Kadowitz PJ (1984) Association between cyclic GMP accumulation and acetylcholine-elicited relaxation of bovine intrapulmonary artery. J Pharmacol Exp Ther 228: 682-690
6. Furchgott R (1983) Role of endothelium in responses of vascular smooth muscle. Circ Res 35: 557-573
7. Rubanyi GM, Romero JC, Vanhoutte PM (1986) Flow-induced release of endothelium-derived relaxing factor. Am J Physiol 250: H1145-H1149
8. Olesen SP, Clapham DE, Davies PF (1988) Haemodynamic shear stress activates a K_+ current in vascular endothelial cells. Nature 331: 168-170
9. Cooke JP, Rossitch E Jr, Andon NA, Loscalzo J, Dzau VJ (1991) Flow activates an endothelial potassium channel to release endogenous nitrovasodilator. J Clin Invest 88: 1663-1671
10. Oates JA, Fitzgerald GA, Branch RA, Jackson EK, Knapp HR, Roberts LJ (1988) Clincal implications of prostaglandin and thromboxane A2 formation. N Engl J Med 319: 689-698
11. Frangos JA, Erskin SG, Chintire LV, Ives CL (1984) Flow effects on prostacyclin production by cultured human endothelial cells. Science 227: 1477-1479
12. Ludmer PL, Selwyn AP, Shook TL, Wayne RR, Mudge GH, Alexander RW, Ganz P (1986) Paradoxical vasoconstriction induced by acetylcholine in atherosclerotic coronary arteries. N Engl J Med 315: 1046-1051
13. Vita JA, Treasure CB, Nabel EG, McLenachan JM, Fish RD, Yeung AC, Vekshtein VI, Selwyn AP, Ganz P (1990) Coronary vasomotor response to acetylcholine relates to risk factors for coronary artery disease. Circulation 81: 491-497
14. Creager MA, Cooke JP, Mendelsohn ME, Gallagher SJ, Coleman SM, Loscalzo J, Dzau VJ (1990) Impaired vasodilation of forearm resistance vessels in hypercholesterolemic humans. J Clin Invest 86: 228-234
15. Nitenberg A, Valersi P, Sachs R, Dali M, Aptecar E, Attali JR (1993) Impairment of coronary vascular reserve in and ACH-induced coronary vasodilation in diabetic patients with angiographically normal coronary arteries and normal left ventricular systolic function. Diabetes 42: 1017-1025
16. Johnstone MT, Creager SJ, Scales KM; Cusco JA, Lee BK, Creager MA (1993) Impaired endothelium-dependent vasodilation in patients with insulin-dependent diabetes mellitus. Circulation 88:2510-2516
17. Treasure CB, Manoukian SV, Klein JL, Vita JA, Nabel EG, Renwick GH, Selwyn AP, Alexander RW, Ganz P (1992) Epicardial coronary artery responses to acetylcholine are impaired in hypertensive patients. Circ Res 71: 776-781
18. Panza JA, Quyyumi AA, Brush JE, Epstein SE (1990) Abnormal endothelium-dependent vascular relaxation in patients with essential hypertension. N Engl J Med 323: 22-27
19. Nitenberg A, Antony I, Foult JM (1993) Acetylcholine-induced coronary vasoconstriction in young, heavy smokers with normal coronary arteriographic findings. Am J Med 95: 71-77
20. Yeung AC, Vekshtein VI, Krantz DS, Vita JA, Ryan TJ Jr, Ganz P, Selwyn AP (1991) The effect of atherosclerosis on the vasomotor response of coronary arteries to mental stress. N Engl J Med 325: 1551-1556

21. Okumura K, Yasue H, Matsuyama K, Ogawa H, Morikami Y, Obata K, Sakaino N (1992) Effect of acetylcholine on the highly stenotic coronary artery: difference between the constrictor response of the infarct-related coronary artery and that of the noninfarct-related artery. J Am Coll Cardiol 19: 752 - 758
22. Bogaty P, Hackett D, Davies G, Maseri A (1994) Vasoreactivity of the culprit lesion in unstable angina. Circulation 90: 5 - 11
23. Leung WH, Lau CP, Wong CK (1993) Beneficial effect of cholesterol-lowering therapy on coronary endothelium-dependent relaxation in hypercholesterolemic patients. Lancet 341: 1496 - 1500
24. Treasure CB, Klein JL, Weintraub WS, Talley JD, Stillabower ME, Kosinski AS, Zhang J, Boccuzzi SJ, Cedarholm JC, Alexander RW (1995) Beneficial effects of cholesterol-lowering therapy on the coronary endothelium in patients with coronary artery disease. N Engl J Med 332: 481 - 487
25. Anderson TJ, Meredith IT, Yeung AC, Frei B, Selwyn A, Ganz P (1995) The effect of cholesterol lowering and antioxidant therapy on endothelium-dependent coronary vasomotion. N Engl J Med 332: 488-493
26. Levine GN, Keaney JF Jr, Vita JA (1995) Cholesterol reduction in cardiovascular disease: clinical benefits and possible mechanisms. N Engl J Med 332: 512 - 521
27. Vita JA, Keaney JF Jr, Loscalzo J (1996) Endothelial dysfunction in vascular disease. In: Loscalzo J, Creager MA, Dzau V (eds) Vascular medicine, 2nd edn. Little Brown, Boston, pp 245 - 263
28. Laurent S, Brunel P, Lacolley P, Billaud E, Annier B, Safar M (1988) Flow-dependent vasodilation of the brachial artery in essential hypertension: preliminary report. J Hypertens 6: S182 - S184
29. Laurent S, Lacolley P, Brunel P, Laloux B, Pannier B, Safar M (1990) Flow-dependent vasodilation of brachial artery in essential hypertension. Am J Physiol 258: H1004 - H1011
30. Safar ME, Peronneau PA, Levenson JA, Toto-Moukouo JA, Simon AC (1981) Pulsed Doppler: diameter, blood flow velocity and volumic flow of the brachial artery in sustained essential hypertension. Circulation 63: 393 - 400
31. Anderson EA, Mark AL (1989) Flow-mediated and reflex changes in large peripheral artery tone in humans. Circualtion 79: 93 - 100
32. Celermajer DS, Sorensen KE, Gooch VM, Spiegelhalter DJ, Miller OI, Sullivan ID, Lloyd JK, Deanfield JE (1992) Noninvasive detection of endothelial dysfunction in children and adults at risk of atherosclerosis. Lancet 340: 1111 - 1115
33. Celermajer DS, Sorensen K, Ryalls M, Robinson J, Thomas O, Leonard RB, Deanfield JE (1993) Impaired endothelial function occurs in the systemic arteries of children with homozygous homocystinuria but not in their heterozygous parents. J Am Coll Cardiol 22: 854 - 858
34. Sorensen KE, Celermajer DS, Georgakopoulos D, Hatcher G, Betteridge DJ, Deanfield JE (1994) Impairment of endothelium-dependent dilation is an early event in children with familial hypercholesterolemia and is related to the lipoprotein (a) level. J Clin Invest 93: 50 - 55
35. Celermajer DS, Sorensen KE, Georgakopoulos D, Bull C, Thomas O, Robinson J, Deanfield J (1993) Cigarette smoking is associated with dose-related and potentially reversible impairment of endothelium-dependent dilation in healthy young adults. Circulation 88: 2149 - 2155
36. Celermajer DS, Sorensen KE, Spiegelhalter DJ, Georgakopoulos D, Robinson J, Deanfield JE (1994) Aging is associated with endothelial dysfunction in healthy men years before the age-related decline in women. J Am Coll Cardiol 24: 471 - 476
37. Sorensen KE, Celermajer DS, Spiegelhalter DS, Georgakopoulos D, Robinson J, Thomas O, Deanfield JE (1995) Noninvasive measurement of endothelium dependent arterial responses in man: accuracy and reproducibility. Br Heart J 74: 247 - 253
38. Celermajer DS, Sorensen KE, Bull C, Robinson J, Deanfield JE (1994) Endothelium-dependent dilation in the systemic arteries of asymptomatic subject relates to coronary risk factors and their interaction. J Am Coll Cardiol 24: 1468 - 1474
39. Celermajer DS, Adams MR, Clarkson P, Robinson J, McCredie R, Donald A, Deanfield JE (1996) Passive smoking and impaired endothelium-dependent arterial dilatation in healthy young adults. N Engl J Med 334: 150 - 154
40. Uehata A, Lieberman EH, Meredith I, Anderson T, Polak J, Ganz P, Selwyn A, Creager M, Yeung A (1992) Noninvasive assessment of flow-mediated vasodilation in brachial arteries: diminished response in young males compared to females. Circulation 86: I - 620
41. Uehata A, Gerhard MD, Meredith IT, Lieberman EL, Selwyn AP, Creager M, Polak J, Ganz P, Yeung AC, Anderson TJ (1993) Close relationship of endothelial dysfunction in coronary and brachial artery. Circulation 88: I - 618
42. Lieberman EH, Uehata A, Polak J, Ganz P, Selwyn AP, Creager MA, Yeung AC (1993) Flow-mediated vasodilation is impaired in the brachial artery of patients with coronary disease or diabetes mellitus (Abstr.). Clin Res 41: 217A
43. Gerhard MD, Roddy M-A, Creager SJ, Creager MA (1993) Aging reduces endothelium-dependent vasodilation in humans (Abstr.). Circulation 88: I - 369
44. Lieberman EH, Knab ST, Creager MA (1994) Nitric oxide mediates the vasodilator response to flow in humans. Circulation 90: I - 138
45. Lieberman EH, Gerhard MD, Uehata A, Walsh BW, Selwyn AP, Ganz P, Yeung AC, Creager MA (1994) Estrogen improves endothelium-dependent, flow mediated vasodilation in post menopausal women. Ann Intern Med 121: 936 - 941
46. Anderson TJ, Uehata A, Gerhard MD, Meredith IT, Knab S, Delagrange D, Leiberman EH, Ganz P, Creager MA, Yeung AC, Selwyn AP (1995) Close relation of endothelial function in the human coronary and peripheral circulations. J Am Coll Cardiol 26: 1235 - 1241
47. Corretti MC, Plotnick GD, Vogel RA (1995) Technical aspects of evaluating brachial artery endothelium-dependent vasodilatation using high frequency ultrasound. Am J Physiol 268: H1397 - H1404
48. Levine GN, Frei B, Koulouris SN, Gerhard MD, Keaney JF Jr, Vita JA (1996) Absorbic acid reverses endothelial vasomotor dysfunction in patients with coronary artery disease. Circulation 96: 1107 - 1113
49. Kool MJF, Hoeks APG, Struyker Boudier HAJ, Reneman RS, Van Bortel LMAB (1994) Short- and longterm ef-

fects of smoking on arterial wall properties in habitual smokers. J Am Coll Cardiol 22: 1881–1886
50. Corretti MC, Plotnick GD, Vogel RA (1995) Correlation of cold pressor and flow-mediated brachial artery diameter responses with the presence of coronary artery disease. Am J Cardiol 75: 783–787
51. Joannides R, Haefeli WE, Linder L, Richard V, Bakkali EH, Thuillez C, Luscher TF (1995) Nitric oxide is responsible for flow-dependent dilatation of human peripheral conduit arteries in vivo. Circulation 91: 1314–1319
52. Hornig B, Maier V, Drexler H (1996) Physical training improves endothelial function in patients with chronic heart failure. Circulation 93: 210–214
53. Tagawa T, Imaizumi T, Endo T, Shiramoto M, Harasawa Y, Takeshita A (1994) Role of nitric oxide in reactive hyperemia in human forearm vessels. Circulation 90: 2285–2290
54. Pallares LCM, Deane CR, Baudouin SV, Evans TW (1993) Strain gauge plethysmography and Doppler ultrasound in the measurement of limb blood flow. Eur J Clin Invest 24: 279–286
55. Lipsitz LA, Bui M, Stiebeling M, McArdle C (1991) Forearm blood flow response to posture change in the very old: non-invasive measurement by venous occlusion plethysmography. J Am Geriatr Soc 39: 53–59
56. Gilligan DM, Panza JA, Kilcoyne CM, Waclawiw MA, Casino PR, Quyyumi AA (1994) Contribution of endothelium-derived nitric oxide to exercise-induced vasodilation. Circulation 90: 2853–2858
57. Meredith IT, Yeung AC, Weidinger FF, Anderson TJ, Uehata A, Ryan TJ Jr, Selwyn AP, Ganz P (1993) Role of impaired endothelium-dependent vasodilation in ischemic manifestations of coronary artery disease. Circulation 87: V56–V66
58. Dodge JT, Brown BG, Bolson EL, Dodge T (1992) Lumen diameter of normal human coronary arteries; influence of age sex anatomic variation, and left ventricular hypertrophy or dilation. Circulation 86: 232–246
59. Vogel RA, Corretti M, Plotnick GD (1995) Changes in flow-mediated brachial artery vasoactivity with lowering of desirable cholesterol levels in healthy, middle-aged men. Am J Cardiol 77: 37–40

Intracoronary Ultrasound Imaging

D. Hausmann, M. Sturm, E. Blessing, A. Mügge, and P. J. Fitzgerald

Introduction

In contrast to conventional angiography, intravascular ultrasound is a technique that provides tomographic, cross-sectional images of the vessel lumen and wall. The first ultrasound catheter was designed more than 20 years ago, but the increasing use of coronary balloon angioplasty and the development of other interventional devices in the 1980s renewed the interest in intravascular ultrasound imaging [1]. As fluoroscopy and angiographic images are indispensable elements of the ultrasound examination, intravascular ultrasound should not be considered as an alternative to angiography but rather as a complementary imaging technique.

The use of intravascular ultrasound imaging is no longer restricted to research, but is emerging as an important diagnostic technique of daily clinical application in interventional cardiology [2]. Experience in recent years clearly indicates that this technique has several advantages over other imaging modalities used for coronary imaging; however, it has not been proven in randomized trials whether the increase in diagnostic information from the use of this technique also leads to improved patient outcome.

Technical Background

Ultrasound transducers convert electrical energy into ultrasound and vice versa by virtue of the intrinsic properties of the piezoelectric transducer material. The transducer is activated by an electrical impulse and vibrates at a characteristic frequency. These brief burst are reflected ("backscattered") by the surrounding tissue and return to the transducer which generates an electrical impulse in the transducer. The signal is then modified and transformed into a graphic display. Currently available intravascular ultrasound systems are based on two different catheter designs: mechanical and phased-array transducers. *Mechanical systems* are single imaging element devices that have either a rotating mirror that directs the ultrasound beam to the transducer or a rotating transducer. Rotation is provided by a flexible cable traveling through the catheter and connected to an external motor drive. This allows circumferential scanning of the ultrasound beam and acquisition of two-dimensional images. *In solid-state systems,* multiple elements are located in a cylindrical array at the tip of the catheter and are activated in sequences to produce a two-dimensional image. The solid-state approach has the advantage that no parts in the catheter are moving, whereas most mechanical systems provide better image quality.

Image resolution is a direct function of transducer frequency, i.e., higher frequencies yield better resolution. However, the penetration depth of the ultrasound field is also dependent on the transducer frequency, so that in practice transducers of 20–30 MHz are used for coronary imaging, whereas 10–20 MHz are appropriate for peripheral arteries. The outer diameter of the coronary ultrasound catheters currently ranges between 2.9 and 3.5 French. In solid-state systems, the guidewire runs coaxially through the catheter shaft and therefore no wire artifact appears on the image. Mechanical catheters are usually delivered with a wire running along the transducer ("rapid exchange" modus). Recently, a mechanical catheter with a distal lumen that can house either the transducer core (during the imaging procedure) or the guidewire (during placement of the catheter) has been introduced. This design is especially attractive because (a) the wire artifact in the imaging plane is avoided, (b) the pullback of the transducer core (instead of the entire catheter shaft) is more accurate for precise longitudinal measurements, and (c) trauma to the vessel is minimized.

The resolution of the system is a major factor in image quality. Resolution is defined as the minimal distance between two points that can be discriminated and is influenced by both the catheter aperture and the transducer frequency. Axial resolution of the system is always better than lateral resolution, indicating that structures aligned on a radial beam from the transducer can be discriminated with greater accuracy than structures positioned in the lateral direction. Eccentric placement of the ultrasound catheter in the vessel significantly degrades image quality, because relatively more structures are influenced by lateral resolution than with the cathered centered.

In addition to the conventional two-dimensional display of ultrasound images, systems for three-dimensional reconstruction have been designed. For this purpose, ultrasound images are acquired during a timed pullback of the ultrasound catheter through a vessel segment; a constant pullback speed of 0.5–1.0 mm/s is usually obtained using a motor-driven device. The ultrasound cross-sectional images acquired during the pullback are processed by the computer and reconstructed into a visual display. These displays allow different operator-controlled views of the imaged segment. Three-dimensional reconstruction of ultrasound images may improve the assessment of structures in which cross-sectional *and* longitudinal perspectives are useful, such as in dissections or deposits of calcium. For guidance of coronary stenting, three-dimensional views may be especially useful to assess lesion length, location of side branches, and relative degree of stent expansion. Recently, an approach to obtain spatially correct three-dimensional reconstruction has been proposed [3]. For this technique, data from electrocardiogram (ECG)-gated biplane cinefluoroscopy are incorporated into the ultrasound reconstruction to allow for more anatomically correct images.

Imaging Procedure

Initial Setup and Imaging

Intravascular ultrasound imaging is similar to interventional procedures; therefore, it should only be performed by or under personal supervision of a fully trained invasive cardiologist. A guiding catheter with a diameter of 8 French (inner diameter, 0.84–0.86 in.) should be used to house the ultrasound catheter and to allow for additional contrast injections. A total of 10 000 U heparin should be given before intracoronary imaging is performed; administration of intracoronary nitroglycerin (0.1–0.3 mg) is also a standard approach in many centers. At least one coronary angiogram before and after the ultrasound procedure is required for documentation.

The ultrasound imaging procedure depends to some degree on the type of ultrasound equipment used. In mechanical catheters, air has to be removed from the space between the imaging element and the surrounding sheath by flushing. The ultrasound catheter has to be connected to the ultrasound processing equipment; in mechanical systems, the catheter is also connected to the motor drive which rotates the mirror or imaging element. The ultrasound imaging catheter is then advanced over the wire into the vessel. As soon as the ultrasound catheter leaves the tip of the guiding catheter, the settings for gain, compression, and reject should be adjusted meticulously until an ultrasound image with an optimal dynamic range is obtained. The ultrasound image should allow reliable differentiation between the different layers of the vessel wall: in the near field, the time-gain control should be reduced to deemphasize the blood backscatter, and in the far field the gain should be gradually increased. If no optimal image can be obtained, the catheter should not be advanced further into the coronary vessels because of the potential risk of catheter-passage without the benefit of obtaining adequate information from the study. If an optimal image can be obtained, the ultrasound catheter can be further advanced into the target segment under careful fluoroscopic guidance. Recordings on videotape are made for off-line analysis. Calibration markers are superimposed on the image for diameter and area measurements. The recordings should be accompanied by spoken text indicating the location of the ultrasound transducer for off-line analysis. In our experience, display of the ultrasound images on the overhead monitor, e.g., side by side with the angiogram, has been very helpful. It is also our practice that an additional person in the catheterization laboratory is dedicated to image optimization, spoken commentary and documenting of the ultrasound recordings.

Orientation in the coronary artery is essential for ultrasound imaging and is often a source of errors. For *longitudinal orientation* in the vessel, branch points should be identified on the ultrasound image and the position should be documented using fluoroscopy with and without contrast injection. Visualization of veins may also provide orientation. The most precise longitudinal orientation, however, is provided by a motorized pullback of the catheter with and without three-dimensional reconstruction of the images. For *rotational orienta-*

tion, fluoroscopy provides no help, and three-dimensional reconstruction of the ultrasound images is also misleading due to potential rotation of the catheter during the pullback. Instead, anatomical landmarks can be used for rotational orientation. For imaging the left system, the transducer is positioned at the bifurcation with the left anterior descending artery coming off at the 3 o'clock position and the circumflex artery at the 9 o'clock position. When the left anterior descending artery is imaged, the diagonal branches come off between 8 and 12 o'clock and the septals come off at 6 o'clock; when the circumflex artery is imaged, the obtuse marginal vessels come off between 12 and 6 o'clock. In the right coronary artery, the image is usually oriented so that the marginal branches come off at 9 o'clock.

Technical Problems and Potential Complications

Ultrasound catheters are stiff in the region of the imaging element, and advancing the catheter to the target segment can be a problem when curved segments have to be crossed. Although smaller catheter designs are now available, it can still be difficult to cross very tight lesions, especially those with superficial calcium deposits. Crossing tight lesions with the ultrasound catheter may cause a certain amount of Dottering effect (mechanical expansion). Furthermore, imaging of the very distal portion of coronary vessels is limited by the size of the imaging catheter. Another technical problem with mechanical systems can be that, despite intensive flushing before insertion of the ultrasound catheter, the intravascular image can still be impaired by air bubbles. Bending or kinking may occur when ultrasound catheters with a relatively short monorail tip are advanced too rapidly or forcefully into the vessel.

Intravascular ultrasound imaging prolongs the catheterization procedure by approximately 10 min and requires an additional person during the imaging procedure to optimize the image settings. When intravascular ultrasound imaging is performed during diagnostic catheterization procedures, the additional use of heparin and insertion of larger sheaths (e.g., 8 French) slightly increases the discomfort and/or risk to the patient.

Potential acute complications of intracoronary ultrasound imaging are spasm, thrombus formation, occlusion, and dissection of the vessel; in addition, placement of the ultrasound catheter into tight lesions can cause reversible myocardial ischemia. A multicenter, "multi-catheter" registry on acute complications of intracoronary ultrasound has been established recently by our group [4]. A total of 2207 ultrasound procedures performed in transplant patients and in patients with native coronary disease with and without intervention were collected from 28 centers. Minor complications that were clearly related to ultrasound imaging were observed in six (0.3%) patients (one dissection, three acute occlusions, one thrombus formation, and one embolism). Handling of these complications should be similar to what is recommended for patients during interventional procedures. First, an attempt to seal the dissection by balloon inflation (standard or perfusion balloon) should be performed. Depending on the severity and clinical significance of the dissection, stenting or bypass surgery should be considered. In the multicenter survey, major complications were caused by ultrasound imaging in only three (0.1%) patients (all three patients had myocardial infarction) [4]. All major complications occurred during interventional procedures. Spasm is the most frequent complication during ultrasound imaging, occurring in up to 3% of patients. Spasm may not only be seen at the tip of the catheter, but also more distally. Removal of the ultrasound catheter is often necessary in the presence of distal spasm because adequate coronary perfusion is crucial in these cases.

Whether manipulation of the ultrasound catheter in the coronary vessels may cause chronic injury resulting in acceleration of the progression of atherosderosis and/or changes in endothelial function remains uncertain at this point. Pinto et al. [5] found no evidence of reduction in lumen dimensions in vessels undergoing intravascular ultrasound imaging; however, quantitative angiography was used in this study to assess serial changes in lumen dimensions and thus the degree of plaque progression may not have been assessed accurately.

Interpretation of Intracoronary Ultrasound Images

Normal Coronary Arteries

The center of the intravascular ultrasound image is a black area produced by the imaging element itself. The surrounding lumen of the vessel shows a weak, speckled echo pattern caused by reflection of the ultrasound beam from red blood cells. The intensity of the blood backscatter increases with the ultrasound frequency used. Furthermore, backscatter is influenced by blood flow velocities, with blood backscatter being highest in areas of low flow velocity [6]. Depending on the type of ultrasound equipment used, the image in a small arc of the circumference is significantly attenuated by an artifact of the catheter strut and by the guidewire running along the imaging element. The basis for the ability of intravascular ultrasound to discriminate between different layers of the coronary vessel wall is their difference in acoustic properties at 20 – 30 MHz. The media of coronary arteries (muscular type) contains only small amounts of elastin and collagen; this contributes to the relatively echolucent appearance of the media as compared to the adventitia and intima. On the ultrasound scan, the media therefore appears as a dark band. Only these different characteristics of the vessel wall layers allow identification of the outer border of atherosclerotic plaque [7]. The internal elastic lamina is a highly reflective structure; it may even cause a "blooming" effect with overrepresentation of the internal elastic lamina on the ultrasound scan. Since the truly "normal" intima consists only of a single cell-layer and is usually too thin to be delineated, the first inner layer of the vessel wall on an ultrasound image at 20 – 30 MHz is the internal elastic lamina. Thickening of the intima is a mechanism that begins at birth and may already be detectable by histology or intravascular ultrasound in otherwise healthy young adults [8]. Intima thickness in early childhood is approximately 50 µm and increases to 200 – 250 µm by the age of 40 years. Whether intimal thickening per se is a pathologic feature therefore remains unclear. For clinical routine it appears appropriate to consider a coronary vessel wall as "normal" if no three-layer appearance is present or if the layer of the intima/internal elastic lamina is represented only by a thin line of less than <200 µm [7].

Atherosclerotic Coronary Arteries

Qualitative Assessment

Atherosclerosis of the vessel wall leads to thickening of the intima layer (Fig. 1) and, in the presence of advanced disease, thinning of the media. The media, which is the major component of the normal vessel wall, is substantially attenuated in areas of overlying plaque, probably because of primary atrophy or as a result of intravasation of the plaque [9]. Intravascular ultrasound studies with histologic validation have shown that media thickness in the absence of atherosclerotic lesions is approximately 0.6 mm, decreasing to 0.1 mm in the area of advanced plaque [10]. Since detection of the outer border of the atherosclerotic plaque relies on identification of echolucent media, moving the ultrasound proximal and distal into areas of less media attenuation may be useful in cases with advanced plaque and no clear media layer.

A major advantage of intravascular ultrasound imaging compared to other imaging techniques is its ability to differentiate plaque composition; this provides important information both for the natural history of the disease and for the response of the plaque to interventions. According to studies comparing in vitro ultrasound images of human atherosclerotic vessels and the corresponding histologic specimen, accurate differentiation between soft, fibrous, and calcified plaque is possible [11, 12]. *Calcified plaques* are brightly reflective on the ultrasound scan and show a dropout of the image peripheral to the calcium deposit. As a result, visualization of vessel wall structures in this area, in particular the outer border of the plaque, is difficult. In the far field, reverberations of the calcium rim can sometimes be seen; this artifact is caused by repeat-

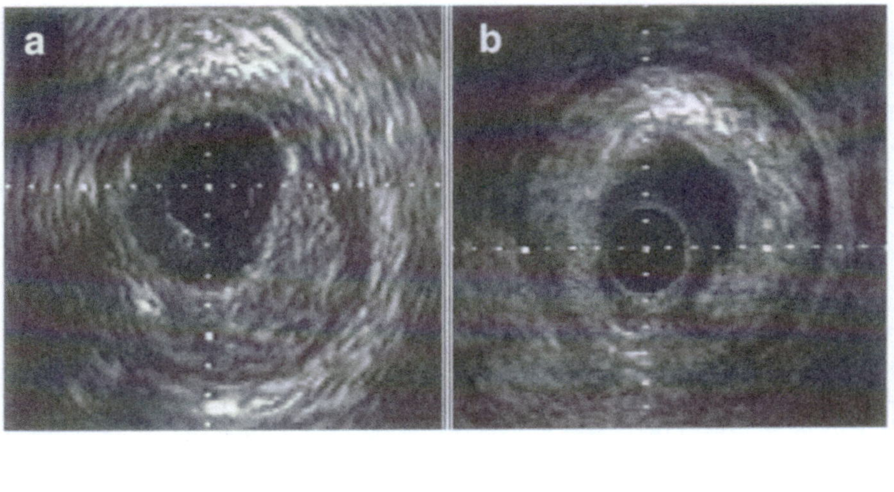

Fig. 1a, b. Intracoronary ultrasound imaging in atherosclerotic coronary arteries. An eccentric, noncalcified plaque demonstrated by ultrasound imaging. Note the three-layer appearance of the vessel wall with the echolucent zone representing the media. Concentric, noncalcified plaque. Calibration, 0.5 mm

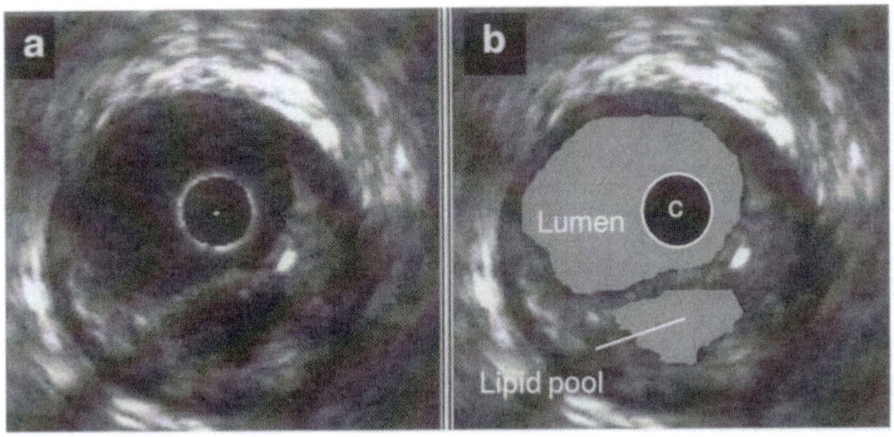

Fig. 2a, b. Intravascular ultrasound image of an echolucent, intramural structure (possibly representing a lipid pool) in the mid-portion of the left anterior descending artery. The patient had unstable angina pectoris. The ultrasound image shows a large residual lumen (4.0 × 3.2 mm); the angiogram (not shown) revealed only mild lumen stenosis at this site. An eccentric plaque with an echolucent, intramural structure and a thin cap can be seen. Cartoon image indicating the area of the vessel lumen and the area of the lipid pool. *C*, catheter.

ed reflection of the returning ultrasound signal. *Fibrous plaques* also show a bright echo on the ultrasound image, but usually cause no intense shadowing; however, depending on transducer characteristics, thick layers of fibrous plaque may also lead to dropout. *Soft plaque* is less reflective and causes no shadowing of peripheral structures. Localized lipid deposits, often occurring within fibrous tissue, are also hypoechoic structures and in favorable cases can be detected by ultrasound imaging [13] (Fig. 2). A major limitation of currently available intravascular ultrasound imaging systems is the difficulty in differentiating thrombotic material in the vessel lumen from soft tissue or from areas of low blood flow velocity [14]. One characteristic feature of fresh thrombus is the "scintillating" appearance; however, organized thrombus may appear very similar to soft plaque. The surface of fresh thrombus is often irregular, and in some cases "footprints" of the ultrasound catheter can be observed on the surface of the thrombus. Nevertheless, differentiation between thrombus and lipid-rich plaque is better with angioscopy because of the high image resolution and color capabilities.

Branch points, bifurcations, and outer parts of bends often show marked intima proliferation due to changing shear stresses in these areas. In a recent study, Kimura et al. [15] showed that atheromas in the very proximal left anterior descending artery are located opposite the circumflex takeoff and maintain eccentricity across a wide range of vessel stenoses.

Tissue characterization during intravascular ultrasound may be helpful to distinguish plaque types and thrombotic material. This approach is based on analysis of the backscattered ultrasound signal, which reveals greater information than the display of the gray scale image alone. Fitzgerald et al. [16] have shown that thrombus and soft plaque are characterized by different radiofrequency signals and that this method may improve the recognition of different tissue types.

Quantitative Assessment

Besides the qualitative assessment of plaque composition, intracoronary ultrasound has the advantage that it allows cross-sectional two dimensional measurements of the vessel lumen and wall dimensions. Compared to histology, this technique has been shown to provide reliable measurements of lumen area and diameter as well as wall thickness of arteries [12, 17, 18]. In cross-sectional images, quantitative measurements include planimetry of lumen and plaque area and measurement of lumen diameters and plaque thickness. The percent age of plaque stenosis calculated fromm the plaque area and total vessel area. The internal elastic lamina is the anatomic outer border of the plaque. However, with intravascular ultrasound imaging, it is often difficult to clearly identify this structure due to fibrous changes in the inner third of the media. In contrast, the external elastic lamina can easily be defined in most cases; thus, a plaque-media complex is often measured rather than the plaque area alone. In calcified plaque, delineation of the outer border of the plaque is limited due to shadowing artifacts; accurate plaque measurements may be possible only with a calcium arc or less than < 90°–120°.

The lumen diameter of the left main coronary artery measures 3–5 mm, and the proximal left circumflex and left anterior descending arteries have a lumen diameter of 2–5 mm. Due to the number of side branches, significant tapering can be observed in the two branches of the left coronary artery. The right coronary artery measures 2 – 6 mm in the proximal portion and is characterized by minor tapering up to the crux cordis.

Recently, automated lumen measurements have been performed in intravascular ultrasound images comparable to quantitative coronary angiography [19]. An algorithm for detection of the lumen-plaque interface based on gray scale analysis has been developed and validated in animal experiments [19]. Automated detection of the outer border of the plaque (plaque-media interface) is technically more challenging due to the fact that differences in the acoustic properties of these structures are small.

Quantitative measurements in ultrasound images have so far been limited to cross-sectional vessel images. However, due to the diffuse pattern of coronary atherosclerosis, two-dimensional images are not sufficient to quantify the extent of atherosclerosis in an entire segment or vessel, especially in view of the potential role of intravascular ultrasound to assess serial changes in the disease (regression studies). Consequently, indices of "plaque volume" have been developed. For this purpose, a third dimension has to be introduced into the calculations by a timed catheter pullback. In a recent study, such an approach was used to describe the extent of atherosclerosis in patients with familar hyperlipidemia and to correlate the findings with the degree of lipid abnormalities [20].

Pitfalls in Image Interpretation

Ultrasound images are generated in an orthogonal direction to the catheter, and image acquisition therefore depends on the angle between the catheter and the vessel to be imaged. Nonorthogonal placement of the ultrasound catheter in the vessel lumen causes image distortion [21]. Another technical problem in mechanical transducers can be that air bubbles in the catheter housing attenuate image quality. Thorough flushing before and, if necessary, during placement of the catheter in the vessel is mandatory. In some patients with intensive plaque calcification, shadowing of deeper structures limits image interpretation; such dropout has to be differentiated from other phenomena, such as air bubbles in the imaging catheter or dissections. Another problem is that, in mechanical catheters, failure to achieve precise rotation can result in nonuniform rotational distortion (NURD) of the ultrasound image.

Blood backscatter intensity increases in areas of low blood flow velocity [6], such as dissections or when blood flow is reduced from occlusion of tight lesions by the ultrasound catheter itself. In these cases, lumen and vessel wall structures can show similar acoustic properties and delineation of the vessel wall can be difficult. Intracoronary injection of echogenic agents can increase the blood backscatter intensity, allowing correct delineation of the vessel wall surface [22].This approach may be clinically useful for detection of inappropriate stent apposition, delineation of postinterventional dissections, or identification of intramural echolucent structures [23].

Since quantitative measurements in intravascular ultrasound images are usually performed on the basis of visual interpretation, subjective judgement can be a source of significant measurement variability [24]. Whereas plaque quantification and plaque thickness show significant variability, lumen measurements are usually associated with the lowest measurement variability. However, parameters derived from several lumen measurements show more variability. In a recent study [25], measurements of the degree of stent expansion (derived from lumen area proximal and distal to the stent and the lumen area in the stent) by two investigators showed a correlation of only $r = 0.76$. Further studies are needed to prove the accuracy and reproducibility of quantitative intravascular ultrasound. Automated image measurements (comparable to quantitative coronary angiography) may help to further reduce the variability of ultrasound measurements.

Diagnostic Applications

Comparison with Angiography

For many years now, quantitative coronary angiography has been the "gold standard" for assessment of intracoronary dimensions, providing accurate and reproducible measurements of intraluminal diameters [26, 27]. Despite its widespread acceptance, coronary angiography has many inherent limitations. Contrast angiography only show a picture of the luminal contour; however, even in patient with "normal" coronary angiographic findings, significant amounts of atherosclerotic plaque have been demonstrated by histology [28 – 30], epicardial echocardiography [31], and intracoronary ultrasound imaging [32–34]. This fundamental problem remains even with further refinement of the angiographic techniques (multiple orthogonal views, videodensitometry, digital subtraction technique). The angiographic image also has inherent limitations in the assessment of the severity of stenosis in eccentric coronary artery lesions and in the estimation of luminal dimensions in the presence of vessel tortuosity or overlap [28, 35].

In several studies, intravascular ultrasound and histologic measurements of lumen area, vessel area, and plaque area showed a dose correlation [12, 36, 37]. Moreover, in vitro ultrasound also showed high accurrency in measurements of cylindrical phantoms of known dimensions [36]. However, non-coaxial alignment of the catheter was found to cause geometric overestimation of lumen size. This non-coaxial alignment of the transducer within the lumen results in a more elliptical than orthogonal cross-sectional imaging plane, leading to overestimation of both diameters and areas. Nevertheless, small-sized coronary arteries prevent significant malalignment of the transducer [21]. However, this potential source of error should be remembered when taking measurements in tortuous coronary segments or in large ectatic vessels (C. Di Mario 1996, personal communication).

In contrast to angiography, intravascular ultrasound provides transmural images of coronary arteries in vivo with visualization of location, distribution, and magnitude of atherosclerotic plaque [12, 38, 39]. Comparisons between quantitative angiography and intracoronary ultrasound measurements have shown high correlations in luminal diameter and cross-sectional area of nondiseased coronary arteries [32, 40–42], but less agreement in atherosclerotic diseased vessels [32, 42–44]. For example, several in vivo studies have reported a very poor correlation between angiographic and intravascular ultrasound measurements of luminal dimensions after percutaneous transluminal coronary angioplasty [41, 42, 45, 46]. A similar pattern has been reported in several studies comparing ultrasound and quantitative angiographic measurements after other coronary interventions, such as directional and rotational atherectomy and stenting [47–49]. Table 1 summarizes the results of eight clinical studies in which quantitative angiography and intravascular ultrasound measurements of human coronary arteries were compared.

In several studies, luminal dimensions measured by ultrasound and angiography in normal and atherosclerotic vessels and in coronary segments after perentaneous transluminal coronary angioplasty (PTCA) have shown alternating systematic bias. However, despite these contradictary reports, most studies suggest that intravascular ultrasound may be superior to contrast angiography because of the ability to directly visualize the irregular lumen border [42, 46, 50, 51].

Glagov et al. [28] first described compensatory enlargement of human atherosclerotic coronary arteries in a postmortem histopathologic study. It was hypothesized that vascular remodeling allows plaque to occupy an average of 30%–40% of the coronary vessel cross-section before luminal encroachment occurs [28–30, 52]. This delay of luminal nar-

Table 1. Lumen measurements in normal, atherosclerotic, and postinterventional coronary arteries; correlation between intravascular ultrasound and quantitative angiographic measurements

Reference	Correlation coefficient	Parameter	Direction of bias
Undiseased coronary arteries			
Nissen et al. [33]	0.92	MLD	
St. Goar et al. [40]	0.86	MLD	IVUS > QCA*
Werner et al. [41]	0.86	MLD	IVUS > QCA*
De Scheerder et al.[42]	0.92	MLD	IVUS > QCA**
Diseased coronary arteries			
Nissen et al. [33]	0.77	MLD	
Porter et al. [43]	0.59	MLD	
De Scheerder et al [44]	0.47	MLD	IVUS > QCA*
Mintz et al. [44]	0.83	MLD	IVUS > QCA*
Coronary arteries post-PTCA			
Werner et al. [41]	0.48	MLD	
Davidson et al. [45]	0.28	MLD	
De Scheerder et al [42]	0.28	MLD	IVUS > QCA*
Haase et al. [46]	0.47	CAS	IVUS > QCA*

PTCA, percuatenous transluminal coronary angioplasty; MLD, minimal luminal diameter, CAS, cross-sectional area; IVUS, intravascular ultrasound; QCA, quantitative coronary angiography.
* $p < 0.01$.
** $p = 0.04$.

rowing may be the reason why coronary angiography is an insensitive method for detection of early atheromatous thickening of the arterial wall. Compensatory enlargement of human arteries has been confirmed by intravascular ultrasound in vivo [53–56] and is believed to be more pronounced in soft plaque than in calcified lesions [57]. Vascular remodeling appears to be a phenomen only in native arteries, since intravascular ultrasound demonstrated the absence of compensatory entlargement in saphenous vein bypass grafts [58]. However, some studies suggest that there is great variability of remodeling in atherosclerotic coronary arteries [59]. A recent study using intravascular ultrasound imaging of human femoral arteries demonstrated that focal failure of compensatory enlargement may contribute to severe arterial luminal narrowing [60]. It is generally accepted that the early atherosclerotic disease process can be studied in vivo using intravascular ultrasound in a manner not achievable with any other imaging modalities [61].

Angiographic detection of lumen narrowing is based on comparison of a lesion with a reference segment that is considered to be normal. Recent intravascular ultrasound studies indicate that atherosclerotic plaque is ubiquitous in angiographically normal coronary artery reference segments [61–63]. The reference segment disease tends to parallel the severity of the target lesion disease [61]. This may lead to an angiographic appearance without localized narrowing or to considerable underestimation of the atherosclerotic plaque by angiography. This may be important during intracoronary interventions when reference segments are used for device sizing. Another clinically important site of angiographically silent plaques may be the left main coronary artery [54, 55, 63].

When luminal dimensions are measured by intracoronary ultrasound imaging, the variation in the coronary lumen during the cardiac cyde has to be taken into account. The maximum cross-sectional area is present in the midsystole and the minimum area in the late diastole (C. Di Mario 1996, personal communication). During the cardiac cycle, the cross-sectional area varies by approximately 10% in normal coronary arteries and 5% or less in diseased arteries [64, 65].

Assessment of Coronary Artery Disease

For evaluation of angiographic stenoses of uncertain severity, intracoronary ultrasound is of unequivocal benefit in clarifying the anatomy. Ostial stenoses or stenoses at the origin of large side branches in particular can sometimes be insufficiently visualized by angiography because of vessel overlapping or foreshortening [66]. Furthermore, angiography often underestimates the severity of eccentric lesions as shown by the (Guidance by Ultrasound Imaging for Decision Endpoints) (GUIDE) trial [67]. All noncircular shapes (elliptical, slit-like orifices, D-shaped, star-shaped, cresentic) can cause under- and overestimation when cross-sectional area is determined by angiography [68]. However, cross-sectional area measurements of intracoronary ultrasound are particularly suitable for the assessment of eccentric lesions and are not limited by vessel overlapping or other causes of insufficient angiographic visualization. Very short "napkin-ring" stenoses or insufficient quality of the angiogram because of extreme obesity or emphysema may be another indication for intravascular ultrasound examination. Two prospective trials showed that preinterventional imaging with intravascular ultrasound may influence the subsequent therapeutic strategy in a considerable subset of patients [44, 69].

The criteria for defining a significant stenosis using intravascular ultrasound are not clear (C. Di Mario 1996, personal communication). Unfortunately, both angiography and intracoronary angiography are imaging techniques that are unable to clarify the functional severity of coronary stenoses. Therefore, the ultimate definition of hemodynamically significant coronary stenosis should be left to functional tests, such as flow velocity measurements with intracoronary Doppler or pressure measurements proximal and distal to the stenosis.

Although luminal narrowing and severe stenosis can cause decreases in coronary flow, the severity of vessel stenosis does not reflect its potential to cause acute ischemic syndromes[70, 71]. Analysis of the composition rather than the luminal encroachment of an atheroma is a potential application of intravascular ultrasound. It is now commonly believed that acute ischemic syndromes result from a disruption of lipid-rich atheromatous plaque, setting into action a cascade of pathogenic mechanisms such as platelet activation, increased vasoconstriction, and thrombus formation [70–73]. Plaque rupture has been visualized with intravascular ultrasound following myocardial infarction [74], and echolucent zones, possibly indicating lipid deposits, are a more sensitive indicator of instability than angiographic criteria [34]. Plaques with lipid deposits and a thin fibrous cap are at particular risk for rupture due to mechanical instability [75]. Figure 2 (s. p. 264) shows a echolucent region believed to be lipid deposit.

Unfortunately, identification of these lesions with intravascular ultrasound is difficult, because echolucent lipid deposits can be mimicked by other tissue and are highly dependent on gain and dynamic range settings [76, 77]. In addition, echolucent areas caused by dissections (false lumen) or acoustic dropout can be misinterpreted as lipid lakes. Calcium may be deposited after plaque rupture or thrombosis, and this is thought to represent a more mature point in the natural course of atherosclerotic lesions [76]. Calcified lesions with low lipid content seem to be more stable and are easy to identify by intravascular ultrasound because of their high echogenicity and distal shadowing of underlying tissue. Intravascular ultrasound can accurately assess the arc, length, and distribution patterns (superficial versus deep) of coronary artery calcification [39, 78].

Difficulties arise in identifying intracoronary thrombus by means of intracoronary ultrasound. Although thrombus appears brighter than moving blood, it remains difficult to differentiate acute thrombus from surrounding soft plaque on intravascular ultrasound images. Recently, Chemarin-Alibelli et al. [79] suggested that acute thrombus after myocardial infarction can be identified with high sensitivity if the ultrasound image has a bright, speckled, echogenic appearance that scintillates with movements of the structure.

Identification of older thrombus seems to be more difficult because the speckled appearance is often replaced by a more linear, mildly echogenic pattern. However, in most cases this structure remain mobile with blood flow and slightly protrudes into the arterial lumen [79, 80], making identification possible in many cases.

Another potential diagnostic application of intravascular ultrasound imaging may be the assessment of the natural course of the disease and the effect of medical interventions. During the past decade, it has become obvious that angiographic regression or slowing the progression of coronary atherosclerosis in humans is possible [81–86], especially when intensive lipid-lowering therapy is initiated. All these studies analyzed progression and regression by means of quantitative angiography, and it is clear that intravascular ultrasound may be a useful complementary tool for future regression studies, since it visualizes the entire cross-section of the plaque. Preliminary studies have shown that the changes in atherosclerotic plaque burden can be accurately assessed by intravascular ultrasound [87, 88]. In addition, multiple samples of cross-sectional intracoronary ultrasound images may provide volumetric measurement of luminal and plaque dimensions [89, 90].

Assessment of Transplant Vasculopathy

Accelerated transplant coronary vasculopathy represents one of the major causes of mortality in cardiac transplant recipients beyond the first year after transplantation [91–93]. The incidence of this disease has been estimated at approximately 8%–10% per year following transplantation [94, 95]. The pathology of transplant vasculopathy is characterized by diffuse, concentric intimal proliferation during the early phase of the disease and ultimately becomes manifest as luminal stenosis of epicardial branches, occlusion of smaller vessels, and myocardial infarction. The pathophysiological mechanism of transplant vasculopathy appears to be immune-mediated damage of the microvasculature and the endothelium, ultimately leading to intimal proliferation [96]. Intracoronary ultrasound studies have shown that intimal proliferation occurs mostly during the first 2 years after transplantation, whereas calcification of plaques occurs later [97, 98]. Because cardiac allografts are functionally denervated, major clinical events including myocardial infarction, congestive heart failure, and sudden death usually occur without prodromal angina. Coronary angiography repeated annually has therefore been recommended to monitor transplant vasculopathy progression [91]. However, due to the diffuse nature of transplant vasculopathy and the concentric pattern of intimal thickening, angiography is normal in most cases despite significant intimal thickening [97, 99, 100].

Intracoronary ultrasound appears to be a safe, sensitive, and reproducible method of measuring both intimal proliferation and plaque composition in heart transplant patients [97, 99, 100]. Due to the limitations of angiography, intravascular ultrasound is frequently used to detect vasculopathy at an early stage of the disease. A typical intravascular image of the distal left anterior descending artery in a patient 1 year after transplantation is shown in Fig. 3. Serial studies can be performed at the time of annual catheterization to determine the progression of intimal thickening. Using planimetry tech-

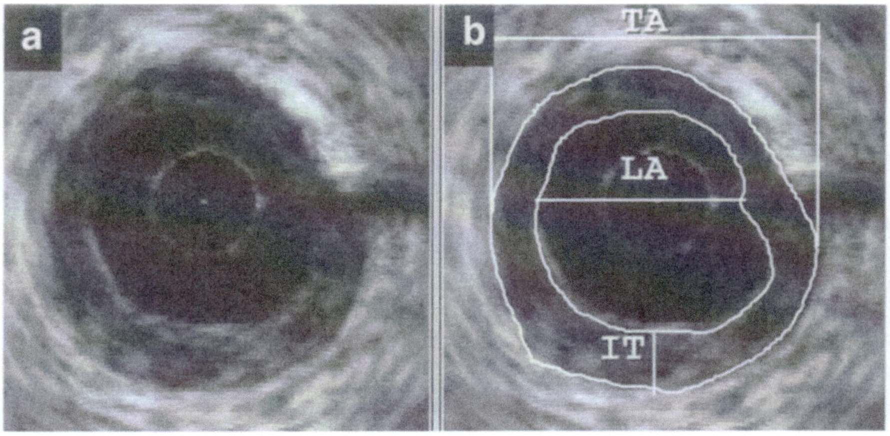

Fig. 3a, b. Intravascular ultrasound image of the distal left anterior descending artery in a patient 1 year after heart transplantation. The angiogram was normal at this site. **a** Intravascular ultrasound imaging shows diffuse intimal thickening. **b** Measurements of total vessel area *(TA)*, initimal thickness *(IT)*, and luminal area *(LA)*

niques and computer software, the intimal thickness and the total vessel and luminal area can be readily measured (Fig. 3) [101]. This approach allows precise monitoring and is essential when studying the early evolution of transplant coronary artery disease and when evaluating possible therapeutic strategies. Use of pravastatin to lower cholesterol levels after cardiac transplantation has shown to be effective in reducing the incidence of coronary vasculopathy as assessed by intracoronary ultrasound measurements [102]. Donor factors may play a role in the etiology of transplant vasculopathy, as highlighted by the correlation of donor age with the disease measured by angiography and intracoronary ultrasound [96, 103]. Identification of factors predisposing to intimal proliferation using intravascular ultrasound has made an important contribution to understanding the pathogenesis of transplant vasculopathy.

In addition to morphologic abnormalities, transplant vasculopathy is associated with changes in vasoreactivity [104–106]. The use of intravascular ultrasound is particularly important, since it can simultaneously study and correlate morphologic and functional vascular changes. It has been shown that endothelial dysfunction precedes intimal thickening and that administration of L-arginine improves the endothelial vasodilator function of coronary conduit if given at an early stage of transplant vasculopathy [105].

Guidance for Intracoronary Interventions

Balloon Angioplasty

Intravascular ultrasound provides the ability to study the relative contributions of different mechanisms of lumen gain during angioplasty, such as plaque compression and tearing, dissection, and stretching of the normal wall [107–109] (Fig. 4). Intravascular ultrasound imaging has now confirmed results of previous pathology studies that demonstrated that the amount of tearing caused by balloon inflation is greater than what can be seen using contrast angiography [32, 110]. In one study, dissections were detected in 50%–70% of patients by ultrasound scanning compared to only 20%–40% by contrast angiography [111]. Depth and extent of dissections after inflation can be detected by intravascular ultrasound in favorable cases; this technique may also identify whether a dissection of only the intimal layers extends into deeper layers.

Besides assessment of dissections *after* angioplasty, intravascular ultrasound has the potential to predict the location of dissection based on pre-interventional plaque characteristics. Two sites in the plaque are predisposed to dissection. First, differences in distensibility are especially high at the edge of an eccentric plaque (between plaque and normal wall segment). At this site, the normal wall is stretched away during inflation and the angulation between the normal wall segment and the plaque creates a dissection plane. Second, the interface between localized calcium deposits surrounding softer tissue is predisposed to tearing during inflation because stress is highest at these points [112]. For detection of localized calcium deposits, ultrasound scanning is far more sensitive than fluoroscopy [78]; in addition, the exact location of the calcium deposits in the plaque can be assessed by intravascular ultrasound, but not fluoroscopy.

Intravascular ultrasound is also able to demonstrate the extent of elastic recoil. Initial data suggest that recoil is greatest in lesions without clear evi-

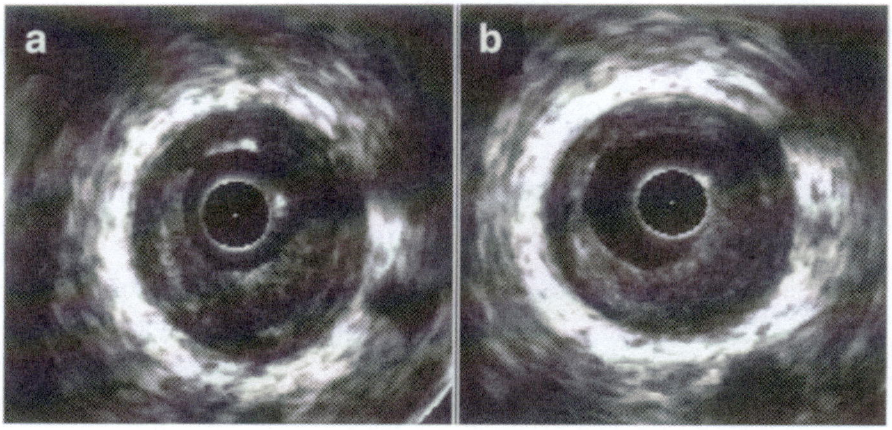

Fig. 4. Before balloon angioplasty, intravascular ultrasound visualizes a noncalcified plaque (lumen area, 2.8 mm^2; plaque area, 12.3 mm^2). After balloon angioplasty, the lumen area has increased to 4.2 mm^2 and the plaque is unchanged (12.0 mm^2). Thus expansion of the vessel was the major mechanism of lumen improvement

dence of tearing [113]. After balloon inflation, the residual lumen of lesions can be precisely identified by ultrasound measurements in order to decide whether additional balloon inflations are required and which balloon size is preferable. As pointed out, previous angiographic comparison with a normal reference segment does not reveal the true potential vessel size; intravascular ultrasound may therefore help to better identify the vessel lumen and the final size of the balloon used.

Recently, combined angioplasty/ultrasound imaging devices have been developed. A design using a multiple element device combined with an angioplasty balloon has been reported [114]. In multicenter experience of a combined device, decisions in approximately one third of all interventions were revised as a result of the information provided by the ultrasound imaging data [115]. Another design has been reported with a mechanical device mounted at same level as the balloon, allowing for simultaneous ultrasound imaging during balloon inflation [116].

Several studies have analyzed whether postangioplasty ultrasound imaging can predict restenosis. In the GUIDE II trial [117], minimal lumen area, plaque area, and percentage plaque area were significantly associated with a lower restenosis rate, whereas all angiographic and clinical parameters were not predictive of restenosis. Similar results concerning the predictive information of postinterventional ultrasound imaging have been reported from the Washington Heart Center [118]. In contrast to these reports, the Post Intra Coronary Treatment Ultrasound Result Evaluation (PICTURE) trial [119] found no association between postangioplasty qualitative or quantitative data derived from ultrasound imaging and the angiographic restenosis rate. In the Serial Ultrasound Analysis of Restenosis (SURE) trial [120], serial ultrasound measurements obtained after balloon angioplasty or directional atherectomy showed that 83 % of late lumen loss is due to remodeling and 17 % due to an increase in plaque area. Interestingly, 63 % of the increase in plaque area occurred in the first 24 h after the procedure. This calls into question the concept of chronic intimal hyperplasia as the main cause for the increase in plaque area.

In summary, the use of ultrasound imaging during balloon angioplasty is limited to assessing the results of the procedure and to using a larger balloon. The approach to upsizing balloons based on ultrasound findings is being tested in another study [121]. In the initial report of this study, the balloon artery ratio increased from 1.03 ± 0.12 to 1.16 ± 0.14 and the lesion lumen area increased from 3.17 ± 1.07 to 4.52 ± 1.0 mm^2 due to balloon upsizing. However, follow-up data are currently not available and it is not clear whether restenosis rates can be reduced using this technique.

Directional Atherectomy

The cross-sectional image produced by intravascular ultrasound directly shows the quadrants of maximal plaque accumulation and has great potential for guiding interventions intended to selectively remove plaque. Intravascular ultrasound therefore seems to be ideal for evaluation of morphology before and after directional coronary atherectomy. Ultrasound scanning can accurately show the depth and location of the atherectomy cuts (Fig. 5). The extent of this injury may be important for the degree of restenosis after interventions. During angiographically guided directional atherectomy,

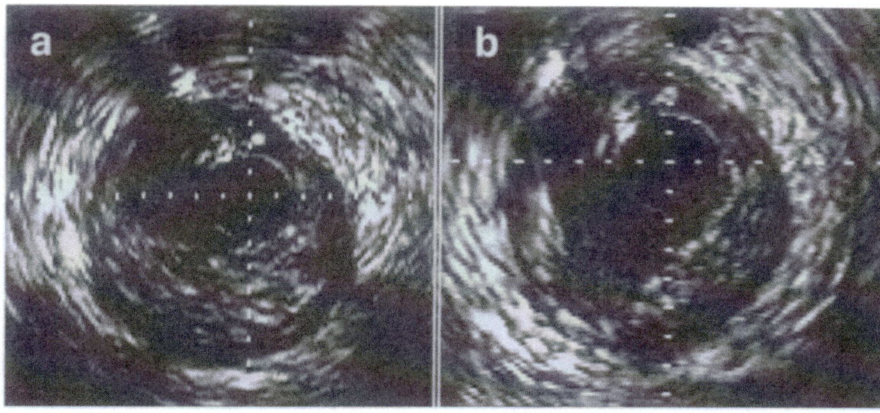

Fig. 5a, b. Intravascular ultrasound imaging before and after directional atherectomy. Eccentric, noncalcified plaque before atherectomy. After atherectomy, the site of the plaque removal (atherectomy cuts) can be demonstrated by intravascular ultrasound. Calibration, 0.5 mm

approximately 50% of interventions show cuts that extend into the media, and one third of the cuts even reach the adventitia. The direction of the atherectomy device in relation to the area of maximal plaque may be clinically important, especially when highly eccentric lesions are treated. Intravascular ultrasound is currently the only technique that can provide rotational orientation. For this purpose, a branch near the target lesion should be identified by ultrasound and the angle to the area of the deepest extent of the plaque measured. The atherectomy device can then be inserted, and by using the branches on angiography as references it can be directed to the maximal plaque accumulation [122]. Baumann et al. [123] introduced this new technique to direct atherectomy cuts by the "reference" cut method.

Calcification of the plaque is among the most important factors determining the success of directional atherectomy. However, conventional contrast angiography is often unable to detect the presence and extent of calcium and provides absolutely no information about the location of calcium in the plaque (deep or superficial). In a study by Fitzgerald et al [124], the effect of directional atherectomy was compared in lesions with no calcium, superficial calcium, and calcium localized deep in the plaque, as assessed by preprocedural intravascular ultrasound imaging. The weight of the tissue retrieved by directional atherectomy was significantly less ($p<0.001$) in lesions with superficial calcium (10.3+5.8 mg) than in lesions with deep calcium (19.7+6.9 mg) or noncalcified lesions (22.5+7.2 mg). Similarly, the vessel lumen after directional atherectomy was smallest in the lesions with superficial calcium [124].

During atherectomy, ultrasound examination may be clinically helpful at different points during the procedure. *Before* the intervention, intravascular ultrasound can be used to confirm the appropriateness of the indication (no or only deep lesion calcium, short length of the stenosis, ideally soft plaques); *between* the atherectomy passes, it can be used to complete plaque removal while avoiding deep cuts in the periadventitial tissue; and *after* atherectomy, it can be used to determine the need for and effect of adjunctive balloon dilatation (used to tack the flaps and smooth irregular wall contours often caused by the atherectomy cuts). The use of intravascular ultrasound during atherectomy frequently results in a more aggressive strategy and leads to a greater extent of plaque removal and a larger minimal lumen diameter, suggesting that ultrasound can overcome some of the limitations of angiographically guided directional atherectomy. The initial results of the Optimal Atherectomy Restenosis Study (OARS) trial [125] confirmed the possibility of achieving an improved immediate result and a high procedural success rate with aggressive ultrasound-guided atherectomy. However, despite these encouraging results, in the first 134 patients evaluated at follow-up the angiographic restenosis rate was approximately 30%, with subsequent target vessel revascularization or major ischemic cardiac events in 20% of patients. More encouraging are the results reported in a smaller, single-center study by Doi et al. [126], showing that in coronary vessels with a reference diameter between 3 and 4 mm the more aggressive approach allowed by direct plaque visualization with intravascular ultrasound leads to a reduction in restenosis rate from 26% (angiographic guidance) to 7% (ultrasound guidance, $p < 0.05$).

Unfortunately, combined ultrasound – atherectomy devices are not yet available for clinical use. Only prototypes have been tested that provide images limited to the quadrants towards which the cutter is oriented [127].

Rotational Atherectomy

Rotational atherectomy is a relatively efficient approach for removing plaque tissue in lesions with superficial calcium. Intravascular ultrasound has demonstrated that, in approximately 75% of patients referred for balloon angioplasty, the target lesions show significant calcification, either deep or superficial in the plaque. In 50% of patients, at least two quadrants of the circumference are covered by calcium [78]. Ultrasound studies have shown that the primary mechanism of lumen enlargement using rotational atherectomy is plaque ablation. Kovach et al. [128] demonstrated a decrease in plaque plus media area (plaque removal), an increase in lumen diameter, no change in external elastic membrane area (no arterial expansion), and a significant decrease in the arc of target lesion calcium. In contrast, adjunctive balloon angioplasty was shown to enlarge the lumen primarily through arterial expansion and not by plaque removal. Typical ultrasound findings after rotational atherectomy included an intimal luminal interface that was distinct and circular and lumen dimensions that were frequently in excess of final bur diameter. Deviations from cylindrical geometry were noted only in areas of calcified plaque manifesting superficial tissue disruption and in areas of soft plaque [78].

In clinical practice intravascular ultrasound may be helpful in the selection of patients for rotational atherectomy. After successful rotational atherectomy, intravascular ultrasound can demonstrate the amount of residual plaque. In our experience, adjunct balloon angioplasty can be performed after rotational atherectomy if intravascular ultrasound has documented major debulking of calcified plaque, indicating lesser likelyhood that a major dissection will occur. A new strategy is to remove calcified plaque by rotational atherectomy prior to stenting ("rota stenting"). Reduction of hard plaque material may result in optimal stent expansion and thus a lower restenosis rate.

Stents

Although previously considered as the gold standard of arterial imaging, angiography does not provide all of the information necessary to completely, accurately, and safely guide stent placement. In general more information about the nature of the underlying lesion is required than angiography can provide. Intravascular ultrasound allows us to better visualize the stent, to determine completeness of expansion, and to see details of stent-vessel wall contact. Furthermore, details of intrastent luminal pathology are required to plan optimal secondary intra- or peristent interventions [128]. Several studies have shown that angiography overestimates the vessel size after stent placement and is incapable of precisely visualizing the details of the stent [129, 130]. However, recent studies showed an improved accuracy of angiography when measurements were performed after using high-pressure implantation technique [131].

Guidance of stent placement is one of the most important applications of intracoronary ultrasound in device assessment. While the metal struts of stents are not usually radiopaque, their echoreflective properties create a distinct appearance on the ultrasound scan; hence the struts can easily be differentiated from the vessel wall. Intravascular ultrasound can therefore be used to recognize suboptimal results after stent placement. Experimental studies with histologic validation have shown that ultrasound measurements of stent dimensions are very accurate. An optimal ratio of stent to vessel size can be obtained with clear and accurate imaging of the location, shape, and degree of arterial pathology [132].

The mechanism of restenosis in stents can also be determined using intravascular ultrasound. The metal struts provide a marker of the original lumen border; thus intimal hyperplasia and mechanical compression of the stent can be differentiated. Based on intravascular ultrasound findings, it seems that the mechanism of restenosis after stent implantation is not chronic mechanical recoil as in other types of interventions, but that intimal hyperplasia or plaque protrusion accounts for lumen reduction within the stent [133, 134].

Intravascular ultrasound can help to identify the morphology and length of dissections. Schrywer et al. [135] reported a case of parallel tract dissection after balloon angioplasty of a restenotic lesion in the right coronary artery. Blessing and colleagues [136] reported a patient with a severe posttraumatic dissection within the left anterior descending artery. The patients subsequently underwent successful stenting of the artery. Furthermore, ultrasound studies have shown that the larger lumen gain with stent implantation in combination with balloon angioplasty as compared to balloon angioplasty alone is probably due to more vessel expansion (and not merely plaque displacement) [137].

Potential uses of intravascular ultrasound imaging prior to stent implantation include accurate measurement of reference vessel dimensions; this may help in appropriate balloon sizing, prevention of overdilatation, and reduction of the number of balloons used. Plaque morphology prior to stenting may also be assessed by intravascular ultrasound. Extensive plaque calcification has been shown to be assodated with less stent expansion, and plaque debulking prior to stenting may be preferred in such cases. Finally, the length of the lesion is often underestimated by angiography and may be more accurately measured by intravascular ultrasound prior to stent deployment. This may result in selection of different stent length.

Assessment of stent placement is currently one of the applications of intravascular ultrasound. Parameters measured by this technique include stent expansion (minimum stent cross-sectional area/average reference cross-sectional area), stent symmetry (ratio of minimum to maximum stent diameter), and strut apposition to the wall (flush axial and radial contact between the stent and vessel wall).

Intravascular ultrasound has been an essential educational tool in the improvement of strategies used for stent deployment. Studies have demonstrated that incomplete apposition of the stent struts (Fig. 6), residual lumen narrowing (Fig. 7), or an irregular eccentric lumen in the stented segment was still present in up to 88% of patients, even though the angiographic result was considered optimal by an experienced operator. This has prompted investigators to develop a more aggressive strategy based on high-pressure balloon dilatation inside the stent [130, 138–140]. Nakamura and colleagues reported their observations from ultrasound imaging during Palmaz-Schatz stent insertion in 63 consecutive patients. Although all patients had a satisfactory angiographic result, 52 patients (80%) showed inadequate stent expansion and required further dilatations. In these 52 patients, the angiographic lesion diameter was 3.12±0.47 mm after the first and 3.61±0.49 mm after final balloon dilatation. The balloon size was 3.7±0.3 mm for the initial and 4.1+0.4 mm for the final dilatations. Inflation pressures were 11.1±1.9 atm during the first and 12.0±2.6 atm during the final dilatations. It was possible to improve stent underexpansion in all cases with repeat balloon dilata-

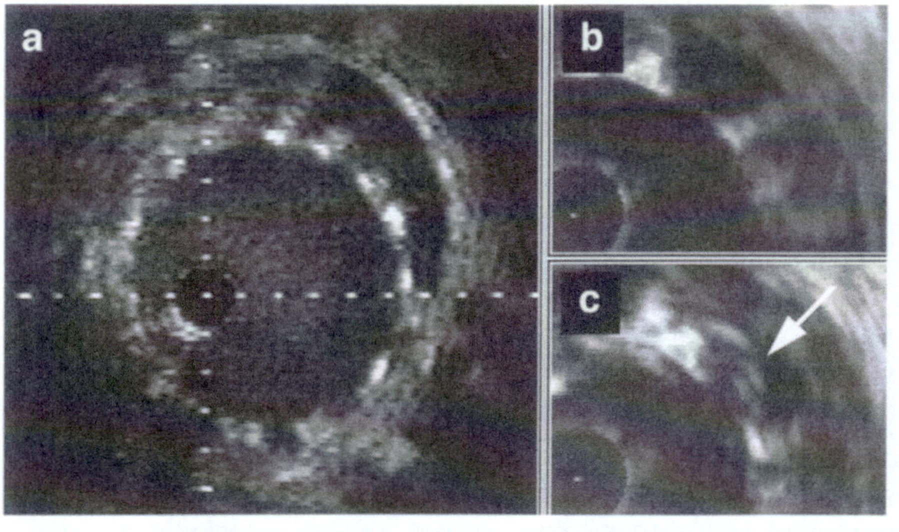

Fig. 6a–c. Intravascular ultrasound imaging after intracoronary stenting. (**a**) Incomplete apposition of the stent struts to the vessel wall (between 12 and 3 o'clock). Calibration, 0.5 mm. (**b**) Detail of an intravascular ultrasound image in another patient with incomplete stent apposition. Same patients as (**c**) After injection of contrast media during intravascular ultrasound imaging, bubbles can be seen between the stent struts and the vessel wall (**arrow**)

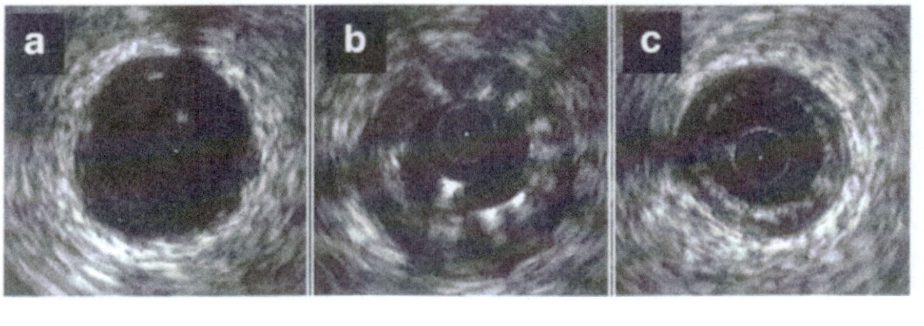

Fig. 7a–c. Intravascular ultrasound imaging after coronary stenting (15-mm Palmaz-Schatz stent) of the left anterior descending coronary artery. To determine the degree of stent expansion, the luminal areas proximal (**a**) and distal (**c**) to the stent are compared with the minimal lumen in the stent (**b**)

tion using larger balloons or higher pressures. Vessel rupture occurred in one patient in whom a balloon was used that was 1.5 mm larger than the distal reference vessel [130]. In the same study, intravascular ultrasound measurements showed that the actual cross-sectional lumen area at the tightest point of the stented segment ranged between 50% and 75% of the expected value (based on balloon size) after the first dilatation and between 61% and 71% after the final dilatation. The minimum lumen diameter within the stented segment was 2.7 ± 0.4 mm after the first dilatation and increased to 3.1 ± 0.5 mm alter the final dilatation. An important manifestation of stent underexpansion was that the lumen cross-sectional area was smaller than the distal reference lumen [130]. Despite angiographically satisfactory results, intravascular ultrasound shows that, in the majority of cases, the stented lumen areas are substantially below the values for the proximal or distal reference segment.

Clinical use of intracoronary stents is impeded by the risk of acute and subacute coronary thrombosis, which occurred in 3%-25% of patients in the era of the non-high-pressure balloon technique. Consequent anticoagulation with heparin, Coumadin (sodium warfarin), and platelet inhibitors was therefore necessary. However, anticoagulation can lead to severe bleeding complications and also significantly prolongs hospital stay. It appears logical that minimizing the exposure of metal struts to the blood by increasing stent expansion may also diminish the risk of thrombosis. Largely due to the pioneering work of Colombo and colleagues, stent thrombosis is now viewed as a mechanical problem that can be prevented by an optimal stent implantation technique eliminating the need for aggressive anticoagulation. Based on their experience, Colombo and coworkers [130, 140] developed criteria for optimal stent placement guided by ultrasound imaging. Using these criteria, the same group [140] studied 191 patients undergoing Palmaz-Schatz stenting in 219 lesions (97% native coronary arteries). The 164 patients with optimal stent placement (according to ultrasound criteria) were subsequently treated only with 250 mg ticlopidine bid for 2 months and aspirin (no heparin or Coumadin). No episodes of acute or subacute stent thrombosis or bleeding complications occurred during a follow-up of 41–153 days.

Whereas Coumadin was considered absolutely mandatory in the era of non-high-pressure balloon technique, antiplatelet therapy now appears to be superior to Coumadin. Schömig and coworkers [141] have shown a benefit of combined antiplatelet therapy with aspirin and ticlopidine compared to conventional anticoagulation therapy (Coumadin) regarding the incidence of cardiac events and hemorrhagic and vascular complications after high-pressure stent implantation. Interestingly, balloons used for implantation were sized by angiographic criteria and intravascular ultrasound was not routinely used by this group [141].

With the use of high-pressure balloon implantation of stents, the incidence of stent thrombosis has been reduced dramatically. In the French registry, the subacute thrombosis rate was 1.6% in 1156 patients using the high-pressure implantation technique without ultrasound control. It is at present unclear whether the use of intravascular ultrasound can further reduce the incidence of subacute thrombosis and randomized trials are not available yet. However, in large series at experienced centers, the thrombosis rate was 0.90% and 0.4% using ultrasound guidance in Milan [140] and Washington [142], respectively. Unfortunately, controlled studies with several thousand patients are needed to prove that intravascular ultrasound guidance can further reduce the rate of subacute thrombosis.

In summary, it is generally accepted that the potential thombogenicity of metallic stents can be substantially diminished by full stent expansion using high pressure and large balloon sizes to optimize in-stent diameter and flow. Clearly, the aggressive use of larger balloons and higher pressure is tempered by the risk of vessel rupture. Randomized studies (e.g., Stent Anticoagulation Regimen Study, STARS) are in progress to determine the value of intravascular ultrasound as an adjunct to stenting and to identify suitable patients for low-intensity anticoagulation regimens.

Optimal ultrasound-guided stent expansion was initially targeted at preventing subacute thrombosis, but this strategy can also help to reduce restenosis. Preliminary studies have shown that intravascular ultrasound-guided stent placement may result in a lower 6-month retenosis rate than the angiographically guided approach (C. Di Mario 1996, personal communication) [143]. A possible explanation for this observation is that ultrasound guidance allows more acute lumen gain than the conventional approach. A randomized trial (Optimization with Intra Coronary Ultrasound to reduce stent stenosis-OPTICUS-trial) will begin enrollment in 1996 to test this hypothesis.

Intravascular ultrasound will likely play an increasingly important role in the development of different prevention strategies for restenosis (e.g., local or systemic pharmacological treatment, radioactivity), since it is capable of performing volumetric plaque measurements inside the stents [143]. A new ultrasound imaging guidewire and three-dimensional online reconstruction may have useful applications in stent implantation in the future [144, 145].

References

1. Yock PG, Johnson EL, Linker DT (1988) Intravascular ultrasound: development and clinical potential. Am J Card Imag 2:185-193
2. Yock PG, Linker DT, Angelsen BAJ (1989) Two-dimensional intravascular ultrasound: technical development and initial clinical experience. J Am Soc Echo 2:296-304
3. Evans JL, Ng KH, Wiet SG, Vonesh MJ, Burns WB, Radvany MG, Kane BJ, Davidson CJ, Roth SI, Kramer BL, Meyers SN, McPherson D (1996) Accurate three-dimensional reconstruction of intravascular ultrasound data. Spatially correct three-dimensional reconstructions. Circulation 93: 567-5
4. Hausmann D, Erbel R, MD, Alibelli-Chemarin MJ et al (1995) The safety of inracoronary ultrasound: multicenter survey of 2207 examinations. Circulation 92: 623-630
5. Pinto FJ, St Goar FG, Gao SZ, Chenzbraun A, Fischell TA, Alderman EL, Schroeder JS, Popp RL (1993) Immediate and one year safety of intracoronary ultrasonic imaging: evaluation with serial quantitative angiography. Circulation 88: 1709-1714
6. Yamada EG, Fitzgerald PJ, Sudhir K, Hargrave VK, Yock PG (1992) Intravascular ultrasound imaging of blood: the effect of hematocrit and flow on backscatter. J Am Soc Echo 5:385-392
7. Fitzgerald PJ, Goar FG, Connolly RJ, Pinto FJ, Billingham ME, Popp RL, Yock PG (1992) Intravascular ultrasound imaging of coronary arteries. Is three layers the norm? Circulation 86:154-158
8. Enos WF, Holmes RH, Beyer J (1996) Coronary disease among united states soldiers killed in action in Korea. Preliminary report. JAMA 256:2859-2862
9. Crawford T, Levene (1953) Medial thinning in atheroma. J Pathol 66:19-23
10. Gussenhoven EJ, Frietman P, The SHK, van Suylen RJ, van Egmond FC, Lancee CT, van Urk H, Roelandt JRTC, Stijnen T, Bom N (1991) Assessment of medial thinning in atherosclerosis by intravascular ultrasound. Am J Cardiol 68: 1625-1632
11. Potkin BN, Bartorelli AL, Gessert JM, Neville RF, Almagor Y, Roberts WC, Leon MB (1990) Coronary artery imaging with intravascular high-frequency ultrasound. Circulation 81: 1575-1585
12. Gussenhoven EJ, Essed CE, Lancee CT, Mastik F, Frietman P, van Egmond FC, Reiber J, Bosch H, van Urk H, Roelandt J, Bom N (1989) Arterial wall characteristics determined by intravascular ultrasound imaging: an in vitro study. J Am Coll Cardiol 14: 947-952
13. Giro EK, Cuenoud HF (1995) Intravascular ultrasound detection of lipid & pools in human coronary arteries. Circulation 92 [Suppl I]: I649
14. Pandian NG, Kreis A, Brockway B (1990) Detection of intraarterial thrombus by intravascular high frequency two-dimensional ultrasound imaging in vitro and in vivo studies. Am J Cardiol 65: 1280-1283
15. Kimura BJ, Russo RJ, Bhargava V, McDaniel M, Peterson KL, DeMaria AN (1996) Atheroma morphology and distribution in proximal left anterior descending coronary artery: in vivo observations. J Am Coll Cardiol 27: 825-831
16. Fitzgerald PJ, Connolly AJ, Watkins RD et al (1991) Distinction between soft plaque and thrombus by intravascular tissue characterization . J Am Coll Cardiol 17: 111A (abstr)
17. Hodgson JM, Graham SP, Savakus AD, Dame SG, Stephens DN, Dhillon PS, Brands D, Sheehan H, Eberle MJ (1989) Clinical percutaneous imaging of coronary anatomy using an over-the-wire ultrasound catheter system. Int J Card Imag 4: 187-193
18. Pandian NG, Kreis A, Brockway B, Isner JM, Sacharoff A, Boleza E, Caro R, Muller D (1988) Ultrasound angioscopy: real-time, two-dimensional, intraluminal ultrasound imaging of blood vessels. Am J Cardiol 62: 493-494
19. Hausmann D, Lundkvist AJS, Friedrich G, Sudhir K, Fitzgerald PJ, Yock PG (1996) Automated border detection during intravascular ultrasound imaging. Echocardiography (in press)
20. Hausmann D, Johnson JA, Sudhir K, MD, Mullen WL, Friedrich G, Fitzgerald PJ, Ports TA, Kane JP, Malloy MJ, Paul G, Yock PG (1996) Angiographically silent atherosclerosis detected by intravascular ultrasound in patients with familial hypercholesterolemia and familial combined hyperlipidemia: correlation with high-density lipoproteins. J Am Coll Cardiol (in press)
21. DiMario C, Madretsma S, Linker D, The SHK, Bom N, Serruys PW, Gussenhoven EJ, Roelandt JR (1993) The angle of incidence of the ultrasonic beam: a critical factor for the image quality in intravascular ultrasonography. Am Heart J 125: 442-448
22. Hausmann D, Sudhir K, Mullen WL, Fitzgerald PJ, Ports TA, Daniel WG, Yock PG (1994) Contrast-enhanced intravascular ultrasound: validation of a new technique for delineation of the vessel wall surface. J Am Coll Cardiol 23: 981-987
23. Hausmann D, Mügge A, Sturm M, Blessing E, Riedel M, Amende I, Lichtlen PR (1996) Intrakoronarer Ultraschall: Diagnostischer Gewinn durch Applikation von Kontrastmitteln? Z Kardiol [Suppl] 2: 267
24. Hausmann D, Lundkvist AJS, Friedrich GJ, Mullen WL, Fitzgerald PJ, Yock PG (1994) Intracoronary ultrasound imaging: intra-and interobserver variability of morphometric measurements. Am Heart J 128: 674-680.
25. Blessing E, Hausmann D, Sturm M, Mügge A, Amende I, Lichtlen PR (1996) Intravaskulärer Ultraschall bei Stent-Implantation: Intra- und Interobservervariabilität der Messungen. Z Kardiol [Suppl] 2: 137
26. Reiber JHC, Serruys PW, Kooijman CJ et al (1985) Assessment of short-, medium-, and long-term variations in arterial dimensions from computer-assisted quantitation of coronary angiograms. Circulation 71: 280-299
27. Mancini GBJ, Simon SB, McGillem MJ, LeFree MT, Friedman HZ, Vogel RA (1987) Automated quantitative coronary arteriography: morphologic and physiologic validation in vivo of a rapid digital angiographic method. Circulation 75: 452-460

28. Arnett EN, Isner JM, Redwood DR, Kent KM, Baker WP, Ackerstein H et al (1979) Coronary artery narrowing in coronary heart disease: comparison of cineangiographic and necropsy findings. Ann Intern 91: 350-356
29. Glagov S, Weisenberg E, Zarins GK, Stankunavicius R, Kolettis GJ (1987) Compensatory enlargement of human atherosclerotic coronary arteries. N Engl J Med 316: 1371-1375
30. Stiel GM, Stiel LSG, Schofer J, Donath K, Mathey DG (1989) Impact of compensatory enlargement of atherozsclerotic coronary arteries on angiographic assessment of coronary artery diseases. Circulation 80: 1603-1609.
31. McPherson DD, Sirna SJ, Hiratzka LF, Thorpe L, Armstrong ML, Marcus ML et al (1991) Coronary arterial remodeling studied by high-frequency epicardial echocardiography: an early compensatory mechanism in patients with obstructive coronary atherosclerosis. J Am Coll Cardiol 17: 79-86
32. Tobis JM, Mallery J, Gessert J, Griffith J, Mahon D, Bessen M et al (1989) Intravascular ultrasound cros-sectional arterial imaging before and after balloon angioplasty in vitro. Circulation 80: 873-882
33. Nissen SE, Gurley JC, Grines CL, Booth DC, McClure R, Berk M et al (1991) Intravascular ultrasound assessment of lumen size and wall morphology in normal subjects and patients with coronary artery disease. Circulation 84: 1087-1099
34. Hodgson J, Reddy D, Suneja R, Nair R, Lesnefsky E, Sheehan H (1993) Intracoronary ultrasound imaging: correlation of plaque morphology with angiography, clinical syndrome and procedural results in patients undergoing coronary angioplasty. J Am Coll Cardiol 21: 35-44
35. Vlodaaver Z, Frech R, van Tassel RA, Edwards JE (1973) Correlation of the antemortem coronary angiogram and post mortem speciem. Circulation 47: 162-168
36. Nishimura RA, Edwards WD, Warnes CA, Reeder GS, Holmes DR, Tajik AJ et al (1990) Intravascular ultrasound imaging: in vitro validation and pathologic correlation. J Am Coll Cardiol 16: 145-154
37. DiMario C, The S, Madretsma S, von Suylen R, Wilson R, Bom N et al (1992) Detection and characterization of vascular lesions by intravascular ultrasound: an in vivo study correlated with histology. J Am Soc Echocardiogr 5: 135-146
38. Hodgson JMB, Graham SP, Sheehan H (1991) Percutaneous intravascular ultrasound imaging: validation of a real time synthetic aperture array catheter. Am J Card Imaging 5: 65-71
39. Mintz GS, Popma JJ, Pichard AD, Kent KM, Satler LF, Chuang YC, Ditrano CJ, Leon MB (1995) Patterns of calcification in coronary artery disease. A statistical analysis of intravascular ultrasound and coronary angiography in 1155 lesions. Circulation 91: 1959-1965
40. St. Goar F, Pinto F, Alderman E, Fitzgerald P, Stadius M, Popp R (1991) Intravascular ultrasound imaging of angiographically normal coronary arteries: an in vivo comparison with quantitative angiography. J Am Coll Cardiol 18: 952-958
41. Werner GS, Sold G, Buchwald A, Kreuzer H, Wiegand V (1991) Intravascular ultrasound imaging of human coronary arteries after percutaneous transluminal angioplasty: morphologic and quantitative assessment. Am Heart J 122: 212-220
42. De Scheerder I, De Man F, Herregods MC, Wilczek K, Barrios L, Raymenants E et al (1994) Intravascular ultrasound versus angiography for measurements of luminal dimensions in normal and diseased coronary arteries. Am Heart J 127: 243-251
43. Porter TR, Sears T, Xie F, Michels A, Mata J, Welsh D et al (1993) Intravascular study of angiographically mildly diseased coronary arteries. J Am Coll Cardiol 22: 1858-1865
44. Mintz GS, Pichard AD, Kovach JA, Kent KM, Sader LF, Javier SP et al (1994) Impact of preintervention intravascular ultrasound imaging on transcatheter strategies in coronary artery disease. Am J Cardiol 73: 423-430
45. Davidson CJ, Sheikh KH, Kisslo KB, Phillips HR, Peter RH, Behar VS, et al (1991) Intravascular ultrasound evaluation of interventional technologies. Am J Cardiol 68: 1305-1308
46. Haase J, Ozaki Y, DiMario C, Escaned J, de Feyter PJ, Roelandt JR, Serruys PW (1995) Can intracoronary ultrasound correctly asses the luminal dimensions of coronary artery lesions? A comparison with quantitative angiography. Eur Heart J 16: 112-119
47. Mintz GS, Potkin BN, Keren G, Satler LF, Pichard AD, Kent KM et al (1992) Intravascular ultrasound evaluation of the effect of rotational atherectomy in obstructive atherosclerotic coronary artery disease. Circulation 86: 1383-1393
48. Laskey WK, Brady ST, Kussmaul WG, Waxler AR, Krol J, Hermann HC et al (1993) Intravascular ultrasound assessment of the results of coronary stenting. Am Heart J 125: 1576-1583
49. DeFranco A, Tuzcu EM, Moliterno DJ, Elliott J, Berkalp B, Franco I et al (1994) Overestimation of lumen size alter coronary interventions: implications for randomized trails of new devices. Circulation 90 [Suppl 4, 2]: 2960
50. Tobis JM, Mallery J, Mahon D et al Intravascular ultrasound imaging of human coronary arteries in vivo. Circulation 83: 913-926
51. Baptista J, DiMario C, Escaned J, Arnese M, Ozaki Y, de Feyter P, Roelandt JR, Serruys PW (1995) Intracoronary two-dimensional ultrasound imaging in the assessment of plaque morphologic features and the planning of coronary interventions. Am Heart J 129: 177-187
52. Zarins CK, Weisenberg E, Kolettis G, Stankunavicius R, Glagov S (1988) Differential enlargement of artery segments in response to enlarging atherosclerotic plaques. J Vasc Surg 7: 386-394
53. Ge J, Erbel R, Zamorano J, Koch L, Kearney P, Görge G et al (1993) Coronary artery remodeling in atherosclerotic disease: an intravascular ultrasonic study in vivo. Coron Art Dis 4: 981-986
54. Hermiller JB, Tenaglia AN, Kisslo KB, Phillips HR, Bashore TM, Stack RS, Davidson CJ 1993) In vivo validation of compensatory enlargement of atherosclerotic coronary arteries. Am J Cardiol 71: 665-668
55. Gerber TC, Erbel R, Görge G, Ge J, Rupprecht HJ, Meyer J (1994) Extent of atherosclerosis and remodeling of the left main coronary artery determined by intravascular ultrasound. Am J Gardiol 73: 666-671
56. Losordo DW, Rosenfield K, Kaufman J, Pieczek A, Isner JM (1994) Focal compensatory enlargement of human arteries in response to progressive atherosclerosis in

vivo documentation using intravascular ultrasound. Circulation 89: 2570 - 2577
57. Mintz GS, Bonner RF, Bouek PC, Kent KM, Pichard AD, Salter LF, Leon MB (1993) Lesion composition determines compensatory vessel responses and plaque accumulation in native coronary artery stenoses: an intravascular study. J Am Coll Cardiol 326 A (abstr)
58. Nishioka T, Luo H, Berglund H, Eigler NL, Kim CJ, Tabak SW, Siegel RJ (1996) Absence of focal compensatory enlargement or constriction in diseased human coronary saphenous vein bypass grafts. Circulation 93: 683 - 690
59. Hausmann D, Mullen WL, Friedrich GJ, Fitzgerald PJ, Yock PG (1994) Variability of remodeling in early coronary atherosclerosis: an intravascular ultrasound study. J Am Coll Cardiol 1A - 484A. 175A
60. Pasterkamp G, Wensing PJW, Post MJ, Hillen B, Mali WPTM, Borst (1995) Paradoxial arterial wall shrinkage may contribute to luminal narrowing of human atherosclerotic femoral arteries. Circulation 91: 1444 - 1449
61. Mintz GS, Painter JA, Pichard AD, Kent MK, Saftler LF, Popma JJ, Chuang C, Buchner TA, Sokolowicz LE, Leon MB (1995) Atherosclerosis in angiographically normal coronary artery reference segments: an intravascular ultrasound study with clinical correlations. J Am Coll Cardiol 25: 1479 - 1485
62. Ge J, Erbel R, Gerber T, Görge G, Koch L, Haude M, Meyer J (1994) Intravascular ultrasound imaging of angiographically normal coronary arteries: a prospective study in vivo. Br Heart J 71(6): 572 - 578
63. Hausmann D, Mügge A, Blessing E, Sturm M, Wolpers HG, Amende I (1996) Angiographic silent plaque in the left main coronary artery. Int J Cardiac Imaging (in press)
64. Murray CD (1962) The physiological principle of minimum work. I. The vascular system and the cost of blood volume. Proc Nate Acad Sci USA 12: 207 - 214
65. Alfonso F, Macaya C, Goicolea J, Hernandez R, Segovia J, Zamorano J, Banuelos C, Zarco P (1993) Angiographic changes induced by intracoronary ultrasound imaging before and after coronary angioplasty. Am Heart J 125: 877 - 880
66. White CJ, Ramee SR, Collins TJ, Jain A, Mesa JE (1992) Ambiguous coronary angiography: clinical utility of intravascular ultrasound. Cathet Cardiovasc Diagn 26: 200 - 203
67. Fitzgerald PJ, Yock, PG (1993) Mechanisms and outcomes of angioplasty and atherectomy assessed by intravascular ultrasound imaging. J Clin Ultrasound 21: 579 - 588
68. McPherson DD, Hiratzka LF, Lamberth WC, Brandt B, Hunt M, Kieso RA, Marcus ML, Kerber RE (1987) Delineation of the extent of coronary atherosclerosis by high - frequency epicardial echocardiography. N Engl J Med 316: 304 - 309
69. Lee DY, Eigler N, Nishioka T, Tabak SW, Forrester JS, Siegel RJ (1995) Effect of intracoronary imaging on clinical decision making. Am Heart J 129: 1084 - 1093
70. Fuster V, Badimon L, Badimon JJ, Chesebro JH (1992) The pathogenesis of coronary artery disease and the acute coronary syndromes. N Engl J Med 326: 1371 - 1375
71. Davies MJ, Richardson PD, Woolf N, Katz DR, Maas J (1993) Risk of thrombosis in human atherosclerotic plaques: role of extracellular lipid, macrophage, and smooth muscle cell content. Br Heart J 69: 377 - 381
72. Davies MJ, Thomas AC (1985) Plaque fissuring the cause of acute myocardial infarction, sudden ischemic death and crescendo angina. 2Br Heart J 53: 363 - 373
73. Richardson P, Davies M, Born G (1989) influence of plaque configuration and stress distribution on fissuring of coronary atherosclerotic plaques. Lancet 2: 941 - 944
74. Zamorano J, Erbel R, Ge J, Görge G, Kearney P, Koch L et al (1994) Spontaneous plaque rupture visualized by intravascular ultrasound. EurHeart J 15: 131 - 133
75. Loree HM, Kamm RD, Stringfellow RG, Lee RT (1992) Effects of fibrous cap thickness on peak circumferential stress in a model atherosclerotic vessels. Circ Res 71: 850 - 858
76. Kimura BJ, Bhargava V, DeMaria AN (1995) Value and limitations of intravascular ultrasound imaging in characterizing coronary atherosclerotic plaque. Am Heart J 130: 386 - 396
77. de Feyter PJ, Ozaki Y, Baptista J, Escaned J, Di Mario C, de Jaegere PT, Serruys PW, Roelandt JR (1995) Ischemia-related lesion characteristics in patients with stable or unstable angina. A study with intracoronary angioscopy and ultrasound. Circulation 92: 1408 - 1412
78. Mintz GS, Douek P, Pichard A, Kent K, Satler L, Popma J, Leon M (1992) Target lesions calcification in coronary artery disease: an intravascular ultrasound study. J Am Coll Cardiol 20: 1149 - 1155
79. Chemarin-Alibelli MJ, Pieraggi MT, Elbaz M, Carrie D, Fourcade J, Puel J, Tobis JM (1996) Identification of coronary thrombus after myocardial infarction by intracoronary ultrasound compared with histology of tissue sampled by atherectomy. Am J Cardiol 77: 344 - 349
80. Frimerman A, Miller HI, Hallman M, Laniado S, Keren G (1994) Intravascular ultrasound characterization of thrombi of different composition. Am J Cardiol 73: 1053 - 1057
81. Blankenhorn DH, Kramsch DM (1989) Reversal of atherosis and sclerosis. The two components of atherosclerosis. Circulation 79: 1 - 7
82. Brown G, Albers JJ, Fisher LD, Schaefer SM, Lin JT, Kaplan C, Zhao XQ, Bisson BD, Fitzpatrick VF, Dodge HT (1990) Regression of coronary artery disease as a result of intensive lipid - lowering therapy in men with high levels of apolipoprotein B. N Engl J Med 323: 1289 - 1298
83. Cashin - Hemphill L, Mack WJ, Pogoda JM, Sanmarco ME, Azen SP, Blankenhorn DH (1990) Beneficial effects of colestipol-niacin on coronary atherosclerosis. A 4-year follow-up. JAMA 264: 3013 - 3017
84. Kane JP, Malloy MJ, Ports TA, Phillips NR, Diehl JC, Havel RJ (1990) Regression of coronary atherosclerosis during treatment of familial hypercholesterolemia with combined drug regimens. JAMA 264: 3007 - 3012
85. Lichtlen PR, Hugenholtz PG, Rafflenbeul W, Hecker H, Jost S, Deckers JW (1990) Retardation of angiographic progression of coronary artery disease by nifedipine. Lancet 335: 1109 - 1113
86. Ornish D, Brown SE, Scherwitz LW, Billings JH, Armstrong WT, Ports TA, McLanahan SM, Gould KL (1990) Can lifestyle changes reverse coronary heart disease? Lancet 336: 129 - 133
87. Gupta M, Connolly AJ, Zhu BQ, Sievers RE, Sudhir K, Sun YP, Parmley WW, Fitzgerald PJ, Yock PG (1992)

Quantitative analysis of progression of atherosclerosis by intravascular ultrasound: validation in a rabbit model. Circulation 86 [Suppl I]: I-518 (abstract)
88. Matar FA, Mintz GS, Douek PC, Leon MB, Popma JJ (1992) Three-dimensional intravascular ultrasound: a new standard for vessel lumen volume measurements? J Am Coll Cardiol 19: 382 (abstr)
89. Roelandt JR, di Mario C, Pandian NG, Li W, Keane D, Slager CJ, de Feyter P, Serruys PW (1994) Three-dimensional reconstruction of intracoronary ultrasound images. Rationale, approaches, problems, and directions. Circulation 90: 1044-1055
90. von Birgelen C, Erbel R, di Mario C, Li W, Prati F, Ge J, Bruining N, Gorge G, Slager CJ, Serruys PW (1995) Three-dimensional reconstruction of coronary arteries with intravascular ultrasound. Herz 20(49): 277-289
91. Gao SZ, Alderman EL, Schroeder JS, Silverman JF, Hunt SA (1988) Accelerated coronary vascular disease in the heart transplant patient: coronary arteriographic findings. J Am Coll Cardiol 12: 334-340
92. Schroeder JS, Gao SZ, Hunt SA, Stinson EB (1992) Accelerated graft coronary artery disease: diagnosis and prevention. J Heart Lung Transplant 11: 258-266
93. Miller LW (1995) Role of intracoronary ultrasound for the diagnosis of cardiac allograft vasculopathy. Transplant Proc 27 (3): 1989-1992
94. Uretsky BF, Murali S, Reddy PS et al (1987) Development of coronary artery disease in cardiac transplant patients receiving immunosuppressive therapy with cyclosporine and prednisone. Circulation 76: 827-834
95. O'Neill BJ, Pfugfelder PW, Singh NR, Menkis AH, McKenzie FN, Kostuk WJ (1989) Frequency of angiographic detection and quantitative assessment of coronary arterial disease one and three years after cardiac transplantation. Am J Cardio 63: 1221-1226
96. Deng MC, Bell S, Huie P, Pinto F, Hunt SA, Stinson EB, Sibley R, Hall BM, Valantine HA (1995) Cardiac allograft vascular disease. Relationship to microvascular cell surface markers and inflammatory cell phenotypes on endomyocardial biopsy. Circulation 91: 1647-1654
97. Rickenbacher PR, Pinto FJ, Chenzbraun A, Botas J, Lewis NP, Alderman EL, Valantine HA, hunt SA, Schroeder JS, Popp RL, Yeung AC (1995) Incidence and severity of transplant coronary artery disease early and up to 15 years alter transplantation as detected by intravascular ultrasound. J Am Coll Cardiol 25: 171-177
98. Chenzbraun A, Pinto FJ, Alderman EL, Botas J, Qesterle SN, Schroeder JS, Valatine HA, Popp RL (1995) Distribution and morphologic features of coronary artery disease in cardiac allografts: an intracoronary ultrasound study. J Am Soc Echocardiogr 8: 1-8
99. St Goar F, Pinto F, Alderman E, Valantine HA, Schroeder JS, Gao ZS, Stinson EB, Popp RL (1992) Intracoronary ultrasound in cardiac transplant recipients: in vivo evidence of "angiographically silent" intimal thickening. Circulation 85: 979-987
100. Ventura HO, Ramee SR, Ashit J, White CL, Collins TJ, Mesa JE, Murgo JP (1992) Coronary artery imagin with intravascular ultrasound in patients following cardiac transplantation. Transplantation. Transplantation 53: 216-219
101. Pinto FJ, Chenzbraun A, Botas J, Valantine HA, St Goar FG, Alderman EL,Oesterle SN, Schroeder JS, Popp RL (1994) Feasibility of serial intracoronary ultrasound imaging for assessment of progression of intimal proliferation in cardiac transplant recipients. Circulation 90 (5): 2348-2355
102. Kobashigawa JA, Katznelson S, Laks H, Johnson JA, Yeatman L, Wang XM, Chia D, Terasaki PI, Sabad A, Cogert GA (1995) Effect of pravastatin on outcomes after cardiac transplantation. N Engl J Med 333 (10): 621-627
103. Botas J, Pinto FJ, Chenzbraun A, St Goar FG, Fischell TA, Alderman EL, Schroeder JS, Valantine HA, Popp RL, Yeung AC (1995) The influence of preexistent donor coronary artery disease on the progression of transplant vasculopathy: an intravascular ultrasound study. Circulation 92 (5): 1126-1132
104. Hausmann D, Mügge A, Fitzgerald PJ, Yock PG, Daniel WG (1993) Nitroglycerin-induced coronary vasodilatation in heart transplant patients is impaired by intimal thickening. J Am Coll Cardiol 21: 334 A (abstr)
105. Drexler H, Fischell TA, Pinto FJ, Chenzbraun A, Botas J, Cooke JP, Alderman EL (1994) Effect of L-Arginine on coronary endothial function in cardiac transplant recipients. Relation to vessel wall morphology. Circulation 89: 1615-1623
106. Heroux AL, Silverman P, Costanzo MR, O'Sullivan J, Johnson MR, Liao Y, McKiernan TL, Balhan JE, Leya FS, Mullen M, Kao WG, Johnson SA (1994) Intracoronary ultrasound assessment of morphological and functional abnormalities associated with cardiac allograft vasculopathy. Circulation 89: 272-277
107. Tenaglia AN, Buller CE, Kisslo KB, Stack RS, Davidson CJ (1992) Mechanisms of balloon angioplasty and directional coronary atherectomy as assessed by intracoronary ultrasound. J Am Coll Cardiol 20: 685-691
108. Potkin BN, Keren G, Mintz GS, Duek PC, Pichard AD, Satler LF, Kent KM, Leon M (1992) Arterial responses to balloon coronary angioplasty: an intravascular ultrasound study. J Am Coll Cardiol 20: 942-951
109. Losordo DW, Rosenfield K, Pieczek A, Baker K, Harding M, Isner JM (1992) How does angioplasty work? Serial analysis of human iliac arteries using intravascular ultrasound. Circulation 86: 1845-1858
110. Honye J, Mahon DJ, Jain A, White CJ, Ramee SR, Wallis JB, Al-Zarka A, Tobis JM (1992) Morphological effects of coronary balloon angioplasty in vivo assessed by intravascular ultrasound imaging. Circulation 85: 1012-1025
111. The GUIDE Trail Investigators (1993) Discrepancies between angiographic and intravascular ultrasound appearance of coronary lesions undergoing intervention. A report of phase I of the GUIDE-trail. J Am Coll Cardiol 21: 118A (abstr)
112. Fitzgerald PJ, Ports TA, Yock PG (1992) Contribution of localized calcium deposits to dissection after angioplasty: an observational study using intravascular ultrasound. Circulation 86: 64-70
113. The GUIDE Trail Investigators (1992) Lumen enlargement following angioplasty is related to plaque characteristics. A report from the GUIDE Trial. Circulation 86 [Suppl I] (abstr)
114. Hodgson JM, Cacchione JG, Berry J et al (1990) Combined intracoronary ultrasound imaging and angioplasty catheter: initial in-vivo studies. Circulation 82 [Suppl III] (abstr)
115. Caccione JG, Reddy K, Richards F, Sheehan H, Hod-

gson JM (1991) Combined intravascular ultrasound/angioplasty balloon catheter: initial use during PTCA. Cathet Cardiovasc Diagn 24: 99-101
116. Isner JM, Rosenfield K, Losordo DW, Rose L, Langevin RE, Razvi S, Kosowsky BD (1990) Combination balloon-ultrasound imaging catheter for percutaneous transluminal angioplasty. Validation of imaging, analysis of recoil, and identification of plaque fracture. Circulation 84: 739-754
117. The GUIDE Trial Investigators (1994) IVUS-determined predictors of restenosis in PTCA and DCA: an interim report from the GUIDE trial, phase II. Circulation 90 [Suppl I] : I-113 (abstr)
118. Mintz GS, Chuang YC, Popma J, Pichard A, Kent KM, Satler L, Bucher T,Griffing J, Leon M (1995) The final % cross-sectional narrowing (residual plaque burden) is the strongest intravascular ultrasound predictor of angiographic restenosis. J Am Coll Cardiol [Suppl] 35 A (abstr)
119. Peters, PICTURE study group (1995) Prediction of the risk of angiographic restenosis by intracoronary ultrasound imaging alter coronary balloon angioplasty. J Am Coll Cardiol [Suppl] 35 A (abstr)
120. Kimura T, Kaburagi S, Tashima Y, Mobuyoshi M, Mintz GS, Popma J (1994) Geometric remodeling and intimal regrowth as mechanisms of restenosis: observation from the serial Ultrasound Analysis of Restenosis (SURE) Trial. J Am Coll Cardiol 92 [Suppl I] : 365 (abstr)
121. Stone GW, Linnemeier T, Goar F, Mudra H, Sheehan H, Hodgson J (1996) Improved outcome of balloon angioplasty with intracoronary ultrasound guidance-core lab angiographic and ultrasound results from the CLOUT study. J Am Coll Cardiol 27 [Suppl II] : 155A (abstr)
122. Kimura BFJ, Fitzgerald PJ, Sudhir K, Amidon TM, Strunk BL, Yock PG (1992) Guidance of directed coronary atherectomy by intracoronary ultrasound imaging. Am Heart J 124: 1365-1369
123. Baumann RP, Yock PG, Fitzgerald et al (1995) "Reference cut" method of intracoronary ultrasound guided directional coronary atherectomy: intial and six month results. Circulation 92 [Suppl I]: I-546.
124. Fitzgerald PJ, Mühlberger VA, Moes NY et al (1992) Calcium location within plaque as a predictor of atherectomy tissue retrieval: an intravascular ultrasound study. Circulation 86 [Suppl I]: I-516 (abstr)
125. Simonton CA, Leon MB, Kuntz RE, Popma JJ, Hinohara T, Bersin RM, Yock PG, Wilson H, Cutlip DE, Baim DS (1995) Acute and late clinical and angiographic results of directional atherectomy in the Optimal Atherectomy Restenosis Study (OARS). Circulation 92: I-545
126. Doi T, Tamai H, Ueda K, Hsu YS, Ono S, Kosuga K, Tanaka S, Wang M, j Motohara S, Uehata H (1995) Impact of intracoronary ultrasound-guided directional atherectomy on restenosis. Circulation 92: I-545.
127. Fitzgerald PJ, Belef M, Connolly AJ et al (1995) Design and initial testing of an ultrasound-guided directional atherectomy device. Am Heart J 129: 593-598
128. Kovach JA, Mintz GS, Pichard AD, Kent KM, Popma JJ, Satler LF, Leon MB (1993) Sequential intravascular ultrasound characterization of the mechanisms of rotational atherectomy and adjunct balloon angioplasty. J Am Coll Cardiol 22: 1024-1032
129. Mudra H, Klauss V, Blasini R et al (1994) Ultrasound guidance of Palmaz-Schatz intracoronary stenting with a combined intravascular ultrasound balloon catheter. Circulation 90: 1252-1261
130. Nakamura S, Colombo A, Gaglione A, Almagor Y, Goldberg SL, Maiello L, Finci L, Tobis JM (1994) Intracoronary ultrasound observations during stent implantation. Circulatio 89: 2026-2034
131. Blasini R, Schuhlen H, Mudra H, Walter H, Paloncy R, Schalkhausser F, Zitzmann E, Hartmann F (1995) Angiographic overestimation of lumen size after coronary stent placement: impact of high pressure dilatation. Circulation 92 [Suppl I): I-223 (abstr)
132. Cavaye DM, Tabbara MR, Kopchok GE, Termin P, White RA (1991) Intraluminal ultrasound assessment of vascular stent deployment. Ann Vasc Surg 5: 241-246
133. Painter JA, Mintz GS, Wong SC, Popma JJ, Pichard AD, Kent KM, Satler LF, Leon MB (1995) Serial intravascular ultrasound studies fall to show evidence of chronic Palmaz-Schatz stent recoil. Am J Cardiol 75: 398-400
134. Dussaillant GR, Mintz GS, Pichard AD, Kent KM, Satler LF, Popma JJ, Wong SC, Leon MB (1995) Small stent size and intimal hyperplasia contribute to restenosis: a volumetric intravascular ultrasound analysis. J Am Coll Cardiol 26: 720-724
135. Schryver TE, Popma JJ, Kent KM, Leon MB, Eldredge S, Mintz GS (1992) Use of intracoronary ultrasound to identify the true coronary lumen in chronic coronary dissection treated with intracoronary stenting. Am J Cardiol 69: 1107-1108
136. Blessing E, Wolpers HG, Hausmann D, Mügge A, Amende I Posttraumatic myocardial infarction with severe coronary intimal dissection documented by intravascular ultrasound. J Am S Echo (in press)
137. Burckhard-Meier C, Albrecht D, Kaspers S, Füssl R, Sechtem U, Höpp HW, Erdmann E (1994) Mechanismen der Lumenzunahme bei PTCA und Stent-Implantation: Vergleichende Untersuchung mit intrakoronarem Ultraschall. Z Kardiol 83 [Suppl I]: 139A (abstr)
138. Goldberg SL, Colombo A, Nakamura S et al (1994) Benefit of intracoronary ultrasound in the deployment of Palmaz-Schatz stents. J Am Coll Cardiol 24: 996-1003
139. Serruys PW on behalf of the Benestent Study Group (1995) Benestent II Pilot Study: 6 months follow-up phase 1, 2 and 3. Circulation 92 [Suppl I]: I-2589 (abstract)
140. Colombo A, Hall P, Nakamura S et al (1995) Intracoronary stenting without anticoagulation accomplished with intravascular ultrasound guidance. Circulation 91: 1676-1688.
141. Schömig A, Neumann FJ, Kastrati A, Schühlen H, Blasini R, Hadamitzky M, Walter H, Zitzmann-Roth E-M, Richardt G, Alt E, Schmitt C, Ulm K (1996) A randomized comparison of antiplatelet and anticoagulation therapy after the placement of coronary-artery stents. N Engl J Med 334: 1084-1089
142. Wong SC, Hong MK, Chuang YC, Satler LF, Kent KM, Pichard AD, Donovan KM, Morgan KM, Deforty D, Hunn D, Buicher TA, Leon MB (1995) The anti-platelet treatment after intravascular ultrasound guided optimal stent expansion (APLAUSE) trial. Circulation 92 [Suppl I]: I-795 (abstr)
143. Blasini R, Zitzmann E, Schalkhausser F, Paloncy R, Bökenkamp J, Walter H, Hadamitzky M, Neumann FJ, Richardt G, Schmitt C, Alt E, Schömig A (1996) Bedeu-

tung einer IVUS-gesteuerten Optimierung koronarer Palmaz-Schatz Stent Implantation auf den klinischen und angiographischen Langzeitverlauf. Z Kardiol 85 [Suppl II]: 476 (abstr)
144. Von Birgelen C, Di Mario C, Li W, Slager CJ, de Feyter PJ, Roelandt JRTC, Serruys PW (1995) Volumetric quantification by intracoronary ultrasound. In: De Feyter PJ, Di Mario C, Serruys PW (eds) Quantitative coronary imagin. Barjesteh and Meeuwes, Delft, pp 211-223
145. Hall P, Maiello L, Colombo A et al (1995) In vivo evidence that Palmaz-Schatz stents do not recoil immediately following deployment. Circulation 92: I-327 (abstr)
146. Prati F, Di Mario C, Gil R et al (1995) Usefulness of online three-dimensional reconstruction of intracoronary ultrasound for guidance of stent deployment. Circulation 92: I-546

Electron Beam Computed Tomography and Cardiovascular Imaging

J.A. Rumberger

Introduction

Noninvasive or minimally invasive medical imaging has allowed safe, serial assessment of patients with proven or suspected cardiac and/or vascular disease in both in- and out-of-hospital situations. Evaluation of such patients by radionuclide angiography, cardiac perfusion field imaging, transthoracic and transesophageal echocardiography, magnetic resonance imaging (MRI), conventional X-ray computed tomography (EBCT) and peripheral ultrasound is now commonplace in clinical practice. Electron beam computed tomography (EBCT) has emerged as yet another powerful means to examine and quantitate cardiovascular anatomy, function, and flow in patients presenting with a variety of diseases of the heart, coronary arteries, pericardium, and great vessels. The three-dimensional registration of the images provides the clinician with qualitative and quantitative information regarding the patient which aids diagnosis, allows prognostic forecasting, and helps guide or monitor acute and long-term responses to pharmacologic and/or surgical interventions. The purpose of this chapter is to examine the applications of EBCT to cardiovascular imaging and discuss clinically appropriate uses of this advanced imaging modality.

EBCT Design and Operation

A practical understanding of the use of EBCT in vascular imaging requires a thorough comprehension of the inherent versatility of the instrument. This involves knowledge of the scanner specifications, available scanning modes, and the indications for imaging in various planes. The device is manufactured by Imatron, Inc., San Francisco, California and marketed by Siemens AG in the USA and Europe under the name Evolution, and by Imatron under the name Ultrafast-CT in the rest of the world.

In general, image acquisition from conventional X-ray CT requires 1–2 s (although "partial" scans can be obtained from spiral CT in ~600 ms). EBCT scan acquisition on the other hand is done using a rotating electron beam technology accomplished using one of two "sweep" speeds: 50 ms or 100 ms (or multiples of 100 ms if necessary). In this way, scanning involves no mechanical movement of the X-ray source/detector pair (Fig. 1).

Due to the advancement of the electron beam technology, current scanning options include an electrocardiographically triggered, rapid sequence multitslice (2–12 level), 50-ms scan acquisition for studies requiring information from temporal se-

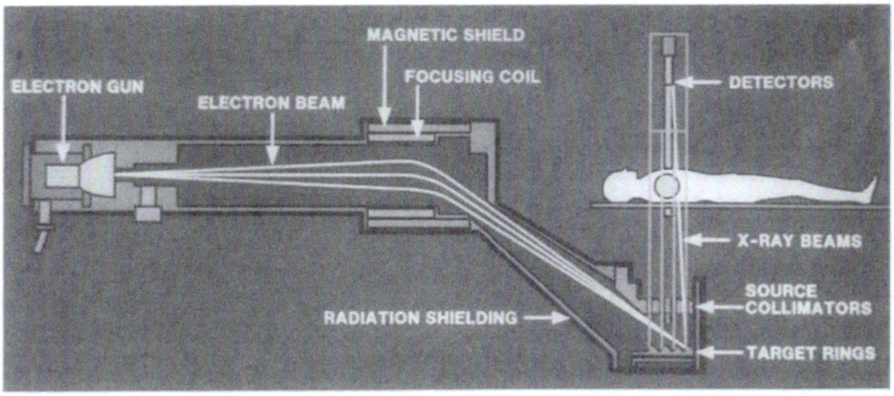

Fig. 1. The EBCT device. Basically, an electron beam is deflected through a series of electromagnets and focused onto one of up to four tungsten target rings which lie beneath the subject. The series of co-planar, stationary detectors lie above the subject. During operation, the electron beam is magnetically deflected, focused to a 1- to 2-mm focal spot, and swept across one of a series of four semicircular (210°) targets that lie beneath the subject. The X-ray transmission data are registered onto a stationary detector system. From these data tomographic reconstructions are performed in a conventional manner using filtered backprojection

quences (e.g., cardiac function and flow) and a single-slice, 100- to 1400-ms acquisition (in steps of 100 ms) for studies requiring improved density and spatial resolution (e.g., coronary calcification and coronary angiography). The tomographic slice thickness is nominally 8 mm for the 50-ms images, but can be 1.5 mm, 3.0 mm, 6.0 mm, or 10.0 mm for the 100-ms images. The sequential scan repetition rate is 17 frames/s for the multislice mode, and up to 12.0 cm of the heart can be scanned in rapid succession. For the "high-resolution" (100-ms) imaging, usually thin sections are acquired one at a time and then the scanning table incremented and the sequence repeated. The specifications of the scanner and the scanning options are given in Table 1.

Table 1. Electron beam computed tomography (EBCT) scanner specifications

	Multilevel mode	Single-slice mode
Number of detectors/tomographic level	432	864
Number of levels/scan	2	1
Number of levels/study	2 – 12	1 – 126[a]
Scan time (s)	0.05	0.1 – 1.4
Slice thickness (mm)	8.0	1.5, 3.0, 6.0, 10.0
Matrix size (number of pixels)	256^2, 360^2	360^2, 512^2
Nominal pixel dimension (for 35 mm reconstruction size)	1.4, 0.97	0.97, 0.68
Maximum number of images/study	160[a]	126[a]

[a] Version 12.2 software.

Electrocardiographic (ECG) triggering (as opposed to manual triggering) is preferred for cardiovascular imaging and can commence at 0%, 40%, or 80% of the measured ECG R – R interval. An analog ECG signal and the timing of each scan are recorded with the scan file header during each acquisition and can be viewed and analyzed independently from the image data. Scanning is performed in one of three modes: cine, flow, or volume. Figure 2 shows an example of ECG scan triggering for each of the three scanning modes.

Basically, the "cine" mode is employed to define time-dependent cardiac cavity and muscle motion, the "flow" mode is employed to follow time-dependent changes in regional vascular opacification which correspond to measurements of local blood flow, and the "volume" mode is used to define static cardiac, coronary, and vascular anatomic information, with or without the use of iodinated contrast.

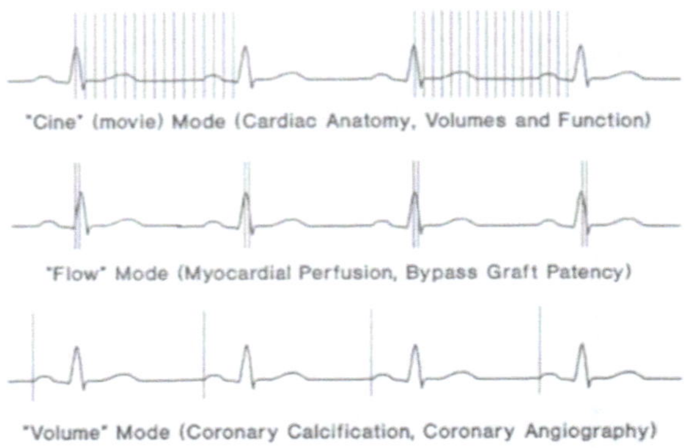

Fig. 2. Types of ECG triggering used for each of the three EBCT scanning modes. Although the multiplane 50-ms and single-plane 100-ms scan speeds can accommodate all three scanning modes, the "cine" and "flow"' modes are most commonly used for multislice imaging while the "volume" mode is exclusively used in single-slice imaging

Standard computed tomographic images of the coronary arteries, aorta, and pulmonary artery are generally obtained from a standard transaxial plane by acquiring images perpendicular to the long axis of the body. This imaging plane is identical to routine positioning for evaluations of the great vessels using conventional computed tomography. However, since the position of the cardiac chambers within the thorax is not parallel to the transaxial plane, it is usually advantageous for the majority of cardiac functional studies to acquire images in a plane different from the standard thoracic/body imaging plane. In two-dimensional echocardiography, the apical four-chamber (apical long axis) and parasternal short axis views generally allow identification of all surfaces of the left ventricle and are complementary in the evaluation of cardiac structure and function. Nearly identical orthogonal views of the left ventricle are routinely obtained by EBCT using variable "slew" (0° – 25°, right or left of center) and "tilt" (up to 15°, head up) of the imaging table and are properly termed "horizontal long axis" and "short axis," respectively. An example of a midventricular short and long axis image pair is shown in Figure 3.

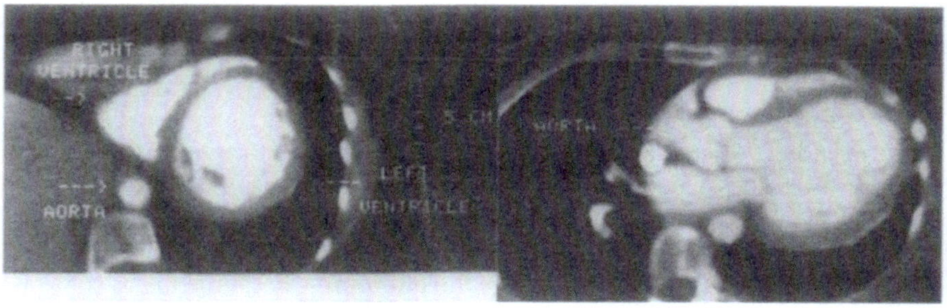

Fig. 3. Example of end-diastolic scan in the "short axis" (transverse cardiac) at the mid-left ventricular level (*left*), and an end-diastolic scan in the "long axis" (horizontal long axis) at the mid-left ventricular level (*right*). These examples are from a patient with a dilated cardiomyopathy. Note that the left ventricle is significantly dilated compared to the normal right ventricle

Applications

EBCT functions as a body scanner and thus is able to perform high-resolution imaging of the thorax and abdomen in much the same fashion as is used for standard and spiral computed tomographic devices. However, patient imaging and thus throughput is much faster than with these conventional instruments. Because of the ability to scan with the ECG trigger, EBCT has, in addition, a number of specific cardiovascular applications, as outlined below.

Right and Left Ventricular Chamber Volumes, Ventricular Function, and Muscle Mass

Aside from a desire to define anatomic information in detail, the potential to provide quantitative data about the size and function of the heart has always been one of the goals of cardiac imaging. EBCT provides a minimally invasive means to determine high spatial, density, and temporal resolution images of the beating heart, quickly and efficiently, at multiple tomographic levels in a known three-dimensional registration. Quantitative right and left ventricular chamber volumes, left ventricular muscle mass, and regional function are determined to a very high degree of accuracy by acquiring polytomographic images of the heart from the left ventricular apex through the right ventricular outflow tract [1, 2]. Up to 12 contiguous tomographic levels (approximately 1.0 cm center-to-center) with 10–20 images each 60 ms through the cardiac cycle can be performed during a single intravenous injection of nonionic contrast medium (version 12.1 software). Studies from a number of laboratories have shown the accuracy of left ventricular muscle mass and left and right ventricular cavitary volumes to be precise to within 5% of the actual values. Thus EBCT remains the most accurate noninvasive method to perform these quantitations. Unlike an MRI, cardiac image quality is nearly universally of excellent quality. Since images are also acquired throughout the cardiac cycle, EBCT can be used to quantify regional ventricular function and wall thickening [3, 4], but also can be used to define characteristics of ventricular systolic function such as ejection fraction [5], contractility [6], and peak rates of systolic emptying as well as early diastolic function [6, 7]. Hajduczok et al. [8] have also confirmed use of the EBCT single-slice mode to measure right ventricular mass to a high degree of accuracy. Additional applications include quantitation of univalvular regurgitation [9], assessment of infarct size [10], and serial studies of cardiac remodeling after infarction [6, 11, 12].

Imaging of the Great Vessels

Recent hardware and software improvements for the EBCT scanner have advanced its ability to conduct comprehensive and diagnostic examinations of the great vessels (pulmonary artery and aorta). Since EBCT does not rely on mechanical motion of the X-ray tube, it does not encounter problems of heat loading (the major limitation of spiral imagers, which can obtain about only about 30 s of continuous imaging at one time). Therefore many images can be acquired over a short period of time; scanning can also be paused for the patient to exhale and then hold his/her breath again and scanning be continued up to a limit of 126 images per data set. For imaging of the great vessels, the scanner is used in the single-slice high-resolution mode. The ability to obtain a single scan in a short time (100 ms at or near end-diastole) has provided superior image quality by decreasing motion unsharpness of any object which moves during scan acquisition. Thus the common streak artifacts seen in thoracic images using conventional and most spiral computed tomographie scans of the heart are absent in properly performed EBCT scans. In addition, because of the speed at which an examination can be done, EBCT is often the examination of choice in our institution in cases of possible aortic dissection when the patient is clinically unstable.

Teigen et al. [13] used EBCT to image the pulmonary vasculature in 60 patients undergoing direct pulmonary arteriography for suspicion of pulmonary embolism. The pulmonary vascular bed was divided into 12 zones and EBCT and angiographic findings were correlated on a patient-by-patient basis for each zone. Thirty-six had both negative EBCT and angiography, where in 15 both were positive. From these data, the sensitivity of EBCT was determined to be 65% while the specificity was 97%; the positive predictive value was 94%, and the negative predictive value was 82%. However, after review of the 9 discordant cases, the sensitivity and specificity of EBCT were found to approach 100% for clinically important acute pulmonary emboli. Additionally, EBCT was equally applicable to depiction of central and peripheral emboli. Currently at our institution, EBCT is used most commonly as a "first-line" diagnostic modality for this application. The advantage of EBCT is that the study can be completed rapidly and safely even in acutely ill patients not felt to be optimal candidates for direct pulmonary angiography. Additionally, it can provide anatomic information not derived from ventilation/perfusion imaging. Recent evidence has also suggested that EBCT can be used also to define pulmonary perfusion abnormalities associated with pulmonary embolization [14].

Coronary Artery Calcification

One of the newest and most clinically promising applications for EBCT is one that employs concepts which have been used clinically for a number of years; that is, the diagnosis of focal coronary artery disease by defining the presence of discrete calcification of the involved coronary arteries. It is well known that coronary artery disease is the major cause of mortality in the world and it is evident that early detection or identification of coronary artery disease, especially in asymptomatic individuals, may allow interventions which could limit this mortality. The detection of coronary artery calcium using fluoroscopy has been reported for a number of years and has been shown to have prognostic value for future coronary syndromes [15].

A calcium scoring system was devised originally by Agatston et al. [16] for review of the high-resolution (3-mm-thick, 100-ms, ECG-triggered, contiguous) EBCT images. Unlike the majority of applications for EBCT, no contrast administration is necessary to visualize the proximal coronary vessels in patients due to the surrounding relatively low density fat in the anterior and interventricular grooves. Standard computed tomographic image display assigns a CT number of –1000 to air (lung), a CT number of 0 to water, and a CT number of +1000 to dense bone. The maximum CT number of the nonopacified blood and myocardium is on the order of 100 CT units. Here a CT density (or Hounsfield number) greater than 130 is commonly used as a threshold to define the absence or presence of discrete coronary calcification. The areas of coronary artery calcium are rapidly definable, even to the untrained observer (Figure 4).

More than 30 articles have been published in the past several years specifically addressing the appli-

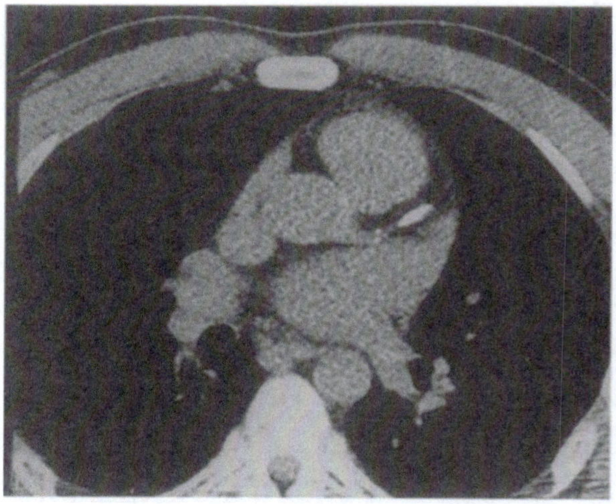

Fig. 4. A single-level, 100-ms, ECG-triggered, 3-mm-thick, noncontrast EBCT scan taken at the base of the left ventricle in a 52-year-old woman with chest pain and a family history of coronary disease. Anatomic details show the aorta (*center of image*), portions of the basal tight ventricle (*anterior and to the right of the aorta*), right and left atria (*left and posterior to the aorta,* respectively), and proximal portions of the left main and left anterior descending coronary arteries. The discrete high-density material to the right of the aorta is intramural calcification of the proximal left anterior descending coronary artery. Localization of the coronary calcification is facilitated by the relatively low (*dark area*) X-ray density of the surrounding epicardial fat. At selective coronary angiography, she was found to have an 80% narrowing of the mid-left anterior descending coronary artery

cation of EBCT-quantified coronary calcium as it relates to histopathologic studies as well as in patients undergoing clinically indicated coronary arteriography for the diagnosis of coronary disease. Simons et al. [17] performed EBCT scanning on dissected coronary vessels from autopsy hearts and compared the extent of coronary artery calcium with paired histologic sections. This study showed that coronary calcium could not be used to absolutely quantify stenosis severity on a segment-by-segment basis and that atherosclerosis can be seen in the absence of discrete calcium at the same anatomic site. However, the presence of "significant" coronary disease (≥75% area, or approximately ≥50% diameter stenosis) was found in only 2.5% of individual coronary segments with no detectable calcium by EBCT scanning. In a clinical study by Breen et al. [18] from a group of 100 patients under the age of 60 who underwent both diagnostic coronary angiography and EBCT, the absence of identifiable coronary calcium had a negative predictive value of 100% in ruling out the presence of any lesions with greater than 50% diameter stenosis. However, although a totally negative EBCT study may have important clinical implications, a recent study by Fallovollita suggested that this degree of accuracy may not been seen in all patient groups [19]. Additionally, although the "calcium score" increases in direct proportion to the increasing severity of coronary atherosclerotic disease, it appears to correlate only loosely with the degree of luminal narrowing found during angiography.

Two recent reports from the Mayo Clinic, one a histopathologic study [20] and the other a clinical study [21], have shown that EBCT coronary calcium has a similar predictive value in men and women for evaluating coronary luminal narrowing. A summary of the results regarding sensitivity and specificity of EBCT coronary calcium for detecting coronary disease as defined by clinical coronary angiography is given in Table 2.

Finally, a recently published study by Rumberger et al. [22] has emphasized that the total area of coronary artery calcification detected by EBCT is linearly correlated with the total area of histologic coronary artery plaque on a segmental, individual coronary artery, and whole coronary artery system basis. However, the total areas of coronary calcification underestimate the total associated coronary plaque areas. Thus, identification of calcium by EBCT scanning demonstrates only the "tip of the atherosclerotic iceberg." Additionally, this study reconfirmed that coronary plaque is not always associated with coronary calcification as detected with X-ray computed tomography. These data suggest that there may be a specific coronary plaque area required for demonstration of coronary calcium, and in small plaques, the calcium is either not present or is undetectable by this methodology.

Table 2. Sensitivity, specificity, predictive values, and standard errors for EBCT detection of coronary calcium (any area >0.52 mm²) and arteriographic disease severity[a]

	Any arteriographic disease[b]		Significant arteriographic disease[c]	
	Women (%)	Men (%)	Women (%)	Men (%)
Sensitivity	97±3	94±3	100±0	98±2
Specificity	38±12	35±10	66±8	57±8
Positive Predictive Value	85±6	89±4	46±8	66±6
Negative Predictive Value	91±9	79±9	100±0	95±5

[a] Reproduced with permission from [21]. Based on EBCT coronary calcium scans and results from coronary arteriography in 86 men and 50 women.
[b] Presence of at least minimal luminal irregularities.
[c] Presence of any luminal stenosis representing ≥50% diameter narrowing.

The two major clinical applications for coronary calcium "screening" with EBCT, based largely on the results given above, is in the identification of patients with premature coronary disease who are asymptomatic but deemed "high-risk" by virtue of various risk factors, and for the evaluation of the patients with atypical type chest pain syndromes in which a negative scan virtually rules out the presence of significant coronary disease and a positive scan suggests further evaluation may be necessary.

Assessment of Bypass Graft Patency

Assessment of coronary artery bypass graft patency using computed tomography was first reported more than a decade ago. These principles were used by researchers in the largest multicenter trial to date which examined the application of EBCT in the "flow" mode to define patency of mammary and saphenous bypass grafts compared to direct angiography [23]. Subsequent improvements in methodology and scanning techniques have shown the overall sensitivity to detect a patent graft to currently be on the order of 94%–96%. This subject was most recently discussed by Stanford et al. [24] and compared with other imaging modalities in determining directly or indirectly the patency of bypass grafts.

Three-Dimensional Anatomy and Reconstruction

X-ray computed tomography, like MRI, acquires digital format data in parallel tomographic images which are thus suitable for three-dimensional image processing and display for quantification of cardiac and peri-cardiac anatomy.

Precise localization and quantitation of left ventricular aneurysms has been attempted with radionuclide and contrast angiography relying significantly on geometric simplifications and/or assumptions. Lessick et al. [25] used EBCT in eight patients to characterize size, shape, and function of anterior fibrous left ventricular aneurysms and the surrounding unaffected myocardium. Using 3D reconstruction methods they examined wall (myocardial) thicknesses, regional thickening and motion analysis, meridional and circumferential curvatures, surface normals, surface area, and regional wall stress indices. They determined that fibrous ventricular aneurysms were characterized by a large, nonthinned region of nonfunctioning myocardium surrounding the thin true aneurysmal area and its transitional border zone. Between the normally functioning myocardium and the aneurysm they determined an intermediate zone which was of normal wall thickness but with reduced function, possibly due to its low radius of curvature and high stress index.

Spiral computed tomography has been shown to have potential for angiography of both the peripheral and of the abdominal vasculature. The advantages of this approach is that true three-dimensional angiograms can be obtained during a single contrast injection; but because of cardiac motion, CT angiography of the heart has not been previously thought possible. However, a recent publication from the University of Erlangen, Germany, has opened the way for a new potential application for EBCT in noninvasive coronary angiography. Mosage et al. [26] studied 27 patients with EBCT who also underwent conventional coronary arteriography. Contiguous 3-mm-thick EBCT scans were acquired during a single breath-hold, commencing at the root of the aorta with 2-mm table overlap during intravenous injections of nonionic contrast medium (120–160 ml). A 15-cm-field of view was used and thus "effective" voxel dimensions for the three-dimensional reconstructions were 0.35 mm × 0.35 mm × 1.0 mm. In this preliminary study, 9 out of 11 (82%) high-grade stenoses and 5 out of 5 (100%) occlusions in the proximal left anterior descending coronary artery as identified by selective arteriography were found on review of the EBCT scans. Five patients who underwent selective angioplasty after arteriography underwent repeat scanning with EBCT. In each case, the improvements in the arterial lumen dimensions were definable in the EBCT images. In addition, 3 of 5 (60%) high-grade stenoses were also visualized in the right coronary artery. However, recognition of stenoses of the left circumflex was not possible. It was presumed that, even with acquisition times of 100 ms, the rapid motion of the proximal left circumflex in the atrio-

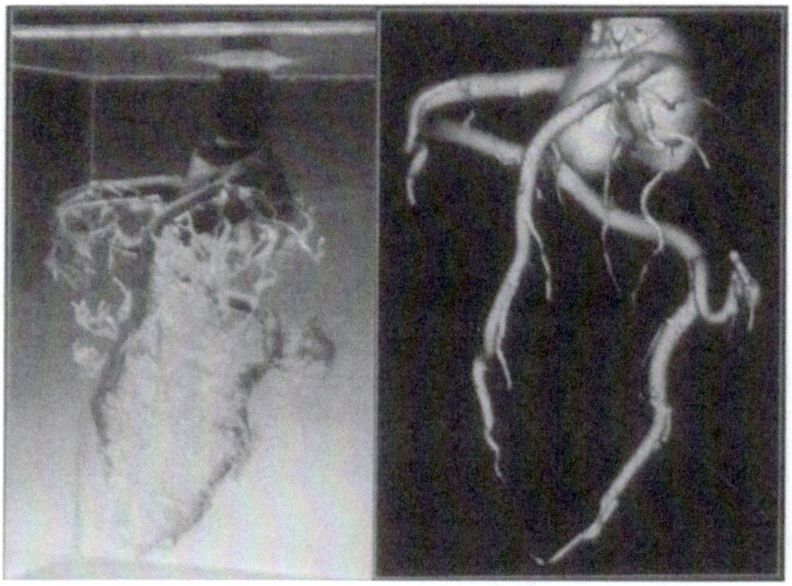

Fig. 5. Photograph of a Plexiglas cast of the coronary arteries of the horse (*left*) and a shaded surface display three-dimensional reconstruction of the cast following from the base of the heart through the apex. The subsequent three-dimensional images were reconstructed using commercially available software

ventricular groove resulted in motion unsharpness in this area. Additionally, these authors feel that with intravenous injections, the opacification of the great cardiac vein, which also traverses the atrioventricular groove, may have resulted in some difficulty in separating arterial from venous opacifications. An example from our laboratory of a three-dimensional reconstruction using EBCT of a plastic cast of the coronary arteries is shown in Fig. 5.

Obviously, more work is required in this area. However, the potential has been shown for EBCT coronary angiography to become a potent adjunct to conventional, invasive coronary angiography, especially when performed in conjunction with noninvasive visualization of mural coronary artery calcified plaque.

Limitations of EBCT

EBCT offers a means to define quantitative aspects of the heart, coronary arteries and great vessels in a direct, extremely reliable, and noninvasive fashion. However, the advantages must be weighed against some of the drawbacks. Subjects are exposed to radiation and most imaging requires the use of intravenous iodinated contrast. The average integrated radiation body dose for a complete cardiac function study is on the order of that received from a standard abdominal computed tomographic scan [27]; for imaging of the coronary arteries, pulmonary artery, and aorta it is significantly less. Although this level of radiation is only one-quarter to one-tenth of that of a standard contrast ventriculogram, pulmonary angiography, coronary angiogram, or aortogram, the need for the EBCT study must be weighed against the minimal but real risk to the patient. The issue regarding the use of intravenous contrast media is often discussed but the risk to the patient is small if consideration is given to excluding patients with elevated creatinine or a history of contrast allergy.

These limitations to EBCT, however, must in turn be weighed against the high likelihood of completion of a satisfactory cardiovascular examination (>95% in our laboratory) and the convenience to the patient (most exams can be completed in 30 min with only moderate cooperation and minor discomfort).

Summary and Conclusions

The clinical impact of obtaining a variety of quantitative cardiac and vascular data from a single medical imaging modality is significant as well as probably cost-effective. Not infrequently, invasive angiography, along with several noninvasive or minimally invasive techniques such as radionuclide angiography, scintillation perfusion scanning, two-dimensional echocardiography, and conventional computed tomography or MRI, are required to fully assess cardiac size, function, perfusion, and/or pathology of the great vessels. In selected patients, EBCT offers the potential to assess such anatomic and functional aspects during a single session. As discussed, the methods of data acquisition employed, the orientation of the imaging planes, and the analysis of the images are designed specifically to answer the clinical questions posed on a per subject basis. There are presently only about 70 EBCT scanners in operation worldwide. However, there is intense interest in this method, largely due to the unique aspects of cardiac and coronary imaging possible.

The future role of diagnostic EBCT in cardiovascular medicine is complementary to conventional methods and offers additional versatility with respect to unique imaging of the heart and great vessels. Given these considerations, it is proper to use EBCT, not in the unnecessary duplication of examinations made using other cardiovascular imaging methods, but as a complementary examination in selected patients, or as a primary noninvasive imaging tool in circumstances that involve unique applications.

References

1. Feiring AJ, Rumberger JA, Skorton DJ, Collins SM, Higins CB, Lipton MJ, Ell S, Marcus ML (1985) Determination of left ventricular mass in the dog with rapid acquisition cardiac CT scanning. Circulation 72: 1355–1362
2. Reiter SJ, Rumberger JA, Feiring AJ, Stanford W, Marcus ML (1986) Precision of right and left ventricular stroke volume measurements by rapid acquisition cine computed tomography. Circulation 74: 890–900
3. Feiring AJ, Rumberger JA, Reiter SJ, Collins SM, Skorton DJ, Rees M, Marcus ML (1988) Sectional and segmental variability of left ventricular function: experimental and clinical studies using ultrafast computed tomography. J Am Coll Cardiol 12: 415–425
4. Lanzer P, Garrett J, Lipton MJ, Gould R, Sievers R, O'Connell W, Botvinick E, Higgins CB (1986) Quantitation of regional myocardial function by cine computed tomography: pharmacologic changes in wall thickness. J Am Coll Cardiol 8: 682–692

5. Rumberger JA (1991) Quantifying left ventricular regional and global systolic function using ultrafast computed tomography. Am J Cardiac Imaging 5: 29 – 37
6. Hirose K, Reed JE, Rumberger JA (1995) Serial changes in left and right ventricular systolic and diastolic mechanics during the first year after an initial left ventricular Q-wave myocardial infarction. J Am Coll Cardiol 25: 1097 – 1104
7. Rumberger JA, Weiss RM, Feiring AJ, Stanford W, Hajduczok Z, Rezia K, Marcus ML (1989) Patterns of regional diastolic function in the normal human left ventricle: an ultrafast-CT study. J am Coll Cardiol 13: 119 – 125
8. Hajduczok Z, Weiss RM, Marcus ML, Stanford W (1990) Determination of right ventricular mass in humans and dogs with ultrafast computed tomography. Circulation 82: 202 – 212
9. Reiter SJ, Rumberger JA, Stanford W, Marcus ML (1986) Quantitative determination of aortic regurgitant volume by cine computed tomography. Circulation 76: 728 – 735
10. Weiss RM, Stark CA, Rumberger JA, Marcus ML (1990) Identification and quantitation of myocardial infarction or risk area size with cine-computed tomography. Am J Cardiac Imaging 4: 33 – 37
11. Rumberger JA, Behrenbeck T, Breen JR, Reed JE, Gersh BJ (1993) Non-parallel changes in global chamber volumer and muscle mass during the first year following transmural myocardial infarction in man. J Am Coll Cardiol 21: 673 – 682
12. Hirose K, Shu NH, Reed JE, Rumberger JA (1993) Right ventricular dilatation and remodeling the first year after an initial transmural wall myocardial infarction. Am J Cardiol 72: 1126 – 1130
13. Teigen CL, Maus TP, Sheedy PF II, Stanson AW, Johnson CM, Breen JF, McKusick MA (1995) Pulmonary embolism: diagnosis with contrast-enhanced electron-beam CT and comparison with pulmonary angiography. Radiology 194: 313 – 319
14. Hoffman EA, Tajik JK, Petersen G, Reiners TJ, Thompson BH, Stanford W (1995) Perfusion deficit vs anatomic visualization in detection of pulmonary emboli via electron beam CT (Abstr). Circulation 92: I – 312
15. Detrano RC, Wong ND, Weiyi T, French WJ, Georgiou D, Young E, Brezden OS, Narahara KA, Brundage BH (1994) Prognostic significance of cardiac cine-fluoroscopy for coronary calcific deposits in a high risk, asymptomatic population. J Am Coll Cardiol 24: 354 – 358
16. Agatston AS, Janowitz WR, Hildner FJ, Zusmer NR, Viamonte M, Detrano R (1990) Quantification of coronary artery calcium using ultrafast computed tomography. J Am Coll Cardiol 15: 827 – 832
17. Simons DB, Schwartz RS, Edwards WD, Sheedy PF, Breen JF, Rumberger JA (1992) Noninvasive definition of anatomic coronary artery disease by ultrafast CT: a quantitative pathologic study. J Am Coll Cardiol 20: 1118 – 1126
18. Breen JF, Sheedy PF, Schwartz RS, Stanson AW, Kaufmann RB, Moll PP, Rumberger JA (1992) Coronary calcification detected with fast-CT as a marker of coronary artery disease: works in progress. Radiology 185: 435 – 439
19. Fallovollita JA, Brody AS, Bunnell IL, Kumar Y, Canty JM (1994) Fast computed tomography detection of coronary calcification in the diagnosis of coronary artery disease. Comparison with angiography in patients <50 years old. Circulation 89: 285 – 290
20. Rumberger JA, Schwartz RS, Simons DB, Sheedy PF, Edwards WD, Fitzpatrick LA (1994) Relations of coronary calcium determined by electron beam computed tomography and lumen narrowing determined at autopsy. Am J Cardiol 73: 1169 – 1173
21. Rumberger JA, Sheedy PF, Breen JR, Schwartz RS (1995) Coronary calcium as determined by electron beam computed tomography, and coronary disease on arteriogram: effect of patient's sex on diagnosis. Circulation 91: 1363 – 1367
22. Rumberger JA, Simons DB, Fitzpatrick LA, Sheedy PF, Schwartz RS (1995) Coronary artery calcium areas by electron beam computed tomography and coronary atherosclerotic plaque area: a histopathologic correlative study. Circulation 92: 2157 – 2162
23. Stanford W, Brundage BH, MacMillan R, Chomka EV, Bateman TM, Eldridge WJ, Lipton MJ, White CW, Wilson RF, Johnson MR, Marcus ML (1988) Sensitivity and specificity of assessing coronary artery bypass graft patency with ultrafast computed tomography: results of a multi-center trial. J Am Coll Cardiol 12: 1 – 7
24. Stanford W, Rooholamini M, Rumberger JA, Marcus ML (1988) Evaluation of coronary bypass graft patency by ultrafast CT. J Thorac Imaging 3: 52 – 55
25. Lessick J, Sideman S, Azhari H, Marcus M, Grenadier E, Beyar R (1991) Regional three-dimensional geometry and function of left ventricles with fibrous aneurysms: a cine-computed tomography study. Circulation 84: 1072 – 1086
26. Mosage WEL, Achenbach S, Seese B, Bachmann K, Kirchgeorg M (1995) Coronary artery stenoses: three-dimensional imaging with electrocardiographically triggered, contrast agent-enhanced, electron-beam CT. Radiology 196: 707 – 714
27. McCollough CH, Zink Fe, Morin RL (1994) Radiation dosimetry for electron beam CT. Radiology 192: 637 – 643

Intravenous Coronary Angiography with Synchrotron Radiation

W.-R. Dix, C.W. Hamm, and W. Kupper

Introduction

In modern units for coronary angiography, the contrast in the images can be enhanced using digital subtraction angiography (DSA) in temporal subtraction mode (Fig. 1). In this image-processing mode, a number of electrocardiography (ECG-) triggered images are acquired before application of the contrast agent. The mean of these images (i.e., the mask) is subtracted from the images acquired after application of the contrast agent, thus enhancing the vascular structures containing iodine. The resulting images are of high quality, permitting definite luminographic evaluation of the coronary arteries. The images visualize coronary arteries including their bifurcations down to a diameter below 1 mm.

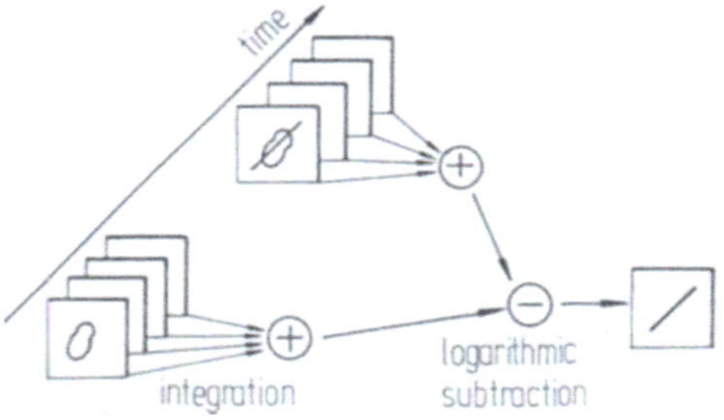

Fig. 1. Principle of digital subtraction angiography (DSA) in temporal subtraction mode

Unfortunately, there is a certain risk with selective coronary angiography due to the introduction of the catheter into the arterial system. This risk can be diminished considerably if the contrast agent is introduced into the veins. However, three problems for the imaging of the coronary arteries then arise:

1. Because after intravenous injection the contrast agent traverses the superior vena cava, the chambers of the right heart, the pulmonary arteries and veins, the chambers of the left heart, and the aorta before it enters the coronary arteries, it is diluted by a factor of 40 – 50 compared to selective coronary angiography. The bolus of the contrast agent is correspondingly elongated. Conventional X-ray units do not allow imaging of this small contrast of the diluted contrast agent in the coronary arteries because of the low signal-to-noise ratio (SNR).
2. Due to the fast motion of the heart, it is not possible to use DSA in temporal subtraction mode if small structures need to be imaged following injection of the contrast agent. The mask and the image, which are taken before and after injection of the contrast agent, are not spatially matched for subtraction. Thus in temporal substraction mode DSA can only be used for large vascular structures, such as the abdominal aorta. Even in ECG triggered images, the spatial resolution is low, typically in the range of 3 – 5 mm. Only structures such as the left ventricle or bypasses can be resolved in most cases with intravenous injection and ECG-triggered DSA in temporal subtraction mode.
3. Due to simultaneous filling of the coronary arteries, cardiac chambers, and the great vascular structure following intravenous contrast application, the coronary arteries are obscured against the background. If, for example, the contrast agent is intravenously injected within 2 s at a rate of 15 ml/s, then the pulmonary veins, left chambers, and the aorta are filled with contrast agent at the same time as the coronary arteries.

The first two problems can be overcome using dichromography.

Dichromography

Dichromography is another form of DSA, namely DSA in energy subtraction mode. In this method, the energy dependence of the X-ray absorption of the contrast agent, usually iodine, is utilized to obtain the two images required for subtraction. In order to obtain different iodine contrast, the discontinuity of the absorption at the *K*-edge is used (Fig. 2).

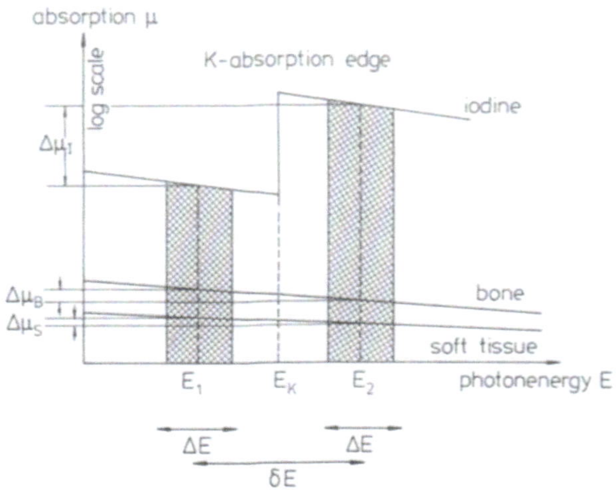

Fig. 2. Energy dependence of the absorption in the region of the *K*-edge (E_K) of iodine (*I*) at 33.17 keV. *S*, soft tissue; *B*, bone; *E*, photon energy. δ *E* (energy separation) <300 eV; Δ *E* bandwidth, *shaded area* <250 eV

This means that one image is acquired with a monochromatic X-ray energy below the *K*-edge of iodine (mask) and the other with an energy above the *K*-edge. By performing a logarithmic subtraction, the subtracted image should contain exclusively the iodine image, i.e., the image of the arterial structure. The absorption coefficient for X-rays above the *K*-edge is approximately sixfold higher than that below. For an energy separation of the two monochromatic X-ray beams of 300 eV, the sensitivity for iodine is 10 000 times higher than for soft tissues. This X-ray absorption difference allows intravenous application of the contrast agent for coronary artery imaging. The two images are taken simultaneously when the contrast agent fills the coronary arteries. Because the images are acquired simultaneously they match, and small iodinated structures can be enhanced by logarithmic subtraction.

The superposition of structures is inherent to all projectional imaging. In order to minimize this problem, the bolus of the contrast agent must be as short as possible. A short bolus typically provides 2 s when the coronary arteries are opacified optimally. However, because the arrival time of the contrast agent depends on the patient's hemodynamics and differs widely, it must be determined before the investigation is started.

The idea for dichromography was originally proposed in 1953 by Jacobson [1]. However, all efforts to use the method by filtering the monochromatic X-ray beams out of the spectrum of conventional X-ray units failed due to insufficient flux. Therefore, work on dichromography was not continued, until synchrotron radiation laboratories were installed with large storage rings in which electrons or positrons are accelerated. From synchrotron radiation sources, the flux per unit solid angle in the region of the *K*-edge of iodine is higher by a factor 10^4–10^7 than that from high-power rotating anode generators. The energy spectrum of synchrotron radiation is continuous, allowing freedom in selection of beam energies. Furthermore, the radiation is inherently highly collimated, allowing adequate spatial separation between the beamline components. Nevertheless, it took about 15 years to develop components which can select sufficient monochromatic flux out of the white synchrotron radiation beam.

Parameters

Contrast Media

For standard selective coronary angiography, iodine is a well-suited contrast agent because of the high concentration available and because the conventional X-ray units work with voltages up to 150 kVp. For dichromography, the high concentration of iodine is also an advantage. However, a disadvantage of iodine is the relatively low energy at the *K*-edge (33.17 keV), which means that tissue penetration is low. The absorption length in soft tissue is only 2.1 cm. A different element with higher *z* and the *K*-edge at higher energy could reduce the radiation dose to the patient without reducing the SNR in the images. A contrast agent containing gadolinium (Gd) used for magnetic resonance imaging (MRI) provides an example. The energy at the *K*-edge of Gd is 50 keV.

The skin dose *K* per subtraction image (two energy images) [2] is given by:

$$K = 2\Phi_0 E\left(\frac{\mu_a}{\varrho}\right)_S \quad (1)$$

where *E* is photon energy at the *K*-edge and $\left(\frac{\mu_a}{\varrho}\right)_S$ is the energy absorption coefficient of soft tissue (strongly energy dependent). The photon flux Φ_0 in front of the patient is determined by:

$$\Phi_0 = 4\left(\frac{SNR}{(\Delta\mu\varrho_I c_I)}\right)^2 \frac{1}{\varepsilon F} exp\left(\Sigma_j\left(\frac{\mu}{\varrho}\right)_j c_j\right) \quad (2)$$

Table 1. Material constants for 33.17-keV photons

	$\frac{\mu}{\varrho}$ (cm²/g)	ϱ (g/cm³)	μ (cm⁻¹)
Iodine	6.55 (for E_1) 35.9 (for E_2)	0.01	0.07 0.36
Soft tissue	0.33	1	0.33
Bone tissue	0.65	1.4	0.91
Lung tissue	0.31	0.16 (inspirium) 0.35 (expirium)	0.05 0.11

μ/ϱ, mass absorption coefficient; ϱ, density; μ, linear absorption coefficient

Table 2. Mass densities (c_j), change in absorption coefficients (Δμ/ϱ), and contrast (Δμ/ϱ) × c

	c_j (g/cm²)	$(\frac{\Delta\mu}{\varrho})_j$ (cm²/g)	$(\frac{\Delta\mu}{\varrho})_j\, c_j$
Iodine	0.001	28.9	0.029
Soft tissue	20	−0.0033	−0.066
Bone tissue	3	−0.0135	−0.04

Energy separation (δE) = 300 eV bracketing the K-edge of iodine at 33.17 keV.

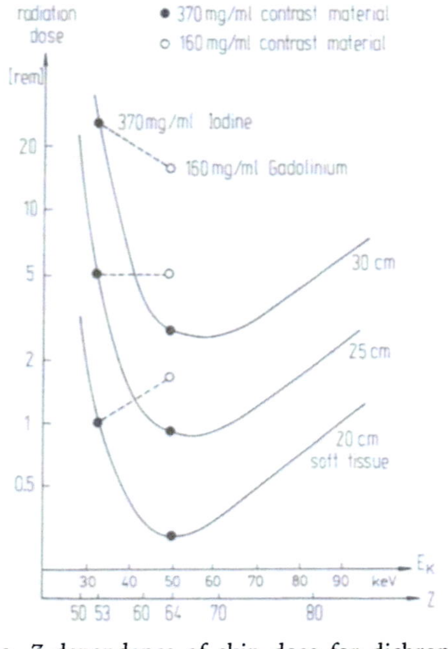

Fig. 3. Z dependence of skin dose for dichromography. *Black circles*, 370 mg contrast medium/ml; *white circles*, 160 mg contrast medium/ml. E_K, energy of the K-edge

where ε is the detector efficiency, F the pixel size, $(\frac{\mu}{\varrho})_j$ the energy-dependent mass absorption coefficients (Table 1), and c_j the mass densities (Table 2); j denotes different materials (I, iodine; S, soft tissue; B, bone).

For dichromography, Fig. 3 shows the z-dependence of the skin dose K for 20, 25, and 30 cm of soft tissue and a concentration of the contrast agent of 370 mg/ml. The other parameters are as follows: SNR=3, c_I = 0.001 g/cm², ε = 0.6, F = 0.25 mm², and $(\mu_a/\varrho)_S$ = 0.106 cm²/g.

Contrast material with an iodine concentration of 370 mg/ml is available. Contrast materials with 370 mg Gd/ml would be better with respect to the radiation dose for the patients (Fig. 3, closed circles). Unfortunately, at present Gd contrast material is only available at a concentration of 78 mg/ml. A concentration of 156 mg/ml will become available in the near future (Fig. 3, open circles). However, presently the application of Gd containing contrast agent is limited to 0.2 ml/kg body weight.

Other contrast agents with higher z elements are not known. Thus all systems for dichromography are at present optimized for the K-edge of iodine.

Mass Density

With a concentration of iodine in the contrast material of 370 mg/ml, a bolus injection of 20 ml contrast agent over 1–2 s into the brachial vein results in a concentration of approximately 10 mg iodine/ml in the aorta and the coronary arteries.

Because coronary arteries greater than 1 mm in diameter are of clinical interest, arteries down to this diameter must be clearly visible in the resulting images. Assuming the above-mentioned concentration of iodine, its mass density in arteries 1 mm in diameter is 1 mg/cm².

During the early years, 30 ml contrast agent was administered at a rate of 15 ml/s via a catheter into the superior vena cava for investigations in patients. This resulted in measured concentrations of iodine in the aorta and the coronary arteries between 8 and 20 mg/ml. The differences in concentration arose from differences in cardiac output. In addition, due to the predominantly diastolic blood flow in the coronary arteries, the contrast enhancement depended on whether the image was taken in diastole or in systole.

In 1994, we began to use contrast agent injections into the subclavian vein. A concentration of 9–15 mg iodine/ml was measured in the aorta and in the coronary arteries. In 1995, catheters were abandoned, and direct injections into the brachial vein are now performed.

Spatial Resolution

In order to image arteries 1 mm in diameter, a spatial resolution of at least 0.5 mm^{-1} is necessary. In fact, the first detectors had a pixel size of 0.5 × 0.5 mm^2. From a technical point of view, it is not a major problem to reduce the size of the pixels, but a linear decrease in the pitch increases the patient dose quadratically because the number of photons per pixel has to be maintained in order to preserve the SNR in the images.

Images of coronary arteries with different resolution, taken with conventional angiography, showed that a resolution of 0.5 mm^{-1} is adequate to visualize stenoses of 70% and greater in arteries 1 mm in diameter. However, images from detectors with different resolutions showed that a higher resolution is preferable [3, 4].

As a compromise, the detectors which are installed for investigation of patients now have a pixel size of 0.4 × 0.4 mm^2 in Hamburg [5] or 0.25 × 0.50 mmm^2 in Brookhaven [3]. The detector planned for the system in Grenoble [6] will have a pixel size of 0.35 × 0.35 mm^2.

Dynamic Range

The dynamic range is defined as maximal output signal divided by noise. The noise includes both quantum noise and electronic noise.

For the signals from the detector digitized to 65536 gray levels (16-bit) and for material constants as indicated in Table 1, a typical example for the distribution of the gray values is given in Table 3.

In the example, a ratio of approximately 60 has been calculated for the transmission through areas dominated by lung tissue to those dominated by bone tissue, respectively. This number represents the theoretical upper limit. In clinical settings, we measured ratios between 14 and 42, depending on the projection angles employed. Furthermore, in practice it is not feasible to adjust the system in such a way that the highest gray values coincide with the upper limit (in the example corresponding to 65536 gray values).

Table 3. Gray values behind different tissues (example)

Tissue	Below *K*-edge	Above *K*-edge	Difference
10.0 cm soft tissue + 12.0 cm lung tissue	65536	65536	–
20.0 cm soft tissue	4404	4404	–
17.5 cm soft tissue + 2.5 cm bone tissue + 0.1 cm iodine	1025	997	28
10.0 cm soft tissue + 5.0 cm lung tissue + 2.5 cm bone tissue + 5.0 cm iodine	6737	1580	5157
10.0 cm soft tissue + 5.0 cm lung tissue + 2.5 cm bone tissue + 5.1 cm iodine	6690	1524	5166

Because the SNR in the images after logarithmic subtraction must be at least 3, the SNR in the energy images should be at least 6. In the example, a coronary artery with a diameter of 1 mm behind 17.5 cm soft tissue and 2.5 cm bone provides a signal of 28 gray values (3%). From these numbers, the dynamic range (D) must be at least 65536 (maximal output signal):4.7 (noise), i.e., 14000:1. The given dynamic range is only valid if the coronary arteries are not superposed on other iodinated structures. If the arteries are superposed on a 5-cm-thick structure-like ventricle or aorta, the dynamic range must be at least 43000:1 (see Table 3).

Because the noise due to electronics should be lower than the quantum noise, the detectors should have an even higher dynamic range.

Selection of Imaging Mode

From the physician's point of view, two-dimensional image recording would be desirable. However, commercially available area detectors (image converter/TV systems) are not suitable for dichromography, mainly because the dynamic range is too low (approximately $D = 900:1$).

Therefore, specially constructed line scan detectors are now installed in most of the systems for dichromography, though they are much slower and more expensive. They have the advantage that the background from scattered X-rays is reduced compared to two-dimensional detectors. In addition, as all systems are now installed in synchrotron radiation beams, line detectors are preferable because they optimally match the fan beam geometry of synchrotron radiation sources, which have very small vertical divergences [e.g., 0.12 mrad (full width half maximum, FWHM) at the angiography beamline at the Hamburg Synchrotron Radiation Laboratory, HASYLAB].

In existing storage rings, the flux is sufficient for dichromography with line scan detectors, but not for two-dimensional detectors. The detectors have the disadvantage that the patients must be moved vertically through the monochromatic X-ray beams, which might seem to make the investigation uncomfortable; however, from our experience it is not. A system which allows movement of the monochromatic beam instead would require an unreasonable technical effort.

In order to avoid fast-moving mechanics such as switching monochromators or beam switchers, two-line detectors are used; these simultaneously record the two lines with different energies. This also has the advantage that it makes better use of the photon flux than a one-line detector.

Temporal Resolution

Image sequences taken with the help of invasive angiography show that the coronary arteries move with high speed. During one heart beat, there are two slow-motion phases with a duration of about 250 ms each and two fast-motion phases of about the same duration. For example, in the right anterior oblique (RAO) 30° projection, the coronary arteries move up to 2 cm/s in the slow-motion phase and up to 6 cm/s in the fast-motion phase.

When using a line scan system, one has to determine how fast the scan must be completed to avoid artifacts due to cardiac motion. By taking subsequent lines from subsequent images of an angiography sequence, we composed new images which show the simulation of images with different line scan speed in different phases of the heart motion [2]. As a result, in images taken during the fast-motion phase of the heart, the distortions of stenoses in coronary arteries are too large, and images therefore have to be taken in the slow-motion phase of the heart. With the intended image size of $12.5 \times 12.5\ cm^2$, a spatial resolution of $0.4\ cm^{-1}$ and a duration of the slow-motion phase of the heart of 250 ms, the exposure time per line must not exceed 0.8 ms. The vertical scan rate must be 50 cm/s, and the patient's seat must be ECG-triggered.

Assuming a pixel size of $0.4 \times 0.4\ mm^2$ and allowing a shift of the structures of interest from one energy image to the image with the second energy of maximal 15% of the pixel size, during the slow-motion phase of the heart the time delay between the exposure of the same pixel in the two images must not exceed 3.2 ms and 1.1 ms in the fast-motion phase of the heart.

Energy Bandwidth

With good approximation, the energy separation δE of the two mean values E_1 and E_2 of the probing beams, but not their bandwidth ΔE, influences the signal height in the subtracted image, as long as ΔE is less than or equal to δE. The change in mass absorption coefficient is given by the following relations:

Iodine:

$$\left(\frac{\Delta\mu}{\varrho}\right)_I = (29.4\ cm^2/g - 1.67 \times 10^{-3} \times \delta E\ cm^2/g \times eV) \tag{3}$$

Soft tissue:

$$\left(\frac{\Delta\mu}{\varrho}\right)_S = -1.1 \times 10^{-5} \times \delta E\ cm^2/g \times eV) \tag{4}$$

Bone tissue:

$$\left(\frac{\Delta\mu}{\varrho}\right)_B = -4.5 \times 10^{-5} \times \delta E\ cm^2/g \times eV) \tag{5}$$

Table 2 lists typical values for $\delta E = 300$ eV. For an energy separation of 300 eV, the signal from artifacts due to edges of soft tissue and bone exceeds the signal of the smallest iodine structure (1 mm coronary artery with $1\ mg/cm^2$). As these contrasts differ in sign, they can be distinguished by visual inspection. The maximal envisaged energy separation in the different systems is 300 eV. This leads to a maximal bandwidth of the quasimonochromatic beams of $\Delta E \leq 250$ eV safely avoiding the K-edge region, or $\Delta E/E \leq 7.5 \times 10^{-3}$.

Flux

For an energy separation of 300 eV, a 1-mm-thick vessel with a mass density of $1\ mg/cm^2$ of iodine shows a 3% difference between the two images. For an SNR of 3, the quantum noise in the subtracted image must not exceed 1%, or 0.5% in the unsubtracted image, if the electronic noise and other uncertainties in the system are small in comparison (about 0.1%).

The formula [2] for the registered photons in one pixel and a given SNR for the subtracted image

$$N = 4 \times \left(\frac{SNR}{(\Delta\mu\varrho)_I c_I}\right)^2 \tag{6}$$

shows that in order to obtain the noise limit of 0.5% in the energy images, 40 000 photons per pixel must be registered. For a pixel size of $0.4 \times 0.4\ mm^2$ and 20 cm soft tissue using Eq. 2 and $\varepsilon = 0.8$, this leads to $\Phi_0 = 2.3 \times 10^8$ photons/mm^2 in front of the patient. Therefore, an intensity of 2.9×10^{11} photons/($mm^2 \times s$) must be available.

If, for example, 2.5 cm of the 20 cm soft tissue are replaced by bone tissue (see Table 3), the numbers for flux and intensity increase by a factor of 4 in order to maintain a SNR of 3 for a 1-mm-thick artery. If, on the other hand, the intensity is kept constant, behind 2.5 cm bone and 17.5 cm soft tissue an SNR of 3 is achieved for 2-mm-thick arteries only.

Experience with investigations of patients [7, 8] showed that 2.7×10^{11} photons/(mm^2×s) in front of the patient and a scan speed of 50 cm/s represent a satisfactory compromise allowing acquisition of diagnostic images of the distal parts of the coronary arteries at acceptable radiation dose levels to the patient.

If the delivered intensity from the source is lower than the above-stated values, a longer exposure time per line must be envisaged. Longer exposure times, however, prevent complete image acquisition within the slow-motion phase of the heart. Currently, only the system NIKOS (Nicht-invasive Koronarangiographie mit Synchrotronstrahlung) in Hamburg allows an exposure time of 0.25 s per image.

For two-dimensional detectors, a further increase of the flux in front of the monochromator by a factor of about 300 is necessary in order to obtain the same SNR in the pixels as in line scan systems.

Radiation Dose

A flux of 3×10^{11} photons/(mm^2×s) corresponds to a skin dose rate of 33 GY/s (see Eq. 1). At a speed of 50 cm/s for the vertical scan and a beam height of 0.4 mm in front of the patient, the time of exposure per line is 0.8 ms. This results in a skin dose per monochromatic beam of 26 mGy or a skin dose of 52 mGy per subtracted image. The number is in very good agreement with measurements with thermoluminescence dosimeters (TLD) on the chest of the patients. For the given conditions, we measured 50 mGy, including the dose from backscattered X-rays (about 20%).

A value of 50 mGy/subtracted image is taken as the upper limit for investigations in Hamburg. In Brookhaven, this limit is 70 mGy/subtracted image, but all investigations were performed with approximately 50 mGy. The total skin dose per investigation must not exceed 350 mGy in Brookhaven, including the dose from the patient's preparation with the fluoroscopy unit, and 300 mGy in Hamburg. In order to obtain the total skin dose, the dose of all images is summed up, even if the entrance areas of the beam do not overlap because of the different projection angles. These numbers are comparable to standard doses delivered in conventional invasive angiography procedures. The dose for selective angiography of the human heart was determined to be 360 mGy skin dose on average [9]. Of course, with this dose in conventional angiography, a sequence of images is taken, providing information about the flow dynamics of the contrast material.

The numbers are valid for the skin dose only, which can be measured simply. From this monochromatic skin entry dose, the effective dose, which is the important quantity for radiation safety, can be

Table 4. Conversion factors from skin entry dose to effective dose

Patient	Factor
Male	0.010
Female, X-ray entering the patient from the back	0.016
Female, X-ray entering the patient from the front	0.020

33.17-keV X-rays in a 12×12-cm^2 area, beam centered to the heart in the left anterior oblique (LAO) 30° projection.

Table 5. Parameters for dichromography with a line scan system

Parameter	Value
Contrast agent	370 mg iodine/ml
Concentration of iodine in coronary arteries	8–20 mg/ml
Mass density of iodine in coronary arteries of 1 mm in diameter	0.8–2.0 mg/cm^2
K-edge of iodine	33.17 keV
Absorption length in soft tissue	2.1 cm
Bandwidth of the monochromatik beams	≤250 eV
Signal of a 1-mm coronary artery	3%
Signal-to-noise-ratio (SNR)	≥3
Statistical noise	≤1%
Electronic noise	≤0.3%
Dynamic range of detector	≥40 000:1
Exposure time per line	≤1 ms
Exposure time per image	≤250 ms
Speed of the vertical scan	50 cm/s
Delay for the same pixel (E_1 and E_2), slow-motion phase	≤3.2 ms
Spatial resolution	≥0.5 mm^{-1}
Intensity in front of the patient	3×10^{11} photons/(mm^2×s)
Skin dose per subtracted image	≤50 mGy
Effective dose per subtracted image (male patient)	≤0.5 mGy

calculated [10]. Detailed attenuation calculations based on anatomical models are weighted by the tissue-weighting factor for each tissue or organ in the path of the beam. The tissue weighting factors are taken from the ICRP Publication 60 [11]. The numbers for the effective dose are about a factor of 50–100 less than those of the skin dose. Conversion factors from skin entry dose to effective dose are given in Table 4.

For example, a skin dose of 50 mGy in a male patient corresponds to an effective dose of 0.5 mGy. The difference in women is due to the large tissue weighting factor for breast tissue.

The parameters for dichromography described in this section are summarized in Table 5.

Line Scan Systems

Worldwide, several line scan systems for dichromography are under development. Only two of these systems – that at the National Synchrotron Light Source (NSLS) [8] and the system NIKOS at HASYLAB [7] – currently allow investigation of patients. The two setups are very similar in principle, and the quality of the resulting images is comparable. As an example, version III of the NIKOS system is shown in Figs. 4 and 5. The components of the NIKOS III system are described below.

In principle, all line scan systems consist of six main components: (1) a wiggler installed in a storage ring, (2) a two-beam monochromator for the diffraction of the two monochromatic X-ray beams, (3) a safety system, (4) fast scanning device, (5) a two-line detector, and (6) a computer system.

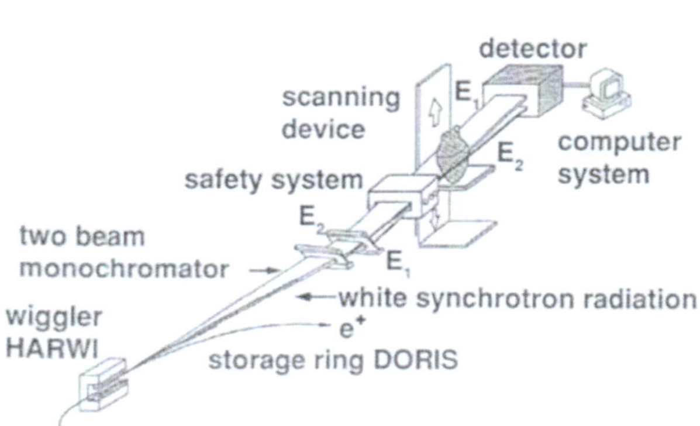

Fig. 4. Experimental setup of the NIKOS III system. E_1 and E_2 are the two mean values of the probing beams (see text for details)

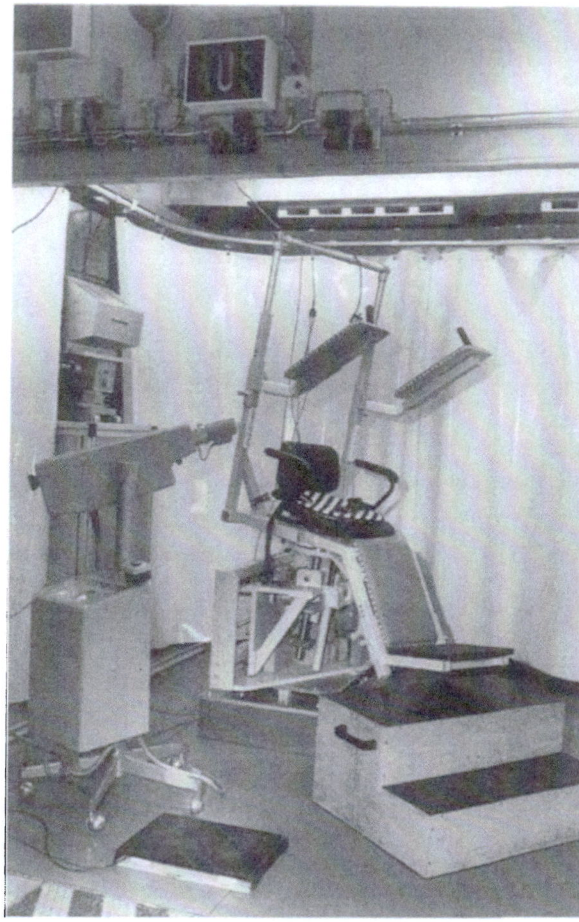

Fig. 5. X-ray cabin

Wiggler

The NIKOS III system is installed in the wiggler beamline W2 of the storage ring DORIS (Doppelring-Speicher) at DESY (Deutsches Elektronen-Synchrotron) in Hamburg. During investigation of patients, DORIS is operated at an energy of 4.5 GeV, with a current of 39–126 mA.

A wiggler is a magnetic structure in a straight part of the storage ring which forces the positrons in the ring on a curved path. Thus the intensity of the synchrotron radiation is enhanced compared to radiation from bending magnets in the ring. The enhancement depends on the number of poles of the wiggler and its magnetic field. The 20-pole wiggler HARWI (Hard X-Ray Wiggler) for NIKOS III [12] has a length 2.4 m plus 0.12 m for the end poles. After installation of a variable vacuum chamber in 1993, the minimal magnetic gap is now 30 mm high and the maximum field strength amounts to 1.26 T. The wiggler was constructed following the hybrid design proposed by Halbach [13]. The permanent-magnet pieces are made from $Co_{17}Sm_2$ (Koermax 200) and the soft-iron pieces from Vacoflux 50. The parameters of the wiggler were chosen to form a strong source of hard X-rays fulfilling the special needs of coronary angiography, i.e., a broad beam and high flux at 33 keV.

The critical energy E_c is given by

$$E_c = 0.665 \times E^2 \times B \tag{7}$$

where E is the energy of the storage ring in GeV and B is the field of the wiggler in tesla. For the above-mentioned conditions, the critical energy is 17.0 keV. E_c is near the optimal value between $1/3 \times E_K$, energy of the K-edge), which is optimal for economic reasons, and $2/3 \times E_K$, which gives minimal heat load [14].

The total power of the wiggler P_{tot} is 4 kW for an I of 100 mA in the storage ring. With 0.2-mm-thick C, 1-mm Be, and 1-mm Al absorbers together with collimators, the power is reduced to 0.6 kW at the entrance of the monochromator.

The horizontal opening angle α with

$$\alpha = \frac{0.955 \times B \times \delta_n}{E} \tag{8}$$

is 6.4 mrad. The periodical length of the wiggler (δ_n) is 24 cm.

The ratio of photons with an energy of 99 keV in the white synchrotron beam to 33-keV photons of r_2 is 0.019. This ratio is of interest because the presence of the harmonics (66 keV, 99 keV, and 132 keV; see below) degrades the image quality, since these X-rays are far less attenuated by the body and thus contribute to the background (beam hardening).

Monochromator

The two monochromatic X-ray beams are diffracted out of the white synchrotron radiation beam by the monochromator. Perfect Si or Ge crystals are mounted in the monochromator. Following Bragg's law

$$n \times \lambda = 2 \times d \times sin\Theta \tag{9}$$

where d is the lattice plane spacing in the crystal, λ is the wave-length of X-ray photons, and Θ is the reflection angle; 33.17-keV photons (λ = 0.374 Å) and the higher harmonics are diffracted when Θ is 3.42° in Si(111). Thus the beam rises with 6.84° behind the monochromator. Furthermore, the two monochromatic beams with energy E_1 and E_2 differ slightly in angle, causing difficulties in the subtraction of bone structures at the front and at the back of the patient simultaneously.

In the early years of patient investigations, one crystal in Bragg reflection geometry was installed for each monochromatic beam. The two Ge (111) crystals split the white synchrotron radiation beam; one diffracts the X-rays with energy E_1 from the upper part, and the other those with energy E_2 from the lower part. The crystals are cut asymmetrically in order to increase the flux. Nevertheless, the flux was insufficient for human imaging when the parameters given in Table 5 were used.

Therefore, an entirely new concept for the monochromator was proposed [15]. This dual-energy bent-crystal monochromator in Laue transmission geometry allows focusing providing efficient use of the white synchrotron radiation beam. Calculations based on a lamellar model of a Laue crystal predicted that a bent Si(111) crystal could provide about a factor of 10 more photons at the iodine K-edge than Bragg reflection geometry. These theoretical predictions were confirmed with the first test installations.

The NIKOS system employs two crystals in the transmission geometry at slightly different Bragg angles to create the two beams of different energies [16]. The Si crystals are double-T shaped and cut asymmetrically. An angle of asymmetry of 35.26° with the (111) reflection is used. The crystals are installed in a He-filled housing. Their thin, central diffracting parts are 0.5 mm thick, 12 mm high, and 113 mm wide. The thick upper and lower bars with a cross-section of 4.5×5.5 mm^2 make the crystals rigid in the horizontal direction and provide efficient cooling. The bottom bar is glued onto a water-cooled copper block and the top bar onto a cooling tube that also carries one lever spring at each side to allow for vertical bending. With a bending radius of 10.3 m, the two diffracted beams are vertically focused to the patient sitting 3.8 m behind the monochromator. In front of the monochromator, the white synchrotron radiation beam is 1.6–2.6 mm high (see below). At the patient, the two monochromatic beams are 120 mm wide and 0.5 mm high, and at the detector 1.0 mm high. They have a bandwidth (ΔE) of 190–270 eV and an energy separation (δE) of 325 eV. The two monochromatic beams must be completely separate in the detector. Therefore, the beams cannot cross within the patient, but about 50 cm in front, leading to an undesired vertical separation of the two beams at the patient.

The flux was measured to be 3.3×10^{11} photons/($mm^2\times s$) for 90-mA current in the storage ring DORIS. The maximal current in DORIS has been increased continuously and now reaches 120 mA; a current of 200 mA is foreseen. Therefore, the system is no longer the limiting factor for the intensity as before; instead, the limiting factor is now the upper limit of the radiation dose to the patient at 2.7×10^{11} photons/($mm^2\times s$). The flux is adjusted to this number by reduction in the height of the white synchrotron radiation beam at the entrance of the monochromator.

For the Ge (111) reflection at the iodine *K*-edge, the harmonic at 66 keV is suppressed, but the harmonics at 99 keV and at 132 keV can still be identified. Therefore, a substantial effort has been expended to understand the effects of the harmonics and to develop algorithms to remove them from images.

Safety System

The most obvious of the safety concerns is the radiation dose to the patient. For a standard scan with the parameters given in Table 5, a dose rate of 64 Gy/s was estimated. For this reason, a safety system with redundancy is indispensable.

The monochromator is installed in a separate room in front of the room with the scan seat. The rooms are lead shielded, and the white beam is stopped in a water-cooled tungsten absorber within the monochromator. Therefore, only the monochromatic beams can enter the room where the patient is investigated.

Two main risks have to be considered whenever a patient is exposed to the beam:

1. The monochromator can drift to lower energies, thereby increasing the dose rate due to stronger absorption and the increasing flux in the spectrum.
2. The scanning device can move at a slower speed than allowed.

The monochromatic beams have to pass two slits and three fast shutters within the safety system. Therefore, small changes in the vertical angle and, correspondingly, in the energy by more than 200 eV result in a complete annihilation of the beams. An increased dose rate due to stronger absorption is impossible.

A possible change in the scanning speed remains the main hazard during the exposure. The speed is permanently measured by two angular encoders which are coupled to the moving part of the scanning device. The pulses generated by these encoders reset continuously running time counters. If the time between subsequent pulses is too long, two fast-beam shutters are activated, which close the beamline within less than 9 ms. The fast-beam shutter is composed of two bars made of tantalum which form a 4-mm slit. A rotation of the bars will close the two monochromatic beams simultaneously. The energy for closing the shutter in an emergency is stored in a preloaded spring, released by an electromagnet. A third identical beam shutter is closed and opened under computer control by a bidirectional turning magnet.

During human study runs, the shutters are also closed if the patient rises from the scan seat, or if the physician leaves the podium he has to stand on if he wishes to stay in the X-ray cabin. (The physician can choose whether to be with the patient in the cabin or remain outside.)

The skin entry dose to the patient has to be measured with TLD on the chest of each patient. The measurements of the ionization chambers in the safety system are only used to predict the dose. The physician has to confirm the dose before the investigation is begun.

Scan Seat

For the line scan mode, a fast-scanning device is needed. The installed device can move loads of up to 300 kg over a distance of 20 cm with constant speed up to 50 cm/s. The total lift of 40 cm of the device includes another 20 cm for acceleration and deceleration. During human study runs in 1995, the scanning device ran with 45–50 cm/s. Its moving force is generated by a hydraulic system with proportional valves controlled by the computer.

The scanning device is equipped with a seat for the patient. The seat allows a patient rotation of $\pm180°$ about the vertical axis and $\pm20°$ about the lateral axis in order to set the appropriate projection angles. It has been designed to scan the patient with raised arms in order to ease the flow of the contrast agent and to avoid overlap problems with the arms in extreme projection angles. The arms rest on pads where the ECG cables and tubes for the injection pump can be fixed. For a precise positioning of the patient, a light frame is projected onto the patient's body indicating the irradiated area, and the seat can be adjusted (motor-driven) vertically and horizontally relative to this area.

During the vertical scan of the patient, a precise optical scale triggers the readout of the detector.

The spatial distance of the trigger signals is selectable and set to 0.4 mm. Thus the vertical pixel size in the images is defined. As the scan seat moves continuously, the pixels are smeared out in a vertical direction. Thus the vertical resolution is decreased.

The motion of the seat is started 6–24 s after injection of the contrast agent, depending on the transit time of the patient. The start is ECG triggered, which allows physicians to take images in particular phases of the heart. The seat moves up and down once. One image is performed in each direction. The time interval between the two images (center of the image of the first scan to the center of the second) depends on the velocity of the seat and varies from 1.3 to 2.0 s depending on the scan speed.

Detector

A two-line detector is installed which simultaneously records the two lines with the energy above and below the *K*-edge, respectively. Simultaneous image acquisition is critical to avoid artifacts in the subtraction process. The detector integrates current rather than counting individual photons.

The detector is a fast, low-noise ionization chamber [5, 17, 18]. It has a common drift cathode and for each line a Frisch grid and ^{336}Cu strips as anodes. The 17-μm-thick and 55-mm-long Cu strips are directed along the monochromatic beams. The center-to-center distance of the strips is 0.4 mm, thus defining the horizontal pixel size in the images. These components are embedded in an aluminum pressure vessel, holding the conversion gas at 13 bar. The chamber is filled with 90% Kr gas and 10% CO_2. The 0.5-mm-thick entrance window is made of carbon fiber imbedded in a polyimide matrix. In front of it, a collimator is mounted with two slits of 2.65-mm vertical height each; the center-to-center distance of the slits is 3.65 mm.

The ionization current of each strip is summed up in resettable integrators whose output is transferred in parallel into sample-and-hold registers and afterwards digitized with two 16-bit VME ADC (Analogic DVX 2503) per line. The readout time per line is 0.73 ms.

The dynamic range of the complete detector system was measured to be 39 000:1 (gain 1). The detective quantum efficiency (DQE) of the complete system

$$\mathrm{DQE} = \frac{(SNR_{OUT})^2}{(SNR_{IN})^2}$$

(where SNR_{OUT} is the SNR in the images, SNR_{IN} the SNR in front of the detector, and $(\mathrm{SNR}_{IN})^2$ is the number of photons per pixel) depends on the electronic noise and on the Poisson statistics. It is determined from the noise in the energy images. For 300 000 photons per pixel, the DQE corresponds to a quantum efficiency (QE) for 33-keV photons of 80%; for 20 000 photons per pixel, a DQE of 56% was measured.

The point spread function (PSF) was measured at 0.43 mm (FWHM) for 90% Xe and 10% CO_2 at 10 bar. The modulation transfer function (MTF) is the Fourier transform of the $(\mathrm{PSF})^2$ and gives the resolution of the detector. The calculation gives a MTF of 0.1 at 1 line pair/mm (lp/mm). Up to 4×10^6 photons/ms, no deviation from linearity within $\pm0.5\%$ was observed. A remarkable nonlinearity due to saturation effects in the detector was observed for incident photon fluxes higher than 2.4×10^7 photons/(ms × pixel).

Computer System

The computer system consists of a VAX station 3500 for the coordination of the computer system and for data acquisition. An Alphastation 400 4/233 is used for image processing and presentation, and a PDP 11/73 for control of all the components of the system via CAMAC. The data from the detector is stored in a VME buffer and, after the scans are finished, transmitted to the computer via a FDDI glass fiber link with a transfer rate of 1.1 Mbaud.

Image processing is carried out using Interactive Display Language [19], a commercial image display and processing system.

Clinical Experience

The first human study on coronary angiography after intravenous injection using dichromography with synchrotron radiation was performed in 1986 at the Stanford Synchrotron Radiation Laboratory (SSRL) [20]. The project was moved to the NSLS in Brookhaven, where the first human images were obtained in 1990. So far another 21 patients have been investigated in this facility.

In 1990, human studies were initiated at the HASYLAB using the NIKOS system. A total of 76 investigations of patients have since been performed in Hamburg.

In the beginning, the work on the two systems concentrated on optimizing hardware and software. The quality of the first human images was not suitable for clinical routine evaluations. Thus, in addition to tests of the performance of the different components in the systems, the primary goals have been to establish the imaging parameters, such as the injection parameters and the projection angles, and the medical protocol necessary to obtain clinically useful data. Steady improvements in the imaging hardware and software have occurred. A remarkable increase in image quality has since been achieved, especially since the installation of the bent Laue monochromator at the NSLS and of version III of the NIKOS system in the middle of 1993. The systems in Hamburg and Brookhaven have now reached a level of imaging technology which will allow physicians to begin to develop medical research programs.

Procedure

The procedures for investigation of a patient start with a complete, computer-controlled system check. The check includes hardware tests, calibration of the monochromator, measurements of offset and fixed pattern noise in the detector, safety system tests, and determination of the background due to radiation in the X-ray cabin. Meanwhile, the physician prepares the patient and plans the projections to be imaged. In general, two views per investigation are planned in order to examine various coronary arteries.

The patient is then placed on the scan seat and aligned to the beam by the physician with the aid of a light frame. Each investigation is started with a positioning run with reduced dose. By a set of attenuators and with a velocity of the scan seat which is determined by the current in the storage ring, a reduced skin dose to the patient (of 15 mGy) is prepared. Just before the injection of the contrast agent with 370 mg iodine/ml, the transit time of the patient is measured. Then a total of 5–10 ml contrast agent is injected at 15–22 ml/s. Depending on the measured transit time, the patient's seat starts moving up. As long as the field of interest of 12.5×12.5 cm^2 are moving through the monochromatic beams, the fast-beam shutters are opened. The seat then returns to its original position. The shutters are not opened while the seat moves down, because only one image is taken for the positioning run. With the help of this image, the physician in charge verifies that the anatomy of interest is in the image field. Furthermore, on the base of the data from this run, the speed for the seat without attenuators in the final investigation run is determined in order to keep the skin dose below the limit of 50 mGy per image. In 1995, this speed varied during our investigations between 38 and 50 cm/s.

After eventual correction of the patient's position and a second measurement of the transit time, the investigation run with two scans is started. The contrast agent (20–30 ml) is injected at a rate of 15–22 ml/s into the venous system; in the first patients, this was usually done via a 7F catheter into the superior vena cava, and during recent human study runs in 82% of cases it was injected into the brachial vein via a 7F introducer sheath. The injection volumes and rates are under the careful control of the physicians.

The time between the positioning run and the investigation run is about 10 min in order to allow for the iodine contrast agent to be cleared. Otherwise, the high iodine background would degrade the image quality. For the same reason, the time between two investigation runs must be at least 30 min. This break can be used for an imaging session of another patient.

Projection Angles

Inherent in coronary angiography after intravenous injection of the contrast medium is the superposition of parts of the coronary arteries on larger structures such as the left chambers and the aorta and, depending on the length of the contrast agent bolus, the pulmonary veins. To overcome or at least minimize this problem and to obtain a clear presentation of all parts of the coronary artery, projection angles for the investigation of patients must be found where the artery of interest is projected over a low-contrast background.

In one study, 22 human hearts excised in toto between the first and third day after death were imaged under different angles [21]. It was demonstrated that it is possible to visualize the right coronary artery (RCA) completely without superposition. The best projection angles should be left anterior oblique (LAO) 40° with a caudo-cranial (CC) 20° tilt. For the left anterior descending artery (LAD), an optimal projection angle of RAO 40° with a CC 20° tilt was found. In about 80% of cases, the LAD can be completely imaged without superposition. While for the visualization of the RCA the diastole of the left ventricle is preferable, for the LAD systole is better. The study also demonstrated that it is difficult to visualize the left main stem and the proximal part of the circumflex coronary artery (Cx) clear of other iodine-containing structures. In most cases, the left main stem is superposed on the aorta or left atrium and part of the Cx on the left atrium or left ventricle.

All these findings were confirmed in principle by studies on humans in Hamburg and Brookhaven. The LAO view is excellent for the entire RCA and, as the bolus dilutes, for the left main stem. In Hamburg, an LAO angle of 20°-60° is employed, and in Brookhaven 40°-60°. For the LAD, the RAO view is the standard projection angle. In Hamburg, an RAO angle of 30°-60° and a CC angle of -10° to 10°, and in Brookhaven a RAO angle of 30°-35° are used.

A third view was introduced by the team in Stanford, i.e., the left lateral (LL) projection. This projection allows the visualization of the RCA and LAD at the same time, but in some cases the RCA is superposed on the left ventricle. At the moment when the bolus dilutes, the Cx becomes much more visible.

In addition, in all images the left interior mammary (LIMA) and the right interior mammary arteries (RIMA) could be seen very easily. Some images also show the intercostal arteries.

Transit Time

It is difficult and in some cases impossible to distinguish between coronary arteries and pulmonary veins if only one image per injection of contrast material exists. Identification of these vessels is much easier if a sequence of images is recorded, because the contrast material enters and leaves these vessels at different times. On the other hand, it is not possible to take a long sequence of images after the injection of the contrast material because of the dose per image. Therefore, as a compromise, two images per injection are recorded (at the NSLS, two or three).

In order to minimize the superposition of the coronary arteries on larger structures and pulmonary veins, the bolus of the contrast medium must be as short as possible. A chance then exists that at least the pulmonary veins are free of iodine when the coronary arteries are opacified. However, a short bolus means that the scan of the patient must be started at the optimal time, which depends on the circulation time of the patient. Studies in humans have shown that the transit times, i.e., the time between injection of the contrast agent and its arrival in the coronary arteries, of different patients can vary from 6.8 to 24.6 s. The values depend on the pulse rate of the patient and the cardiac output, which can in some cases change dramatically during the imaging procedure. These changing transit times can influence the quality of the images because the time interval for optimal images is small.

For the RCA in LAO projection, the images must be taken at a Δt of 1 s after the arrival of the contrast agent in the coronary arteries; 2 s later the image quality is no longer satisfactory. For the LAD in RAO projection, a Δt of 2 s is preferable. There are small differences in Δt, depending on whether coronary arteries or aortocoronary venous bypasses (CABC) need to be imaged. For the Cx and the main stem, a Δt of 4 s is a good value, because these vessels are best visualized if the bolus of iodine is more diluted in the large structures such as aorta and ventricles. More experience is necessary before reliable numbers for Δt in relation to projection and coronary arteries can be given. Nevertheless, the exact transit time is of great importance.

Therefore, in the NIKOS system this time is measured with a dye just before each run is started. For this purpose, 5 ml Cardio Green is injected via the same catheter or introducer sheath as used for the contrast agent. With the use of a sensor at the patient's ear and a densitometer, the time between injection of the solution and its arrival in the ear is determined. The measured time corresponds to the transit time.

This procedure has allowed the scan to be recorded at the optimal time in about 70% of cases. More experience with this method will improve this result.

Intravenous Angiograms

Images obtained with NIKOS or at the NSLS have shown a wide range of coronary artery morphologies. Normal arteries have been visualized as well as completely occluded ones or arteries with residual lesions following percutaneous luminal coronary angioplasty (PTCA). Three examples are presented here. Figure 6 shows an intravenous angiogram of a 57-year-old male patient with a body weight of 99 kg.

The image was taken in LAO 60°/CC 7° projection. The scan was started 11.0 s after the contrast agent injection. Thirty milliliters of contrast agent (370 mg iodine/ml) were injected at a rate of 20 ml/s via a 7F pigtail catheter into the superior vena cava. The patient was scanned at a velocity of 50 cm/s

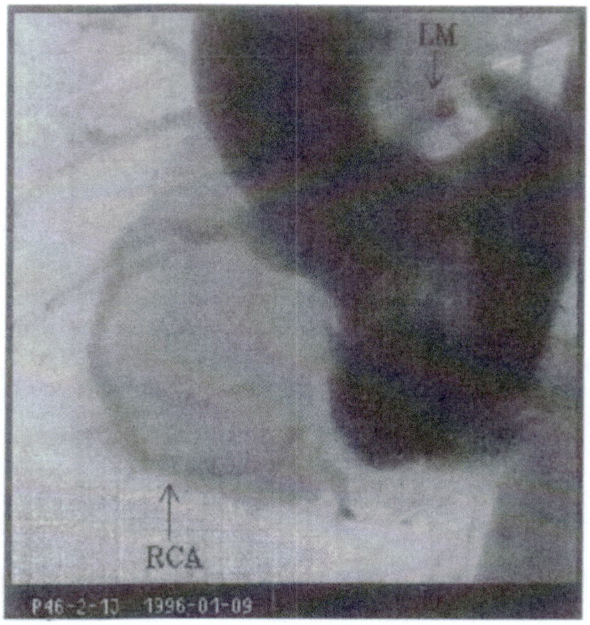

Fig. 6. Intravenous angiogram of the right coronary artery (*RCA*) in left anterior oblique (LAO) 60°/caudocranial (CC) 7° projection. (For parameters, see text) *LM*, Left main stem RCA, Right coronary artery

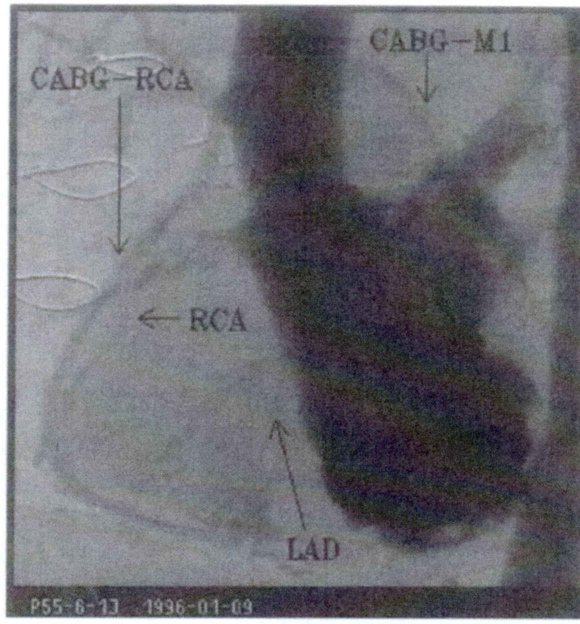

Fig. 7. Intravenous angiogram of vein grafts to the right coronary artery (*RCA*) and marginal branch (*M1*) in left anterior oblique (LAO) 60°/caudocranial (CC) 7° projection. *CABG*, coronary artery bypass graft; *LAD*, left anterior descending artery. (For parameters, see text)

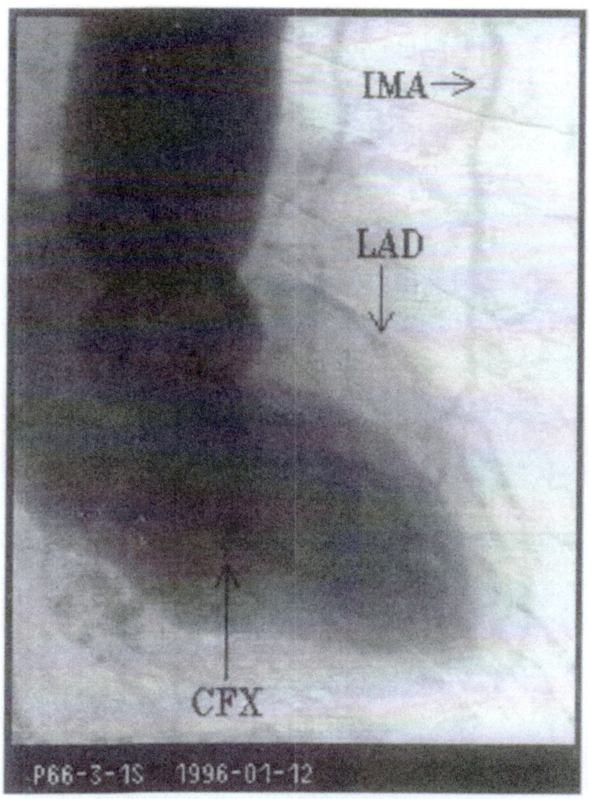

Fig. 8. Intravenous angiogram of the left anterior descending coronary artery (*LAD*) in right anterior oblique (RAO) 60° projection. *IMA*, internal mammary artery; *CFX*, circumflex coronary artery. (For parameters, see text)

corresponding to 0.25 s per image. The machine current in the storage ring was 97 mA. This results in a measured skin entry dose of 50 mGy per image in a field of 12.5×12.5 cm^2, corresponding to an effective dose of 0.5 mGy. The pulse rate of the patient was 82/min. The angiogram clearly shows the RCA, left main stem, and parts of left atrium (LA), left ventricle (LV), aorta, and pulmonary veins.

The second example (Fig. 7) shows the intravenous angiogram of a 58-year-old man (71 kg). The image was taken in LAO 60°/CC 7° projection 16.4 s after the injection. The speed of the scan seat was 49 cm/s. The machine current was 86 mA, and the pulse rate of the patient 69/min. The other parameters for the imaging session were identical to those in the first example.

The angiogram shows the RCA (occluded), LAD (superposed), vein grafts to RCA and marginal branch (M1), parts of the LA, LV, aorta, and pulmonary veins, and the wire structures (WS) of the intervention.

In the third example (Fig. 8), the intravenous angiogram of a 68 year-old woman with a body weight of 68 kg is presented. The image was taken in RAO 60° projection. The scan was started 10.3 s after the contrast agent injection. A total of 20 ml of contrast agent was injected at a rate of 15 ml/s via a 7F introducer sheath into the brachial vein. The patient was scanned at a velocity of 50 cm/s. The machine current in the storage ring was 108 mA. This results in a measured skin entry dose of 50 mGy, corresponding to an effective dose of 1.0 mGy. The pulse rate of the patient was 88/min. The angiogram shows the LAD, internal mammary artery (IMA), and parts of the LA, LV, aorta, and pulmonary veins.

Image Processing

After a scan has been completed, the raw data is transferred to the workstation for display and any desired image enhancement. The image data is corrected for the offset and dark current and normalized with the calibration file taken prior to the patient run. With the calibration file, the pixel-to-pixel variations (fixed pattern noise) are removed. In addition, imperfections of the seat movement are corrected; these are measured during the scan with the help of a precise optical scale and a fast clock. The results are high- and low-energy images. An example is given in Fig. 9, in which the energy images of the subtraction image in Fig. 6 are presented.

Once these corrections and normalizations have been done, the two energy images are subtracted logarithmically, a process which is identical to a division of the two images. During this operation, the two images have to be shifted relative to each other in the vertical and/or horizontal direction. A vertical shift is necessary if the two beams do not cross exactly at the arteries of interest. The system gives the opportunity to determine the value for the shift interactively in order to minimize the artifacts from edges of the ribs at the front and at the back of the patient at the same time. The subtraction is very sensitive to this shift. There can even be a different shift in the same patient and the same system parameters but a different projection angle. A horizontal shift can occur if the two beams have a small horizontal relative divergence, as the beams are produced by two crystals.

The subtraction images are produced instantaneously within a few seconds and are displayed for interpretation by the physician. They serve as a basis for the decision as to how the investigation of the patient should proceed.

In most cases, the resulting subtraction image is presented with a linear scale (Figs. 6–8). Sometimes, the visibility of the coronary arteries is enhanced by a nonlinear gray value transformation, such as a logarithmic or square-root operation or histogram equalization. These transformations, together with further parameters such as positive or negative images or gray level adjustment, can be changed interactively by the physician in order to optimize interpretation of the images. There are no

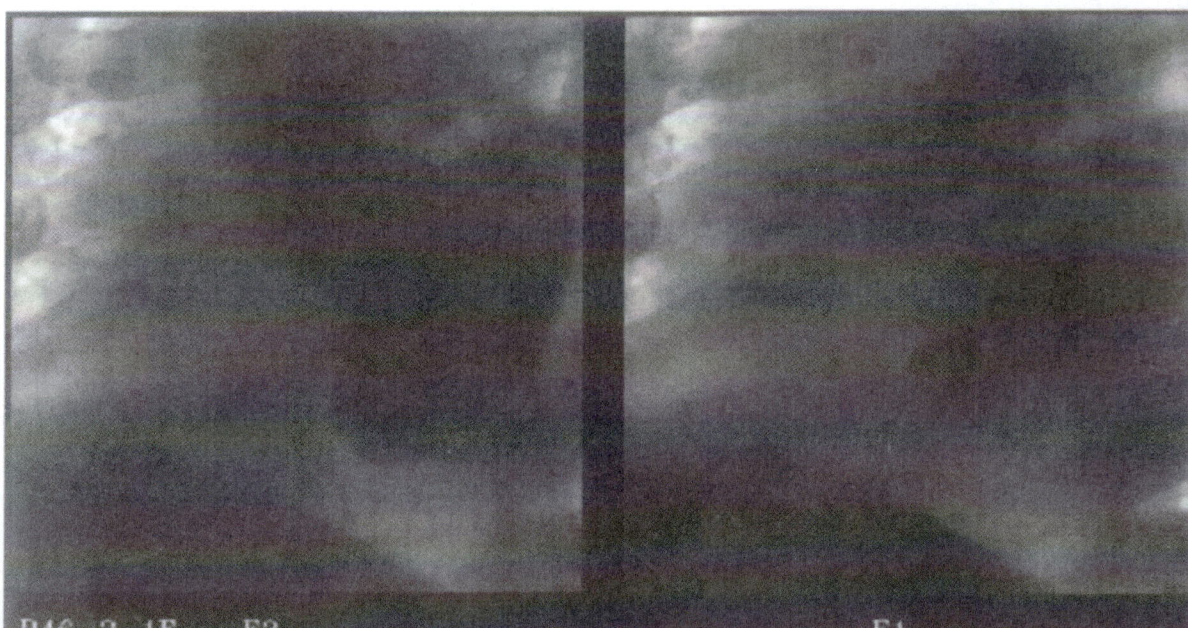

Fig. 9. Energy images of the iodine image in Fig. 6. *Left*, image with energy above the *K*-edge of iodine; *right*, energy below the *K*-edge

fixed rules for the best presentation, because it may change from patient to patient depending on the projection angle, the anatomy of the patient, and the physician's preference.

Iodine Images

The present goal of dichromography is to enable quantitative analysis of the coronary arteries. To this end, an image with the mass density of the iodinated arteries is necessary. This iodine image (Figs. 6, 7) is not identical to the subtraction image (Fig. 8) because of the superposition of different tissues in the projection angiography.

The team at the NSLS mainly developed algorithms for the extraction of the iodine image from the energy images [22, 23]. Since there are two signals which are simultaneously measured, one from a beam above and one from a beam below the *K*-edge, two different mass densities can be calculated for each pixel. One of the images can be iodine and the other can be "water." The "water" image actually contains information on bone and other tissue, even though the absorption coefficients are different. The analysis procedures for the calculation of iodine images include corrections for different detector efficiency below and above the *K*-edge, detector cross-talk from line to line, spurious background signals from other body tissue, and, most importantly, corrections for beam harmonics. The harmonic signal can add significant background to the high- and low-energy images which increases the noise in the absolute iodine image. A large percentage of the detector signal is due to harmonics of the fundamental due to beam hardening in the patient. As any algorithm for removing the artifacts due to harmonics may introduce errors, thus degrading the quantitative results, the systems are optimized in such a way that contamination in the monochromatic beams due to harmonics is as small as possible. Detailed analysis in progress in Brookhaven shows that, for an average-sized patient, the harmonics cause errors in the absolute iodine calculations.

From the iodine mass density image, the relative arterial cross-sectional area can be determined by a line integral across the artery. In general, the values along an artery will be relative. However, under the assumption that the artery has a circular cross-section, the concentration ϱ_I of iodine at a selected position in the artery can be calculated from the subtraction image following the formula

$$\varrho_I = -\frac{\ln S_I S_o}{\Delta\mu \times \Delta x} \tag{10}$$

where S_I ist the signal of the iodine, S_o is the signal of the surroundings of the artery, $\Delta\mu$ is the difference in the linear absorption coefficient at the *K*-edge of iodine, and Δx is the diameter of the artery.

One of the severe limitations of projection angiography is that it is not possible to distinguish a change in the apparent measured cross-sectional area from a change in the angle of the artery relative to the viewing field. Stereoscopic systems [23] might be able to overcome this problem.

A great advantage for analysis is the venous injection technique, which allows uniform mixing of iodine in the blood and provides uniform opacification of the coronary arteries. Except in a few cases in which a subtotal stenosis delays the flow, the concentration everywhere in the heart and the arteries will be the same.

Filter Methods

Because it is essential that all coronary arteries can be imaged, additional image-processing methods must be used to visualize those parts of the coronary arteries which are superposed on large iodinated structures such as the aorta and heart chambers. The main problem is to visualize the proximal part of the Cx superposed on the LV.

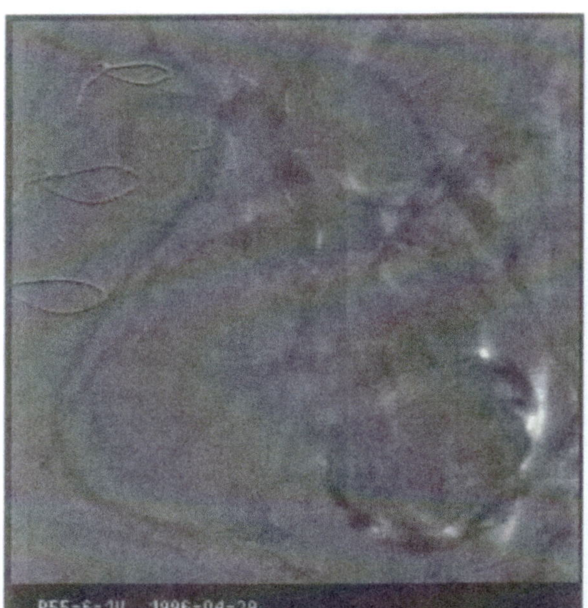

Fig. 10. Unsharp masking image of the iodine image in Fig. 7

A simple but powerful method is the unsharp masking technique. In the first step, the subtraction image is corrected with a wide-range median filter (radius, ρ20 pixels). In the second step, the original subtraction image is divided by the median filtered image. Thus the large structures such as the aorta, LV, and large pulmonary veins are suppressed and small structures are enhanced. Figure 10 shows the unsharp masking images of the iodine image in Fig. 7.

With the unsharp masking method, it is not difficult to see small structures in front of large, thin structures such as the aorta. Unfortunately, the LV is a structured chamber and is not smooth like the aorta. Therefore, an iterative median filter algorithm is necessary to find the optimal filter size for a given Cx.

Edge detection filters such as Laplace or Sobel operators can enhance the arteries of interest but also, for example, the artifacts from ribs. Thus in most cases these filters produce confusing images which are largely uninterpretable. More sophisticated algorithms such as different edge-preserving smoothing methods must be applied to the images. They currently work with phantom images, but are not yet used for images in human study runs.

Summary and Outlook

A further increase in image quality without an increase in the radiation dose to the patient is of great clinical importance. To accomplish this goal, changes in the hardware will be required. An upgraded patient's seat and more powerful computer hardware (VME) for system control will be installed by the end of 1996. More work is still necessary to optimize the functional parameters of the detector, including lower noise, a higher dynamic range, and increased DQE. New sophisticated readout electronics has already been developed for this purpose. The improved parameters will increase the SNR in the images.

Better subtraction images should be available after minimizing contamination due to higher harmonics in the beam.

Many additional details will be improved in the system. However, all these improvements (except the detector electronics) are not expected to increase image quality as much as improvements in hardware during recent years obviously have done. They will mainly increase the reproducibility and stability of the setup, which is an important point in systems that are used for studies in humans.

More gain in image quality is expected from software than from hardware. Work on image processing will be intensified. With new algorithms for edge-preserving smoothing and other contrast enhancement techniques, corrections for higher harmonics in the monochromatic beams, system-dependent corrections, advanced methods for presentation of images, among others, a higher image quality should be achieved. As a result, the quantification of arterial lesions should become possible.

Though the work on hardware and software must be continued over the coming years and will demand great effort, the quality of images from the two systems in Brookhaven and Hamburg, already allows clinical decisions. Therefore, the main aspect of the work within the next 2–3 years will be optimization of the parameters for the investigation of patients without degradation of image quality.

The following parameters will be evaluated in detail.

1. The best projection angles for imaging of all coronary arteries with a minimum of superposition on large iodinated structures
2. The best-suited phase of the heart cycle for the images
3. The optimum scan time relative to the measured transit time, depending on projection angle and coronary artery of interest
4. The image acquisition rate, depending on projection angle and coronary artery of interest
5. The minimum volume of contrast agent
6. The maximum rate for injection of contrast agent in order to obtain a short bolus
7. The effect of injecting into the brachial vein instead of the superior vena cava
8. The dependence of the image quality on the X-ray flux in order to determine the minimum dose

The aim of determining these parameters and effects is to visualize all three main coronary arteries including their branches down to those 1 mm in diameter after intravenous injection without a catheter into the brachial vein. Though some effort will be necessary to reach this goal during this first phase of medical research, the benefit to the patient is potentially substantial. Work will concentrate on follow-up after medical interventions to allow noninvasive investigations by intravenous coronary angiography instead of selective coronary angiography.

In a second phase, dichromography will be validated against selective coronary angiography in human studies. As the technology opens up the possibility of doing serial examinations, basic research on the natural history of coronary artery disease and study of the effects of therapeutic interventions will also become possible.

In parallel, new advanced initiatives in technology are underway which promise to advance imaging capabilities even more. Initial tests for the development of a stereoscopic system have been performed [24]. This would allow spatial reconstruction of the vessels and would present a more accurate visualization of the anatomy. A second method to obtain depth information would be to take two consecutive images with the patient orientation changed between them, which will be possible using the new scan seat at the NSLS. Although not truly stereoscopic, this would allow clarification of projection-dependent ambiguities.

The NSLS is to develop a system to gate image acquisition from signals related to the position of the iodine contrast agent bolus in the patient and the ECG. For this purpose, the logarithmically subtracted images must be displayed in real time, with each line being processed and displayed in 1 ms or less. Development of a high-speed optical fiber data, image, and voice link is also planned for communication between the NSLS, the SUNY Health Sciences Center, and other institutions. The team at the European Synchrotron Radiation Facility (ESRF) plan to replace iodine by a different contrast agent with higher *K*-edge in order to reduce the dose to the patient.

Systems for dichromography are now based on storage rings in large laboratories. The method can be validated at these few institutions at existing beamlines. However, in order for the technology to become widespread, and therefore of greater value to the general population, compact sources of X-rays with sufficient flux must be developed. Except for the source itself, all other components of the systems are inexpensive in comparison to routinely used advanced medical equipment, such as magnetic resonance imaging (MRI) or computed tomography (CT) devices. Some Japanese heavy industrial companies are proposing synchrotron radiation facilities for medical applications [25]. These are dedicated storage rings with a diameter of about 13 m. At the NSLS, collaboration [26] has led to the development of another approach, in which X-rays are to be produced with a characteristic line X-ray source driven by a compact, electrostatic electron accelerator. The system includes a rotating anode and a capillary optic.

Much more work needs to be done before this method is established as a routine diagnostic tool in the medical field. We have come a long way since the idea of dichromography was first suggested in 1953, but with the presentation of the first images from clinically relevant human studies, an important milestone has been reached.

References

1. Jacobson, B (1953) Dichromatic absorption radiography, dichromography. Acta Radiol 39: 437–452
2. Graeff W, Dix W-R (1991) NIKOS – non-invasive angiography at HASYLAB. In: Ebashi S, Koch M, Rubenstein E (eds) Handbook on synchrotron radiation, Vol. 4. Elsevier Science, Amsterdam, pp 407–430
3. Thompson AC, Lavender WM, Chapman D, Gmür N, Thomlinson W, Rosso V, Schulze C, Rubenstein E, Giacomini JC, Gordon HJ, Dervan JP (1994) A 1200 element detector system for synchrotron-based coronary angiography. Nucl Instr Meth Phys Res A347: 545
4. Chapman D, Thomlinson W, Gmür NF, Dervan JP, Stavola T, Giacomini J, Gordon H, Rubenstein E, Lavender W, Schulze C, Thompson AC (1995) Effects of spatial resolution and spectral purity on transvenous coronary angiography images. Rev Sci Instr 66(2): 1329–1331
5. Menk RH, Dix W-R, Graeff W, Illing G, Reime B, Schildwächter L, Tafelmeier U, Besch HJ, Großmann U, Langer R, Lohmann M, Schenk HW, Wagener M, Walenta AH, Kupper W, Hamm C, Rust C (1995) A dual line multicell ionization chamber for transvenous coronary angiography with synchrotron radiation. Rev Sci Instr 66(2): 2327–2329
6. Elleaume H (1994) Les applications du rayonnement synchrotron en recherche médicale, Workshop at the ESRF, Grenoble, 4 February 1994, 1/9
7. Dix W-R, Besch HJ, Graeff W, Hamm CW, Illing G, Kupper W, Lohmann M, Meinertz T, Menk RH, Reime B, Rust C, Schildwächter L, Tafelmeier U, Walenta AH (1994) Coronary angiography with synchrotron radiation. J Phys IV C9 (4): 279–286
8. Thomlinson W, Gmür N, Chapman D, Garett R, Lazarz N, Zeman HD, Brown GS, Morrison J, Reiser P, Padmanabhan V, Ong L, Green S, Giacomini J, Gordon H, Rubenstein E (1992) First operation of the medical facility at the NSLS for coronary angiography. Rev Sci Instr 63: 625–628
9. Westerholt R (1983) Strahlenexposition und Strahlenrisiko von Patient und Personal bei der Herzkatheterisierung und Angiokardiographie Erwachsener – Meßergebnisse bei 100 Untersuchungen. Thesis, University of Hamburg
10. Nordstrom E, Gmür N, Chapman D, Collins M, Thomlinson W (1989) Dose rate to human organs from monochromatic synchrotron beams. BNL Informal Report, BNL-43433
11. ICRP Publication 60 (1990) 1990 recommendations of the International Commission on Radiological Protection. Pergamon, New York
12. Graeff W, Bittner L, Brefeld W, Hahn U, Heintze G, Heuer J, Kouptsidis J, Pflüger J, Schwartz M, Weiner EW, Wroblewski T (1989) HARWI – a hard X-ray wiggler beam at DORIS. Rev Sci Instr 60: 1457–1459

13. Halbach K (1983) J Phys 44: C1 - 211
14. Graeff W (1992) Monochromators. Angiography workshop at the ESRF, Grenoble, 28. January 1992, pp 59 - 68
15. Suortti P, Thomlinson W (1988) A bent Laue crystal monochromator for angiography at the NSLS. Nucl Instr Meth Phys Res A269: 639 - 648
16. Illing G, Heuer J, Reime B, Lohmann M, Menk RH, Schildwächter L, Dix W-R, Graeff W (1995) Double beam bent Laue monochromator for coronary angiography. Rev Sci Instr 66(2): 1379 - 1381
17. Besch HJ, Dix W-R, Großmann U, Heuer J, Langer R, Lohmann M, Menk RH, Schenk HW, Tafelmeier U, Wagener M, Walenta AH, Xu HC (1993) A position sensitive multi channel ion chamber (MCIC) for non-invasive coronaxy angiography with synchrotron radiation. Phys Med IX N.(2 -): 171 - 174
18. Besch HJ, Großmann U, Langer R, Schenk HW, Walenta AH, Dix W-R, Heuer J, Graeff W, Illing G, Lohmann M, Menk RH, Schildwächter L, Tafelmeier U, Kupper W (1994) An imaging ionisation chamber for medical application with synchrotron radiation. SPIE 2278: 30 - 38
19. IDL (Interactive Data Language) Reference Guide (1993) Research Systems, Boulder, Colorado
20. Rubenstein E, Hofstadter R, Zeman HD, Thompson AC, Otis JN, Brown GS, Giacomini JC, Gordon HJ, Kernoff RS, Harrison DC, Thomlinson W (1986) Transvenous coronary angiography in human using synchrotron radiation. Proc Natl Acad Sci USA 83: 9724 - 9728
21. Kupper W, Dix W-R, Graeff W, Steiner P, Engelke K, Glüer CC, Bleifeld W (1988) In: Burattini E, Rindi A (eds) Synchrotron radiation applications to digital subtraction angiography (SYRDA). Società Italiana di Fisica, Bologna, pp. 165 - 170
22. Zeman HD, Moulin HR (1992) Removal of harmonic artifacts from synchrotron radiation coronary angiograms. IEEE Trans Nucl Sci 39(5): 1431 - 1437
23. Chapman D, Schulze C (1993) Arterial cross-section measurements from dual energy transvenous coronary angiography images. Nuclear Science Symposium and Medical Imaging Conference, IEEE Conf Rec, pp 1528 - 1532
24. Schulze C (1994) Stereoscopic synchrotron radiation coronary angiography with bent Laue crystal monochromators. Thesis, University of Hamburg
25. Yokomizo H, Yanagida K, Sasaki S, Harami T, Konishi H, Masahiko K, Ashida K, Harada S, Hashimoto H, Iizuka M, Kabasawa M, Nakayama K, Yamada K, Suzuki Y (1989) Construction of compact electron storage ring JSR. Rev Sci Instr 60: 1724 - 1727
26. Gmür NF, Chapman D, Thomlinson W, Scalia K, Malloy N, Mangano J, Jacob J (1994) NSLS transvenous coronary angiography project advanced technology initiatives. Synch Radiat News 7(5): 34 - 36

Three-Dimensional Reconstruction of Coronary Arteries from X-Ray Projections

S. Grosskopf and A. Hildebrand

Introduction

The gold standard for diagnosis of coronary artery disease remains X-ray angiography, recently combined with intravascular ultrasound (IVUS) [13]. The main advantages of this technique are the high spatial and temporal resolution and good image contrast.

The way the information is presented to the cardiologist influences the accuracy and objectivity of the diagnosis and impact on treatment. In order to improve the diagnostic accuracy, three-dimensional reconstruction from two-dimensional coronary angiograms appears desirable [19].

In this chapter, we will review the three-dimensional reconstruction methodology and outline the novel three-dimensional reconstruction prototype system for coronary arteries, CORRECT (*co*ronary *re*cons*t*ruction), which requires coronary arteriography taken from different views by a cinefilm sequence using a rotating monoplane X-ray system. In order to determine the exact phase of the heart cycle for each image, an electrocardiogram (ECG) is recorded simultaneously.

State of the Art

Existing three-dimensional reconstruction methods differ in the degree of user interaction, the number of required images, and the type of a priori anatomic-morphologic knowledge used during the reconstruction. To facilitate an understanding of the existing methods, the basic ideas will be introduced and the differences discussed.

Reconstruction Methodology

In order to reconstruct an arbitrary object from different views, a universal mathematical model has to be found to represent the object for computations.

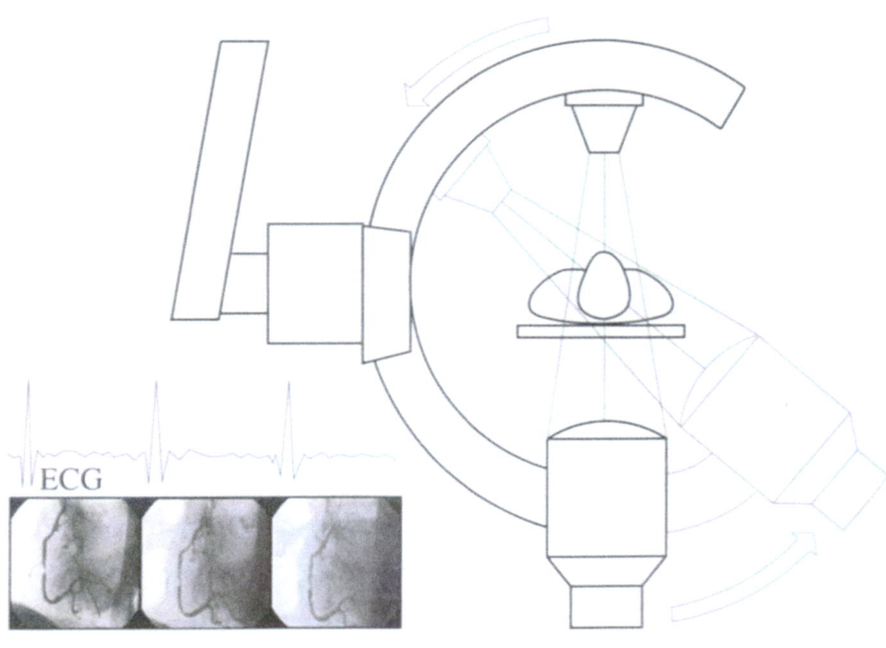

Fig. 1. Image sequence taken during rotation. Simultaneous to the acquisition process, an electrocardiogram (*ECG*) is recorded

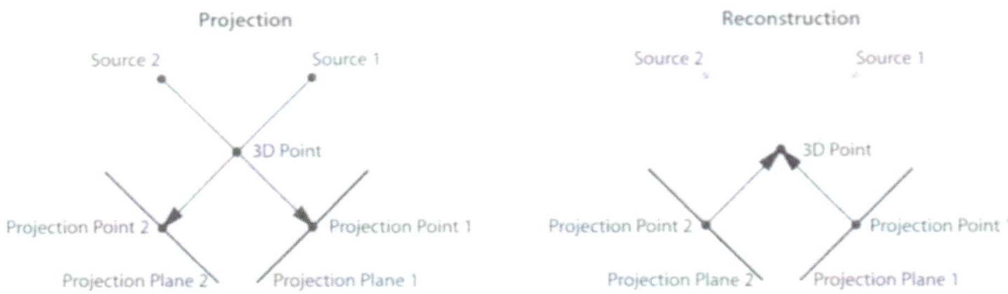

Fig. 2. Reconstruction of a point from two projections

The model may be adapted to an individual object by modification of a set of parameters describing the dimensions, shape, topology, etc. A set of these parameters is denoted as high-level description.

Most models are a collection of a number of primitives, which may be reconstructed individually [4]. By grouping the reconstructed primitives according to the object in the projections, the complete object may be reconstructed. This can only be done under the assumption that the primitives of object do not move in relation to each other, i.e., that the object is rigid.

An example of a simple geometrical primitive is a point. Most objects may be represented by a set of points and their relations, e.g., a cube may be re-pres-
ented by its corner points, which are connected after reconstruction of each individual point. Since the primitive point is important in reconstruction, we will describe the reconstruction of individual points below by way of example.

To reconstruct a point in three-dimensional space from several projections, the same point has to be identified in each of the individual projections. A point in a single projection is projected by a ray leading from the ray's source through the three-dimensional point to the projected point (see Fig. 2). If the position of a source is known, identifiying the point in several projections directly defines the associated rays. The intersection of these rays yields the three-dimensional point.

Since under reality conditions neither the position of the source nor the position of the projected point can be determined without error, the constructed rays normally do not intersect at a single point. The three-dimensional coordinates of the point can only be estimated. The quality of this estimation increases with the number of projections used.

Definition of a Vessel Model

In order to provide a universal mathematical model of the coronary system for computations, due to the morphologic analogy a tree structure has been selected. The root node represents the ostium and each lower node represents a bifurcation.

The vessel sections between two nodes are primitives denoted as segments. The model of the three-dimensional lumen of a vessel segment is divided into further primitives, the centerline and a series of perpendicular slices (Fig. 3). Projected (two-dimensional) vessel segments are described by the centerline and the perpendicular diameters.

As will be discussed below, this model proves to be suitable for reconstruction, since the only points which can be consistently identified and matched in each angiogram are points along the centerline of the vessels.

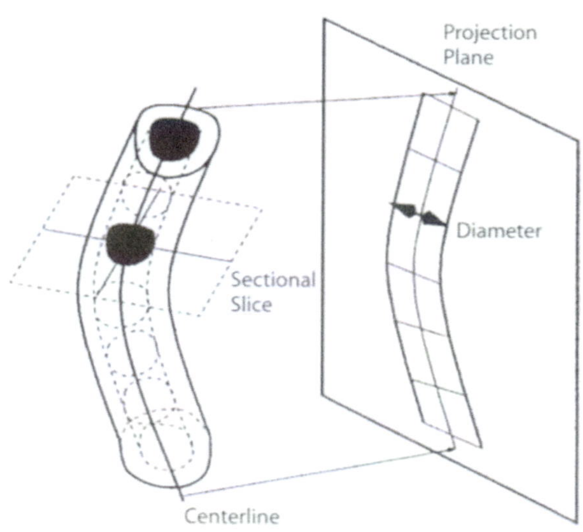

Fig. 3. In three-dimensional representation, a vessel segment is modeled by the centerline and a series of sectional slices, whereas the same vessel segment is represented in two dimensions by a projected centerline and perpendicular diameters

Reconstruction Steps

For the reconstruction of vessels, six tasks are usually performed:

1. Noise reduction
2. Identification of the vessel structure in each view
3. Finding of corresponding vessel segments in different views (matching)
4. Finding of corresponding centerline points in different views
5. Reconstruction of the centerline
6. Reconstruction of the sectional slices

In most cases, preprocessing is included to reduce the noise. The angiograms are then analyzed in order to extract the identical vessel segments from the different projectional images and to build up a high-level description, as defined above.

Reconstruction is performed in two consecutive steps, centerline reconstruction and sectional reconstruction. First, the centerlines of vessel segments are reconstructed, requiring the determination of identical vessel segments, a process denoted as matching (task 3). After the correspondence problem has been solved for the individual segments in all projections, the spatial centerline reconstruction is performed using a number of equidistant points on the projected centerline. To this end, in each view representing the same point of the vessel's centerline in three dimensions has to be identified (task 4). Using the coordinates of these points and the angles between the different projections, the spatial coordinates of the point can be calculated. The spatial centerline is finally obtained connecting the reconstructed three-dimensional points.

The entire process concludes with the reconstruction of the sectional slices from the determined diameters. The problem of a point-based reconstruction of a single slice is that it is ambiguous, since the only points which can be exactly identified in an angiogram are the points delineating the contour of the vessel, i.e. its endothelial edges. An attempt to match these points in different angiograms will fail, since by rotating the X-ray system, new points of the three-dimensional contour of the vessel lumen will appear as contour points in the angiogram. Since the reconstruction problem cannot be solved from the pure input data, i.e., the angiogram, some sort of a priori knowledge is required, as discussed below.

Differences in Application of A Priori Knowledge

For the clinical application of three-dimensional reconstruction methods, a priori anatomic knowledge employed for the reconstruction is crucial and has to be thoroughly defined and evaluated. Two different approaches can be distinguished.

In the first approach (see, e.g., [1, 16, 20]), only a priori knowledge about the morphology of a vessel, e.g., the shape of the sectional slices is considered, whereas in the second approach (see, e.g., [5, 17, 21]) a priori knowledge about the structure and geometry of the coronary system is also considered. The latter approach uses a rule-based system to model the hierarchy, position, and dimensions of the segments and the relative position of the bifurcations.

In the first approach, the user enters a number of points of the entire artery and matches them in different projections interactively, which may be a time-consuming process.

A priori knowledge about the coronary system in the second approach is introduced to recognize and match each vessel segment in the individual views. Recognized subsegments of vessel segments are labeled with their anatomic annotation and grouped into a segment, the matching of segments in different views thus implicitly performed. This approach has the advantage that it requires less user interaction. A major difficulty, however, is posed by the invariance towards pathologic changes of the coronary arteries. For example, complete occlusion of one of the main arteries close to the tree root can prevent correct reconstruction.

Differences in Information Used for Sectional Reconstruction

Another difference lies in the type of information used for sectional reconstruction. While some authors [16, 20] only consider the contours as diameters of the vessels for a geometric reconstruction, others [1] also evaluate the image intensities to reconstruct the sectional slices.

The former assume that the contour points found in an angiogram are in a plane perpendicular to the ray. Using two projections, it is possible to reconstruct the sectional slice as an ellipse, applying the scaled diameters as the main axes. Reconstruction of a sectional slice of a vessel as an ellipse is a valid assumption for approximately 95% of the stenotic vessel segments [3].

In some other approaches, additional information based on the intensity levels of the vessels in angiograms is considered. This approach is called densitometric reconstruction. It is based on the fact that the path of the X-rays through the contrast media-filled vessel lumen correlates with the absorption of X-rays as defined by the Lambert-Beer law. The quality of reconstruction is dependent on the number of projections used and the image quality of the angiograms.

Reconstruction System CORRECT

In order to minimize user interaction and a priori knowledge introduced into the reconstruction process a new method, CORRECT [7], has been developed and implemented.

CORRECT requires a minimum of user interaction, limited to the segmentation of vessels in the initial image of each angiographic sequence. The segmentation result is exploited in the entire series of angiograms to track each individual vessel.

In contrast to the assumption typically made in three-dimensional reconstructions from multiple projections, coronary arteries are not rigid. Due to the deterministic nature of the mobility of the heart with respect to the phase of heart motion, CORRECT uses distinct images, showing the heart at the same phase of the cardiac cycle.

The different processing steps used for reconstructing the three-dimensional geometry of the vessel are shown in Fig. 4 and discussed below.

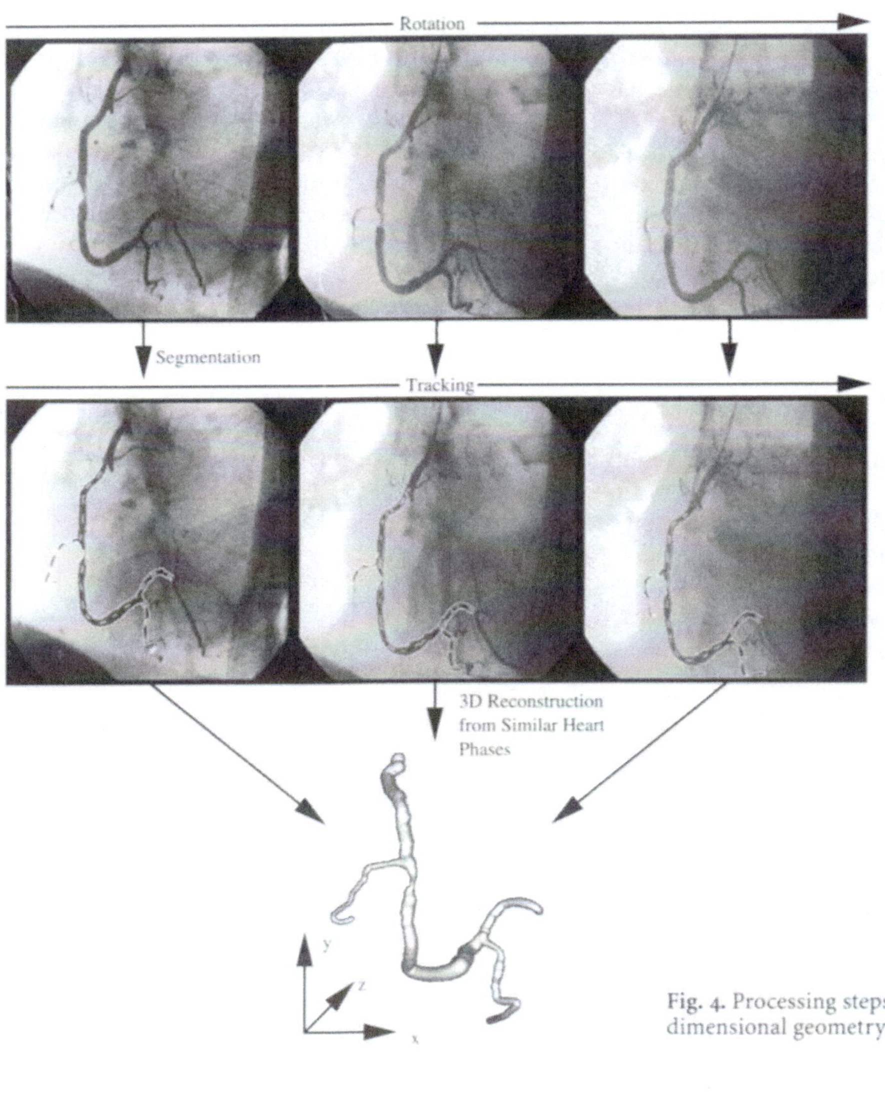

Fig. 4. Processing steps used to reconstruct the three-dimensional geometry of the coronary vessels

Segmentation of Vessel Structure

In order to separate the vessel tree to be reconstructed, the image has to be segmented. The major drawbacks of most of the existing segmentation algorithms are a very limited amount of variation in the input data amenable to processing by a fully automatic algorithm and the necessity of extensive user interaction [2, 8, 10, 15].

CORRECT allows a compromise in which the user only identifies a very small number of points interactively. The segmentation process is separated into two steps: (1) detection of the vessel centerline and (2) evaluation of the vessel contour.

Centerline Detection. Within the initial segmentation step, the centerline of the vessel is detected. This is done by an automatic contour-following algorithm which connects two points given by the user. The algorithm works with a cost-minimizing A^* search tree [14, 18], which proved to be robust against noise and may be fully controlled by the user.

During the definition of the centerlines of a vessel tree, the user marks the bifurcation and the end point of each vessel of interest. The hierarchy of the vessel tree is defined within this step.

Contour Evaluation. After detecting the centerlines of all vessels, the contours need to be extracted. For this purpose, a number of scan lines orthogonal to the centerline are selected. The image intensities of these scan lines are obtained by an equidistant sampling of the scan lines [3].

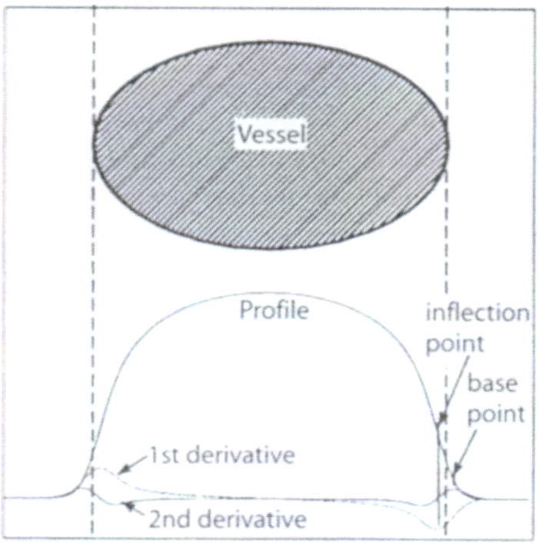

Fig. 5. Projection of a vessel according to the Lambert-Beer law

By a detail analysis of the intensity profiles of the coronary vessels, it has been determined that the border of the vessel can be described by a point which lies between the first and the second derivation of the scan line intensity values (see Fig. 5) [12]. To determine the complete contour, the individual contour points are connected.

Tracking Vessel Structure

Tracking the vessels means adapting the two-dimensional vessel model to each image. Within each tracking step, the centerline of a vessel is represented by a snake. Snakes [11] are curves used for image processing tasks which are able to change shape, driven by quasi-forces of an image (e.g., they may be attracted to contours of an object within an image). An internal tension of the curve is resistant against highly angled curvatures. After a starting position is given for a snake, it is adapted to an image by relaxation to an equilibrium of the force and tension.

The definition of the forces moving the snakes depends on the application area. Within the reconstruction system CORRECT, the centerlines of the two-dimensional vessel models are attracted to areas of the image which are similar to the area of the previous image. The similarity is calculated by a gray level correlation of rectangular areas, centered at the centerline. This approach has to be sound. However, the presence of significant shadows in the background of the vessels may introduce a positioning error in each tracking step (see Fig. 6).

For this reason, each tracking step includes an adjustment [6], made by improving the centerline and the contours. To increase the accuracy of the tracking, a final smoothing process using snakes is applied. The result of the tracking method using adjustment and smoothing is shown in Fig. 7.

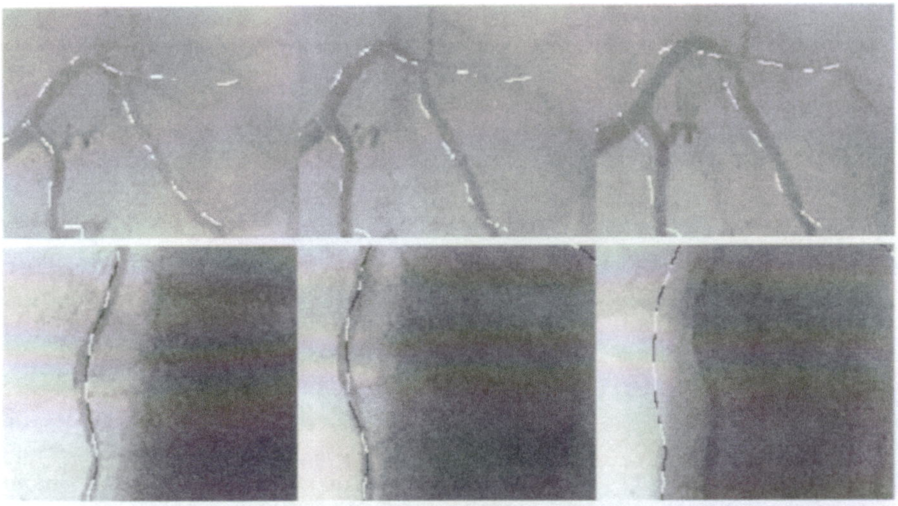

Fig. 6. Tracking by snakes (without adjustment) in two sequencies, each consisting of 15 images (images 4, 8, and 15 are shown)

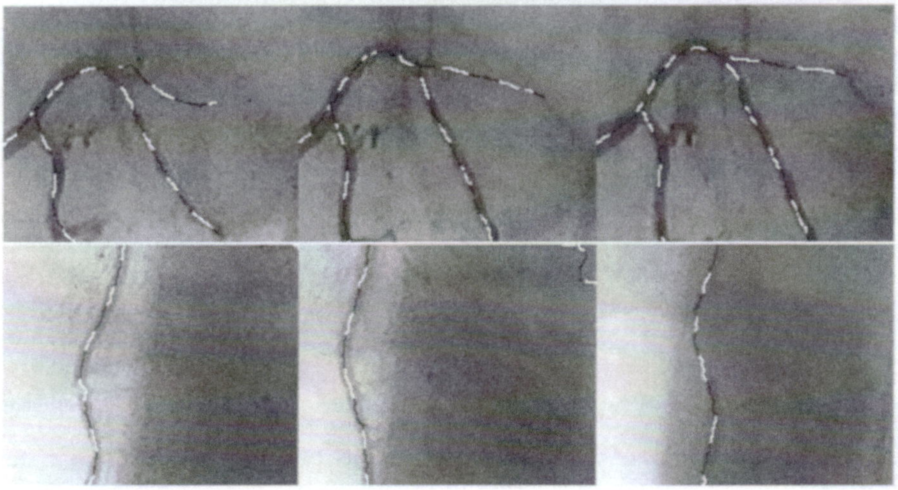

Fig. 7. Tracking in two sequences, each consisting of 15 images (images 4, 8, and 15 are shown)

Reconstruction of the Three-Dimensional Geometry

Reconstruction is based on the extracted vessel tree structures, the known relative orientation (i.e., the angle) of the projections, and the imaging parameters of the X-ray system. Three-dimensional reconstruction is performed from images of identical heart phases. It begins with two projections of the same phase, defining the largest angle.

Within the first step of reconstruction, centerline points of the two projections have to be matched. Artery segments have already been matched in the process of tracking. To match single curve points of the centerline, these points are moved along the curve, minimizing the distance between the rays which projected these points into the image plane. For this purpose the rays are projected into the projection plane of the other projection. The projection is called the epipolar line.

For each pair of matched points, a three-dimensional point can be obtained algebraically [4] from the point which is defined by finding a point close to both rays, ideally their intersection.

In the next step, this first reconstruction result is refined, considering additional projections. Within this step, the distance of the projected points to the centerline of all considered projections is minimized. Figure 8 shows examples of projected centerlines before and after refinement.

Reconstruction is completed by sectional reconstruction scaling the diameters of the two-dimensional vessel description according to depth. The scaled diameters are used to reconstruct the sectional slices as ellipses of the three-dimensional description.

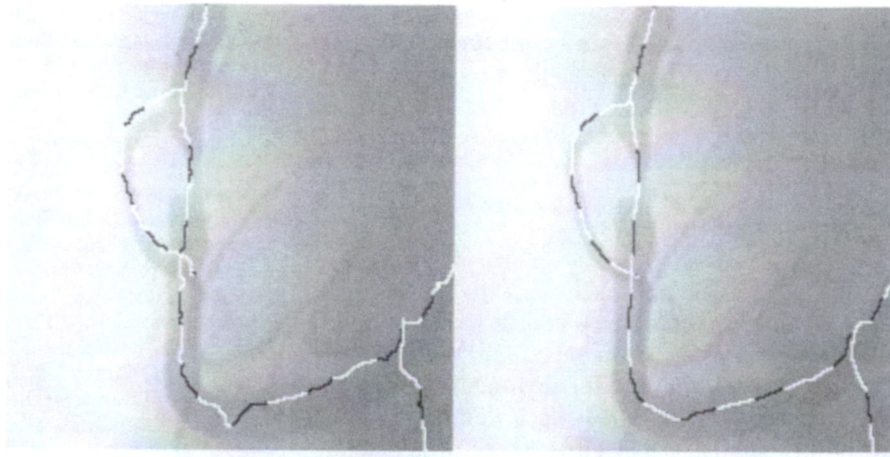

Fig. 8. Projection of the reconstruction result before (*left*) and after (*right*) refinement by snakes

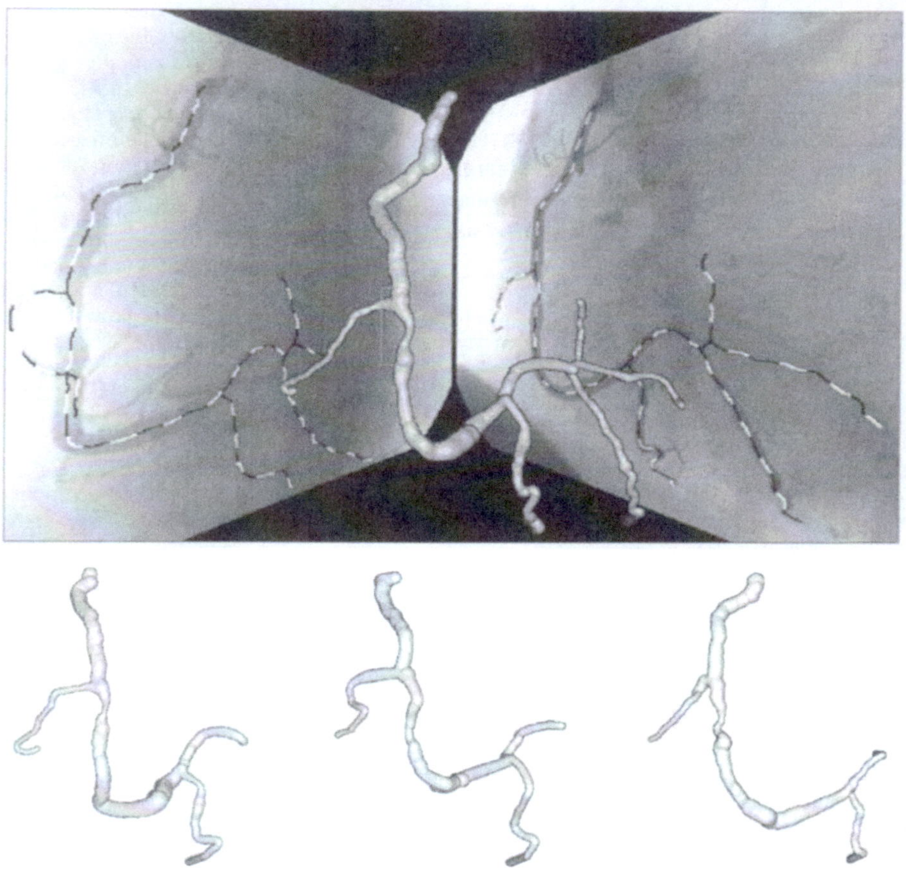

Fig. 9. Reconstructed vessels rendered by the volume rendering system In vivo (Interactive Visualizer of Volume data) [22]. *Top,* combined presentation of the volume-rendered reconstruction result and angiograms. *Bottom,* frames of the three-dimensional simulation

Visualization and Simulation

Since, on the one hand, volume renderers are commonly used to render medical data, e.g., computed tomography (CT), magnetic resonance imaging (MRI), three-dimensional ultrasound, and, on the other hand, volume rendering systems deal with polygonal representations, we decided to create both volumetric and surface representations of the reconstruction result. The voxelizing algorithm gives spheres centered at centerline positions connected by cones. For use in a virtual reality environment, a polygonal model has been created.

In addition to the three-dimensional geometry

of the coronary vessels, the trajectories of distinct points of the vessel are determined during tracking of the vessel structure. As a result, these trajectories can be used to simulate the movement of the vessel caused during the heart beat (Fig. 9, bottom row).

Conclusion and Future Work

In this chapter, a new technique to reconstruct three-dimensional coronary vessels based on a sequence of images has been explained. With a minimum of user interaction, the geometry of the vessels can be determined, using a combination of tracking, epipolar constraints, three-dimensional visualization: In addition, the trajectories which are derived during the tracking step can be used to simulate the real heart beat. CORRECT needs to be validated and further evaluated on vessels in different parts of the human body. Furthermore, the developed techniques will be transferred to virtual reality equipment to prove the performance of the algorithm within the scenario of an operating suite in the year 2000 [9].

References

1. Bao Y (1991) On three-dimensional reconstruction and modelling of coronary arteries from biplane X-ray angiograms. PhD thesis, Technische Universität Berlin
2. Bässmann H, Besslich PW (1989) Konturorientierte Verfahren in der digitalen Bildverarbeitung. Springer, Berlin Heidelberg New York
3. Beier J (1993) Automatische Quantifizierung von Koronarstenosen aus angiographischen Röntgenbildern. Fortschr Ber VDI Reihe 17 Nr 95. VDI, Düsseldorf
4. Faugeras OD (1993) Three-dimensional computer vision: a geometrical viewpoint. Massachusetts Institute of Technology, Cambridge
5. Garreau M, Coatrieux JL, Collorec R, Chardenon C (1991) A knowledge-based approach for 3-D reconstruction and labelling of vascular networks from biplane angiographic projections. IEEE Trans Med Imag 10(2): 122-131
6. Grosskopf S (1994) Entwicklung und Implementierung eines Verahrens zur Rekonstruktion von Herzkranzgefäßen auf d er Basis von angiographischen Projektionen. Dissertation, Technical University of Berlin
7. Hildebrand A, Grosskopf S (1995) 3D reconstruction of coronary arteries from X-ray projections. In: Lemke HU, Inamura K, Jaffe CC, Vannier MW (eds) Proceedings of the computer assisted radiology CAR '95 conference, Berlin. Springer, Berlin Heidelberg New York, pp 201-207
8. Hildebrand A, Neugebauer P (1993) Segmentierung. In: Hofmann GR, Blum C, Hildebrand A et al (eds) Bildverarbeitung und Bildkommunikation. Springer, Berlin Heidelberg New York, pp 173-214
9. Hildebrand A, Neugebauer PJ, Sakas G, Ziegler R (1995) Closing the gap: from computer vision to virtual reality. Tutorial notes: Eurographics Conference, Maastricht, 28. Aug-1 Sept 1995
10. Hofmann GR, Blum C, Hildebrand A, Neugebauer P, Neumann L, Schneider U, Strack R (eds) (1993) Bildverarbeitung und Bildkommunikation. Springer, Berlin Heidelberg New York
11. Kass M, Witkin A, Terzopoulos D (1987) Snakes: active contour models. IEEE 1st international conference on computer vision, pp 259-268
12. LeFree M, Simon SB, Lewis RJ, Bates ER, Vogel RA (1985) Digital radiographic coronary artery quantification. Proceedings, Computers in Cardiology, pp 99-102
13. Leugyel, Greenberg DP, Popp R (1995) Time-dependent three-dimensional intravascular ultrasound. In: Cook R (ed) Computer graphics proceedings. SIGGRAPH, Los Angeles, pp 457-464
14. Neugebauer PJ (1995) Interactive segmentation of denztistry range images in CIM systems for the construction of ceramic inlays using edge tracing. In: Lemke HU, Inamura K, Jaffe CC, Vannier MW (eds) Proceedings of the computer assisted radiology CAR '95 conference, Berlin. Springer, Berlin Heidelberg New York
15. Niemann H (1990) Pattern analysis and understanding. Springer, Heidelberg New York
16. Parker DL, Pope DL, White KS, Tarbox LR, Marshall HW (1986) Three-dimensional reconstruction of vascular beds. In: Bachorach SL (ed) Information processing in medical imaging, pp 414-430
17. Smets C, Suetens P, Oosterlinck A, Van de Werf F (1989) A knowledge-based system for the labeling of the coronary arteries. In: Lemke HU, Inamura K, Jaffe CC, Felix R (eds) CAR '89: computer assisted radiology. Springer, Berlin Heidelberg New York, pp 322-326
18. Vosselman G (1992) Relational matching. Springer, Berlin Heidelberg New York
19. Wahle A, Wellnhofer E, Mugaragu I, Trebeljahr A, Oswald H, Fleck E (1995) Application of accurate 3D reconstruction from biplane angiograms in morphometric analyses and in assessment of diffuse coronary artery disease. In: Lemke HU, Inamura K, Jaffe CC, Vannier MW (eds) CAR '95: computer assisted radiology, Berlin, Germany, 21-24 June 1995. Springer, Berlin Heidelberg New York
20. Wahle A, Oswald H, Schulze G-A, Beier J, Fleck E (1991) 3D reconstruction, modelling an viewing of coronary vessels. In: Lemke HU, Rhodes ML, Jaffe CC, Felix R (eds) CAR '91: computer assisted radiology. Springer, Berlin Heidelberg New York
21. Yachida M, Iwai S, Tsuji S (1984) 3D reconstruction of coronary artery from cine-angiograms based on left ventricular model. In: Proceedings of the 7th International Conference on Pattern Recognition, 30 Juli-2 August, Montreal, pp 1156-1159
22. Sakas G (1993) Interactive rendering of large fields. Vis Comput 9: 425-438

Digital Imaging and Data Integration Technology

T.J. Vogl, T. Diebold, J. Ricke, and H. Kleinholz

Introduction: The Clinical Information Highway

Modern imaging techniques such as computed tomography (CT), magnetic resonance imaging (MRI), ultrasonography, and digital subtraction angiography (DSA) have undergone rapid development in the last few years, proliferating into virtually all branches of modern medicine. In addition to the proliferation of digital imaging technology, the need to handle an enormous amount of other data created by physicians and administrators has profoundly changed hospital and office daily routine. Unfortunately, the spread of computing in medicine, including advances in communication technology, has not quite kept pace. Efficient transfer and storage of medical knowledge and data is the single most important prerequisite for top-class, yet economically affordable medicine in the future. Computing services promise to improve the quality of treatment, to simplify physicians' tasks, and to reduce costs. To demonstrate the potentials of computing in medicine, we present in this chapter the evolving concept of the filmless, fully digitalized Department of Radiology, including digital manipulation of examination results and replacement of conventional archiving. Remote access to patient-related data and immediate, loss-free transfer of information will also be discussed.

The Filmless Department of Radiology

Although the currently practiced solutions in digital data transfer, ranging up to the fully digitalized department of radiology, are still proprietary, communication standards for information transfer between computing modalities of different manufacturers have been proposed and in some cases already developed. To review the solutions that already exist today for efficient computer-assisted data management in medicine, we will describe scalable digital data transfer instrumentations ranging from digital image processing for radiologists to remote access to the mass storage necessary for fully digital communication and archiving in hospitals and offices. We will then outline potential future communication standards and network solutions and briefly summarize the imaging procedures available and their impact on vascular imaging.

Digital Versus Analog Image Acquisition

In radiology departments with conventional equipment, examinations are usually documented by analog media, such as films and printouts, which are sensitive to exposure to radiation. Analog images generated in this way serve as documentation and can be read and stored. Any modification of image characteristics or of the examination technique have to be done before the examination ist carried out. If the results are inappropriate, the entire examination has to be repeated, causing an increase in radiation exposure for patient and staff as well as additional costs. Modern imaging modalities such as DSA, CT and MRI are typically semi- or fully digitalized. Digital information can be visualized, processed after acquisition, and manipulated on a monitor, increasing diagnostic efficacy and avoiding repeat examinations. For documentation and archiving, complete studies and/or selected images with individually adjusted parameters (window, center, contrast) are stored digitally and analog films or prints are generated when needed.

The filmless Department of Radiology implies fully digitized image acquisition and processing. This includes an enormous memory capacity for online access to archives with information transfer, and allows image modification long after the examination was carried out. Ideally, viewing stations at various locations in all parts of a hospital or practice should allow authorized display and visualization of patient data, including the images, at all times. As an extension of this in-hospital or in-office concept, external networking would allow extensive servicing of external collaborators, including

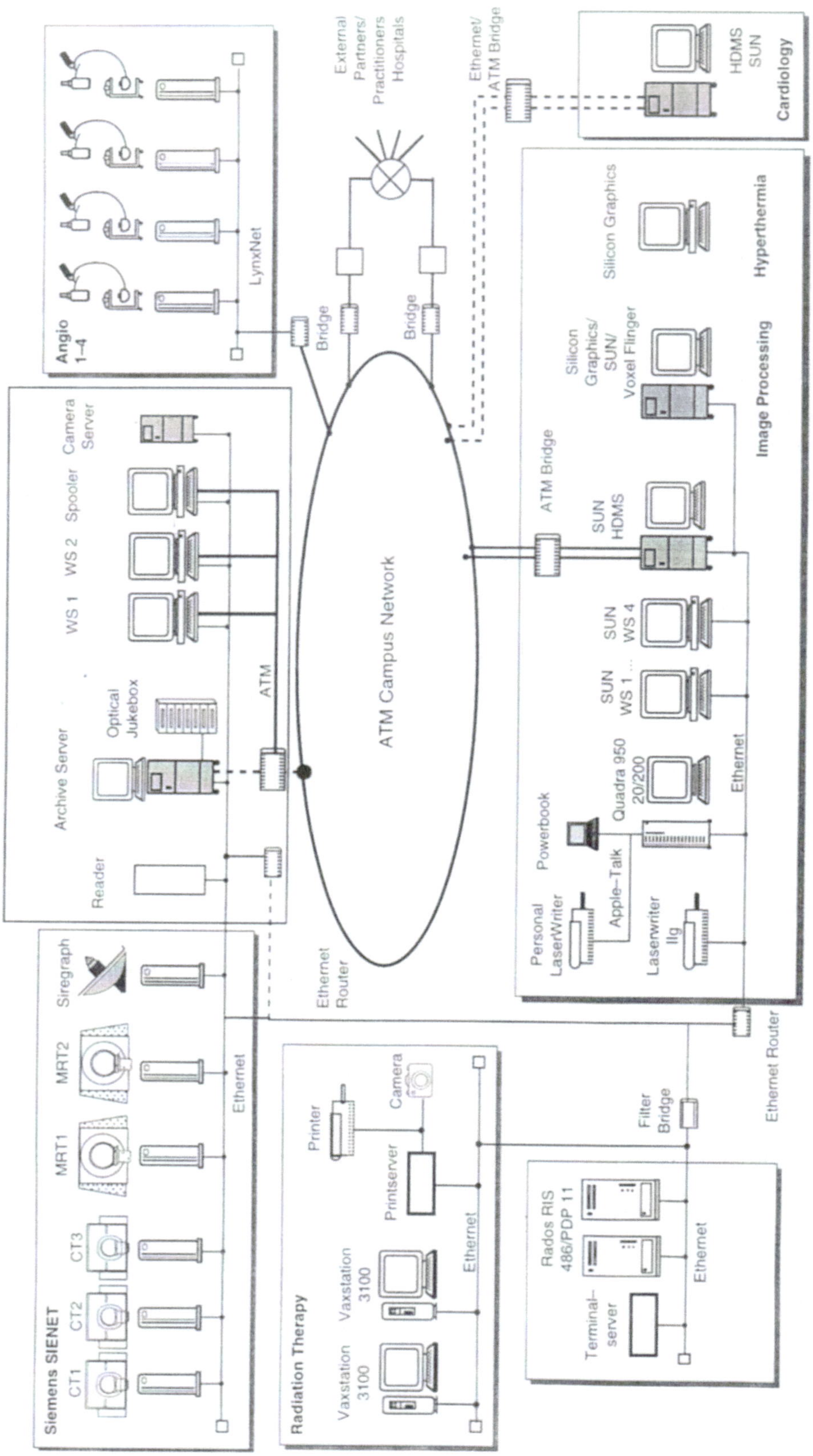

Fig. 1. Requirements of a filmless department of radiology

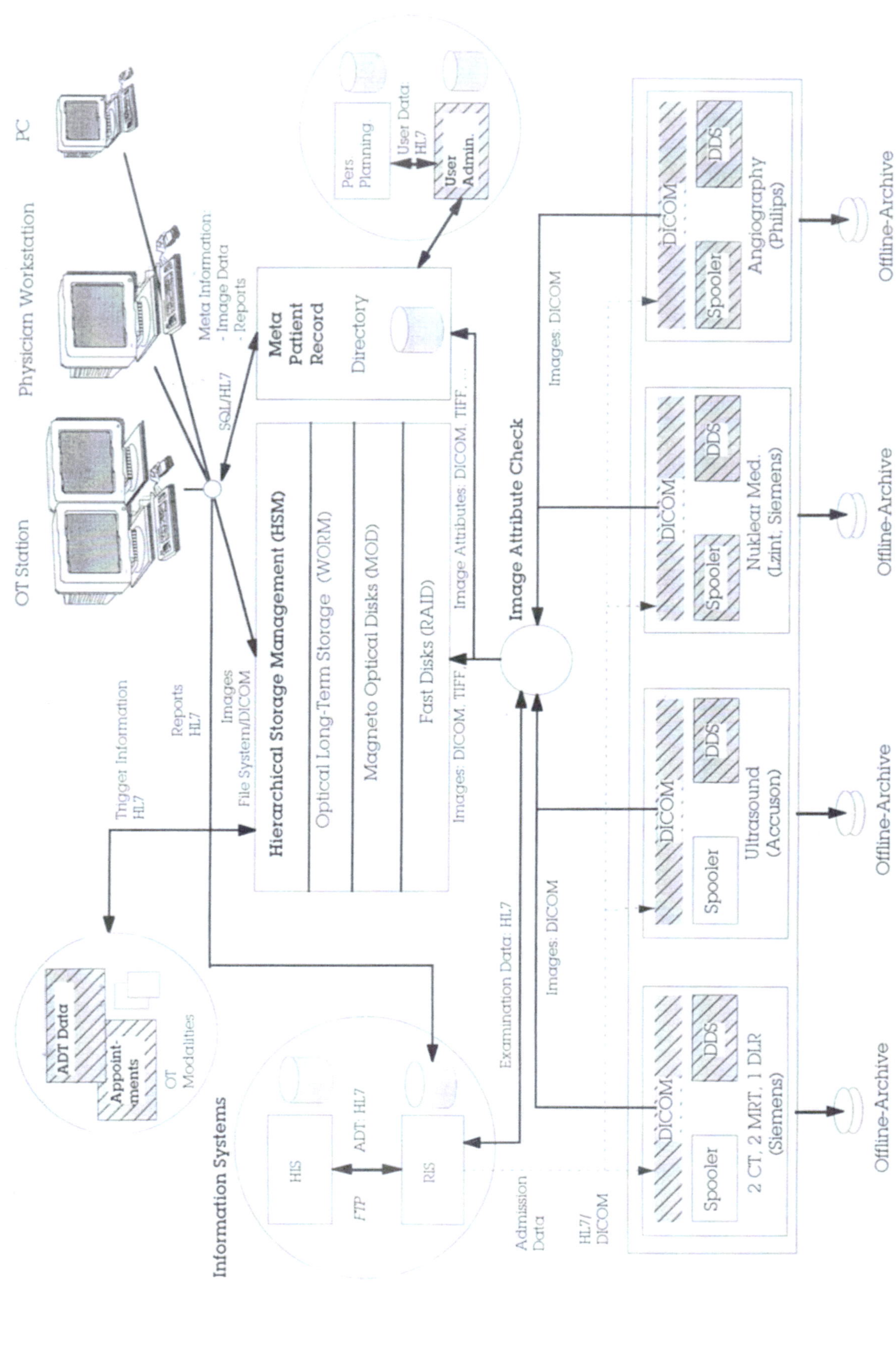

Fig. 2. Interlinkage between the filmless department of radiology and other information systems in the hospital

teleconsultations. In summary, what is needed for the filmless department of radiology (Fig. 1) are fully digitized information sources, a digital infrastructure (like the Ethernet or ATM network), a digital archive, and a number of viewing stations at various key points of the institution. Figure 2 adds to the scenario of a fully digitized department of radiology, the interlinkage of electronic patient records. A file server (in the center of the figure: in this case HSM by Hewlett Packard) adds its image data, retrieved via individual spoolers, to the electronic patient record directory, the "Meta Patient Record." This directory contains patient-specific information from administration systems and all other information systems of a hospital. Visualization of patient data or images is possible on either PCs or workstations.

Medical Equipment and Image Processing Facilities

Recent advances in computer technology have not only affected fringe areas of medicine, but have already penetrated the working day of every physician in mainstream medicine. Today, in the vast majority of medical facilities in Germany, computers are routinely used at the very least for word processing and book-keeping purposes, with integration of digital image data just beginning.

Commercial solutions available to fulfill these simple function are usually PC-based, whereas large-scale workstations are used in the area of image processing. In addition, advances in computer technology have enabled widespread introduction of new, noninvasive imaging modalities, particularly in vascular diagnostics. While digital angiography remains the "gold standard" in the imaging of vascular diseases, increasingly, noninvasive imaging methods such as ultrasonography, spiral CT, and MRI are evolving into viable alternatives. Besides their noninvasiveness, other advantages of the newer vascular imaging techniques are becoming recognized, such as visualization of the vessel walls, their relationship with surrounding tissues, and 3D vascular image reconstructions.

3D image reconstructions can be performed by various postprocessing algorithms, the most frequently used being the maximum intensity projection (MIP) modes and the more complex "ray tracing" surface reconstruction modes. Both these reconstruction techniques utilize 2D datasets for 3D reconstructions. In CT, spiral technique with an effective slice thickness of 1–4 mm and 100–250 ml contrast medium is essential for 3D reconstruction. In MR angiography examination sequences are performed without contrast medium. In both imaging modalities postprocessing is performed after the examination, taking approximately 3 min for a routine MIP reconstruction and up to 30 min for a complex surface reconstruction, depending on the algorithm selected. If a routine MIP reconstruction is of low quality and needs to be improved, manual segmentation of the original dataset, excluding data outside the region of interest (ROI), is done. After this ROI dataset is loaded into a program and the reconstruction is started. A typical example of this limitation of routine MIPs is CT of

Table 1. Clinical routine in neuroradiology

		CT		MRI			
	Ultrasound (Doppler)	Plain/enhanced CT	MIP/surface reconstruction	Plain/enhanced MRI	MRA	MIP/surface reconstruction	DSA
Malformations:							
Vascular (aneurysms)		x/xxx	xx/xx	xx/xxx	xxx	xxx/x	xxxx
Nonvascular (teratoma)		xx/xx	xx/–	xxx/xxx	xxx	xx/–	xxx
Degenerative diseases:							
Arteriosclerosis, aneurysms	xx	xx/xx	xx/xx	xxx/xxx	xx	xxx/xx	xxxx
Infarctions:							
Ischemic	x	xx/–	x/–	xxx/xxx	xxx	xxx/xx	xxx
Hemorrhagic	x	xxxx/–	x/–	xxx/xxx	xxx	xx/–	xxxx
Inflammatory diseases	x	xx/xx	x/–	xxx/xxx	xxx	xx/–	xxxx
Tumors	xx	xx/xxx	x/–	xxx/xxxx	xxx	xxx/xx	xxx
Trauma	x	xxxx	x/xxx	xx/x	x	xx/xx	–

CT, Computed tomography; MRI, magnetic resonance imaging; MRA, magnetic resonance angiography; MIP, maximum intensity projection; DSA, digital subtraction angiogtraphy.
x, Fair; xx, good; xxx, very good; xxxx, gold standard; –, no indication.

Table 2. Clinical routine imaging in head and neck radiology

		CT		MRI			
	Ultrasound (Doppler)	Plain/enhanced CT	MIP/surface reconstruction	Plain/enhanced MRI	MRA	MIP/surface reconstruction	DSA
Malformations:							
Vascular (hemangioma)	xx	x/xx	xx/x	xxx/xxxx	xxx	xxx/xxx	xxxx
Nonvascular (dermoid)	xx	xx/xx	xx/–	xxx/xxxx	x	x/x	x
Degenerative diseases:							
Occluding atherosclerosis	xxx	x/xx	xx/xx	x/x	xxx	xx/–	xxxx
Inflammatory diseases	xx	x/xx	xx/–	xx/xxx	xxx	xx/–	xxx
Tumors	xx	x/xx	xx/–	xxx/xxxx	xx	xxx/x	xxx
Trauma	xx	xxx/xxxx	x/xxx	xx/x	x	xx/xx	–

Table 3. Clinical routine imaging in cardiovascular radiology

		CT		MRI			
	Ultrasound (Doppler)	Plain/enhanced CT	MIP/surface reconstruction	Plain/enhanced MRI	MRA	MIP/surface reconstruction	DSA
Malformations:							
Vascular (arteria lusoria)	xx	x/xx	xx/xx	xxx/xxx	xxx	xxx/xxx	xxxx
Nonvascular (lymphangioma)	x	xx/xx	x/–	xxx/xxxx	xx	xx/x	–
Degenerative diseases:							
Aneurysms/dissections	xxx	xx/xx	xxx/xxx	xxx/xxx	xxx	xxx/xxx	xxxx
Inflammatory diseases	x	xx/xx	x/–	xx/xxx	xxx	xx/–	xxx
Tumors	x	xx/xxx	xxx/–	xxx/xxx	xxx	xxx/xx	xxxx
Trauma	x	xxx/xxxx	x/–	xx/x	x	xx/xx	–

Table 4. Clinical routine in abdominal radiology

		CT		MRI			
	Ultrasound (Doppler)	Plain/enhanced CT	MIP/surface reconstruction	Plain/enhanced MRI	MRA	MIP/surface reconstruction	DSA
Malformations:							
Vascular (aplasia of inf. v. cava)	xxx	xx/xx	xx/–	xxx/xxx	xxx	xx/–	xxxx
Nonvascular (lymphangioma)	xx	xx/xx	xx/–	xxx/xxxx	xx	xx/–	–
Degenerative diseases:							
Aneurysms	xxx	x/xx	xx/xxx	x/xx	xxx	xx/xxx	xxxx
Inflammatory diseases	xx	x/x	xx/–	xx/xxx	xxx	xx/–	xxx
Tumors	xx	xx/xxx	xx/–	xxx/xxx	xxx	xx/–	xxxx
Trauma	x	xxx/xxxx	x/–	xx/x	x	xx/xx	–

Table 5. Clinical routine in pelvic radiology

		CT		MRI			
	Ultrasound (Doppler)	Plain/enhanced CT	MIP/surface reconstruction	Plain/enhanced MRI	MRA	MIP/surface reconstruction	DSA
Malformations:							
Vascular (arteriovenous shunts)	xxx	xx/xx	xx/–	xx/xxx	xxx	xx/–	xxxx
Nonvascular (lymphangioma)	xx	xx/xx	xx/–	xxx/xxxx	xx	xx/–	–
Degenerative diseases:							
Occluding arteriosclerosis	xxx	x/x	xx/–	x/xx	xxx	xx/xxx	xxxx
Inflammatory diseases	xx	x/x	xx/–	xx/xxx	xxx	xx/–	xxxx
Tumors	xx	xx/xxx	xx/–	xxx/xxx	xxx	xx/–	xxxx
Trauma	x	xxx/xxxx	x/–	xx/x	x	xx/xx	–

Table 6. Clinical routine in peripheral radiology

		CT		MRI			
	Ultrasound (Doppler)	Plain/enhanced CT	MIP/surface reconstruction	Plain/enhanced MRI	MRA	MIP/surface reconstruction	DSA
Malformations:							xxx
Vascular (arteriovenous shunts)	xxx	xx/xx	xxx/–	xxx/xxx	xxx	xxx/xxxx	–
Nonvascular (lymphangioma)	xx	xx/xx	xx/–	xxx/xxxx	xx	xx/–	
Degenerative diseases:							
Aneurysms, arteriosclerosis	xxx	x/xx	xxx/xxx	x/xx	xxx	xx/xxx	xxxx
Inflammatory diseases	xxx	x/x	xx/–	xx/xxx	xxx	xx/–	xxx
Tumors	xx	xx/xxx	xx/–	xxx/xxx	xxx	xx/–	xxxx
Trauma	x	xxx/xxxx	x/–	xx/x	x	xx/xx	–

the carotid arteries. While MR angiographic studies of this area display only the arterial vessels at high signal intensity, in CT examinations the contrast-enhanced vessels have to be distinguished from bony structures, which also have a high signal intensity. While MIP reconstructions of CT datasets are still experimental in most institutions, they have become routine in MR angiography, though they still have their limitations. As to 3D surface reconstructions, the situation is almost the reverse. In CT, musculoskeletal 3D surface reconstructions have already become routine in many institutions. Experiences of vascular surface reconstructions are still limited with both CT and MRI, but vascular surface reconstructions from CT datasets are now becoming routine. Tables 1–6 give an overview of the different imaging modalities and 3D reconstruction techniques used in vascular diagnostics.

Databases, Communication Standards, and Networks

The costs of digital archiving depend on the number and heterogeneity of the integrated modalities and the storage capacity required. The terms "distributed computing" and "open systems" have attracted increasing attention in the attempt to improve cost-effectiveness. "Distributed computing" implies a change in computing structures from monolithic applications to integration of heterogeneous independent media such as PCs, file systems, and databases. "Open systems" support this trend, by allowing decentralized computing, assuring interoperability and true communication within networks [8, 12]. To permit flawless communication between systems, communication standards have to be implemented. For medical image format, digital imaging communications in medicine DICOM [1, 2] has become an increasingly recognized standard among the manufacturers of medical imaging technology. Other standard formats, such as tagged image file format (TIFF) or graphic interchange format (GIF), will probably remain in use for image visualization and display.

However, since transformation of data and changes in data configurations are necessary to comply with these formats, loss of information cannot be ruled out. Compression modi like widespread JPEG offer a higher transmission rate at the same cost since they save on the amount of data to be transmitted. Regarding the communication of user information in open systems (administration, patient identification), standards are selected depending on the size and structure of the overall system. For radiology department requirements, computing systems (PC, standard workstation) with multimedia standards such as object linking and embedding (OLE) or application programming interface (API) (for communication among different PC programs) serve any kind of information management well [4]. However, large-scale applications and "desktop standards" are no longer sufficient. For large-scale applications, a number of standards have been discussed with HL7 evolving into the upcoming standard [7, 9].

Due to the enormous amount of bits and bytes a hospital generates (up to an estimated 20 Tbit/year for a major hospital), semi-online applications using optical storage media have been developed to reduce hardware costs (Fig. 2). Even a radiology department alone generates a reasonable amount of data particularly from imaging devices requiring expensive optical storage media. In practice, modern storage media may hold patient-related data online for a number of years, whereas older data are labeled and archived. To retrieve the original data, the appropriate disk needs to be inserted in the system (Fig. 2). To allow integration of imaging modalities, computer workspaces, and digital storage facilities, a departmental network is needed. Key issues are data transmission, capacity, and affordability.

For high-efficiency data transmission in a complex environment with sophisticated workstations, ATM (asynchronous transfer mode) is emerging as the most promising technology, especially when installed as high-speed communication on optical fiber. ATM allows multimedial information transfer with integrated audio, video, text, graphics, fixed images or other digital data, but it is substantially more expensive than conventional networks such as Ethernet, which in the past few years has been widely accepted and has become a standard application. Compared with the maximal data transmission rate of 2,4 Gbit/s of ATM, which is limited to use on optical fiber, Ethernet performs at a maximum of 10 Mbit/s on either optical fiber or copper cable. Ethernet can still be effectively used in smaller departments where overload from too many users and modalities is unlikely [3, 6, 11, 14]. Full external communication data transmission via optical fiber will probably not be available even in the next 10 years, however, due to the lack of infrastructure. Satisfactory data transmission rates at 2 × 64 Kbit/s, including the option of video transmission for teleconsultations [3, 10], are offered by digitalized public telephone lines such as the worldwide standard ISDN (Integrated Services Digital Network).

Further Issues in Digital Imaging and Data Integration Technology

One of the important issues in the reliable and efficient use of computer aids in medicine is preservation of the integrity of data being transferred. Loss of information has to be excluded not only during data transfer but also on display on screen. For example, any conventional images such as standard chest X-rays carry large amounts of information. Not only must all this information be completely digitalized, but the capacity of the monitors used for display also has to match the information density of the original image (e.g., number of pixels). As to image manipulation tools, it must be ensured that previously archived information cannot be deleted or changed when being "returned" after access.

Because of its major advantages in regard to such things as cost efficiency and handling, digital data acquisition and processing will become standard in all areas of medicine in the near future [13]. Alongside the availability of this powerful technology, several problems need to be addressed expeditiously, e.g., the legal aspects of handling digital data. In most countries, no legal regulations exist regarding the security of patient data. The storage of images or other patient-related data on digital sources without analog backup currently faces a similar legal vacuum, although public discussion has already begun. Special applications such as 3D segmented MIP and surface reconstructions of MR angiographic or CT datasets will enable noninvasive assessment of the human vasculature. The resulting reconstructions may afterwards be transferred from universities to smaller hospitals and centers, or even vice versa, by computer networking, allowing complex operative maneuvers even at hospitals without their own MRI or spiral CT unit.

Conclusions

As a result of the proliferation of digital and computerized technology, two major developments in vascular medicine can be expected in the near future. First, imaging modalities such as Doppler ultrasonography, spiral CT and echo planar MRI will improve substantially. The temporal and spatial resolution of these modalities will increase, probably making visualization of small vessels such as the coronary arteries on CT and/or MRI possible in the future. The manipulation of acquired datasets and images will also be improved and simplified, such that physicians will be able to obtain 3D reconstructions routinely. Second, integration of networks will allow free exchange of data among medical facilities, making teleconsulting a daily routine.

References

1. American College of Radiology and National Electronic Manufacturers Association (ACR-NEMA) (1988) ACR-NEMA standard V. 2.0. ACR (Standards publication no. 300.1988)
2. American College of Radiology and National Electronic Manufacturers Association (ACR-NEMA) (1993) Digital image and communications in medicine (DICOM). I. Introduction and overview: version 3.0. ACR (NEMA standards publication PS3.1)
3. Bocker P (1987) ISDN – Das dienstintegrierte digitale Nachrichtennetz. Konzept, Verfahren, Systeme. Springer, Berlin Heidelberg New York
4. Brockschmidt K (1994) Inside OLE 2. Microsoft

5. CEN/TC 251/PT 011 EHCRA (1994) Electronic healthcare record architecture, first interim report. State University Gent, Belgium
6. Fuchs S, Kleinholz L, Ohly M et al (1995) Broadband telemedicine applications: experiences and results of the ARUBE project. Proc European Symposium on Advanced Networks and Services, Amsterdam 1995
7. Kleinholz L (1994) Integrated medical application. In: Fleck E (ed) Open systems in medicine. IOS, Amsterdam
8. Kleinholz L, Ohly M (1994) Multimedia medical conferencing: design and experience in the BERMED project. Proc IEEE Multimedia Computing and Systems, Boston
9. Kleinholz L (1991) Multimedia documents. In: Fleck E (ed) Open systems in medicine. IOS, Amsterdam
10. Kleinholz L, Ohly M, Ricke et al (1995) Multimedia medical conferencing: standards, products, ATM, ISDN, and other technical perspectives. Proc CAR, Berlin
11. McConnell J (1988) Internetworking computer systems. Interconnecting networks and systems. Prentice-Hall Englewood Cliffs
12. Ohly M (1994) Realization of an open distributed management system. In: Fleck E (ed) Open systems in medicine. IOS, Amsterdam
13. Ricke J, Kleinholz L, Hosten N et al (1995) Computer conferencing support in radiology – how economic viability will make it the radiologist's workspace of the next decade. Proc IMAC, Oahu
14. Siegmund G (1993) ATM – Die Technik des Breitband-ISDN. Decker, Heidelberg
15. Vogl TJ (1994) MR-Angiographie und MR-Tomographie des Gefäßsystems. Klinische Diagnostik. Springer, Berlin Heidelberg New York
16. Vogl TJ, Diebold T, Bergman C et al (1993) MRI in the pre- and post-operative assessment of tracheal stenosis due to pulmonary artery sling. J Comput Assist Tomogr 17(6): 878–886

Part II: Diagnostics of Vascular Diseases: Work-in-Progress

Section II: Laboratory Methods

Genetic and Molecular Biology Techniques for the Assessment of Vascular Disease

M.P.M. de Maat, P.H.A. Quax, and V.W.M. van Hinsbergh

Introduction

The health of the circulatory system depends largely on proper functioning of the heart and the vessel wall. The cells in the vessel wall, in particular smooth muscle and endothelial cells, respond to humoral factors, such as growth factors, hormones, and cytokines, and interact with adjacent cells and with their extracellular matrix. Changes in these interactions may cause dysfunctioning of the vascular cells resulting in, among other things, arteriosclerosis, hypertension, thrombosis, or vascular leakage. In comparison with coagulation factors and lipoproteins, which are constituents of plasma and can be determined in the peripheral blood, the functioning of the vessel wall cells is less easy to evaluate from plasma or serum samples. Only a limited number of secretion products, usually from the endothelium, can be assayed in the blood, e.g., von Willebrand factor, tissue-type plasminogen activator, endothelin, and plasminogen activator inhibitor-1. In addition, a number of indirect measurements, such as determination of blood pressure and flow, can be used. However, determination of a specific change in vascular cells requires biochemical studies of vessel biopsy specimens, or can be deduced from the efficacy of pharmacological intervention.

The introduction of molecular cell biology to vascular research has greatly increased the possibilities of studying the expression and regulation of genes in vascular cells. Once factors contributing to vascular functioning have been recognized, and even before that, molecular genetic assays can be used to identify specific defects in the coding sequences of proteins or in the nucleotide sequences that regulate the synthesis of these genes. In particular, the introduction of restriction enzymes and the polymerase chain reaction (PCR) has enabled the determination of alterations in the composition of specific DNA sequences in a small number of cells. These techniques allow assessment of genetic aspects of vascular functioning by procedures that are fairly noninvasive for the patient, such as venipuncture.

Although molecular genetics technology can identify genomic loci involved in a disease even without any knowledge of the function of these loci, most genetic approaches focus on candidate genes. Candidate genes for vascular disease can for example be genes that are involved in lipoprotein metabolism or that are expressed in the diseased vascular tissue in a different way than in the unaffected blood vessel wall. Molecular biology technology again appears useful in identifying such genes. The differential display technique can reveal genes that are specifically expressed or repressed in a diseased tissue. Furthermore, in situ hybridization makes it possible to localize enhanced gene expression in vascular tissue. Molecular biology technology not only enables the understanding and diagnosis of diseases which depend on single or multiple genes, but it also provides fascinating techniques which allow the manipulation of gene expression in experimental animals. Furthermore, it offers new potential applications for the prevention and therapy of cardiovascular disease.

This chapter describes methods by which to determine mutations and DNA polymorphisms responsible for or associated with altered expression or composition of proteins in the vessel wall, followed by a survey of several techniques used in molecular vascular biology to determine the expression and synthesis of proteins in the vessel wall. Finally, it briefly deals with transgenetics, a potent set of tools which are becoming very useful in the evaluation and confirmation of defects in vascular functioning, and site directed gene transfer in the vessel wall.

Determination of Genetic Factors Contributing to Vascular Dysfunction

Mutations and DNA polymorphisms

The expansion of molecular biology techniques in the past decade has already contributed considerably to our understanding of the relation between human genetics and diseases. Molecular defects directly responsible for some familial cardiovascular disorders, such as Marfan syndrome, supravalvular aortic stenosis, and a number of dyslipoproteinemias, have been identified. Such molecular defects, resulting in the synthesis of an abnormal protein, are called mutations. However, most DNA sequence alterations in the genome do not cause the synthesis of abnormally functioning proteins. Neutral DNA sequence variations also occur and reside within genes mainly in the noncoding regions, the introns. These neutral DNA variations are called DNA polymorphisms. In contrast to mutations, which are relatively rare, allelic variations detected by DNA polymorphisms occur with high frequency in general population (>1%). This makes the DNA polymorphisms suitable for genetic analysis of diseases in which several factors interact. Indeed, some DNA polymorphisms do appear to be associated with a disease. This is usually explained by a fairly close physical linkage of the DNA polymorphism to a functional mutation elsewhere. In such cases the polymorphism is a genetic marker by which a disease-predisposing region of the genome can be identified. For example, a significant association has been reported between risk for cardiovascular disease and a DNA polymorphism in the noncoding part of the gene encoding tissue-type plasminogen activator (t-PA), but this DNA polymorphism did not influence the plasma t-PA concentration [82]. Similarly, associations between DNA polymorphisms and cardiovascular disease have been described for other products of vascular cells, such as angiotensin converting enzyme (ACE), the ACE receptor, and endothelial-type nitric oxide synthese [31, 70, 74].

The distinction between DNA polymorphisms and mutations is not always unequivocal. Some polymorphisms cause only minor changes in the gene products, without significant implication. Because these benign changes are not directly responsible for disorders, they are also called DNA polymorphisms. For example, a variation in DNA may result in the replacement of an amino acid in the protein, and this amino acid change (e.g., factor VII MspI polymorphism with glutamine 353 to arginine [22, 38]) results in a charge difference of the protein without changing its activity. There are also some polymorphisms known in the promoter region, and there are indications that these polymorphisms influence the transcription of the gene. For example, smoking increases the plasma fibrinogen levels more strongly in individuals with the A^{-455} allele of the G/A^{-455} fibrinogen β-gene polymorphism than in individuals who have only the common G^{-455} allele [10, 23].

Whenever a polymorphism is physically linked to a disease locus, the genotype may have clinical significance, even if the DNA variation is not functional. Soon after molecular techniques became widely available, the magnitude of heterogeneity in the noncoding genomic fraction among different individuals was recognized and this became the starting point for the study of DNA polymorphisms in clinical investigations. The first DNA polymorphisms recognized were called restriction fragment length polymorphisms (RFLP), refering to the fact that the fragments displayed different molecular sizes after digestion of the DNA with one or more restriction enzymes. An RFLP locus usually has two possible alleles. Subsequently, other DNA polymorphisms were observed with a much greater variability. Examples are variable number of tandem repeats (VNTR) loci and microsatellite loci. These hypervariable DNA regions are stably inherited and give a size pattern of DNA fragments unique to each person.

Southern Hybridization Analysis

The traditional way to analyze RFLP loci has been the Southern hybridization analysis [64]. In this technique 10–20 μg total genomic DNA is incubated with a restriction enzyme. After separation of the resulting DNA fragments of different sizes by electrophoresis in agarose gels, the DNA is transported (Southern blotting) in a single-stranded form to a more robust nitrocellulose or nylon filter. The filter is then incubated with a single-stranded ^{32}P-labeled probe, usually part of the cDNA of the gene of interest. The unbound radiolabeled probe is removed by a stringent washing procedure and the filter is exposed to an X-ray film. After developing the film the length of the DNA fragments which have bound the radiolabeled probe can be determined and the genotype is assessed. Although this technique has been valuable in identifying mutants underlying cardiovascular disease, such as defective LDL receptor mutants [28], the technique has been largely abandoned because it consumes large amounts of genomic DNA.

Polymerase Chain Reaction

In the past decade, the use of thermostable polymerases, such as *Taq* (*Thermophilus aquaticus*) DNA polymerase, in the PCR technique has led to an exponential growth of the use of this technique in molecular biology [63], while Southern blotting has become rarely used. PCR is a process that enables the amplification of a small DNA fragment a few hundred base pairs to 10 kilobase pairs, or even up to 35 kilobase pairs with spezial adaptations [2] up to a million-fold in vitro [50, 62, 71]. Figure 1 depicts this process schematically. The principle is that DNA is heated to a temperature at which the two strands come apart. Subsequently, the temperature is lowered so that specific primers (oligonucleotides) can bind (annealing step). On each single strand, a new complementary strand can then be formed. PCR is based on a continuous repetition of these steps (denaturation, primer annealing, and extension). At the start of the PCR reaction, the excess of primers over target DNA is about 5×10^7. Therefore, the binding of primers is favored over reannealing of the DNA strands, and the amplification is exponential. Later, after a number of amplification cycles, the primer excess gets smaller and the PCR reaction levels off. Because each step theoretically results in a doubling of DNA, 30 cycles give a 2^{30} amplification. The size and composition of the amplified DNA can subsequently be evaluated directly or after digestion with a restriction enzyme. This can be done by agarose electrophoresis (if a size difference is the determinant). Modifications of this procedure also allow the detection of single nucleotide mutations (see below).

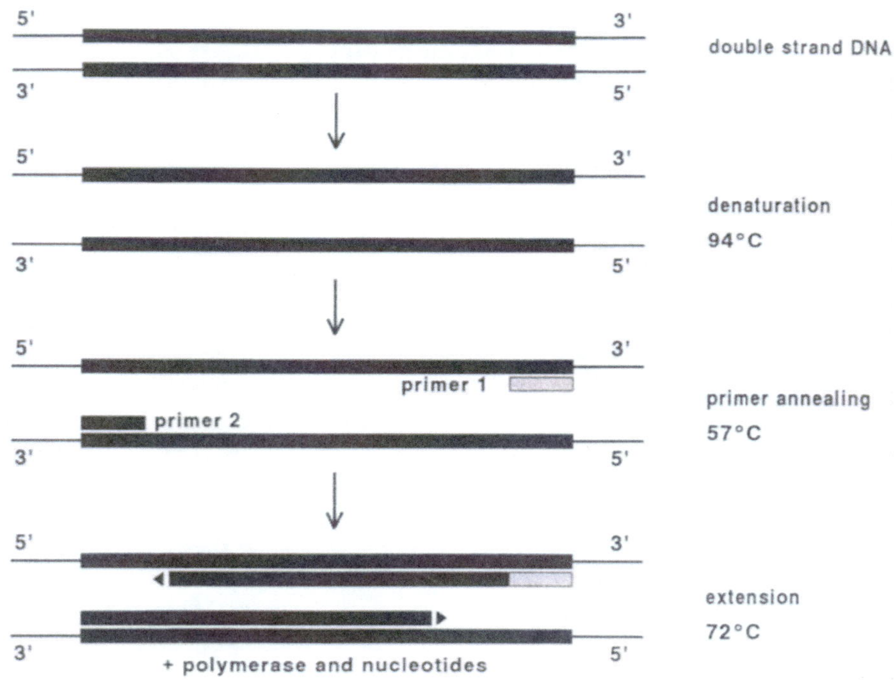

Fig. 1. The polymerase chain reaction (PCR) allows amplification of a targeted DNA sequence. After separation of the DNA strands at high temperature (5 min at temperatures between 90°C and 96°C; step 1), the temperature is lowered so that specific primers can bind (step 2). These primers are small DNA fragments, usually about 20 nucleotides. The two primers anneal to their complementary sequences in the DNA which flank the target sequences. The primers thereby define the DNA fragment that will be amplified. When the primers are bound to the DNA they function as the starting point for the DNA polymerase to synthesize a new strand of DNA, which is complementary to the original template. The annealing temperature is a few degrees below the melting temperature (T_m), the temperature at which 50% of the DNA is denatured, and depends on the relative number of C/G and A/T pairs, which are bound by three and two hydrogen bonds, respectively. If the temperature is just below the T_m the binding of the primer will be most specific, since each mismatch between the two stands will give a reduction in the T_m of about 5°C. A temperature of a few degrees below T_m is chosen, because then sufficient binding is obtained that is also specific. In the next step (step 3), the primer-directed extension, the temperature is increased again to between 65°C and 75°C, which is the optimal temperature for the *Taq* DNA polymerase. A complementary strand of new DNA is synthesized by enzyme-mediated addition of nucleoside triphosphates onto the 3' ends of each primer. This process is repeated in the PCR reaction. In each PCR cycle the DNA is doubled. The temperatures indicated are arbitrary and depend on the particular composition of the DNA strands

Practical Aspects of PCR

Genomic DNA for PCR

For PCR 20 ng to 1 μg of genomic DNA is needed. Several procedures have been described for the isolation of DNA from whole blood. In these methods first the red cells are removed by lysing the blood cells for 30 min on ice in a lysis buffer containing 3.0 mol/l aminonium chloride, 0.2 mol/l $KHCO_3$, and 0.02 mol/l EDTA (pH = 7.4), after centrifugation (10 min 550 × *g*) the white-cell pellet is incubated with 20 mg/ml proteinase-K or pronase in a nuclear lysis buffer [75 mmol/l NaCl, 25 mmol/l EDTA, 0.5% (w/v) SDS, pH = 7.4]. The proteins are then precipitated by adding 0.3 volume of 8 mol/l ammonium acetate and gently inverting the tube. After centrifugation 1 volume of isopropanol is added to precipitate the DNA, which is then washed in 70% ethanol and dissolved overnight in sterile water or Tris/EDTA buffer (10 mmol/l Tris-HCl, 1 mmol/l EDTA, pH = 7.4). The concentration and purity of the DNA can then be determined by measuring the extinctions at 260 and 280 nm. The ratio of these extinctions is a measure of the purity of the DNA. A ratio of about 1.8 is indicative of pure DNA, a lower ratio indicates that there is some protein contamination, in which case another precipitation step is advisable. The extinction at 260 nm can be used to calculate the DNA concentration. (An extinction of 1 at 260 nm corresponds to 50 μg/ml). The salting-out with 8 mol/l ammonium acetate can be replaced by a salting-out step with 6 mol/l NaCl [48] or a phenol-chlorophorm extraction [1].

Although it is known that hemoglobin inhibits the amplification of DNA, reports have been published that it is also possible to omit the extraction of DNA and to PCR directly from blood [45, 57]. PCR with DNA obtained from mouth-swabs [46], urine [75], or buccal mouth wash-outs [40] has also been described.

Equipment and Consumables

Several companies sell equipment for PCR nowadays, e.g., Perkin-Elmer Cetus (Norwalk, CT, USA), Hybaid (Middlesex, UK), MJ Research Inc. (Cambridge, MA, USA). Most thermal cyclers have a heating block that undergoes programmed heating and cooling cycles. There are also pieces of apparatus that move a PCR plate between heat blocks at the various required temperatures (Stratagene, Cambridge, UK).

The most important consumables for PCR are microcentrifuge tubes or 96-well plates and pipette tips. The buffers, pipette tips and microcentrifuge tubes used for PCR are autoclaved before use (45 min, 1 bar) to destroy any proteolytic enzymes. Traditionally, microcentrifuge tubes were used for PCR. These tubes need to have a thin wall to improve the rates of heating and cooling. Lately, the use of 96-well plates has been becoming more and more popular (Hybaid, Middlesex, UK). Especially for studies of large populations, working with 96-well plates and multichannel pipettes improves the throughput of the assays. When digestion of the PCR product with restriction enzymes is part of the protocol, the enzyme may be added directly to the PCR product and this also is done more efficiently with 96-well plates. In our experience, contamination of DNA from one well to another in a 96-well plate is negligible, but the use of several blanks, spread over the plate, is advisable.

PCR Reagents

The PCR protocols resemble each other closely. Usually, the reaction volume is 25 μl for microtiter plates and 25–100 μl for microcentrifuge tubes. The reaction mix contains (1) target DNA, (2) the primers that flank the area to be amplified, (3) the *Taq* polymerase enzyme, (4) deoxynucleotides to be incorporated in the newly formed DNA strands, and (5) a buffer. On top of the reaction mix, liquid paraffin is added to prevent evaporation during the PCR.

The *Taq* polymerase is the enzyme most used for PCR. It was the first available thermostable polymerase for PCR. Other polymerases, e.g. *Pwo* polymerase from *Pyrococcus woesei* and *Pfu* polymerase from *Pyrococcus furiosus* [2], are now also available. They exhibit proofreading capacity, which, reduces the mistake rate during PCR and by which the amplification of guanine-cytosine-rich areas is easier. These enzymes are also capable of amplifying much larger fragments than *Taq* polymerase. Amplification of fragments up to 35 kilobase pairs is within reach [2].

Pitfalls and Controls

Because PCR is such a sensitive technique there is a strong risk of reagent or sample contamination. The contamination may be due to exogenous previously amplified sequences or DNA from the skin of the technician. Ideally the work with the sample DNA should be done in a laminar flow hood and separated from the laboratory where the PCR reaction is performed, i.e., with separate supplies of pipettors, pipette tips, tubes, and reagents. A set-up like this is not always achievable, but several routine precautions can be taken to reduce the risk of contamination. When new reagents are made, they should be aliquoted so that when a contamination is suspected, all reagents can be replaced. Disposable gloves should be worn, especially when working with the sample DNA. These disposable gloves should be changed frequently. Furthermore, in each PCR experiment, several control reactions should be used. The first is a blank, where distilled water is added instead of template DNA. There should not be any product in this reaction. If there is some PCR product, it means that one of the reagents is contaminated, and often this is the water. Other controls are samples with known genotypes. On each gel, a basepair ladder (DNA markers of different sizes) should be added, and comparing the size of the PCR product with this standard is another control.

Another component that has to be considered is the accuracy of the DNA polymerase, i.e., the number of errors produced per added nucleotide. For *Taq* polymerase the error rate for base substitution is 1/9000 and that for frameshift is 1/41 000 per nucleotide polymerized [69]. This accuracy is influenced by a high deoxynucleotide triphosphate (dNTP) concentration, since this drive is the enzymatic reaction in the direction of DNA synthesis, thereby decreasing the amount of error discrimination in the extension step. A low dNTP concentration will therefore increase the accuracy. The accuracy of the reaction can also be improved by optimizing the $MgCl_2$ concentration, the cycle number, and the reaction times [13].

Detection of PCR Products

Some PCR products can be detected directly after electrophoresis by ultraviolet illumination of ethidium bromide-stained gels (details of electrophoresis are given below). Figure 2 shows two examples of such polymorphisms. A DNA polymorphism

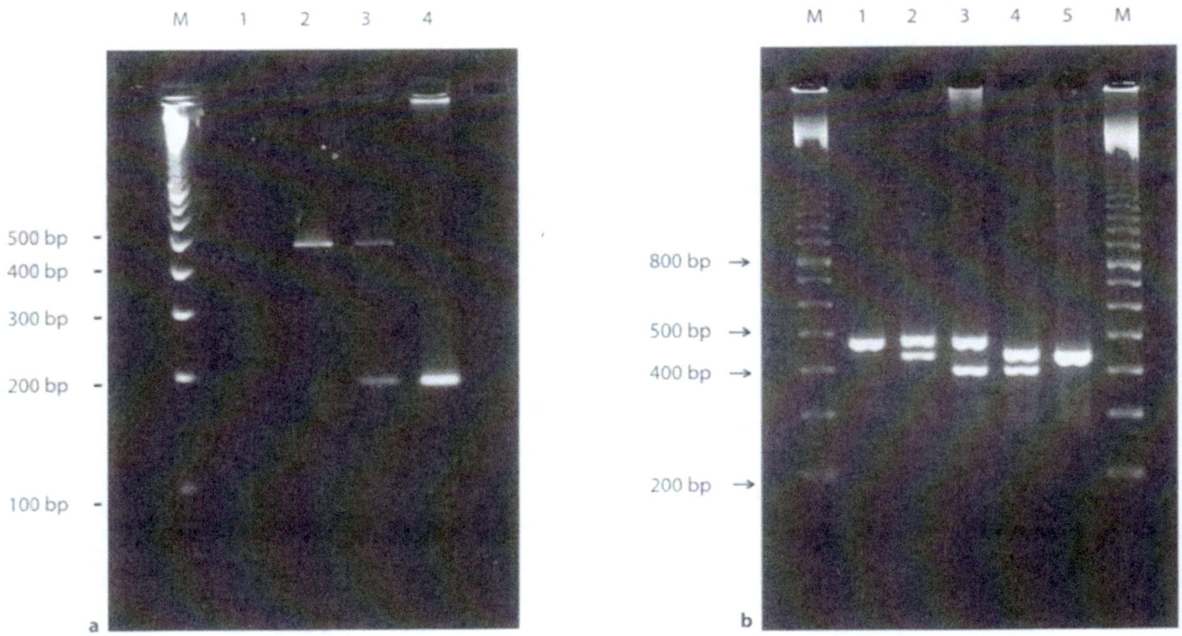

Fig. 2a, b. Detection of PCR products after agarose gel electrophoresis. **a** PCR products of the ACE polymorphism. Two DNA polymorphisms with different molecular weights are obtained after cleavage of the PCR product with a restriction enzyme. *Lane M:* Marker DNAs of different sizes; *lane 1:* negative control; *lanes 2–4:* genotypes I/I, I/D, and D/D, respectively. **b** PCR products of the factor VII-HVR4 polymorphism. The polymorphism has three form with five, six or seven repeat units. *Lane M:* Makers; *lanes 1–5:* PCR product fragments of homozygotes with only seven repeat units (*lane 1*) or only five repeat units (*lane 5*); *lanes 2–4:* Products of heterozygotes with both six and seven repeat units (*lane 2*), both five and seven repeat units (*lane 3*) or both five and six repeat units (*lane 4*). The DNA fragments are visualized by ultraviolet illumination after intercalation of ethidium bromide into the DNA strands

with two alleles is represented by an insertion/deletion polymorphism in the ACE gene (Fig. 2a). The HVR4 polymorphism in intron 7 of coagulation factor VII [44] is characterized by a different number of a 37-basepair repeat unit, of which four alleles are presently known. Figure 2b shows three of these alleles. More frequently the PCR product does not contain an insertion/deletion polymorphism but a single basepair substitution. In that case, incubation of the PCR product with a restriction enzyme is often part of the detection procedure. Restriction enzymes, which originally were part of the defense system of many bacteria against introduction of foreign DNA, e.g., by viruses, can cut a specific DNA sequence, usually with about 6-basepair specificity. The names of restriction enzymes are derived from the bacteria from which they are isolated, e.g., EcoRI from *Escherichia coli* and BclI from *Bacillus caldolyticus*.

When a PCR product with only 1 basepair difference in length is studied, e.g., the 4G/5G polymorphism of plasminogen activator inhibitor Type-1 (PAI-1) [9] or the 5G/6G polymorphism of stromelysin [77] the difference cannot be detected on an agarose gel, but allele-specific oligonucleotide (ASO) hybridization may be used. Each PCR fragment is blotted (using dot-blotting) on two nitrocellulose filters. One filter is then incubated with a labeled probe that specifically binds the one allele, the other filter with a labeled probe that specifically binds the other allele. By carefully selecting the hybridization conditions, specific binding of the two probes can be achieved. The probe can be labeled with ^{32}P, but nonradioactive labeling with digoxygenine (DIG) (Boehringer Mannheim, Germany) is also possible.

Another possible detection method for polymorphisms is allele-specific primer (ASP) amplification. In this procedure, two PCR procedures are performed that each detect the presence of one of the alleles. One consensus primer is used and two allele-specific primers that bind to one of the two possible polymorphic sites. When a specific PCR product is detected, after analysis by gel electrophoresis and hybridization, it means that the primer of that specific PCR product bound to the polymorphic site and that the accompanying specific allele is present (Fig. 3). Combining the results of the two PCR procedures identifies the genotype. Obviously, a control fragment must be amplified in the same PCR mixture to indicate that absence of the allele-specific PCR product is not a false negative result. This procedure is much faster than procedures that include restriction enzyme digestion or ASO hybridization. ASP procedures have recently been described for PAI-1 and factor V DNA polymorphisms [35, 43].

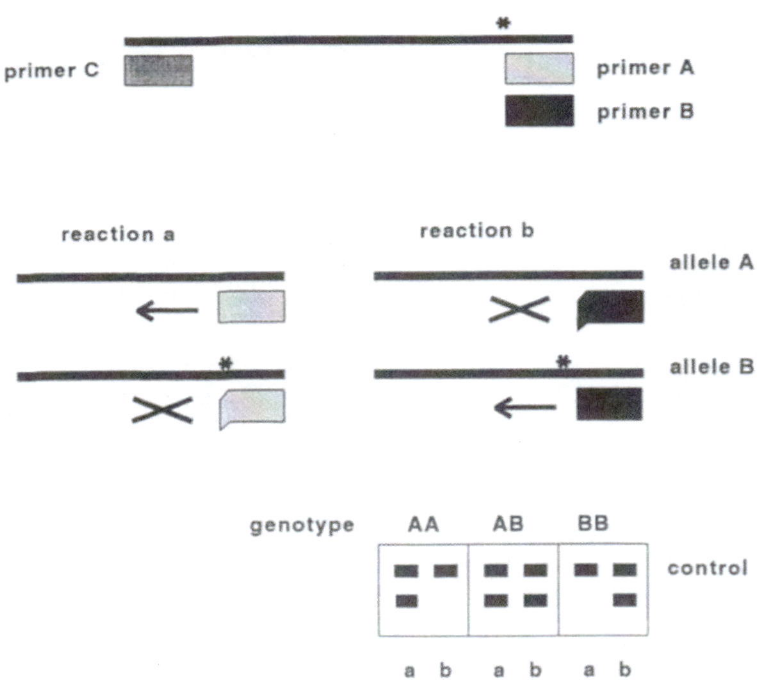

Fig. 3. Allele-specific primer amplification (ASP). At the *top* of the figure the gene of interest is depicted with the site of the polymorphism indicated with an *asterisk*. The *middle* part of the figure depicts the annealing of the sequence-specific primers to the two alleles. Amplification only occurs when the annealing is optimal. At the *bottom* electrophoreses has been performed; the AA genotype is characterized by a band in the *a* lane only; the heterozygous genotype (AB) is characterized by bands in the *a* and *b* lanes, while the homozygous BB has a strand in the *b* lane only

Electrophoresis and Mutation Analysis

DNA is negatively charged at pH = 8.4 and it therefore runs to the anode. Double-strand DNA does this with a mobility that is dependent on the fragment size. For the separation of DNA fragments the standard medium is agarose. The choice of concentration of agarose in the gel depends on the length of the fragment that is being studied. Most commonly used are concentrations between 0.7% (w/v) for fragments ranging from 0.8 to 10 kilobase pairs and 2% (w/v) agarose for fragments ranging from 0.1 to 3 kilobase pairs.

For DNA electrophoresis the submarine system is the most commonly used. The agarose is dissolved in Tris-borate-EDTA (TBE; 50 mmol/lö Tris-HCl, 50 mmol/l. H_3BO_3, 1 mmol/l Na_2EDTA) by boiling in a microwave oven. The gel is run in a horizontal direction with a layer of ±5 mm of buffer on top of the gel. The advantages of this system are ease of pouring and sample loading, and support for the gel from below.

It is very convenient to have some ethidium bromide (±0.1 μg/ml gel) present in the gel. Since ethidium bromide intercalates with the DNA helix and fluoresces strongly, it is possible to visualize the DNA under ultraviolet light (309 nm). A photograph of the gel can then be taken, or the gel can be scanned and analyzed using computer software. Ethidium bromide is mutagenic. Recently other dyes (e.g., SYBR Green) have become available. A sample containing DNA fragments of known sizes is usually included as a marker to enable estimation of the size of the DNA fragments (such markers are commercially available).

For the detection of single-base substitutions, which often underlie mutations, several adaptations of the electrophoresis procedure have been developed. In particular, denaturing gradient gel electrophoresis and heteroduplex formation are suitable techniques to screen disease-associated mutations in large numbers of patients. Denaturing gradient gel electrophoresis uses the conversion of double-strand DNA obtained by PCR into single-strand DNA by an increasing gradient of a denaturing agent in the gel and the fact that DNA migrates differently during agarose electrophoresis than double-strand DNA [47]. This technique has been successfully used to screen patients for defects in their LDL-receptor gene, the most frequent determinant of familial hypercholesterolemia [42]. Heteroduplex formation uses a special "hydrolink" gel to detect single-base mismatches in double-strand DNA [33]. Another technique to analyze mutations is single-strand conformation polymorphism (SSCP), which uses the fact that under denaturing conditions small differences can exist in the electrophoretic mobilities of single-strand DNAs of equal size but with a change in their nucleotide sequence [61]. Mutation analysis has been very useful in studies regarding different aspects of cardiovascular disease. It has provided insight in various cardiovascular diseases varying from the generation of cardiac malformations to hypertension, from heart insufficiency to atherosclerosis. For example, large numbers of mutations are presently known for the LDL receptor [28], which causes most cases of familial hypercholesterolemia, and for apolipoproteins [65], many of which contribute to various types of dyslipoproteinemias. Mutations in the genes for angiotensinogen can contribute to hypertension [30]. A defect in the coding region of fibrillin, a protein that connects collagen fibres, underlies Marfan's disease.

Determination of Proteins and mRNA in Vascular Tissue

Genetic analysis of genes contributing to a disease can be done without knowing the specific defect underlying the disease. However, understanding the causes of the disease will need knowledge of the structure, function, and regulation of the gene products involved. Through studies on biopsy specimens of blood vessels from patients and unaffected controls, specific products can be identified which are associated with the disease. Information about the amounts of mRNA and protein expressed in a diseased vessel can be obtained from biochemical studies on tissue extracts or via analysis of tissue sections by immunohistochemistry and in situ hybridization. For example, the presence of stromelysin and collagenases in aneurysm tissue and atherosclerotic plaques as determined by immunohistochemistry and in situ hybridization suggest a contribution of these matrix-degrading proteinases to the weakening of the vessel wall [11, 19]. Alternatively, a number of changes in the production of growth factors [5, 76], structural proteins, such as osteonectin [20], various receptors [56, 59], and changes in cell proliferation [21] may be involved in the development of atherosclerosis. Some of them may be secondary responses of the disease, while others may be the reflection in a genetic sensitivity towards an exaggerated response. Intervention studies and studies in transgenic animals can provide further indication that the altered protein expression and the disease are causally related.

Determination of Specific mRNAs in Tissues

To determine whether a particular gene is expressed in vascular tissue, the RNA or protein can be extracted from the tissue. This requires specific precautions because RNA is rapidly degraded by RNases. To prevent RNA degradation the tissue is usually immediately frozen in liquid nitrogen or in cooled isopentane (–160°C); the frozen tissue is ground in a mortar (pre)cooled with liquid nitrogen, and dissolved in a solution that blocks all RNase activity. The procedure described by Chomczynski and Sacchi [8] is frequently used for RNA extractions from vascular cells, with good results. Excellent RNA preparations are also obtained when small pieces of frozen tissue are extracted directly. To that end, the frozen tissue is mixed with an extraction solution (RNAzol B, Cinna/Biotecx) and an aliquot of glass beads (1 mm diameter), and heavily shaken in a Mini-Beadbeater apparatus (Biospec Products) at 4°C. Subsequently, the RNA is collected from the mixture by chloroform and isopropanol extraction. The RNA can subsequently be separated by agarose gel electrophoresis, blotted, and hybridized with a ^{32}P-labeled cDNA, and the amount of hybridized radiolabeled cDNA can be quantified in a phospho-imager or by exposure of the hybridized blot to a suitable film (Northern blotting analysis).

Often, when only a small specimen of tissue is available and the total amount of RNA obtained is limited, a specific mRNA can be be determined (semi)quantitatively using a so-called RT-PCR analysis. To this end, the mRNA is transcribed into cDNA by reverse transcriptase (RT). Subsequently, specific oligonucleotides primers are added and a PCR is started (see above). The PCR product is subsequently blotted on a filter and can be quantified as described above.

An alternative to RT-PCR is nuclear acid sequence-based amplification (NASBA). NASBA, also known as self-sustained sequence replication (3SR), also amplifies nucleic acids [34]. In this method synthesis of cDNA with the enzyme reverse transcriptase and cDNA-dependent transcription of RNA alternate. The method works with both DNA and RNA but seems to work best with direct RNA detection. An advantage of this technique is that it does not require alternate changes in temperature. A disadvantage is that little experience is available at present with this technique, whereas ample experience exists with RT-PCR.

Using RT-PCR the increased expression of a number of genes in the atherosclerotic plaque have been demonstrated, such as apolipoprotein E, PAI-1, and growth factors. Nowadays, the identification of specific gene expression in affected tissues is done by differential display analysis, which compares a large number of genes simultaneously, or by in situ hybridization, which recognizes the cell types that contain the mRNA investigated (see below).

Differential Display Analysis

Recently, so-called differential display analysis has been introduced [41]. This is a very elegant technique for analyzing the differences in gene expression between two tissues, e.g., a diseased and a normal blood vessel. Basically, differential display analysis is based on RT-PCR analysis of all mRNAs present in a tissue, and subsequent comparison of expressed mRNAs in the two tissues. The displayed differences in mRNA expression may point to the genes involved in the disease, independently of whether the gene has been identified before or not. It is currently applied in many fields of investigation, e.g., in analyzing specific genes which are induced by angiotensin II [15], and in identifying the specific expression of genes in the downstream anastomosis of prosthetic arterial grafts [25].

In Situ Hybridization and Immunohistochemistry

Localization of mRNA can be done by in situ hybridization, if information regarding the cell types that synthesize a specific mRNA in a disease is required. In this technique a ^{35}S-labeled cDNA probe is made and hybridized with the mRNA in a tissue slice. Usually 2- to 5-μm sections of snap-frozen tissues are used, but 4% formaldehyde-fixed and paraffin-embedded tissue sections can also be used. Precautions have to be taken that the mRNA is not degraded. A ^{35}S-radiolabeled probe is preferentially used, because the radiation range of ^{35}S is shorter than that of ^{32}P or ^{125}I, resulting in better resolution. The specific activity of ^{35}S is higher than that of ^{3}H, but the sensitivity of the assay is still limited by the specific activity that can be obtained for ^{35}S. Therefore, if only a few copies of mRNA are expressed in a cell, they are difficult to detect. It is expected that in the next few years techniques will be developed which combine in situ hybridization with PCR [58]. To that end, the PCR reaction must proceed on a solid support, otherwise the original localization of the mRNA is lost. By in situ hybridization the expression of many types of mRNA has been demonstrated in the arteriosclerotic plaque, which are absent in the unaffected artery, such as growth factors including platelet-derived growth factor mRNA [76] and basic fibroblast growth factor [5], and the proteases stromelysin-1 mRNA [27], collagenase and gelatinase B [19], and the thrombin receptor in smooth muscle cells [56].

The presence of a specific mRNA is usually accompanied by the synthesis of the protein that is translated from this mRNA. However, exceptions occur, in which no synthesis of a specific protein is found despite of elevated levels of its encoding mRNA. Immunolocalization, although semiquantitative, is the preferred technique to demonstrate the presence of proteins in the vessel wall. It has the advantage that it reveals the localization of the protein in the tissue. A disadvantage is that protein antigen is detected, and that it is difficult to estimate whether the protein is in an active or an intact form, or is inactivated or partially degraded. The use of monoclonal antibodies, which recognize specific "sensitive" epitopes of the protein can be helpful in overcoming this problem. By this method many proteins have been demonstrated in the arteriosclerotic plaque and aortic aneurysms which are absent in the unaffected artery. They comprise growth factors, cytokines, monocyte chemotactic protein-1, tissue factor, activation markers for monocytes and lymphocytes [26]. Use of specific antibodies, e.g., against proliferating cell nuclear antigen (PCNA), which is an essential cofactor for DNA polymerase-δ and recognizes replicating cells, can give additional information regarding the proliferation of specific cells [29]. Because the ultrastructure of the tissue slice and the reactivity of the antibody with the antigen to be determined are influenced by the fixation procedure, special care has to be taken to select the appropriate fixation procedure, or, if this is not possible, to select an antibody that reacts in the tisslie slices that are available.

Transgenic Animals and Site-Directed Modulation of Gene Function

Transgenic animals

The association of altered synthesis of a specific protein with the occurrence of a vascular disease does not prove that the protein is causally involved in the disease, because it may also be expressed as a consequence of the disease. Evidence of a causal relationship can sometimes be obtained by pharmacological intervention studies, but often it cannot. The recent availability of techniques to generate transgenic animals, in which a certain gene is overexpressed or deleted, appears to be a major step forward in the evaluation of the role of proteins in vascular disease [12, 68]. These techniques have several advantages. Firstly, the expression of proteins with unknown functions can also be changed. Secondly, thus far unknown functions of a protein or gene can be detected and analyzed. Thirdly, animal models can be made in which certain genetic factors contributing to a multifactorial disease can be controlled. This makes it possible to study other contributing factors better. Fourthly, a gene with a defective function can be introduced. If the protein coded for by this gene has a dominant trait, as has for example been shown for certain human apolipoprotein mutants in transgenic mice, its effect on the metabolism of the animal and its blood vessels can be studied [4, 73]. Finally, a gene can be completely "knocked out," i.e., no functional protein can be formed in these animals. The technique of homologous recombination in murine embryonic stem cells allows selective mutation or disruption of genes in mice. This technique has been used to evaluate the role of many proteins in cardiovascular development, atherosclerosis, and vascular remodeling after injury. Formation of normal blood vessels was disturbed in mice lacking integrins or vascular endothelial cell growth factor receptors [17, 66]. Severe atherosclerosis occurs in mice lacking apoliprotein E [4]; intimal thickening after injury is reduced in mice lacking urokinase-type plasminogen activator and enhanced in mice deficient in PAI-1 [6]. A complication in the use of transgenic animals, especially in the case of the "knock out" animals, is that several of the induced protein deficiencies, or certain proteins in homozygous or even in heterozygous animals, cause early death of the embryo. In order to evaluate the effect of such proteins in later stages of development or in specific adult tissues, conditional transgenic expression has to be achieved [16]. This means that the gene for the specific protein is activated or silenced under specific conditions, e.g., because it is placed behind an inducible promoter, such as the metallothionein promoter or a tetracycline-sensitive promoter [18]. The recognition of cell-type-specific promoters also makes it possible to study the expression of an altered gene in that particular cell type. For example, endothelial cell-specific expression has been demonstrated using the promoter region of *tie* [37].

Gene Transfer in the Vessel Wall

An alternative for the manipulation of gene expression in normal and transgenic animals is direct modulation of gene expression in vivo by gene transfer. Gene transfer can be performed in an artery segment using special devices which allow a site-specific delivery of gene, e.g., a double-balloon catheter [51] or a pluronic gel that is applied to the adventitial side of a vessel segment [67]. A variety of gene transfer techniques are available to modulate gene expression in vascular cells. On the one hand, a gene can be inactivated by antisense oligonucleotides [3, 67]. On the other hand a foreign gene can be introduced in vascular cells by using an expression plasmid bearing the gene of interest flanked by a eukaryotic promoter and polyadenylation signal. This plasmid is transfected into the cell via liposomes or after incorporation in adapted viruses [24, 39, 52].

The successful use of antisense oligonucleotides to inhibit the proliferation of smooth muscle cells in animals has been reported by several groups. In these studies predominantly genes have been used which are thought to be involved in the cell cycle, i.e., *c-myc* [3], *c-myb* [67], *cdc2* [49] kinase, and PCNA [49]. Indeed, by the use of antisense oligonucleotides against cell division cyclin 2 (*cdc2*) kinase or the proto-oncogene *c-myb*, intimal hyperplasia and thus formation of restenotic lesions can be significantly inhibited (up to 95%) in animal models. A successful application in human vascular disease has still to be demonstrated.

Adenovirus-mediated gene transfer is also a very efficient method for modulation of gene expression in the vessel wall in vivo. Using adenoviral vectors and a site-directed delivery device, endothelial cells can be transfected in vivo very efficiently. In injured vessel, too, the medial smooth muscle cells can easily be transduced using this approach.

Selective gene transfer into the arteries of experimental animals has been demonstrated by several groups using plasmids in liposomes or in modified viruses. Overexpression of one of three growth factors, acidic fibroblast growth factor (aFGF), platelet-derived growth factor (PDGF), or transforming growth factor-β (TGFβ), caused intimal thickening in pigs, but each intimal thickening had its own specific characteristics [53–55]: PDGF induced smooth muscle accumulation, aFGF both smooth muscle cell proliferation and angiogenesis, whereas accumulation of matrix proteins was the dominant trait of $TGF\beta_1$-induced lesions. Another approach is the selective elimination of dividing cells [7, 60].

Although the ability to genetically alter endothelial and vascular smooth muscle cells hold promises in providing insight into a variety of processes such as restenosis and angiogenesis, it should be emphasized that there are still many unanswered questions regarding its applicability in vivo and its safety,
efficiency, and selectivity.

Future Perspectives

We have described molecular biological techniques and how they can contribute to an understanding of the etiology and diagnosis of vascular diseases. The versatility of recombinant DNA technologies makes it likely that further rapid developments will take place. Progress in the human genome project will substantially facilitate future genetic studies. Furthermore, it should be mentioned that many other applications, such as the preparation of recombinant proteins, techniques for studying gene regulation, and the use of combinatorial libraries (phage display) to prepare competitive receptor ligands contribute to the rapidly expanding field of vascular biology and medicine.

References

1. Adeli K, Ogbonna G (1990) Rapid purification of human DNA from whole blood for potential application in clinical chemistry laboratories. Clin Chem 36: 261–264
2. Barnes WM (1994) PCR amplification of up to 35 kb DNA with high fidelity and high yield from lambda bacteriophage templates. Proc Natl Acad Sci USA 91: 2216–2220
3. Biro S, Fu YM, Yu ZX, Epstein SE (1993) Inhibitory effects of antisense oligonucleotides targeting c-myc mRNA on smooth muscle cell proliferation and migration. Proc Natl Acad Sci USA 90: 654–658
4. Breslow JL (1993) Transgenic mouse models of lipoprotein metabolism and atherosclerosis. Proc Natl Acad Sci USA 90: 8314–8318

5. Brogi E, Winkles JA, Underwood R, Clinton SK, Alberts F, Libby P (1993) Distinct patterns of expression of fibroblast growth factors and their receptors in human atheroma and nonatherosclerotic arteries. Association of acidic FGF with plaque microvessels and macrophages. J Clin Invest 92: 2408-2418
6. Carmeliet P, Collen D (1994) Evaluation of the plasminogen/plasmin system in transgenic mice. Fibrinolysis 8: 269-276
7. Chang MW, Barr E, Seltzer J, Jiang YQ, Nabel GJ, Nabel EG, Parmacek MS, Leiden JM (1995) Cytostatic gene therapy for vascular proliferative disorders with a constitutively active form of the retinoblastoma gene product. Science 267: 518-522
8. Chomczynski P, Sacchi N (1987) Single-step method of RNA isolation by acid guanidinium thiocyanate-phenol-chloroform extraction. Anal Biochem 162: 156-159
9. Dawson SJ, Wiman B, Hamsten A, Green F, Humphries S, Henney AM (1993) The two allele sequences of a common polymorphism in the promoter of the plasminogen activator inhibitor-1 (PAI-1) gene respond differently to interleukin-1 in HepG2 cells. J Biol Chem 268: 10739-10745
10. De Maat MPM, de Knijff P, Green FR, Thomas AE, Jespersen J, Kluft C (1995) Gender-related association between β-fibrinogen genotype and plasma fibrinogen levels and linkage disequilibrium at the fibrinogen locus in Greenland Inuit. Arteriosclerosis Thromb Vasc Biol 15: 856-860
11. Dollery CM, McEwan JR, Henney AM (1995) Matrix metalloproteinases and cadiovascular disease. Circ Res 77: 863-868
12. Dzau VJ, Gibbons GH, Kobilka BK, Lawn RM, Pratt RE (1995) Genetic models of human vascular disease. Circulation 91: 521-531
13. Eckert KA, Kunkel TA (1990) High fidelity DNA synthesis by the Thermus aquaticus DNA polymerase. Nucleic Acids Res 18: 3739-3744
14. Falconer DS, Mackay TFC (1996) Introduction to quantitative genetics, 4th edn. Longman, Harlow
15. Feener EP, Northrup JM, Aiello LP, King GL (1995) Angiotensin II induces plasminogen activator inhibitor-1 and -2 expression in vascular endothelial and smooth muscle cells. J Clin Invest 95: 1353-1362
16. Fishman GI (1995) Conditional transgenetics. Trends Cardiovasc Med 5: 211-217
17. Fong GH, Rossant J, Gerstenstein M, Breitman ML (1995) Role of the flt-1 receptor tyrosine kinase in regulating the assembly of vascular endothelium. Nature 376: 66-70
18. Furth PA, St Onge L, Böger H, Gruss P, Gossen M, Kistner A, Bujard H, Hennishausen L (1994) Temporal control of gene expression in transgenic mice by a tetracycline-responsive promoter. Proc Natl Acad Sci USA 91: 9302-9306
19. Galis ZS, Sukhova GK, Lark MW, Libby P (1994) Increased expression of matrix metalloproteinases and matrix degrading activity in vulnerable regions of human atherosclerotic plaques. J Clin Invest 94: 2493-2503
20. Giachelli CM, Bae N, Almeida M, Denhardt DT, Alpers CE, Schwartz SM (1993) Osteopontin is elevated during neointima formation in rat arteries and is a novel component of human atherosclerotic plaque. J Clin Invest 92: 1686-1696
21. Gordon D, Reidy MA, Benditt EP, Schwartz SM (1990) Cell proliferation in human coronary arteries. Proc Natl Acad Sci USA 87: 4600-4604
22. Green F, Kelleher C, Wilkes H, Temple A, Meade T, Humphries S (1991) A common genetic polymorphism associated with lower coagulation factor VII levels in healthy individuals. Arteriosclerosis Thromb 11: 540-546
23. Green F, Hamsten A, Blomback M, Humphries S (1993) The role of beta-fibrinogen genotype in determining plasma fibrinogen levels in young survivors of myocardial infarction and healthy controls from Sweden. Thromb Haemost 70: 915-920
24. Guzman RJ, Lemarchand P, Crystal RG, Epstein SE, Finkel T (1993) Efficient and selective adenoviral-mediated gene transfer into vascular neointima. Circulation 88: 2838-2848
25. Hamdan AD, Aiello LP, Quist WC, Ozaki CK, Contreras MA, Phaneuf MD, Ruiz C, King GL, LoGerfo FW (1995) Isolation of genes differentially expressed at the downstream anastomosis of prosthetic arterial grafts with the use of mRNA differential display. J Vasc Surg 21: 228-234
26. Hansson GK, Jonasson L, Seifert PS, Stemme S (1989) Immune mechanisms in atherosclerosis. Arteriosclerosis 9: 567-578
27. Henney AM, Wakeley PR, Davies MJ, Foster K, Hembry R, Murphy G, Humphries S (1991) Localization of stromelysin gene expression in atherosclerotic plaques by in situ hybridization. Proc Natl Acad Sci USA 88: 8154-8158
28. Hobbs HH, Russell DW, Brown MS, Goldstein JL (1990) The LDL receptor locus in familial hypercholesterolemia: mutational analysis of a membrane protein. Annu Rev Genet 24: 133-170
29. Isner JM, Kearney M, Bauters C, Leclerc G, Nikol S, Pikkering JG, Riessen R, Weir L (1994) Use of human tissue specimens obtained by directional atherectomy to study restenosis. Trends Cardiovasc Med 4: 213-221
30. Jeunemaitre X, Soubrier F, Kotelevtsev YV, Lifton RP, Williams CS, Charru A, Hunt SC, Hopkins PN, Williams RR, Lalouel JM, Corvol P (1992) Molecular basis of human hypertension: role of angiotensinogen. Cell 71: 169-180
31. Katsuya T, Horiuchi M, Chen YDI, Koike G, Pratt RE, Dzau VJ, Reaven GM (1995) Relations between deletion polymorphism of the angiotensin-converting enzyme gene and insulin resistance, glucose intolerance, hyperinsulinemia, and dyslipidemia. Arteriosclerosis Thromb Vasc Biol 15: 779-882
32. Kazazian HH (1989) Use of PCR in the diagnosis of monogenic disease. In: Erlich HA (ed) PCR technology: principles and applications for DNA amplification. Stockton, New York, pp 153-169
33. Keen J, Lester D, Inglehearn C, Curtis A, Bhattacharya S (1991) Rapid detection of single-base mismatches as heteroduplexes on "hydrolink" gels. Trends Genet 36: 460-465
34. Kievits T, van Gemen B, van Strijp D, Schukkink R, Dirck M, Adriaanse H, Malek LT, Sooknanan R, Lens P (1991) NASBA-isothermal enzymatic in vitro nucleic acid amplification optimized for the diagnosis of HIV-1 infection. J Virol Methods 35: 273-286
35. Kirschbaum NE, Foster PA (1995) The polymerase

chain reaction with sequence specific primers for the detection of the factor V mutation associated with activated protein C resistance. Thromb Haemost 74: 874-878
36. Kogan S, Doherty M, Gitschier J (1996) An improved method for pre-natal diagnosis of genetic diseases by analysis of amplified DNA sequences. N Engl J Med 316: 985-990
37. Korhonen J, Lahtinen I, Halmekytö M, Alhonen L, Jänne J, Dumont D, Alitalo K (1995) Endothelial-specific gene expression directed by the *tie* gene promoter in vivo. Blood 86: 1828-1835
38. Lane A, Cruickshank JK, Mitchell J, Henderson A, Humphries S, Green FR (1992) Genetic and environmental determinants of factor VII coagulant activity in ethnic groups at differing risk of coronary heart disease. Atherosclerosis 94: 43-50
39. Lee SW, Trapnell BC, Rade JJ, Virmani R, Dichek DA (1993) In vivo adenoviral vector-mediated gene transfer into balloon-injured rat carotid arteries. Circ Res 73: 797-807
40. Lench N, Stanier P, Williamson R (1988) Simple non-invasive method to obtain DNA for gene analysis. Lancet 1: 1356-1358
41. Liang P, Pardee AB (1992) Differential display of eukaryotic messenger RNA by means of the polymerase chain reaction. Science 257: 967-971
42. Lombardi P, Sijbrands EJG, van de Giessen K, Smelt AHM, Kastelein JJP, Frants RR, Havekes LM (1995) Mutations in the low density lipoprotein receptor gene of familial hypercholesterolemic patients detected by denaturing gradient gel electrophoresis and direct sequencing. J Lipid Res 36: 860-867
43. Mansfield MW, Stickland MH, Grant PJ (1995) Environmental and genetic factors in relation to elevated circulating levels of plasminogen activator inhibitor-1 in Caucasian patients with non-insulin-dependent diabetes mellitus. Thromb Haemost 74: 842-847
44. Marchetti G, Gemmati D, Patracchini P, Pinotti M, Bernardi F (1991) PCR detection of a repeat polymorphism within the F7 gene. Nucleic Acids Res 19: 4570
45. Mercier B, Gaucher C, Feugeas O, Mazurier C (1990) Direct PCR from whole blood, without DNA extraction. Nucleic Acids Res 18: 5908
46. Meulenbelt I, Drog S, Trommelen GJM, Boomsma DI, Slagboom PE (1995) High-yield noninvasive human genomic DNA isolation method for genetic studies in geographically dispersed families and populations. Am J Hum Genet 57: 1252-1254
47. Meyers RM, Maniatis G, Lerman LS (1987) Detection and localization of single base changes by denaturing gradient gel electrophoresis. Methods Enzymol 155: 501-527
48. Miller SA, Dykes DD, Polesky HF (1988) A simple salting-out procedure for extracting DNA from human nucleated cells. Nucleic Acids Res 16: 1215
49. Morishita R, Gibbons GH, Ellison KE, Nakajima M, Vonderleyen H, Zhang LN, Kaneda Y, Ogihara T, Dzau VJ (1994) Intimal hyperplasia after vascular injury is inhibited by antisense Cdk 2 kinase oligonucleotides. J Clin Invest 93: 1458-1464
50. Mullis K, Faloona F (1987) Specific synthesis of DNA in vitro via polymerase-catalyzed chain reaction. Methods Enzymol 155: 335-350
51. Nabel EG (1995) Gene therapy for cardiovascular disease. Circulation 91: 541-548
52. Nabel EG, Platz G, Nabel GJ (1990) Site-specific gene expression in vivo by direct gene transfer into the arterial wall. Science 249: 1285-1288
53. Nabel EG, Yang Z, Liptay S, San H, Gordon D, Haudenschild CC, Nabel GJ (1993) Recombinant platelet-derived growth factor B gene expression in porcine arteries induces intimal hyperplasia in vivo. J Clin Invest 91: 1822-1829
54. Nabel EG, Yang Z, Plautz G, Forough R, Zhan X, Haudenschild CC, Maciag T, Nabel GJ (1993) Recombinant fibroblast growth factor-1 promotes intimal hyperplasia and angiogenesis in arteries in vivo. Nature 362: 844-846
55. Nabel EG, Shum L, Pompili VJ, Yang Z, San H, Shu HB, Liptay S, Gold L, Gordon D, Derynck R, Nabel GJ (1993) Direct transfer of transforming growth factor β1 gene into arteries stimulates fibrocellular hyperplasia. Proc Natl Acad Sci USA 90: 10759-10763
56. Nelken NA, Soifer SJ, O'Keefe J, Vu TKH, Charo SR, Coughlin SR (1992) Thrombin receptor expression in normal and atherosclerotic human arteries. J Clin Invest 90: 1614-1621
57. Newton CR, Kalshaker N, Graham A, Powell S, Gammack A, Riley J (1988) Diagnosis of α_1-antitrypsin deficiency by enzymatic amplification of human genomic DNA and direct sequencing of polymerase chain reaction products. Nucleic Acids Res 16: 8233-8243
58. Nuovo GJ, Gallery F, MacConnell P, Becker J, Bloch W (1991) An improved technique for the in situ detection of DNA after polymerase chain reaction amplification. Am J Pathol 139: 1239-1244
59. O'Brien KD, Allen MD, McDonald TO, Chait A, Harlan JM, Fishbein D, McCarty J, Ferguson M, Hudkins K, Benjamin CD, Lobb R, Alpers CE (1993) Vascular cell adhesion molecule-1 is expressed in human coronary atherosclerotic plaques. Implications for the mode of progression of advanced coronary atherosclerosis. J Clin Invest 92: 945-951
60. Ohno T, Gordon D, San H, Pompili VJ, Imperiale MJ, Nabel GJ, Nabel EG (1994) Gene therapy for vascular smooth muscle cell proliferation after arterial injury. Science 265: 781-784
61. Orita M, Iwahana H, Kanazawa H, Hayasho K, Sekiya T (1989) Detection of polymorphisms of human DNA by gel electrophoresis as single-strand conformation polymorphism. Proc Natl Acad Sci USA 86: 2766-2770
62. Panet A, Khorana HG (1974) Studies on polynucleotides. The linkage of deoxyribonucleotide templates to cellulose and its use in their replication. J Biol Chem 249: 5213-5221
63. Saiki RK, Gelfand DH, Stoffel S, Scharf S, Higuchi R, Horn GT, Mullis KB, Erlich HA (1988) Primer-directed enzymatic amplification of DNA with a thermostable DNA polymerase. Science 239: 487-491
64. Sambrook J, Fritsch EF, Maniatis T (1989) Molecular cloning. A laboratory manual, 2nd ed. Cold Spring Harbor
65. Schonfeld G, Krul ES (1994) Genetic defects in lipoprotein metabolism. In: Goldbourt U, de Faire U, Berg K (eds) Genetic factors in coronary heart disease. Kluwer, Dordrecht, pp 239-266
66. Shalaby F, Rossant J, Yamaguchi TP, Gertenstein M, Wu XF, Breitman ML, Schuh AC (1995) Failure of blood is-

land formation and vasculogenesis in flk-1 deficient mice. Nature 276: 62–66
67. Simons M, Edelman ER, DeKeyser JL, Langer R, Rosenberg RD (1992) Antisense c-myb oligonucleotides inhibit intimal arterial smooth muscle cell accumulation in vivo. Nature 359: 67–70
68. Smithies O, Maeda N (1995) Gene targeting approaches to complex genetic diseases: atherosclerosis and essential hypertension. Proc Natl Acad Sci USA 92: 5266–5272
69. Tindall KR, Kunkel TA (1988) Fidelity of DNA-synthesis by the Thermus aquaticus DNA polymerase. Biochemistry 27: 6008–6013
70. Tiret L, Tirat B, Visvikis S, Breda C, Corvol P, Cambien F, Soubrier F (1992) Evidence, from combined segregation and linkage analysis, that a variant of the angiotensin I-converting enzyme (ACE) gene controls plasma ACE levels. Am J Hum Gen 581: 197–205
71. Towbin JA (1995) Polymerase chain reaction and its uses as a diagnostic tool for cardiovascular disease. Trends Cardiovasc Med 5: 175–185
72. Van der Bom JG, de Knijff P, Bots ML, Haverkate F, Holman A, Kluft C, Grobbee DE (1995) Polymorphism of the blood clot lysis enzyme tissue-type plasminogen activator is associated with myocardial infarction. Circulation 92 Suppl: 1–30
73. Van Vlijmen BJM, van den Maagdenberg AMJM, Gijbels MJJ, van der Boom H, HogenEsch H, Frants RR, Hofker MH, Havekes LM (1994) Diet-induced hyperlipoproteinemia and atherosclerosis in apolipoprotein E3-Leiden transgenic mice. J Clin Invest 93: 1403–1410
74. Wang XL, Sim AS, Badenhop RF, McCredie RM, Wilkken DEL (1996) A smoking-dependent risk of coronary artery disease associated with a polymorphism of the endothelial nitric oxide synthase gene. Nature Med 2: 41–45
75. Wenham PR (1992) DNA-based techniques in clinical biochemistry: a beginner's guide to theory and practice. Ann Clin Biochem 29: 598–624
76. Wilcox JN, Smith KM, Williams LT, Schwartz SM, Gordon D (1988) Platelet-derived growth factor mRNA detection in human atherosclerotic plaques by in situ hybridization. J Clin Invest 82: 1134–1143
77. Ye S, Watts GF, Mandalia S, Humphries SE, Henney AM (1995) Preliminary report: genetic variation in the human stromelysin promotor is associated with progression of coronary atherosclerosis. Br Heart J 73: 209–215

Part II: Diagnostics of Vascular Diseases: Work-in-Progress

Section III: Future Perspectives

Integrated Approach to Cardiovascular Medicine

P. Lanzer

Introduction

Cardiovascular diseases (CVD) are the primary cause of morbidity and mortality in industrialized countries. In 1993, 440896 people (49.14% of total) died from CVD in Germany, including 184487 (20.56%) and 105767 (11.79%) patients with coronary artery and cerebrovascular disease, respectively. In comparison, during the same period of time 219764 people (24.49%) died of cancer [1].

The exact costs associated with treatment, disability, and premature death as a result of CVD in Germany are not known. However, based on indirect indicators, CVD-related expenditure is estimated to exceed several billions of marks per year. In 1993, for example, 2.1 million (15.4%) of all in-hospital treatments (total, 13.8 million) in Germany were due to CVD [2]. In 1992, the largest health insurance company in Germany, the Allgemeine Ortskrankenkasse (AOK), reported CVD as the single most important cause of hospitalization (18.9% of all days spent in hospital). In comparison, 8.5% of all days spent in hospital were due to cancer [3]. Due to the great significance of CVD in medical and economical terms, the choice of an optimum approach to management in CVD patients is mandatory.

Cardiovascular Diseases

Definition

CVD include all diseases of the heart and vasculature, including the arterial, arteriolar, capillary, venular, venous, and lymphatic vessels of all vascular beds. In the early stages, CVD are limited to the cardiocirculatory organ (cardiovascular stage, i.e., limited disease), and only later are the end-organs also involved (end-organ stage, i.e., extended disease). The spectrum of late CVD has been summarized in the International Classification of Diseases (ICD) under a single heading, encompassing numbers 100–199 [4]. Among CVD, the atherosclerotic diseases are by far the most important entity; in 1993, 389813 people died in Germany from atherosclerosis-related causes (88.4% of all CVD-related deaths) [1].

The early stages of clinically silent CVD, i.e., limited disease, have not yet been acknowledged as a disease entity or officially classified. However, full use of the preventive interventional measures can only be made if they are applied during the early (cardiovascular) stages of CVD. As we now have both the necessary tools to diagnose CVD in the early stages and valid preventive principles to successfully intervene, it seems necessary to extend the currently accepted definition of CVD to include the cardiovascular stages.

Interdisciplinary Features

The heart and vasculature constitute a *pathomorphologic, functional,* and *nosologic* unity. In atherosclerotic diseases the *pathomorphologic* unity was documented by landmark autopsy studies conducted in the late 1960s and early 1970s in the United States and Europe [5,6]. In these studies the uniform pathomorphology and the systemic distribution of atherosclerotic lesions were shown (Fig. 1a, b).These findings were later confirmed by numerous clinical observations [7–10].

The *functional* unity is evident from the close interdependence and coupling between the heart and vasculature [11]. The mechanical and biological integrity of the cardiovascular system, as shown in the example of congestive heart failure, has been convincingly demostrated [12], and the systemic nature of vascular endothelial disorders and the similarities in their biologic behavior, as exemplified by endothelial responses to vascular injury [13, 14], also attest to this evidence.

The *nosologic* unity is based on the common pathogenesis and shared clinical features. Thus, for example, regardless of the specific vascular territo-

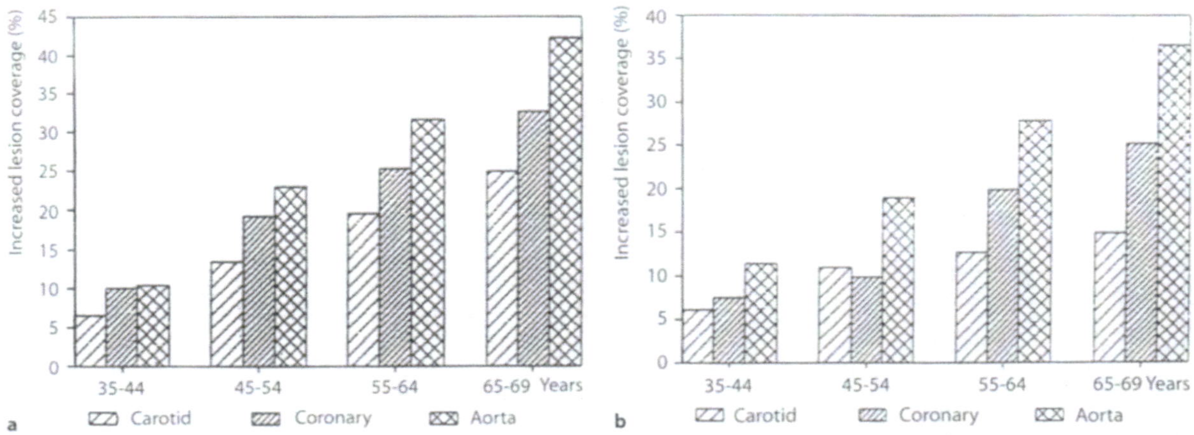

Fig. 1a, b. Extent of coronary, cerebrovascular, and abdominal aortic atherosclerosis (intimal coverage with raised atherosclerotic lesions in % of the examined surface) in **a** men and **b** women. (Adapted from [30])

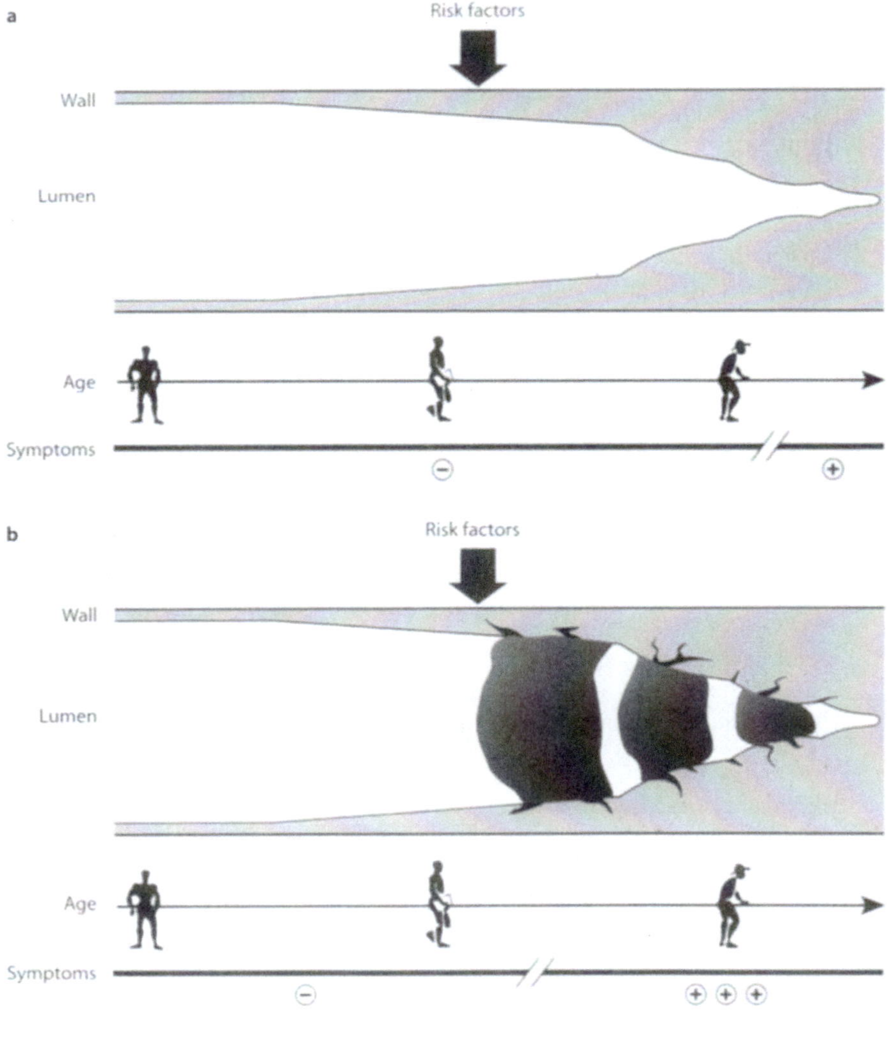

Fig. 2a, b. Progression of cardiovascular disease from the vascular to the end-organ stage. **a** Chronic and **b** chronic-acute progression from the clinically silent cardiovascular stage (limited disease) (⊖) to the clinically manifest end-organ stage (extensive disease) (⊕)

ry the hallmarks of atherosclerotic diseases include common pathogenesis, simultaneous involvement of many vascular beds, an early onset, a long clinically silent course (i.e., limited disease), and late clinical manifestations due to thromboembolic, ischemic, or hemorrhagic endorgan complications (i.e., extended disease, [15–17] Fig. 2 a, b).

The need for an integrated, interdisciplinary approach to cardiovascular medicine is rooted in the emerging common molecular and cellular pathogenesis of CVD [18, 19], in the integral unity of the cardiovascular organs, and in the multiorgan involvement in late stages. In early CVD, optimum management requires close collaborations among cardiovascular specialists and radiologists, lipidologists, hemostasiologists, geneticists, nutritionists, and others. In late CVD, following vascular-related end-organ manifestations, close cooperation among cardiovascular physicians and end-organ specialists, including neurologists, nephrologists, pulmologists, gastro-enterologists, and others is crucial.

In addition to medical factors, the increasingly competitive economical environment has become an important nonmedical driving force to consolidate and integrate modern cardiovascular medicine. Thus, for example, in response to the increasing economic pressures and changing needs, the medical industry has begun to design and manufacture modular, versatile, and universal technologies, which replace former inflexible, closed-off-stand-alone medical systems. Using the latest modular ultrasound (Fig. 3a, b) and integrated angiographic equipment (Fig. 4), complete and comprehensive money-saving noninvasive and invasive one-stop-single-step assessment of the entire cardiovascular system is now feasible.

End-Organ Principle

Management of patients with CVD is now based on the end-organ principle (EP). According to the EP, diagnosis and treatment of CVD is resumed according to clinical manifestations of the vascular-related end-organ disease. At this stage the CVD is already extensive and difficult to treat; mostly, palliative interventions and secondary prevention are employed. CVD is managed by a number of end-organ specialists, including cardiologists and cardiac surgeons (heart), neurologists, neuroradiologists, and neurosurgeons (brain); angiologists, radiologists and vascular surgeons (peripheral skelettal musculature); dermatologists (skin); pulmologists (lungs); nephrologists (kidney); gastroenterologists (visceral organs); urologists and gynecologists (urogenital organs); internists and general practitioners (Fig. 5). In addition, laboratory specialists and lipidologists may be involved.

In treatments based on EP, the end-organs and not the culprit "vasculature" are primarily targeted and therefore the order of causality in CVD is reversed ("effect prior to cause" strategy). The late

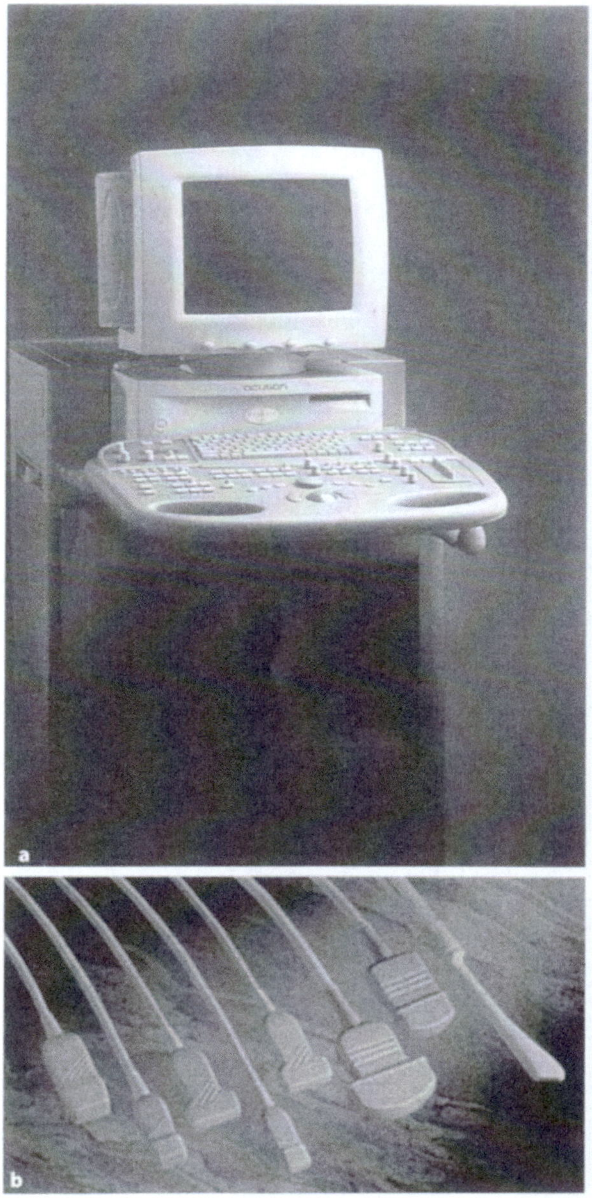

Fig. 3a, b. Modular ultrasound technology. **a** Universal ultrasound machines designed to assess the heart and the entire vasculature. **b** The corresponding transducers

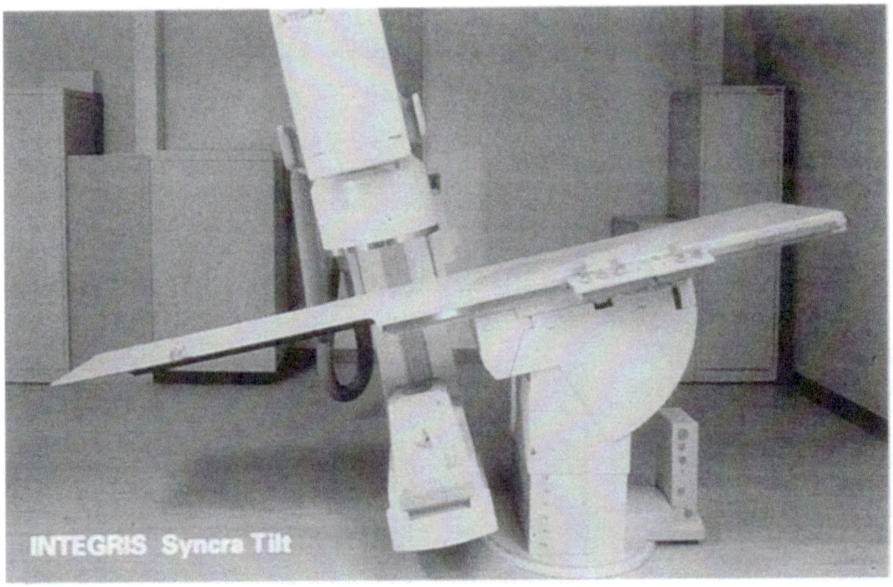

Fig. 4. Universal angiographic equipment. Angiographic unit designed for conventional and interventional evaluation of the entire cardiovascular system, including the heart and all areas of the arterial and venous vasculature

onset of therapy renders both prevention and intervention inefficient.

The main features of CVD management according to the EP include the lack of interdisciplinary coordination, multiple referrals, repeat diagnostic procedures, and fragmented treatments. Late therapy is associated with an increased need for inhospital treatments, prolonged hospitalizations, chronic morbidity, and high mortality. In addition, incosistency in the cardiovascular competence of therapists, as well as excessive dissemination, underutilization, and high operating costs of the expensive technology are typical.

Integrated, Interdisciplinary Principle

The integrated, interdisciplinary principle (IIP) represents a fundamental departure from the EP approach to cardiovascular care. In contrast to the EP, the IIP approach targets primarily the cardiovascular system, aiming to detect early CVD (i.e., limited disease) with the major goal of preventing cardiovascular-related premature death and disability. IIP is characterized by vigorous screening, and primary prevention and interventions prior to the onset of vascular-related end-organ disease. Genetic [e.g., apoprotein E (apo E), apo B, low-density-lipoprotein (LDL)-receptors) [20], metabolic (e.g., carbohydrates, lipoproteins, homocysteine) [21], hemostatic (e.g., fibrinogen, factor V (FV), antithrombin III (ATIII), protein S (PS), protein C (PC)] [22], morphologic (high resolution B-mode sonography) [23], and increasingly functional (high resolution A-mode sonography) [24] screening is employed in the clinical setting. Staged nonmedical, pharmacological, and, where necessary, invasive approaches are selected based on the results of screening. For optimum management of early CVD close collaboration among cardiovascular specialists and radiologists, laboratory specialists (e.g., lipidologists geneticists), nutritionists, and physical therapists is established.

In the management of early and late CVD (i.e., limited and extended disease) the order of causality in CVD is preserved ("cause prior to effect" strategy), rendering both prevention and intervention highly efficient in the majority of patients. For optimum management of late CVD close interdisciplinary links among cardiovascular physicans with end-organ specialists (e.g., neurologists, nephrologists, and pulmologists) (Fig. 6) and radiologists are obligatory.

The main features of CVD management according to IIP are integration of cardiovascular care, functional interdisciplinary coordination, efficient diagnostics, and complete treatments. The early detection and the timely onset of intervention allow the outpatient services to be fully utilized. The IIP management of CVD is further characterized by highly competent cardiovascular therapists, infrequent referrals, optimum utilization of existing resources and rapid transfer of research know-how into clinical benefits [25-27].

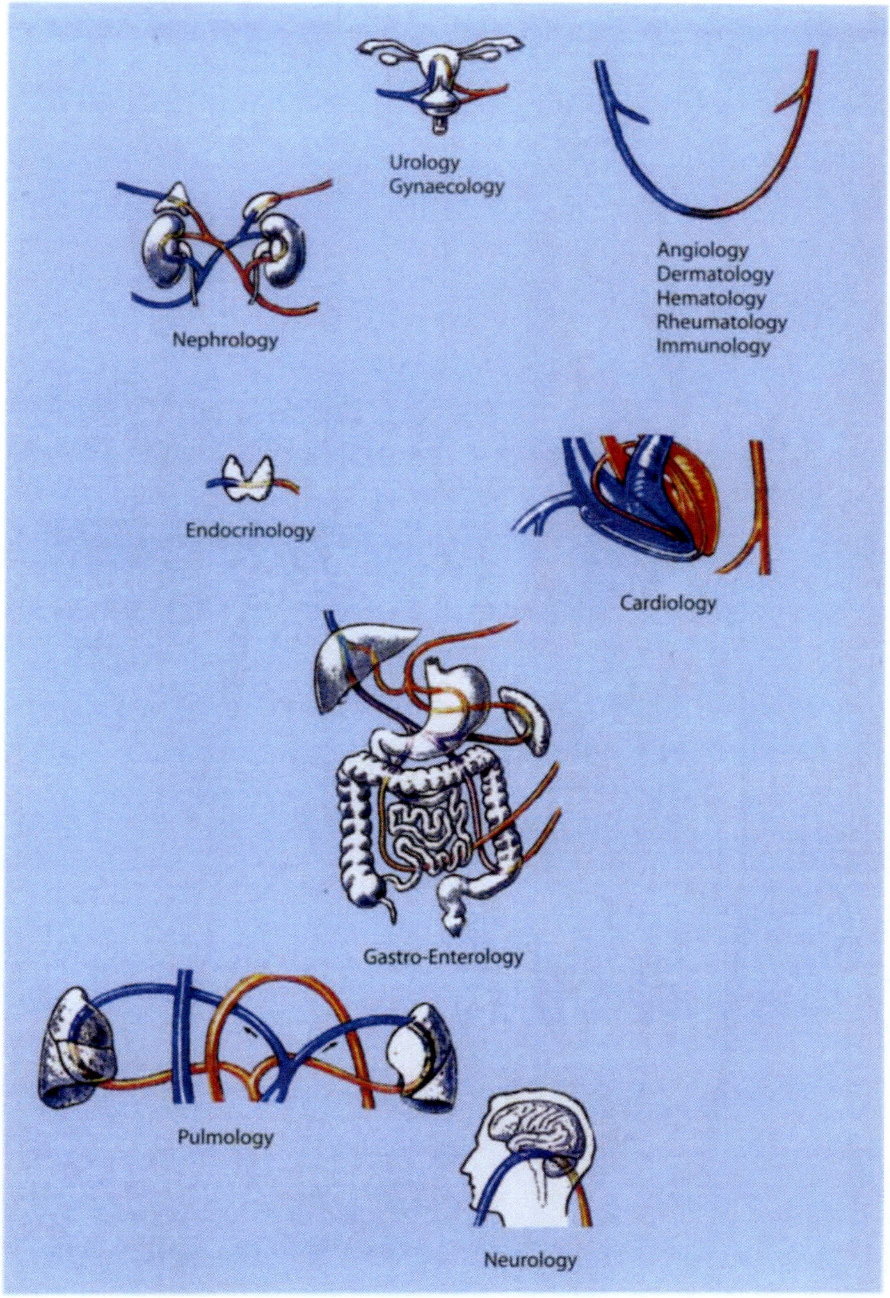

Fig. 5. End-organ principle (EP). Management of diseases of the heart and circulation is primarily end-organ related; patients are treated by end-organ specialists. (Modified from [31])

Two-Stage Model of Cardiovascular Centers

Based on the IIP, a two-stage model of cardiovascular centers (CC) has been designed. Stage I CC will provides services to all outpatients, whereas stage II CC is responsible for all inpatient treatments. All IIP-based CC is fully integrated into the networks of specialized and general medical care.

IIP-based CC treats patients with cardiocirculatory disorders, including those with cardiac and cerebral, coronary, visceral and peripheral, arterial, venous, capillary and lymphatic vascular diseases. In addition, high-risk subjects are screened and treated when necessary.

Initially, IIP CC treatment will be provided by conventionally trained cardiovascular physicians. Ultimately, treatments by comprehensively trained cardiovascular specialists with individual expertise

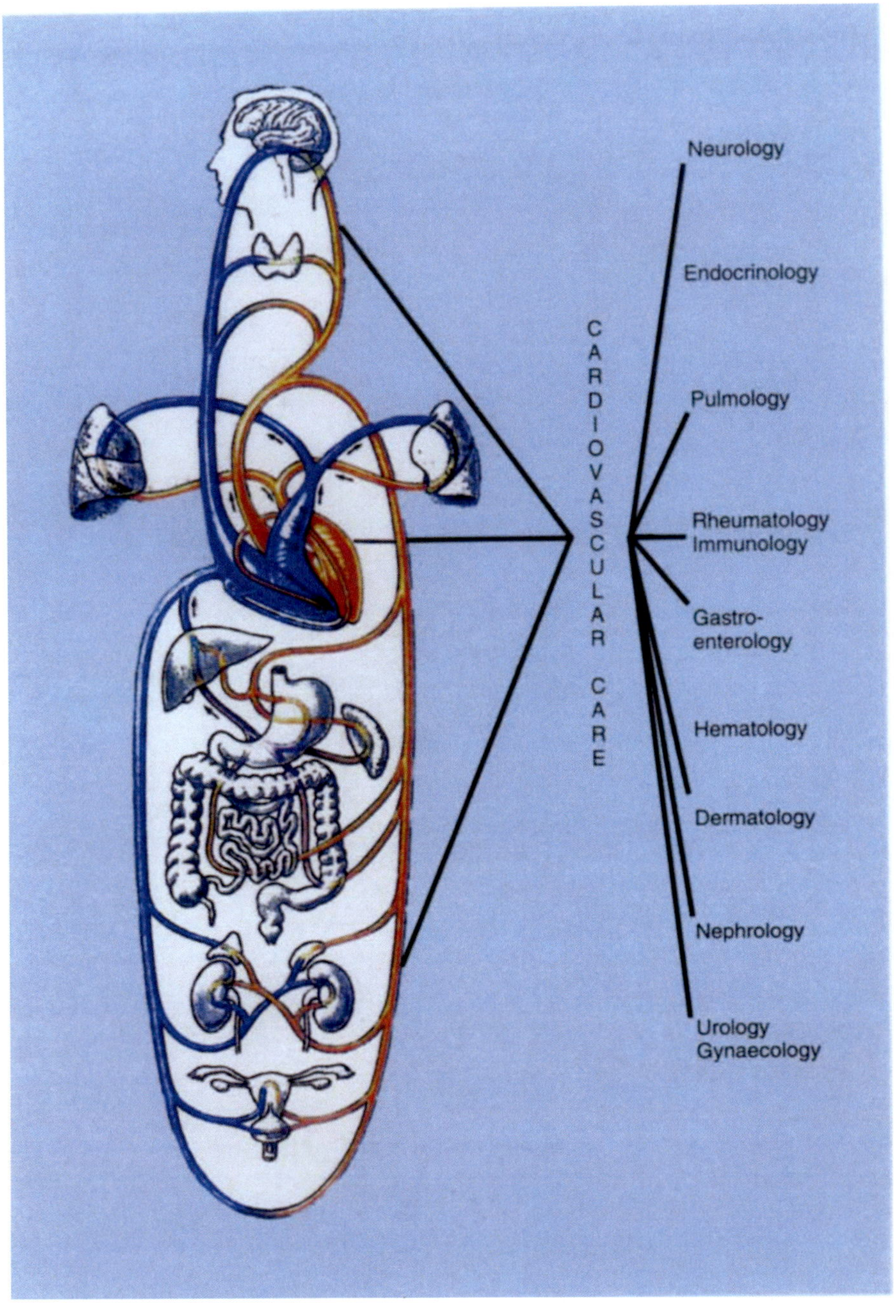

Fig. 6. Integrated, interdisciplinary principle (IIP). Management of diseases of the heart and circulation is primarily related to the cardiovascular organ; patients are treated by cardiovascular specialists (limited and extensive disease) and end-organ specialists (extensive disease). (Modified from [31])

in noninvasive and invasive diagnostics and preventive, conventional, interventional, and surgical therapy are envisioned. Cardiovascular professionals will function as a team providing complete and comprehensive CVD care. The professional expertise of the staff, combined with the patient- and prevention-oriented CC-environment will guarantee a high standard, and accessible and cost-effective cardiovascular care.

Stage I Cardiovascular Centers

Stage I CC represent an integrated extension of the existing conventional outpatient cardiology clinics and facilities. For comprehensive IIP-based cardiovascular care, expansion, restructuring, reorganization, and supplementary staff and equipment will be necessary in most cases [28].

In stage I CC complete and referral-free outpa-

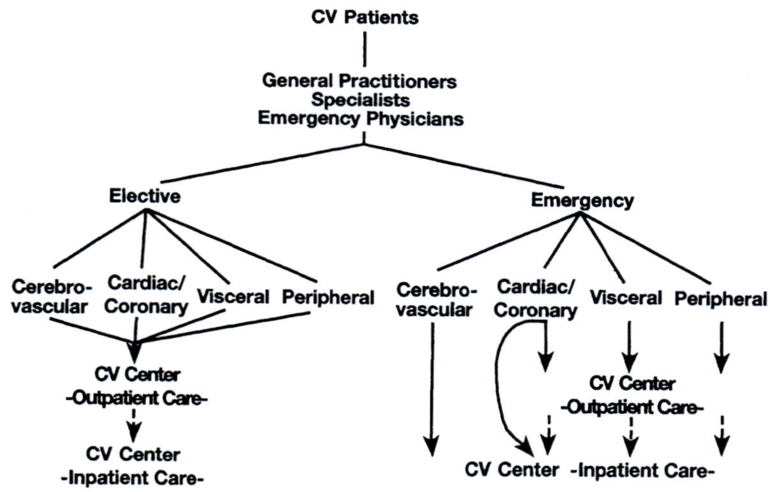

Fig. 7. Referral concepts for elective and emergency patients with diseases of the heart and circulation within the framework of stage I and II cardiovascular (CV) centers

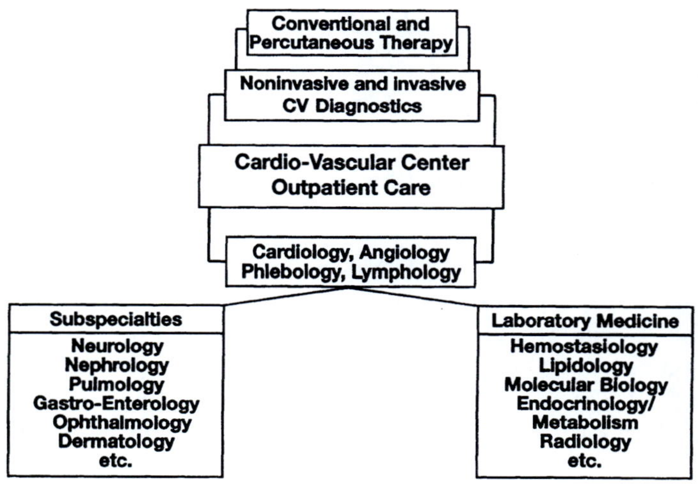

Fig. 8. Organizational structure of integrated, interdisciplinary principle (IIP)-based cardiovascular (CV) center outpatient care facilities (stage I)

tient management of all elective patients with CVD of the heart and the cerebral, coronal, visceral and peripheral arterial, venous and lymphatic circulations will be provided. In addition, all critically ill CVD patients will be treated on an emergency basis. However, definitive and, whenever feasible primary treatment of CVD emergencies will be provided by the stage II CC (Fig. 7). Cardiovascular screening, primary and secondary prevention, and direction of follow-up programs in the communities constitutes an important part of the stage I CC activities.

Owing to the comprehensive cardiovascular competence of stage I CC, noninvasive and invasive diagnostic procedures, conventional, and elective interventional therapeutic measures in all areas of CVD can be performed. On a consultant basis, close collaboration with end-organ subspecialists, radiologists, and laboratory physicians will be established (Fig. 8).

Stage I CC will serve the public and community physicians as primary referral centers for patients with CVD and subjects at risk for CVD. For outpatient treatments, functional networks incorporating the sharing of responsibilities, a high level of communication and continuing education with the referring physicians, prevention and rehabilitation centers will be developed. For inhospital treatments a close collaboration, including sharing of facilities and equipment, will be established between stage I and II CC.

Stage II Cardiovascular Centers

Stage II CC (Fig. 9) represent an integrated extension of the existing conventional cardiology and vascular medical and surgical departments, hospitals, and clinics.

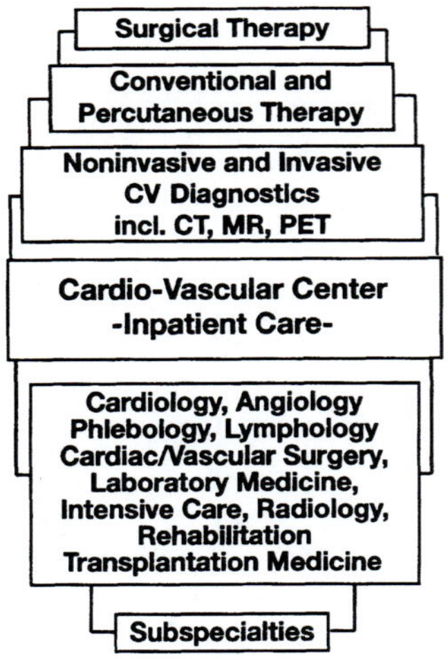

Fig. 9. Organizational structure of integrated, interdisciplinary principle (IIP)-based cardiovascular center outpatient care facilities (stage II). *CT*, computed tomography; *MR*, magnetic resonance imaging; *PET*, positron emission tomography

For extended IIP-based cardiovascular care restructuring, reorganization, and supplementary staff and equipment will also be necessary in these facilities. The costs involved in transforming the conventional institutions into IIP-based stage II CC will depend on existing standards and future assignments. In general, compared to community care stage II CC higher costs will be incurred by establishing teaching and researching stage II CC institutions. To guarantee high-quality care to all patients while controlling the costs and preserving the limited hospital resources access to expensive technology such as computed tomography, positron emission tomography, and magnetic resonance tomography and specialized laboratories will be shared between stand-alone or hospital-integrated stage II CC and other intra- and/or interhospital facilities (28). The creation of centralized, fully digitized, interdisciplinary, nonimaging laboratory and imaging i.e. ultrasonographic and radiographic, hospital departments provides a viable option to cost control in this high technology era.

In stage II CC complete and referral-free inpatient management of all elective and emergency patients with diseases of the heart and all the vascular beds will be provided. The indications for inpatient treatments include all surgical and emergency percutaneous therapies in patients with acute coronary, cerebral, visceral and most peripheral vascular syndromes and in those with chronic, therapy-resistant disease states (e.g., heart failure NYHA stage IV, peripheral arterial disease Fontaine stage IV). For optimum utilization and integration of the out- and inpatient sectors, elective patients will usually be referred to stage II CC by physicians at stage I CC, whereas emergency patients will be referred as required on an emergency basis (Fig.7).

Based on the comprehensive cardiovascular competence of staff and integration in stage II CC the quality of inhospital treatments will improve and the average stay inhospital will decrease. Repeat diagnostics, multiple referrals, and incomplete management due to multiorgan manifestations of the underlying CVD and limited competence at the conventional CVDfacilities will be eliminated.

Stage II CC will serve the public interest in providing an access to high-quality inhospital care to all patients at acceptable costs. They will offer referring physicians, the centers providing inpatient and outpatient rehabilitation and long-term, convalescent care, and other medical facilities the capable and reliable partnership which is critical to success in the increasingly complex area of cardiovascular care (Fig. 10).

Benefits and Advantages of the Integrated, Interdisciplinary Principle

In IIP-based CVD management, the principles of modern, complete, prevention-centered, referral-free, and primarily outpatient-oriented medical care are realized. To assess the impact of the IIP on costs, expediture for EP CVD management and the projected expenditure for IIP CVD management would need to be known. In the absence of precise figures, a direct comparison of the two approaches is, however, not yet possible, and the standard measures of efficacy employed in cost-efficiency analysis in health care, e.g., cost-effectiveness (costs/years of life saved), cost/utility (costs/quality-adjusted life-years), and cost/benefit (costs/costs saved), therefore cannot be used at present. Due to the lack of quantitative data, only general comparisons based on the differences between the two principles will be briefly discussed.

According to the EP approach, CVD are diagnosed and patients treated based on end-organ manifestation corresponding to late-stage disease. The hallmarks of CVD management according to the EP are lack of prevention, late diagnosis, and palliative in-hospital management. This form of therapy is known to be both cost intensive and cost ineffective.

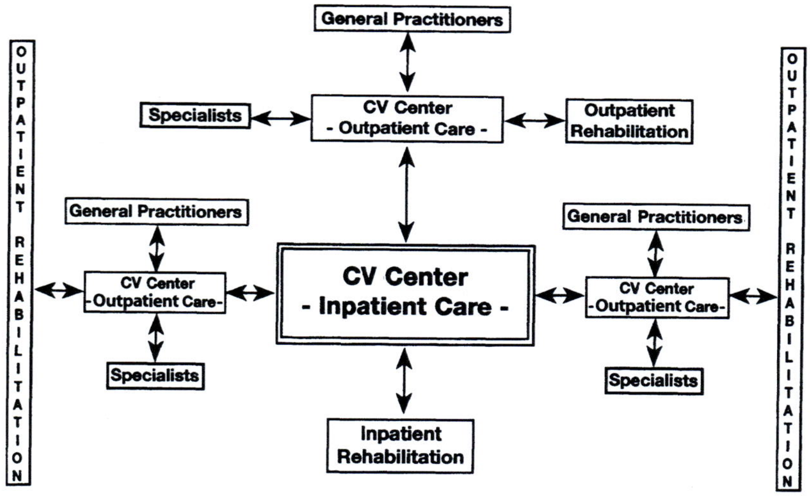

Fig. 10. Central position of stage I and II cardiovasular centers in the management of patients with diseases of the heart and circulation and their integration into the existing structures of medical care

According to the IIP approach, CVD are diagnosed during the early cardiovascular stages (limited disease) prior to end-organ involvement (extended disease). The hallmarks of CVD management according to the IIP are prevention, early diagnosis, and outpatient-based management. This form of therapy is increasingly recognised as cost effective.

CVD treatments based on the EP are carried out by physicians with variable qualifications and expertise in cardiovascular medicine, resulting in unpredictable results and predictably high costs. The systemic character of CVD is not recognized, and single end-organ manifestations in different patients and multiple end-organ manifestations in a single patient are treated in an unrelated fashion. Fragmented and incomplete management is a high-cost, low-benefit approach.

CVD treatments based on the IIP are provided by CVD-trained physicians, resulting in predictable outcomes and predictable costs. The nosologic unity of the cardiovascular organ is recognized and reflected in intra- and interdisciplinarily coordinated management. Unlike the EP, the IIP enables the increasingly complex advanced medical technology to be properly selected and optimally utilized. Multiple diagnostic evaluations, fragmented and incomplete therapies, and suboptimal coordination of the inpatient and outpatient sectors are avoided, resulting in a better outcome at lower costs.

The combination of EP-based low-priority prevention and late therapeutic interventions contribute to the high cardiovascular morbidity and mortality rates and to the high direct and indirect costs.

Due to the preventive and early interventional character of IIP, the quality of life and life expectancy will be improved, and costs will be reduced, particularly those associated with management of end-organ diseases [29].

References

1. Statistisches Bundesamt (1995) Todesursachen 1993. Statistisches Bundesamt, Wiesbaden
2. Statistisches Bundesamt (1995) Erstmals Ergebnisse aus der neuen Krankenhausdiagnosestatistik. Mitteilung für die Presse. Statistisches Bundesamt, Wiesbaden
3. AOK (1995) Krankheitsartenstatistik 1992. AOK-Bundesverband, Bonn
4. Deutscher Ärzte-Verband (1995) Diagnoseverschlüsselung in der Arztpraxis. Fachgruppenbezogene Diagnosekataloge auf der Grundlage der ICD-10. Deutscher Ärzte-Verlag, Cologne
5. McGill HC (1968) The geographic pathology of atherosclerosis. Williams and Wilkins, Baltimore
6. World Health Organization (1976) Atherosclerosis of the aorta and coronary arteries in five towns. WHO, Geneva
7. Hertzer NR et al (1984) Coronary artery disease in peripheral vascular patients. Ann Surg 189: 223–233
8. Hertzer NR (1987) Basic data concerning associated and peripheral vascular patients. Ann Vasc Surg 5: 616–620
9. Gersh BJ et al (1991)Evaluation and management of patients with both peripheral vascular and coronary artery disease. J Am Coll Cardiol 18: 302–214
10. Missouris CG et al (1994) Renal artery stenosis: a common and important problem in patients with peripheral vascular disease. Am J Med 96: 10–14
11. Ter Keurs HEDJ, Tyberg JV (1987) Mechanics of the circulation. Nijhoff, Dordrecht

12. McKelvie RS, Koon KT, McCartney N, Humen D, Montaque T, Yusuf S (1995) Effects of exercise training in patients with congestive heart failure: a critical review. J Am Coll Cardiol 25: 789–796
13. Lüschner TF, Noll G (1995) The endothelium in coronary vascular control. In: Braunwald E (ed) Heart disease: Update 3. Saunders, Philadelphia, pp 1-10
14. Bennett MR, Schwartz SM (1995) Antisense therapy for angioplasty restenosis. Circulation 92: 1981-1991
15. Stary HC (1989) Evolution and progression of atherosclerotic lesions in coronary arteries of children and young adults. Arteriosclerosis Suppl 9: I19-I32
16. Stary HC et al (1992) A definition of the intima of human arteries and of its atherosclerosis-prone regions. Arteriosclerosis Thromb 12: 120-134
17. Woolf N (1982) Pathology of atherosclerosis. Butterworth, London
18. Ross R (1993) The pathogenesis of atherosclerosis: a perspective for the 1990: Nature 362: 801-809
19. Dzau VJ, Gibbons GH, Kobilka BK, Lawn RM, Pratt RE (1995) Genetic models of human vascular disease. Circulation 91: 521-531
20. Dammerman M, Breslow JL (1995) Genetic basis of lipoprotein disorders. Circulation 91: 505-512
21. Shepherd J, Lobbe SM, I Ford, Isles CG, Lorimer AR, MacFarlane PW, McKillip JH, Packard CJ (1995) Prevention of coronary heart disease with pravastatin in man with hypercholesterolemia. N Engl J Med 333: 1301-1307
22. Meade TW, Miller GJ, Rosenberg RD (1992) Characteristics associated with the risk of arterial thrombosis and the prethrombotic state. In: Fuster V, M Verstraete (eds) Thrombosis in cardiovascular disorders. Saunders, Philadelphia
23. Lanzer P, Bond MG (1992) Karotisultraschall in der Früherkennung der Atherosklerose. Dtsch Ärztebl 48: 4096-4105
24. Celerjamer DS, Sorensen KE, Gooch VM, Spiegelhalter DJ, Moller OI, Sullivan ID, Lloyd JK, Deanfield JE (1992) Noninvasive detection of endothelial dysfunction in children and adults at risk of atherosclerosis. Lancet 340: 1111-1115
25. Grace AA, Chien KR (1995) Congenital long QT-syndromes. Toward molecular dissection of arrhythmia substrates. Circulation 92: 2786-2789
26. Marian AJ, Roberts R (1995) Recent advances in the molecular genetics of hyperthrophic cardiomyopathy. Circulation 92: 1336-1347
27. Berina RM, Koeleman BPL, Kosten T, Rosendal FR, Dirvan RJ, de Ronde H, van der Velden PA, Reltsma PH (1994) Mutation in blood coagulation factor V with resistance to activated protein C. Nature 369: 64-66
28. Lanzer P (1995) Interdisziplinär integrierte Herz- und Gefäßzentren: Konzept und Wirtschaftlichkeit. Gesundheitspreis '95 (unpublished data)
29. Goldman L, Gordon DJ, Rifkind BM, Hulley SB, Detsky AS, Goodman DS, Dinosian B, Weistein MC (1992) Cost and health implications of cholesterol lowering. Circulation 85: 1960-1968
30. Bates SR, Gangloff EC (eds) (1987) Atherogenesis and aging. Springer, Berlin Heidelberg New York
31. Ferner H, Staubesand J (eds) (1982) Sobotta Atlas der Anatomie des Menschen. Urban and Schwarzenberg, Munich

Subject Index

FSC
www.fsc.org
MIX
Papier | Fördert
gute Waldnutzung
FSC® C083411

Kolibri 360 GmbH
Ferdinand-Jühlke-Straße 7
99095 Erfurt, Deutschland
produktsicherheit@kolibri360.de